Surgical Techniques in Ophthalmology
Cataract Surgery

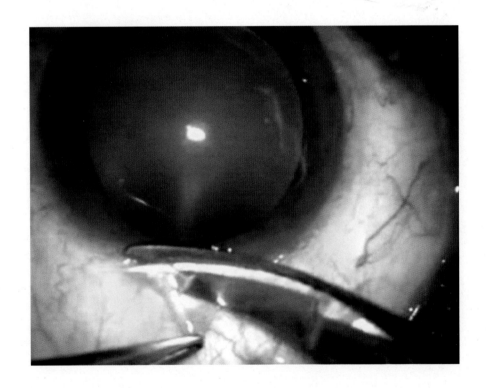

SURGICAL TECHNIQUES IN OPHTHALMOLOGY CATARACT SURGERY

Editors-in-Chief

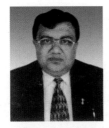

Ashok Garg
MS, PhD, FRSM, ADM, FAIMS, FICA
International and National Gold Medalist
Chairman and Medical Director,
Garg Eye Institute and Research Centre
235-Model Town, Dabra Chowk
Hisar-125005 (India)

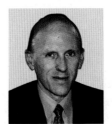

Jorge L Alio
MD, PhD
Professor and Chairman of Ophthalmology
Medical Director
Instituto Oftalmologico De Alicante
Avda. Denia S/n 03016
Alicante, Spain

Foreword

David F Chang

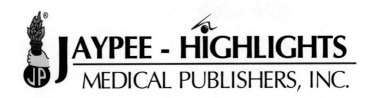

JAYPEE - HIGHLIGHTS
MEDICAL PUBLISHERS, INC.

Editors

Marie Jose Tassignon
MD, PhD
Professor
Department of Ophthalmology
Univesity Hospital Antwerp
Wilrijkstraat 10, B-2650
Edegem (Antwerp), Belgium

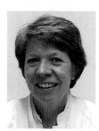

Shui H Lee
MD, FRCS, FAAO
Medical Director of Sunray
Outpatient Aesthetic Multi-specialty
Surgical Center
Medical Director of Central
Square Medical Eye Clinic
Unit 255-4231 Hazel Bridge Way
Richmond B.C. V6X 3L7
Canada

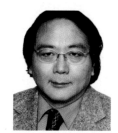

Robert J Weinstock
MD
Director
Cataract and Refractive Surgeon
The Eye Institute of West Florida
148, 12th Street SW
Largo, Florida 33770, USA

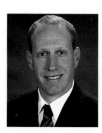

Boris Malyugin
MD, PhD
Professor of Ophthalmology
Chief of Department of
Cataract and Implant Surgery
Dy. Director General
S. Fyodorov Eye Microsurgery
Complex State Institution
Beskudnikovsky blvd 59A
127486 Moscow
Russia

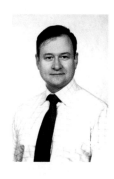

Keiki R Mehta
MS, DO, FIOS
Chairman and Medical Director
Mehta International Eye Institute
147, Shahid Bhagat Singh Road
Colaba Road
Mumbai-400005
India

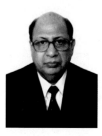

D Ramamurthy
MS
Director
The Eye Foundation
582-A, RS Puram, DB Road
Coimbatore-641002
Tamil Nadu
India

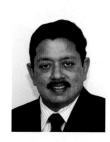

Jerome Jean - Philippe Bovet
MD
Consultant Ophthalmic
Surgeon, FMH
Clinique de I'oeil
15, Avenue du Bois-de-la-Chapelle
CH-1213 Onex
Switzerland

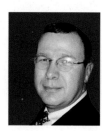

Mahipal S Sachdev
MD
Chairman and Medical Director
Centre for Sight
B-5/24, Safdarjung Enclave
New Delhi-110029
India

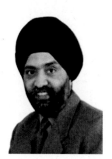

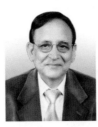
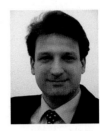
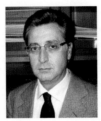
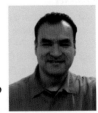
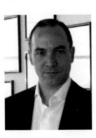
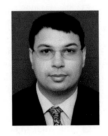

Published by

Jitendar P Vij

Jaypee Brothers Medical Publishers (P) Ltd

Corporate Office

4838/24 Ansari Road, Daryaganj, **New Delhi** - 110002, India, Phone: +91-11-43574357, Fax: +91-11-43574314

Registered Office

B-3 EMCA House, 23/23B Ansari Road, Daryaganj, **New Delhi** - 110 002, India
Phones: +91-11-23272143, +91-11-23272703, +91-11-23282021
+91-11-23245672, Rel: +91-11-32558559, Fax: +91-11-23276490, +91-11-23245683
e-mail: jaypee@jaypeebrothers.com, Website: www.jaypeebrothers.com

Branches

❑ 2/B, Akruti Society, Jodhpur Gam Road Satellite
Ahmedabad 380 015, Phones: +91-79-26926233, Rel: +91-79-32988717
Fax: +91-79-26927094, e-mail: ahmedabad@jaypeebrothers.com

❑ 202 Batavia Chambers, 8 Kumara Krupa Road, Kumara Park East
Bengaluru 560 001, Phones: +91-80-22285971, +91-80-22382956, 91-80-22372664
Rel: +91-80-32714073, Fax: +91-80-22281761 e-mail: bangalore@jaypeebrothers.com

❑ 282 IIIrd Floor, Khaleel Shirazi Estate, Fountain Plaza, Pantheon Road
Chennai 600 008, Phones: +91-44-28193265, +91-44-28194897, Rel: +91-44-32972089
Fax: +91-44-28193231 e-mail: chennai@jaypeebrothers.com

❑ 4-2-1067/1-3, 1st Floor, Balaji Building, Ramkote Cross Road,
Hyderabad 500 095, Phones: +91-40-66610020, +91-40-24758498
Rel:+91-40-32940929, Fax:+91-40-24758499 e-mail: hyderabad@jaypeebrothers.com

❑ No. 41/3098, B & B1, Kuruvi Building, St. Vincent Road
Kochi 682 018, Kerala, Phones: +91-484-4036109, +91-484-2395739
+91-484-2395740 e-mail: kochi@jaypeebrothers.com

❑ 1-A Indian Mirror Street, Wellington Square
Kolkata 700 013, Phones: +91-33-22651926, +91-33-22276404, +91-33-22276415
Fax: +91-33-22656075 e-mail: kolkata@jaypeebrothers.com

❑ Lekhraj Market III, B-2, Sector-4, Faizabad Road, Indira Nagar
Lucknow 226 016 Phones: +91-522-3040553, +91-522-3040554
e-mail: lucknow@jaypeebrothers.com

❑ 106 Amit Industrial Estate, 61 Dr SS Rao Road, Near MGM Hospital, Parel
Mumbai 400 012, Phones: +91-22-24124863, +91-22-24104532,
Rel: +91-22-32926896, Fax: +91-22-24160828 e-mail: mumbai@jaypeebrothers.com

❑ "KAMALPUSHPA" 38, Reshimbag, Opp. Mohota Science College, Umred Road
Nagpur 440 009 (MS), Phone: Rel: +91-712-3245220, Fax: +91-712-2704275
e-mail: nagpur@jaypeebrothers.com

North America Office
1745, Pheasant Run Drive, Maryland Heights (Missouri), MO 63043, USA Ph: 001-636-6279734
e-mail: jaypee@jaypeebrothers.com, anjulav@jaypeebrothers.com

Central America Office
Jaypee-Highlights Medical Publishers Inc., City of Knowledge, Bld. 237, Clayton, Panama City, Panama   Ph: 507-317-0160

Surgical Techniques in Ophthalmology (Cataract Surgery)

First Edition: **2010**

ISBN 978-81-8448-776-3

Typeset at JPBMP typesetting unit
Printed at Nutech Print Services

Dedicated to

- My Respected Param Pujya Guru Sant Gurmeet Ram Rahim Singh Ji for his blessings & motivation.
- My Respected Parents, teachers, my wife Dr. Aruna Garg, son Abhishek and daughter Anshul for their constant support and patiencxe during all these days of hard work.
- My dear friend Dr. Amar Agarwal, a leading International Ophthalmologist from India for his continued support & guidance.

— Ashok Garg

- To Mayca, Jorge, Fernando and Maria Lucia and most especially to my beloved wife Maria, for the hours that were taken from our family life to make this book possible.

— Jorge L Alio

- Nothing will be cherished more than you to come, my first grand child.

— Marie Jose Tassignon

- My father Stephen M. Weinstock, MD. In addition to his tremendous success as an ophthalmologist, he continues to inspire and support me in all that I do. With patience and understanding he has taught me the importance of honesty and balance in my life.

— Robert J Weinstock

- Zena the light of my life.

— Keiki R Mehta

- Yveric, Luc and Fanny Laure.
- Silvio Korol, who was not only a teacher but also an intellectual guide and a friend.

— Jerome Bovet

- My parents for their inspiration, teaching and motivation.
- My brother Peter for his continued support, guidance and inspiration in my professional career.

— Shui H Lee

- To my father Edvard Malyugin for everything and to my wife Natalia for her continuous support and love.

— Boris Malyugin

- To my family, who make it all so worthwhile.

— D Ramamurthy

- My family without whose help it would not have been possible to do book.

— Mahipal S Sachdev

- My dear wife Dr. Indira Dhull and my children Tushar and Chirag.

— CS Dhull

- My wife Lorena and my sons Pier Francesco, Enrico Maria, Massimiliano and Chiara that, with their love and patience, enable me to get energies and ardor for my work.

— Gian Maria Cavallini

- I dedicate this book to India's Talented ophthalmologists, in the fervent hope that they may become increasingly devoted to refractive surgery.

— Roberto Pinelli

- To my son Valentin Aleksandar.

— Bojan Pajic

- I dedicate my work to all the people in the world with ophthalmic diseases, with the best wish that we can improve with this kind of material our quality of care. I also dedicate this opus to Prof. Ashok Garg, because he has trusted in my work many times.

— Arturo Perez-Arteaga

- My parents for everything.
- To Vini my Best friend.

— Cyres K Mehta

Contributors

Ahmad K Khalil MD,PhD
Associate Professor of
Ophthalmology
Saridar Clinic Tower
92, Tahrir St., Dokki
Cairo (Egypt)

AK Grover MD, FRCS
Chairman
Deptt. of Ophthalmology
Sir Gangaram Hospital
Rajender Nagar
New Delhi, India

Albrecht Hennig MD
Lahan Eye Hospital
C/o UMN, P.O. Box 126
Kathmandu, Nepal

Amar Agarwal MS, FRCS, FRC Ophth
Consultant
Dr Agarwal's Eye Hospital
19, Cathedral Road
Chennai-600086, India

Antonio Toso MD
Consultant
Bassano del Grappa City Hospital
Ospedale San Bassiano, Unità
Operativa di Oculistica, 36061
Bassano del Grappa (VI) Italy

Armando Capote MD
Vice Chairman Microsurgery Center
Cuban Institute of Ophthalmology
Ramon Pando Ferrer
Havana, Cuba

A Divya
Consultant
Dr Agarwal's Eye Hospital
19, Cathedral Road
Chennai-600086, India

Arturo Perez-Arteaga MD
Medical Director
Centro Oftalmologico Tlalnepantla
Dr. Perez - Arteaga Vallarta No.42
Tlalnepantla, Centro, Estado de
Mexico 54000, Mexico

Arun C Gulani MD
Director
Gulani Vision Institute
8075 Gate Parkway (W)
Suite 102 and 103, Jacksonville,
Florida-32216, USA.

Ashok Garg MS, PhD, FRSM
Chairman and Medical Director
Garg Eye Institute and Research
Centre
235-Model Town, Dabra Chowk
Hisar-125005 (India)

Athiya Agarwal MD, DO, FRSH
Consultant
Dr. Agarwal's Eye Hospital
19, Cathedral Road
Chennai-600086, India

Bassam El Kady MD, PhD
Clinical Research Fellow
Vissum-Instituto Oftalmologico de
Alicante
Department of Research and
Development, Alicante, Spain

Belkis Rodriguez MD
Microsurgery Centre
Cuban Institute of Ophthalmology
Ramon Pando Ferrer, Havana, Cuba

Bojan Pajic MD,FEBO
Swiss Eye Research Foundation
Eye Clinic Orasis,
Titlisstrasse 44, 5734, Reinach
Switzerland

Boris Malyugin MD, PhD
Professor of Ophthalmology
Chief of Department of Cataract and
Implant Surgery
Dy. Director General
S. Fyodorov Eye Microsurgery
Complex State Institution
127486 Moscow
Beskudnikovsky blvd 59A
Russia

Brigitte Pajic-Eggspuehler MD
Augen Zentrum Pajic (AZP)
Research Institute
Titlisstrasse 44, 5734
Reinach, Switzerland

Carlo Francesco Lovisolo MD
Medical Director
Quattro Elle Eye Center
via Cusani, 7-9, 20121
Milano, Italy

Chandresh Baid MD
Consultant
Dr Agarwal's Eye Hospital
19, Cathedral Road
Chennai-600086, India

Charu Khurana MD
Consultant Ophthalmologist
Centre for Sight
B-5/24, Safdarjung Enclave
New Delhi-110029, India

Chitra Ramamurthy MD
Director
The Eye Foundation
D.B. Road, Coimbatore-641002
Tamil Nadu, India

Cristina Masini MD
Institute of Ophthalmology
University of Modena and Reggio
Emilia via del Pozzo 71-41100
Modena, Italy

CS Dhull MS, PhD FIAO
Director and Senior Professor and
Head
Regional Institute of Ophthalmology
PGIMS, Rohtak-124001 (Haryana)
India

Cyres K Mehta MS, FSVH, FAGE
Director and Consultant
Mehta International Eye Institute
Seaside, 147, Colaba Road
Mumbai-400005, India

D Endriss MD
Department of Congenital Cataract
Cornea and External Eye Diseases
Altino Ventura Foundation and
Pernambuco Eye Hospital
Pernambuco
Brazil

David F Chang MD
Clinical Professor of
Ophthalmology
University of California
762, Altos Oaks Drive, Suite-1
Los Altos, CA 94024
USA

D Ramamurthy MS
Director
The Eye Foundation
D.B. Road
Coimbatore-641002
Tamil Nadu
India

Elizabeth A Davis MD
Minnesota Eye Consultants,
9117, Lyndale Aves
Bloomington
MN 55420
USA.

Frank Goes MD
Director Goes Eye Centre
W.Klooslaan 6 B2050
Antwerp
Belgium

Frederic Hehn MD
Centre de La Vision
Nations - Vision,
23, Boulevard de l'europe
54500, Vandoeuvre
France

Gian Maria Cavallini MD
Director
Institute of Ophthalmology
University of Modena and Reggio
Emilia via del Pozzo 71-41100,
Modena
Italy

Gilles Lesieur MD
32, Place Jean Jaures
81000
Albi-France
060-9706266

GL Arun Kumar MD
Director
Appasamy Eye Hospital and
Research Centre, Aruumbakkam
Chennai
India

I Howard Fine MD, FACS
Oregon Eye Surgery Centre
1550, Oak Street
5, Eugene, OR - 97401
USA

Jasna Ljubic MD
Swiss Eye Research Foundation
Eye Clinic Orasis
Titlisstrasse 44, 5734, Reinach
Switzerland

Jerome Bovet MD
Consultant Ophthalmic Surgeon,
FMH
Clinique de l'oeil
15, Avenue du Bois-de-la-Chapelle
CH-1213 Onex
Switzerland

Jes Mortensen MD
The Eye Department
Orebro University Hospital
SE-701 85 Orebro
Sweden

JJ Rozema MD
Department of Ophthalmology
University Hospital Antwerp
Wilrijkstraat 10, B-2650
Edegem (Antwerp)
Belgium

Jorge Alvarez Marin MD, PhD
Hospital Ntra, Sra. de La
Candelaria,
Ctra. del Rosario s/n
Santa Cruz de Tenerife,
Spain

Jorge L Alio MD, PhD
Instituto Oftalmologico De Alicante
Avda. Denia 111, 03015
Alicante
Spain

Jorg Muller MD
Nova Optik,
Hauptplatz 6, 6431 Schwyz
Switzerland

Kadil Jojo Jr Sinolinding MD, DPBO
Sinolinding Eye Clinic
Desert Ambulatory Referral Center
Cotabato Doctors Clinic Buidling
Sinsuat Avenue
Cotabato City 9600
Philippines

Kayo Nishi MD
Nishi Eye Hospital
Osaka
Japan

Keiki R Mehta MS, DO, FIOS
Chairman and Medical Director
Mehta International Eye Institute
147, Shahid Bhagat Singh Road
Colaba Road
Mumbai-400005
India

Kumar J Doctor MS
Director
Doctor Eye Institute
Spenta Mansion, 1st Floor
S.V. Road, Andheri (West)
Mumbai-400048, India

L Gobin PhD
Department of Ophthalmology
University Hospital Antwerp
Wilrijkstraat 10, B-2650
Edegem (Antwerp), Belgium

LO Ventura MD, PhD
Department of Pediatric
Ophthalmology and Strabismus
Altino Ventura Foundation and
Pernambuco Eye Hospital
Pernambuco
Brazil

Luca Campi MD
Institute of Ophthalmology
University of Modena and
Reggio Emilia
via del Pozzo 71-41100, Modena
Italy

Mahipal S Sachdev MD
Chairman and Medical Director
Centre for Sight
B-5/24, Safdarjung Enclave
New Delhi-110029
India

Marcelino Rio MD
Microsurgery Centre
Cuban Institute of Ophthalmology
Ramon Pando Ferrer, Havana
Cuba

MC Ventura MD
Department of Cataract, Retina and
Vitreous
Altino Ventura Foundation and
Pernambuco Eye Hospital
Pernambuco
Brazil

Marie Jose Tassignon MD, PhD
Professor
Department of Ophthalmology
University Hospital Antwerp
Wilrijkstraat 10, B-2650
Edegem (Antwerp)
Belgium

Mark Packer MD
Oregan Eye Surgery Centre
1550, Oak Street
5, Eugene, OR- 97401
USA

Mohan Rajan DO, DNB
Medical Director,
Rajan Eye Care Hospital
5, Vidyodaya East II Street
T-Nagar
Chennai-600017
India

Neel Desai MD
Cataract and Refractive Surgeon
The Eye Institute of West Florida
148, 12th Street SW
Largo, Florida 33770
USA

Okihiro Nishi MD
Director
Nishi Eye Hospital
Osaka
Japan

Pawel Klonowski MD, PhD
Vissum-Instituto Oftalmologico de
Alicante, Department of Research
and Development, Alicante
Spain

P Kaushik MS
Doctor Eye Institute
Spenta Mansion, 1st Floor
S.V. Road, Andheri (West)
Mumbai-400048
India

Peter Cikatricis MD
Department of Ophthalmology
Royal Hallamshire Hospital
Glossop Road
S10 2JF Sheffield
United Kingdom

Peter G Kansas MD, FACS
Clinical Professor of
Ophthalmology
Albany Medical College
Albany,New York
President
Kansas Eye Surgery Associates
PC 24, Century Hill Drive
Latham, New York
USA

Priye Suman Rastogi MS
Rajan Eye Care Hospital
#5, Vidyodaya East II Street, T-Nagar
Chennai-600017
India

Ranjit S Dhaliwal MS,DOMS
Director
Eye Infirmary
Hira Mahal, Radha Soami Marg
Nabha-147201, Punjab
India

Richard L Lindstrom MD
Minnesota Eye Consultants, PA
710 East, 24th Street, Suite 106
Minneapolis, MN 55404
USA

Richard S Hoffman MD
Oregon Eye Surgery Centre
1550, Oak Street, # 5 Eugene
OR- 97401, USA

Roberto Bellucci MD
Chief of Ophthalmic Unit
Hospital of Verona
University of Verona, Italy

Robert J Weinstock MD
Director
Cataract and Refractive Surgeon
The Eye Institute of West Florida
148, 12th Street SW
Largo, Florida 33770, USA

Roberto Pinelli MD
Director
Instituto Laser Microchirurgia
Oculare, Crystal Palace
Via Cefalonia, 70
25124 Brescia, Italy

Rohit Om Parkash MS
Director
Dr. Om Parkash Eye Institute
117-A, The Mall, Amritsar, India

Sanjay Chaudhary MS
Director,
Chaudhary Eye Centre and Laser
Vision Centre
4802, Bharat Ram Road
Daryaganj, New Delhi
India

Shaloo Bageja MS
Consultant
Deptt. of Ophthalmology
Sir Gangaram Hospital
Rajender Nagar
New Delhi
India

Shilpa Kodkany MS
Doctor Eye Institute,
Spenta Mansion, 1st Floor
S.V. Road
Andheri (West)
Mumbai-400048
India

S Sivagnanam BE
Appasamy Eye Hospital
and Research Centre,
Aruumbakkam
Chennai
India

Simonetta Morselli MD
Director of Anterior Segment
Surgery
Ophthalmic Unit
Hospital of Verona
University of Verona
Italy

Simon Pelloni MD
Institute of Ophthalmology
University of Modena and Reggio
Emilia
via del Pozzo 71-41100, Modena
Italy

Shiao Chang MD
Nishi Eye Hospital
Osaka, Japan

Shui H Lee MD, FRCS,FAAO
Medical Director of Sunray
Outpatient Aesthetic Multi
specialty Surgical Center
Medical Director of Central Square
Medical Eye Clinic
Unit 255-4231 Hazel Bridge Way
Richmond B.C. V6X 3L7
Canada

Soosan Jacob
Consultant
Dr Agarwal's Eye Hospital
19, Cathedral Road
Chennai-600086, India

Sujatha Mohan MD
Rajan Eye Care Hospital
5, Vidyodaya East II Street
T-Nagar, Chennai-600017, India

Sunita Agarwal MS, DO, PSVH
Dr. Agarwal's Eye Hospital
19, Cathedral Road
Chennai-600086, India
15, Eagle Street, Langford Town
Bangalore, India

Sumit Sachdeva MS
Assistant Professor
Regional Institute of
Ophthalmology, PGIMS
Rohtak-124001 (Haryana), India

TKJ Chan FRCOphth, FRCS
Consultant Ophthalmic Surgeon
Department of Ophthalmology
Royal Hallamshire Hospital
Glossop Road
S10 2JF Sheffield
United Kingdom

Vaijayanti Deodhar MS DOMS
Deodhar Eye Hospital
39/25, Erandawane
Karve Road
Pune-411 004, India

Yutaro Nishi MD
Nishi Eye Hospital
Osaka, Japan

Foreword

Complicated cataract cases challenge all ophthalmologists, regardless of their level of experience. Although complex cases may comprise only 5-10% of all patients in a typical cataract practice, much of our continuing surgical education is devoted to solving problems posed by these eyes. As with most challenging problems in medicine and surgery, there is no single approach that works ideally and consistently well for everyone. This is what makes these patients so difficult, and why having an armamentarium of different strategies to select from is prudent.

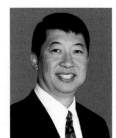

In their new book on Surgical Techniques in Ophthalmology (Cataract Surgery), renowned Editors Ashok Garg and Jorge Alio have assembled an impressive collection of chapters devoted to complex cases and advanced topics in cataract surgery. Equally noteworthy is their lineup of international contributors who have written detailed descriptions of their pearls and strategies. In most cases, these experts have taken a step-by-step approach to describing their techniques, which are illustrated with a generous number of photos and diagrams. The editors have wisely decided to invite multiple authors to describe differing approaches to advanced problems and topics. The geographic diversity of these experts assures that the reader will be exposed to a variety of different techniques and technologies.

There is appropriate emphasis on the removing the dense cataract and multiple contributors describe a wide assortment of strategies ranging from biaxial and coaxial microincisional surgery to several methods of manual small incision extracapsular surgery. The entire gamut of phaco methods is covered as well. Finally, many new and innovative technologies and approaches are introduced in this book. These range from using intraoperative wavefront aberrometry, to glue-fixating IOL haptics to the sclera in the absence of capsular support.

With new technological advances arriving at such a rapid rate, it is a remarkably exciting time to be a cataract surgeon. Of course, these developments challenge us to constantly assimilate and incorporate new ideas and devices. This timely and comprehensive book seeks to provide cutting edge knowledge about advanced cataract surgical topics as clearly as possible. A host of international experts have generously shared their clinical experience and pearls. This reference will undoubtedly benefit all experienced cataract surgeons and their patients.

David F Chang MD
Professor of Ophthalmology
762, Altos Oaks Drive, Suite 1
Los Altos, CA 94024, USA
Ph. 001-650-948-9123
Fax : 001-650-948-0563
E-mail dceye@earthlink.net

Preface

Ophthalmic Surgery technology has undergone rapid advancements and innovations in last two decades. From Modest and conventional surgical techniques in early eighties, now it has become high-tech surgery with least indoor stay and excellent visual outcomes. Microincision surgery in both anterior and posterior segments, corneal and lenticular refractive surgery, modern keratoplasty techniques, pediatric and strabismus surgery, oculoplastic and reconstructive surgery and stem cell transplantation have entirely changed the scenario in ophthalmic surgery today.

Modern ophthalmic surgery is a vast subject. It is important for ophthalmologists to master various surgical steps in the ophthalmic surgery procedures of their interest. There are very few qualities international *Surgical Techniques in Ophthalmology* books which can teach and guide the ophthalmologists to master various surgical techniques properly. Keeping in view of this factor, we have conceptualized the present series of *Surgical Techniques in Ophthalmology* books which shall contain 8 volumes. These volumes shall cover all aspects of ophthalmic surgery in a comprehensive and easy-to-read format. These volumes shall focus on especially Cataract surgery, Corneal and Lenticular Refractive surgery, Glaucoma surgery, Corneal surgery, Retinal surgery, Pediatric surgery, Oculoplastic and Reconstructive surgery, Strabismus and Neuroophthalmic surgery. A panel of International Eminent ophthalmologists are contributing chapters in these volumes for the benefit of ophthalmologists worldwide.

First volume deals with all important topics of cataract surgery. In this volume, International cataract experts show surgical steps of various cataract surgery techniques, management of complex cataracts, complications and recent advances in cataract surgery technology in a lucid manner.

Our gratitudes are due to Shri Jitendar P Vij (CEO), Mr. Tarun Duneja (Director-Publishing) and all staff members of our publisher M/s Jaypee Brothers Medical Publishers (P) Ltd. who took keen interest in this project and for speedy completion of this mega task.

We expect that present series of *Surgical Techniques in Ophthalmology* books shall serve as quick look reference books for ophthalmologists worldwide to sharpen their surgical skills.

— Editors

Contents

Section II: Management of Complicated Cataracts and Cataract Surgery Complications

Section III: Advances in Cataract Surgery Techniques and Technology

Chapter 1

Pearls and Tricks in Congenital Cataract Surgery

Simonetta Morselli, Roberto Bellucci (Italy)

INTRODUCTION

The definition of congenital cataract is the evolutive opacification of the crystalline lens that causes limitation of the visual acuity. This type of opacity can be present at birth or it can develop in the first three months of life. This type of cataract is called "early developmental" cataract. The incidence of the congenital cataract is 0.4 % of the total population. It is an important blindness factor for babies, that accounts from 20 to 38% of the total blindness.[1] The management of this disorder has long challenged clinicians, but the past few decades have seen significant changes in the approach and in the management, due to the information gathered from basic scientific and clinical research.[2-3] The most important visual loss is mainly attributable to amblyopia, that is caused from stimulus deprivation with the additional factor of ocular rivalry in unilateral disease. Thus, enhanced understanding of critical periods of visual development led to surgical intervention for dense cataract being deemed necessary within the first 3 months of life, and possibly as early as the first 6 weeks in unilateral disease.[3] The need to ensure early detection and to allow prompt treatment has resulted in the implementation of various strategies, it is recommended to carry out population screening examinations of newborn examination in many countries.

Diagnosis

The diagnosis is very easy when a complete cataract is present at birth because of the visible leukocoria. When the cataract is posterior and not progressing to the anterior lens layers, the white color of the pupil cannot be detected easily and the diagnosis can be very late, when nistagmus or strabismus appears. Unfortunately, the visual deprivation in the first month of life creates a sensorial obstacle that causes amblyopia, nistagmus and strabismus.

PREOPERATIVE PEARLS

Pupil Dilation

The dilation of the pupil is a very important factor for congenital cataract surgery. The mydriasis is very difficult to obtain and to maintain during surgery. In our experience this type of mixture works very well: 1 mL of phenylephrine 10 % and tropicamide 0.5 % + 1 mL of atropine 1% diluted in the same syringe with 8 cc of saline water. Apply 1 drop every 15 min, starting two hours before surgery and until the pupil is dilated. To maintain the mydriasis inject 0.5 mL of adrenaline into the 500 mL BSS bottle used during surgery.

IOL Implantation

We plan to implant in babies from birth and onwards, because we had negative experiences in the compliance with glasses or with contact lenses after surgery. The type of IOL implantation at the time of cataract surgery is one of the most critical points in congenital cataract surgery. Polymethylmethacrylate (PMMA) IOLs have been successful in pediatric eyes; however, the capsular and inflammatory responses remain a problem.[5-11] Now the AcrySof IOLs made of flexible hydrophobic acrylic material are available (Alcon Laboratories, Forth Worth, Texas), with favorable outcome when used in children. Out of the AcrySof family, the 5.5 mm optic lens seems the most apt to small babies. Until recently, the 5.5 mm optic AcrySof IOL was available only in a 3-piece design with PMMA haptics (MA30 BM), with a total diameter of 12.5 mm. Now also the single piece AcrySof SA30AL IOL is produced, with the same optic diameter and overall length (Fig. 1).

IOL Power Calculation

Preoperative values of axial length and corneal curvature are rarely available in patients with congenital cataracts. Therefore

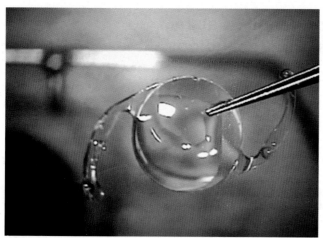

Fig. 1: AcrySof SA30AL IOL is available. This model has a 12.5 mm overall diameter and 5.5 mm optic diameter

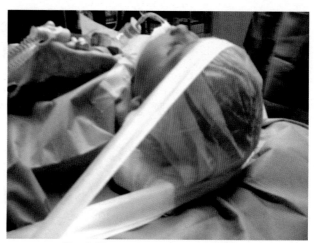

Fig. 2: The baby head must be fixed with an adhesive strip to the operating bed

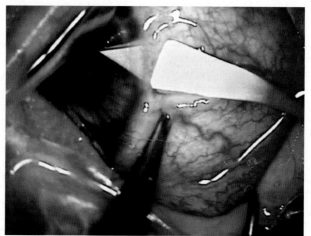

Fig. 3: The incision is created at 12 o'clock under a conjunctival flap

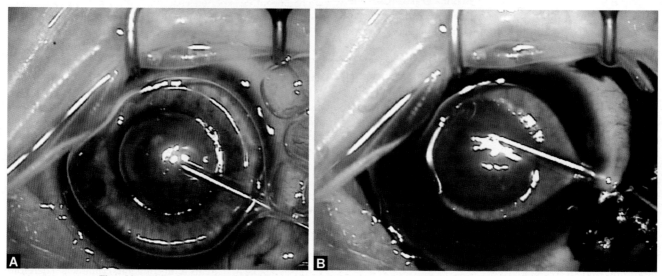

Figs 4A and B: Aspirate 1 ml of methylene blue in an insulin syringe with an air bubble, inject the air bubble first and then methylene blue, with the same syringe through the side port incision

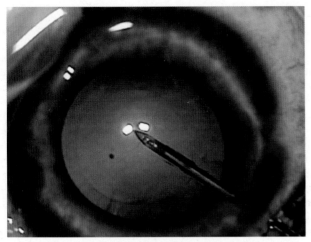

Fig. 5: A small hole in the center of the posterior capsular bag with a needle

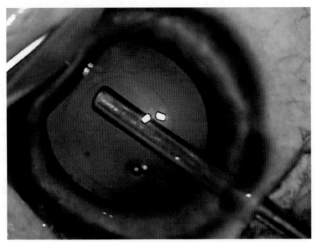

Fig. 8: Anterior vitrectomy is mandatory

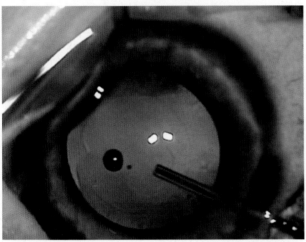

Fig. 6: Inject the viscoelastic between the anterior surface of hyaloid and the posterior surface of the capsular bag

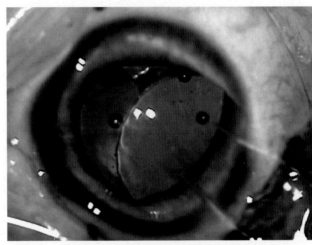

Fig. 9: The IOL is inserted with the injector or with the forceps trying to inject the first in the sulcus

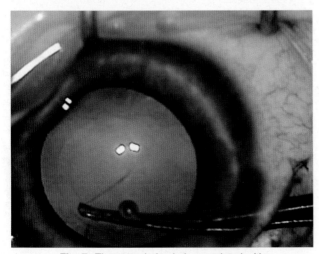

Fig. 7: The capsulorhexis is completed with 'Coridon forceps'

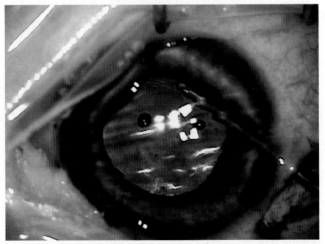

Fig. 10: The optical plate of the IOL is incarcerated behind the two capsules

these values have to be obtained under general anesthesia immediately before surgery. K readings are not easy to obtain even under general anesthesia because a portable corneal topographer is necessary. In addition, the K readings can change during the growth of the eye. Therefore it could be convenient to base the IOL power calculation not on the K readings but only on the axial length. We select the IOL power with reference to the rules of Dr Dahan for babies less than one year old. If the axial length is about 20 mm we select a +25 D IOL, if it is about 19 mm we implant a +26 D, if the length is about 18 mm we implant a +28 D IOL. If the axial length is between 21mm and 23 mm the power of the IOL will be equal to the axial length value +1D per mm exceeding 21.[5] If the axial length is longer than 24 mm the power implanted will be equal to the axial length value -1D per mm exceeding 24.[12]

GENERAL ANESTHESIA

The anesthesiologist must be skilled in general anesthesia in very young patients. The use of curare is mandatory to have the eye in natural position and not in the "Bell phenomenon position". The baby's head must be fixed with an adhesive strip to the operating bed; two rolled cloths help to immobilize the head (Fig. 2).

SURGICAL PEARLS AND TRICKS

We pass a suture through the superior rectus muscle and fix it with 'Pean forceps' to modulate the position of the eye as the surgeon requires during the various steps of the surgery.

The main incision is created at 12 o'clock under a conjunctival flap (Fig. 3).

At least one side-port incision is also created. At the end of the surgery it is mandatory to close the incisions with 10/0 vicryl.

The use of methylene blue under an air bubble is very helpful to color the anterior capsule before performing anterior capsulorhexis. Aspirate 0.5 mL of the methylene blue dye into an insulin syringe, followed by 0.5 mL of filtered air. Inject the air bubble first and then the methylene blue, to avoid any collapse of the anterior chamber: The air will empty the anterior chamber and the dye will be injected onto the capsule without touching the endothelium (Figs 4A and B). Use high molecular weight and cohesive viscoelastic substance to help performing capsulorhexis. The newborn capsule is very elastic and needs to be perforated by a 30G needle. The rhexis tear tends to escape toward the equator because of this elasticity, like it happens in pig eyes in wet-labs.

Posterior capsulorhexis is easier if you do not overfill the capsular bag with viscoelastic substance. A small hole in the center of the posterior capsule with a 30G needle (Fig. 5) helps creating space to inject allows viscoelastic injection between the anterior hyaloid surface and the posterior surface of the posterior capsule (Fig. 6).

The posterior capsulorhexis is completed with 'Corydon forceps' (Fig. 7).

Anterior vitrectomy is mandatory (Fig. 8).

The IOL is inserted with the injector or with the forceps trying to inject the first loop into the ciliary sulcus (Fig. 9).

This is usually difficult because the operated eye is very soft at this moment. The second loop is positioned in the sulcus with a manipulator. The optical plate is then pushed under the posterior capsulorhexis, so while the loops remain in the sulcus, the optical plate is incarcerated behind the two capsules (Fig. 10).

Doing this maneuver the capsular bag remains closed and there is less opportunity for the remaining lens cells to proliferate and to create secondary cataract. The IOL remains stable and centered into the eye. The vitreous body stays behind the IOL and the capsular bag. With this method of IOL implantation, we experienced less inflammation and less synechiae between the IOL and the iris. In the postoperative, it is mandatory to maintain the pupil dilated with omatropine applied twice a day at least for one month to reduce inflammation and to prevent posterior synechiae.

REFERENCES

1. Nelson LB, Ullman S: Congenital and developmental cataracts; chapt 74; Clinical Ophthalmology by Duane- jeger. Harper-Rown, Philadelphia, 1987.
2. Nihalani BR, Vasavada AR. Single piece Acry-Sof intraocular lens implantation in children with congenital and developmental cataract. J Cataract Refract Surg 2006;32(9):1527-34.
3. Wiesel TN. Postnatal development of the visual cortex and the influence of environment. Nature 1982;299:583-91.
4. Maurer D, Lewis TL. In: Simons K (Ed). Early Visual Development, Normal and Abnormal. New York: Oxford University Press 1993;454-84.
5. Wilson ME. Intraocular lens implantation: Has it become the standard of care for children? [Guest editorial] Ophthalmology 1996;103:1719-20.
6. Dahan E, Salmenson BD. Pseudophakia in children: precautions, technique, and feasibility. J Cataract Refract Surg 1990;16:75-82.
7. Buckley EG, Klombers LA, Seaber JH, et al. Management of the posterior capsule during pediatric intraocular lens implantation. Am J Ophthalmol 1993;115:722-28.
8. Wilson ME, Apple DJ, Bluestein EC, Wang X-H. Intraocular lenses for pediatric implantation; biomaterials, designs, and sizing. J Cataract Refract Surg 1994;20:584-91.
9. Dahan E, Drusedau MUH. Choice of lens and dioptric power in pediatric pseudophakia. J Cataract Refract Surg 1997;23:618-23.
10. Vasavada AR, Trivedi RH. Role of optic capture in congenital cataract and intraocular lens surgery in children. J Cataract Refract Surg 2000;26:824-31.
11. Vasavada AR, Trivedi RH, Singh R. Necessity of vitrectomy when optic capture is performed in children older than 5 years. J Cataract Refract Surg 2001;27:1185-93.
12. Dahan E. Lens implantation in microphtalmic eyes of infant. Eur J Impl Refr Surg 1989,1:9-11.

Chapter 2

Cataracta Juvenilis and Congenital Lens Subluxation Surgical Procedure

Bojan Pajic, Brigitte Pajic-Eggspuehler, Jasna Ljubic, Jörg Müller (Switzerland)

INTRODUCTION

A visual acuity of 0.32 or less would suggest that cataract surgery is indicated. The decrease may be due to the cataract, amblyopia or a combination of these. The onset of strabismus or nystagmus related to visual deprivation is another indication for surgery. Some children who are very young or delayed developmentally may never subjectively provide a measured visual acuity. In these cases, the ophthalmologist's clinical Judgment following assessment of the size, laterality of the cataract, will indicate if and when cataract surgery should be performed.

Children with a complete monocular congenital cataract should have surgery performed before 3 months of life.[1] Although there was emphasis at one time on operating and rehabilitating children immediately after birth[2] it is now considered prudent to wait a week or two for the infant to become stable medically, to initiate diagnostic evaluations, and to have sufficient time to initiate appropriate pediatric and anesthesiology consultations to ensure the safety of the administration of general anesthesia.[3] If cataracts involve both eyes, surgery should be performed on the eye with the denser opacity. Once this eye has recovered, (usually 2 to 3 weeks), cataract surgery should be performed on the fellow eye.

Once a decision has been made to perform cataract surgery, the next consideration is selection of the method of optical rehabilitation that will be used. For patients with monocular cataracts, aphakic spectacles are not practical. Before 1 year of age, use of contact lens rehabilitation is suggested. After 1 year, an intraocular lens could be considered (Tables 1 and 2). In patients with bilateral cataracts, contact lens rehabilitation is recommended before 1 or 2 years. Once the eye becomes mature or the child becomes resistant to contact lenses or glasses, secondary implants can be considered.[4, 5]

THE CATARACT PROCEDURE

Children younger than 6 months have their pupils dilated with 0.5 cyclopentolate (Cyclogyl) and 2.5 phenylephrine (Neosynephrine) drops applied twice, 5 minutes apart a half hour prior to coming to the operating room. Use of stronger concentrations of phenylephrine in children may cause elevated blood pressure and irritability of the myocardium. Older children will accept stronger concentrations of these mydriatic agents. Once anesthesia has been administered, axial length determinations can be performed using an A scan probe. If the lens is opaque, a standardized B scan can be performed. The corneal curvature is measured using one of several intraoperative handheld keratometers. If an IOL is going to be used, the pseudophakic lens power calculation can be made while the patient is being propped.

Glaucoma is a problem that occurs in 25 to 31 % of children who have a congenital cataract.[6-8] Presurgical and frequent

---

Table 1: Indications for use of an IOL in children

- Unilateral cataract
- Age 1-8 years old with a unilateral congenital cataract, expected or proven contact lens failure
- Age 1-17 years old with an acquired cataract with previously known adequate vision
- Unilateral developmental cataract age 1-17 years old
- Unilateral traumatic cataract
- Bilateral cataracts
- Patient older than 3 or 4 years of age
- Radiation induced cataracts
- Dry eyes
- Large amplitude nystagmus
- Eyelid scars

Table 2: Relative contraindications for pediatric IOL implantation

- Age less than 1 year
- Microphthalmia
- Microcornea (<9.0 mm cornea)
- Glaucoma
- Inflammation
- Aniridia
- Dislocated lens

postsurgical measurements of the intraocular pressure should be made with similar instrumentation, as Perkins applanation tonometer, Tonopen or Schiotz tonometer, so that valid comparison of the pressure can be made.

CATARACT SURGERY, WITHOUT PLACEMENT OF AN INTRAOCULAR LENS

We initially used a scleral frown incision. The advantage of a self-sealing, no stitch incision in a child is not a consideration since most surgeons will suture all wounds for safety. Children will often rub their eyes following surgery.

A small peritomy or fornix based conjunctival flap is opened with a Vannas scissors. Entry is made into the anterior chamber using a 2.8 mm keratome for performing frown incision. Viscoelastic is introduced into the anterior chamber with an at tempt to make the lens-iris diaphragm bow posterior and become somewhat concave. Care should be exercised not to exaggerate this since an increase in the ocular pressure can occur and the vascular supply to the retina could be compromised. A needle with a bent tip is used to engage and tear the central portion of the anterior capsule (Fig. 1). With frequent regrasping of the flap and tearing toward the center of the lens while watching for radial tears, a continuous curvilinear capsulorhexis is attempted (Fig. 2). This is a very difficult procedure to accomplish in patients younger than 4 years. If there is evidence of extension of the tear radially and it threatens to go to the equator of the lens, this procedure should be abandoned and the remainder of the capsule should be removed with a high frequency capsulotomy device. The lens substance in children is soft and hydrodissection and hydrodelineation are in some cases not performed. The suction part of ultrasound device can be to remove the anterior lens cortex and the lens nucleus (Fig. 3). Ultrasound is rarely necessary. Once the nucleus has been aspirated, the peripheral lens cortex is removed from the fornices of the lens with an I/A Tipp (Fig. 4). It is best to have linear control of the suction pressure so that remnants of lens cortex can be engaged and then teased from the lens capsule without tearing the capsule. If the child is older than 5 or 6 years and will cooperate for a Nd:YAG laser capsulotomy, the posterior lens capsule, if it is clear, is left intact. However, if the child is too young or problems are anticipated with a Nd:YAG laser capsulotomy, a posterior (Fig. 5) capsulectomy and anterior vitrectomy (Figs 6A and B) should be performed using a suction cutting instrument. Attention to the size and location of the capsular opening is important. Care should be taken to make the anterior lens capsule opening slightly larger than the posterior lens capsule opening. The capsule leaflets will later fuse and form a baffle or a ring of support that may be important for stability of an IOL, if a secondary implant is required later. The pupil should be dilated frequently and kept moving to prevent iris-lens capsule adhesions from forming. The anterior chamber is reestablished with balanced solution saline (BSS) and an iridectomy may be considered. If the child is at low risk for developing glaucoma or the iris is vascular, the surgeon may elect not to perform an iridotomy or an iridectomy. However, in patients with uveitis and in some patients with traumatic cataracts, performing an iridotomy or iridectomy may be prudent. The incision may be self-sealing by design but it is safer to close all wounds in children with a 10-0 suture.

Postoperative care consists of drops and a shield. I prefer not to use a bandage dressing. Atropine 0.5% is used in children younger than 6 months of age and 1% atropine drops are used twice a day in eyes of children older than 6 months. An antibiotic steroid combination such as Tobradex may be used or Ocufloxacin combined with a steroid such as Prednisolone acetate can be used during the postoperative period. The eye is shielded for 3 days and the patient is usually seen within 48 hours following surgery. Topical medications are discontinued when inflammation has subsided. This is usually 2 or 3 weeks following surgery. Refraction is performed at this time and repeated frequently. Once the refraction is stable, contact lens or spectacle correction is prescribed.

CATARACT SURGERY WITH LENS IMPLANTATION

Patients with monocular cataracts who are older than 2 year or those who are contact lens resistant or those with inadequate family support to provide reliable and consistent application and removal of contact lenses are candidates for an IOL (Tables 1 and 2). The lens style should be biconvex and have a 6 to 6.5 mm optic diameter optic that has a UV coating. The haptics are angulated and should be between 12 and 13.5 mm in diameter with soft C or J loop configuration. Usually PMMA or acrylic IOL are used as lens material. Measures should be taken to select a lens of appropriate power for the age of the child. Replacement of an IOL that has been placed in the eye of a child is difficult. Adhesions between the IOL and the lens capsule will be fibrotic and replacement or explanation of the lens will be difficult and hazardous. If possible the power selection should be one that is appropriate for a lifetime. There are a few studies that have evaluated the growth of the eye of primates and humans following cataract surgery with and without an IOL. The studies issue conflicting information on the growth patterns of the eye.[9-16] In children with dense lens opacities, the eye may have a longer than expected axial length. Other studies have shown that growth of the eye is reduced following implantation of a lens. Other studies have shown that the aphakic eye continues to elongate axially so that the correction of aphakia reduces with time even until age 20. We set as our goal to achieve a refractive error in adulthood that produces 1.50 D or less of anisometropia. In children younger than 2 years of age, the power selected should provide a final power that is close to the power that the fellow eye is expected to achieve. For example, if the fellow eye in a 2-year-old has a piano refractive error and the child has a traumatic cataract, it would be assumed that the power of the sound eye would eventually develop a myopic refractive error of about –2.00 D. If we calculated a lens power of +20.00 to achieve a piano refractive error in the injured eye, we would reduce the lens calculated power by –2.00 D and implant a +18.00 lens. Between 2 and 8 years of age, the lens power would be reduced by 1.50 D. In children older than 8 years of age, the refractive error is calculated to match the fellow eye (Figs 7 and 8).

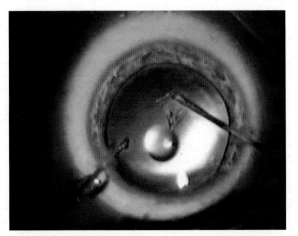

Fig. 1: Opening the capsule anterior with a insulin needle to perform a capsulorhexis

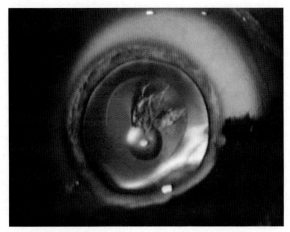

Fig. 2: Continuous curvilinear capsulorhexis

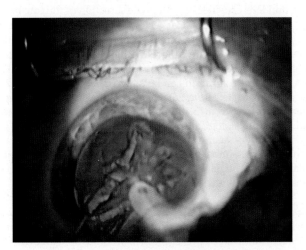

Fig. 3: Removing the anterior lens cortex and the lens nucleus with ultrasound

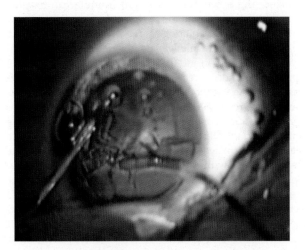

Fig. 4: Lens cortex is removed from the fornices of the lens with an I/A Tip

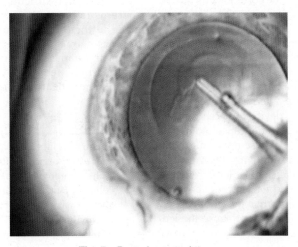

Fig. 5: Posterior capsulotomy

IMPLANTATION OF AN INTRAOCULAR LENS

The technique used to implant an IOL is a modification of the procedure used to remove a cataract without an IOL. Style and power of the lens are selected and confirmed by the surgeon. This will facilitate maneuvering instruments in the anterior chamber. When implanting a PMMA 6.5 mm optic lens, a fornix based conjunctival perimetry is made. A frown incision is constructed at the mid-limbal position and entry is made into the anterior chamber with a keratome. Viscoelastic is introduced to partially fill the anterior chamber. A bent needle is used to puncture the anterior lens capsule and a capsulorhexis is performed with a needle or capsulorhexis forceps. The lens material is removed as described in the previous section. After all cortical remnants are removed the posterior lens capsule is polished. A posterior capsulectomy combined with a small anterior vitrectomy using a vitrecome or similar suction cutting instrument is performed. If one desires, the sleeve can be removed and a separate irrigation cannula can be placed through a stab incision in the peripheral cornea. Viscoelastic is introduced into the anterior chamber. Viscoelastic is used to separate the lens capsule leaflets. The lens is irrigated with a balanced salt solution and the inferior haptic is inserted into the capsular bag under direct visualization. The superior haptic is grasped with a nontooth forceps and, with gentle pressure, is inserted into the superior lens capsular bag (Fig. 9). The lens is then dialed into position with a Sinsky hook so the lens is centered and the haptics are positioned with a 3 and 9 o'clock orientation. If the lens capsule has a radial tear that precludes lens placement within the capsular bag, the haptics may be alternatively placed in the ciliary sulcus. The haptics must both be either in the capsular bag or both in the ciliary sulcus. One in each position will cause decentration and possible iris capture. The frown incision is adapted for security with one or two 10-0 sutures. Viscoelastic is aspirated with the vitrectome suction unit from the anterior chamber (Fig. 10). An iridotomy may be performed at this time. If the surgery has been uneventful and the patient is at low risk for developing glaucoma, an iridotomy or iridectomy is not performed. When the posterior lens capsule is clear and the patient of 6 age or more with a good cooperationof the child, we will leave it intact. We are fortunate to have access to the microruptor three Nd:YAG laser to treat capsular opacification.[17] Alternative methods to "manage" the posterior capsule are to complete the lens implantation and then make a separate pars plana or a pars plicata incision. An irrigation cannula is inserted into the anterior chamber and an vitrectome or similar suction cutting device is placed through the pars plana incision to perform a posterior capsulotomy and removal of the anterior vitreous.[18] We use a capsulorhexis technique to open the posterior capsule with a consecutive anterior vitrectomy. The anterior capsule leaflet is reflected and a Utrata forceps is inserted behind the lens but above the surface of the posterior capsule to perform a posterior capsule capsulorhexis. A further modification is to prolapse the lens optic through the posterior capsule opening in effort to block lens epithelial cell migration in an effort to reduce the formation of secondary membranes.[19, 20] These maneuvers are technically difficult to perform and there is an increased risk for creating a radial tear in the capsule which may cause the lens to decenter.

SURGICAL TECHNIQUE OF CONGENITAL LENS SUBLUXATION

The aim of the novel surgical technique is to preserve the capsule with implanting the IOL in the bag.

In Figure 11 the preoperative situation of a congenitale lens subluxation can be seen. The lens edge of the subluxated lens induces an aberration of higher order, which is heavily to correct with glases or contact lenses (Fig. 12). The Capsulorhexis we perform with a needle or/and forceps (Fig. 13). After the hydrodissection (Fig. 14) a capsular ring have to be implanted in the capsular bag (Fig. 15). With low energy of phacoemulsification (Fig. 16) the lens content can be take away following irrigation and aspiration (Fig. 17) The IOL implantation in the bag (Fig. 18) leeds to a better centration, but it is still not sufficient (Fig. 19). The suture is fixed anterior and posterior the IOL haptic, capsular ring and lens capsule (Fig. 20) in the direction of the calculated optimal, main mathematical vector (Fig. 21). The next step is to prepare a scleral pocket 1 mm from the limbus (Fig. 22). With a insulin needle the suture is placed in the area of the scleral pocket (Fig. 23). A consecutive suture fixation can be done using a (Fig. 24). A perfect centration can be stated after surgery (Fig. 25), even after 1 year later (Fig. 26). The advantage of the novel surgery method is a long-term fixation and centering of chamber posterior IOL at the physiological space. The capsule is adherent with the ciliary body after months. The known disadvantages of the aphakia and chamber anterior IOL could be avoid. The surgical treatment of a congenital lens subluxation is sophisticated surgery method which shows excellent results.

CONCLUSION

Early identification and prompt surgical treatment of pediatric cataracts followed by prescription of accurate optical correction and amblyopia treatment will ensure the best visual result. Pre-existing eye conditions, absence of the fovea, undetected retinal problems, late onset glaucoma, secondary membrane formation, and difficulties in treatment of amblyopia are concerns to the treating ophthalmologist. Progress has been made in the management of children with cataracts. Three decades ago, cataract surgery for children with unilateral complete cataracts was not a consideration. Results that are reported now frequently yield visual acuities better than 0.5 and in some patients, high levels of binocular function are being reported.

REFERENCES

1. Cheng KP, Hiles DA, Biglan AW, Pettapiece MC. Visual results after early surgical treatment of unilateral congenital cataracts. Ophthalmology 1991;98:903-10.
2. Beller R, Hoyt CS, Marg E, Odom JV. Good visual function after neonatal surgery for congenital monocular cataracts. AmJ Ophthalmol 1981;91:559-65.
3. Woelfel SK, Brandon BW. Anesthesia for the pediatric ophthalmology patient. In: Tasman W, Jaeger EA (Eds):

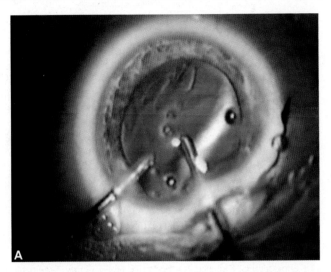

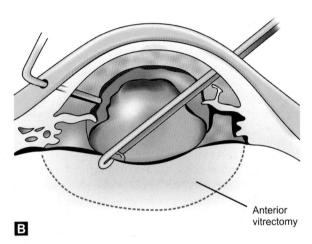

Figs 6A and B: Anterior vitrectomy

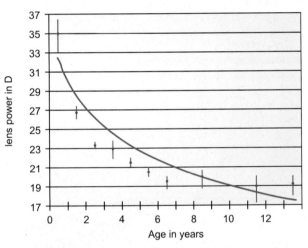

Fig. 7: Lens power attitude correlated with age

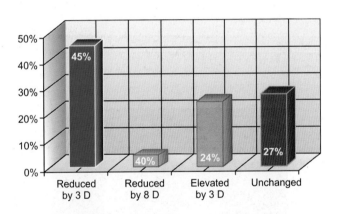

Fig. 8: Corrections error after 2 years of age

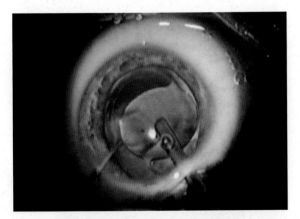

Fig. 9: IOL insertion in the capsular bag after a posterior capsulorhexis and anterior vitrectomy

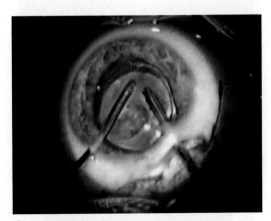

Fig. 10: Viscoelastic evacuation with the vitrectome suction unit

Duane's Clinical Ophthalmology. Philadelphia: Lippincott Raven; 1995;l-l7.

4. DevaroJM, Buckley EG, Awner S, SeaberJ. Secondary posterior chamber intraocular lens implantation in pediatric patients AmJ Ophlhalmol 1997;123:24-30.

5. Biglan AW, Cheng KP, Davis JS, Gerontis CC. Secondary intraocular lens implantation after cataract surgery in children. Am J Ophthalmol 1997;123:224-34.

6. Simon JW, Mehta N, Simmons ST, et al. Glaucoma after pediatric lensectomy/vitrectomy. Ophthalmology 1991;98:670-74.

7. Mills MD, Robb RM. Glaucoma following childhood cataract surgery. J Pediatr Ophthalmol Strabismus 1994;31:355-60.

8. Johnson CP, Keech RV. Prevalence of glaucoma after surgery for PHPV and infantile cataracts. J Pediatr Ophthalmol Strabismus 1996;33:14-17.

9. Lambert SR, Drack AV. Infantile cataracts. Surv Ophthalmol 1996;40:427-58.

10. Raviola E, Wiesel TN. An animal model of myopia. N EnglJ Med 1985;312:609-15.

11. Von Noorden OK, Lewis RA. Ocular axial length in unilateral congenital cataracts and blepharoptosis. Invest Ophth Vis Sci 1987;4:750-52.

12. Fernandes A. Aphakia, pseudophakia and occlusion: effects on postnatal axial eye elongation in a monkey model. In Collier E, Taylor D, Lambert S (Eds): Congenital Cataracts. London: Landes Co, 1994;189-99.

13. Rasolly R, Ben Ezra D. Congenital and traumatic cataract. The effect on ocular axial length. Arch Ophthalmol 1988; 106: 1066-68.

14. Moore BD. Changes in the aphakic retraction of children with unilateral congenital cataracts. J Pediatr Ophthalmol Strabismus 1989;26:290-95.

15. Sinsky RM, StoppelJO, Amin PA. Ocular axial length changes in a pcdiatric patient with aphakia and pseudophakia. J Cataract Refract Surg 1993;19:787-88.

16. Kora Y, Inatomi M, Fukado Y, Mammon M, Yaguchi S. Long-term study of children with implanted intraocular lenses. J Cataract Refract Surg 1992;18:485-88.

17. Atkinson CS, Hiles DA. Treatment of secondary posterior capsular membranes with the Nd:YAG laser in a pediatric population. Am J Ophthalmol 1994;18:496-501.

18. Buckley EG, Klombcrs LA, SeaberJH, Scalisc-Gordy A, Minzter R. Management of the posterior capsule during pediatric intraocular lens implantation. Am J Ophthalmol 1993;15:722-28.

19. Gimbel HV, Ferensowicz M, Raanan M, DeLuca M. Implantation in children. J Pediatr Ophthalmol Strabismus 1993:30:69-79.

20. Parks MM. Posterior lens capsulectomy during primary cataract surgery in children. Ophthalmology 1983,90:344-45.

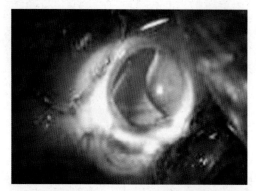

Fig. 11: Lens subluxation preoperative

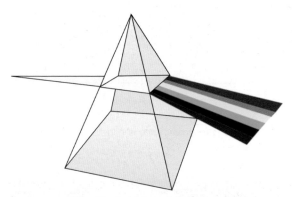

Fig. 12: Induction of aberration

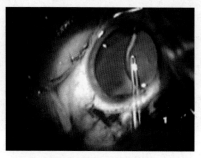

Fig. 13: Capsulorhexis

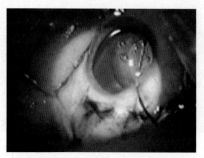

Fig. 14: Hydrodissection

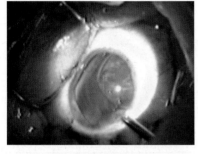

Fig. 15: Capsular ring

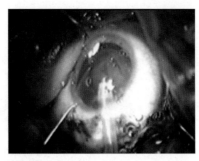

Fig. 16: Phacoemulsification

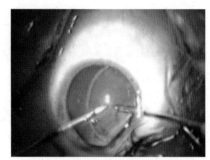

Fig. 17: Irrigation / Aspiration

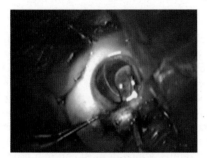

Fig. 18: IOL implantation

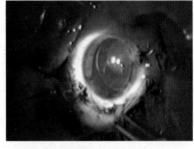

Fig. 19: Insufficient centration

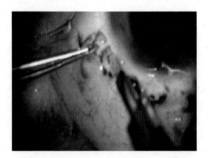

Fig. 20: Scleral pocket preparation

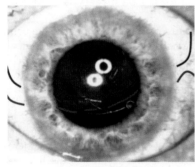

Fig. 21: Target suture area

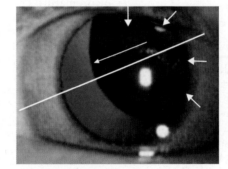

Fig. 22: Target zone vector calculation

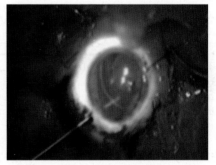

Fig. 23: Suture placing

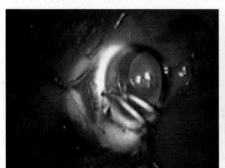

Fig. 24: Suture fixation

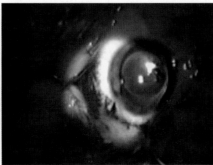

Fig. 25: Perfect centration

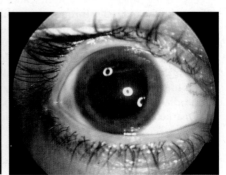

Fig. 26: Result after one year

Chapter 3

Congenital Cataract Surgery

Ventura MC, Ventura LO, Endriss D (Brazil)

INTRODUCTION

Congenital cataract is one of the leading causes of childhood blindness, representing an enormous problem in terms of human morbidity, economic loss, and social burden. It has been estimated that one out of 3.000 children has or develops optically significant lens opacities that need surgery early in life. Fortunately, many advances have been made in preventing, diagnosing and management of pediatric cataracts over the last ten years. Advances in surgical technique and optical rehabilitation specially seem to have significantly improved the prognosis for visual function in these children. Nevertheless, early diagnosis and prompt therapy are necessary to maximize visual function in children with congenital cataract.

TREATMENT IN CONGENITAL CATARACT

Treatment of congenital cataract is challenge in pediatric ophthalmology. Therapeutic approach must consider extension of lens opacity, age of the patient at onset, duration of visual deprivation, monocular versus binocular involvement and type of cataract.

A comprehensive ophthalmic assessment is vital as it influences the management plan. Careful examination of the cataract morphology, along with associated findings, is frequently helpful in determining the etiology and prognosis. Formal evaluation of visual function can be particularly difficult in very young infants. Visual significance of a cataract can be assessed by the red reflex through the undilated pupil with the retinoscope. The retinoscope demonstrates, by retroillumination, not only the absolute area of the lens opacity, which appears black against the red reflex, but also optical distortion extension produced by adjacent areas of what may appear to be clear cortex. Dense ocular opacities greater than 3 mm in diameter are visually significant. Opacity smaller but with marked surrounding cortical distortion may also induce low vision (Fig. 1).

Children are born with an immature visual system and, for normal visual development to occur, they need clear, focused images to be transmitted to the higher visual centers. There is a level of urgency on treating childhood visual impairment. In congenital cataract surgery should be performed early enough to prevent amblyopia, but not too early in order to reduce the likelihood of secondary glaucoma. Most authors advocate that surgery should be performed between the sixth and eight week of life for the best prognosis. Bilateral cases require surgery first in the eye with poorer vision, with surgery for the second eye within one week, except in cases of life risk, when both eyes should be operated on at the same day. Infants with dense bilateral congenital cataract should undergo cataract surgery before the onset of nystagmus, which in most children occurs after the first ten weeks of life. The presence of preoperative nystagmus is a predictor of a poor visual outcome. In the case of premature child, the timing of surgery is adjusted to chronological age (Fig. 2).

In children with acquired progressive opacities, such as posterior lenticonus or lamellar cataracts, the visual outcome depends on the age of the patient at onset and the duration of visual deprivation. Children whose lenses are relatively clear during the first six months of life may develop excellent acuity even if the lens opacity is not detected and treated until two or even three years of age (Fig. 3).

Congenital cataract may be associated with posterior hyperplastic primary vitreous (PHPV). In this case, there is increased tissue reactivity and the visual results following surgery are variable, depending largely on the degree of posterior segment involvement (Fig. 4).

In cases of partial cataracts, especially unilateral developmental cataracts of uncertain visual significance, a trial of pupil dilatation and occlusion therapy may be worthwhile. Several other important covarying factors and conditions affect visual outcome, such as correction of refraction, visual stimulation, presence of intraocular lenses, postoperative complications, nystagmus, strabismus, and coexisting ocular as well as systemic abnormalities.

IOL POWER IN CONGENITAL CATARACT

It has been well- documented that infants, on average, are hyperopic and that the hyperopia gradually decreases during infancy and early childhood. These natural changes in refractive error are presumed to reflect finely regulated eye growth. The process is known as emmetropisation. The rate of change appears to be most rapid in the first 12 months.

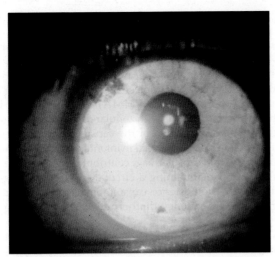

Fig. 1: Cataract polar <3 mm, with normal visual acuity

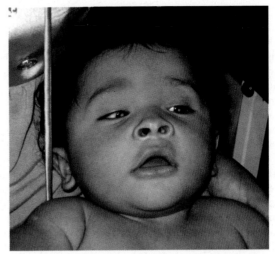

Fig. 2: Eleven-month-old child with bilateral total cataract

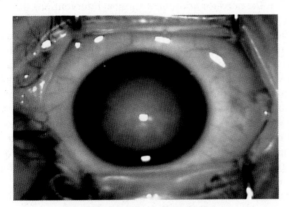

Fig. 3: Complete congenital cataract

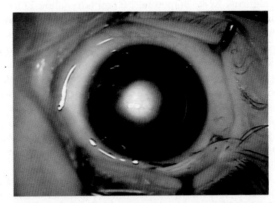

Fig. 4: Congenital cataract associated with posterior hyperplastic primary vitreous (PHPV) in a three-month-old child

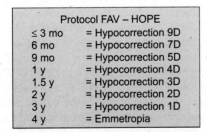

Protocol FAV – HOPE	
≤ 3 mo	= Hypocorrection 9D
6 mo	= Hypocorrection 7D
9 mo	= Hypocorrection 5D
1 y	= Hypocorrection 4D
1.5 y	= Hypocorrection 3D
2 y	= Hypocorrection 2D
3 y	= Hypocorrection 1D
4 y	= Emmetropia

Fig. 5: Protocol used for selection of the IOL power mo= months; D= diopters; y= years

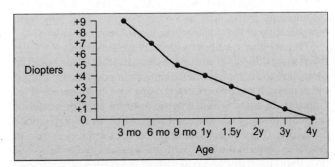

Fig. 6: Postoperative residual hypermetropia expected according to the Protocol FAV-HOPE, 1994 mo = months; y = year

The IOL power prescription depends on the child's age, with allowances made for predicted future growth of the eye and the resulting myopic shift. In accordance with other authors, we use undercorrecting the emmetropic calculation with the induced hyperopia corrected by spectacles that are adjusted throughout life.

In our experience, IOL power is best calculated with the Holladay II formula. The target postoperative refraction is emmetropia by the age of four, which was the initial protocol, adopted since 1994 and adjusted according to the age of the child (Figs 5 and 6).

The IOL power is calculated according to the refraction of the fellow eye if the child is pseudophakic or had unilateral cataract, avoiding an anisometropia more than 2D. The advantage of providing a correction closer to emmetropia during early childhood is if the overcorrection is not worn, the reduced blur in this eye may result in less developing amblyopia.

SURGICAL TECHNIQUE

Preoperatively, the pupil is dilated with tropicamida 1% and phenylephrine 2.5%. Sometimes, 0.1ml adrenaline 1/1000 is used into the anterior chamber to complete the pupil dilatation.

The procedure involves a superior 3.2 mm scleral tunnel incision, approximately 1.0 mm from the limbus that is dissected into clear cornea. Scleral tunnel incisions decrease the frequency of iris prolapse into the wound during surgery and assist the surgeon in preventing collapse of the anterior chamber, which occurs with greater frequency in the soft eyes of children. Furthermore, we use scleral incision rather than clear cornea incision because the Descemet's membrane high elasticity in children can provide a poor apposition of the wound, in our experience.

A viscoelastic substance is injected into the anterior chamber to resist effectively the increased tendency for anterior chamber collapse due to decreased scleral rigidity and a positive vitreous pressure. This approach helps to maintain a deep anterior chamber facilitating attempts of manual anterior capsulorhexis.

The elasticity of the pediatric lens capsule can pose problems for cataract surgeons. During cataract surgery, the anterior capsulotomy shape, size, and edge integrity affect long-term centralization of the capsular-bag-fixated intraocular lens.

The anterior continuous circular capsulorhexis (CCC) is much more difficult in young eyes than in adults and should be controlled and completed, remaining an important edge during the surgery. It can be performed using an Utrata forceps (Figs 7 and 8). In cases within intense anterior and/or posterior capsular fibrosis we are routinely using a radiofrequency diathermy (Easy Rhex, Loktal Medical Electronics, made in Brazil) to perform the CCC, with good results and lower costs. (Figs 9 and 10). It involves coagulation and cutting of the capsule using a high-frequency probe, providing a safe, regular and predictable capsulorhexis. The capsulotomy size and shape are controlled by the surgeon as the tip is moved along a circular path. We have not observed any fragility of the capsule (Figs 11 and 12). This procedure is also suitable in cases of mature cataract in which there is no red reflex, in eyes with small pupil and especially for surgeons with low experience in capsulorhexis. The tryphan-blue staining is also an important and secure way to perform the CCC. (Figs 13A and B)

The lens cortex and nucleus are commonly aspirated with an irrigation-aspiration handpiece (Fig. 14). Implantation of a polymethyl methacrylate (PMMA) endocapsular ring, commonly used in patients with zonular dialysis, promotes the expansion and stabilization of the capsular bag. This endo-capsular tension ring is also used in infantile cataract in attempt to provide a stable capsular bag, contributing to keep the free visual axis and maintaining a circular, central and regular capsulorhexis. The posterior capsulotomy is also performed using the radiofrequency diathermy (Easy Rhex) (Figs 15 and 16).

We advocate performing a primary posterior capsulotomy combined with an anterior vitrectomy in all eyes of children under four years of age, via anterior approach. The posterior capsulotomy should be around 4.0 mm in diameter and the anterior vitreous is removed to ensure a clear visual axis and prevent the need for additional surgical interventions during a long-term follow-up, due to secondary cataract (Fig. 17).

The risk of posterior capsule opacification (PCO) in children, when the posterior capsulotomy is not performed, may be as high as 95%, and it is a major obstacle to visual rehabilitation following pediatric cataract extraction. The younger the patient, the more rapid the opacification, and finally disturbance of the visual functions. One approach that has been suggested to prevent PCO, is capturing the IOL optic through the posterior capsule opening while the haptics remain in the bag (posterior capsulorhexis with optic capture). However, capturing the optic through posterior capsulorhexis without anterior vitrectomy did not always ensure a clear visual axis.

The confection of a primary posterior capsulorhexis (PPC) is not enough to maintain a clear visual axis because the anterior hyaloid offers a scaffold for lens epithelial cell (LEC) migration and regeneration. Thus, an anterior vitrectomy is necessary. Therefore, even with anterior vitrectomy the visual axis may be reoccluded, especially when the posterior capsulorhexis is too small. In brief, primary posterior capsulotomy with anterior vitrectomy allows a clear visual axis, facilitating visual rehabilitation, and decreases the reoperation rate.

The best place to implant the intraocular lens is into the capsular bag; this is true for adult and to a more extent for child eyes. In-the-bag IOL implantation could provide a good centralization and reduce the change of PCO. Even in the presence of a round posterior capsulotomy, positioning an IOL within the bag is easily achievable in these children's eyes if the edges of the capsulotomy are freed from formed vitreous (Figs 18A and B). Some surgeons who are reluctant of inserting the IOL in the presence of a posterior capsulotomy suggest performing a posterior capsulotomy after placing the IOL within the bag using the vitrectomy probe, either by way of the limbus or by way of the pars plana. Others advocate the use of Nd:YAG laser after surgery. In younger children, Nd:YAG laser

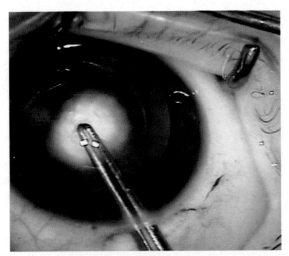

Fig. 7: Utrata forceps used to perform the anterior continuous circular capsulorhexis

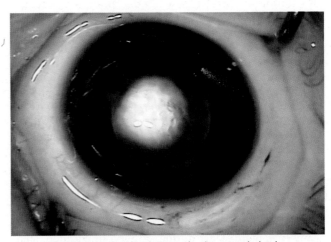

Fig. 8: Anterior continuous circular capsulorhexis

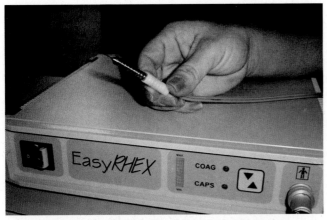

Fig. 9: Radiofrequency diathermy (Easy Rhex, Loktal Medical Electronics, made in Brazil). Used to perform the continuous circular capsulorhexis

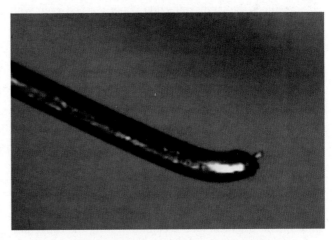

Fig. 10: Easy Rhex high-frequency probe

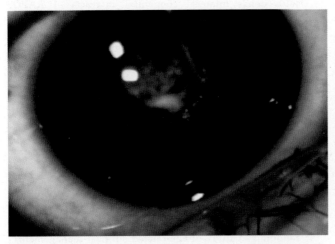

Fig. 11: Anterior continuous circular capsulorhexis in a case within intense anterior capsular fibrosis performed using a radiofrequency diathermy (Easy Rhex)

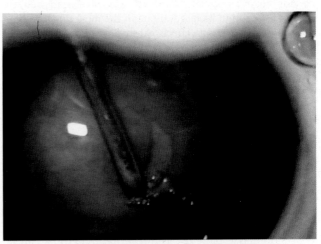

Fig. 12: Trypan-blue staining for security of continuous circular capsulorhexis

capsulotomies often close and require a surgical membranectomy or repeated laser treatment. This is because of a possible transformation of residual LECs into myofibroblasts, which use the anterior vitreous face and the posterior surface of the IOL as a scaffold. Furthermore, this procedure is not without risks, and requires the child collaboration, almost unavailable in very young patient.

There has been growing tendency to use acrylic IOL. We use a single foldable acrylic IOL in all cases: AcrySof Type 7B (Alcon), with an optic diameter of 5.5 mm and a haptic diameter of 12.5 mm. It has been postulated that acrylic IOL induces less cellular reac-tion and is more adhesive to the capsular bag than PMMA IOL. It is believed that the biomaterial and biomechanical properties of the acrylic IOL help reduce the frequency of secondary membrane formation. Foldable IOLs are implanted through smaller incisions than PMMA lenses, so the anterior chamber is more stable during surgery. In addition, small incisions incite less inflammation, and lower surgically induced astigmatism.

Sometimes the target refraction is not reached even with the highest power available in the IOL styles used in the patients. Thus, the residual refraction is corrected with glasses, in bilateral or unilateral cataracts. Some authors suggested the use of piggyback IOLs when high degrees of dioptric power are needed. They state that this technique improves visual outcome by providing a portion of refractive correction in a more permanent location (inside the eye), and by avoiding periods of uncorrected aphakia. In these cases an IOL is placed in the capsular bag and a second IOL in the ciliary sulcus. A second surgery is inevitable to remove the IOL of the ciliary sulcus. A single undercorrected IOL implanted in the bag, and the residual refraction corrected by spectacles is generally preferred by the majority of pediatric surgeons.

Recently a pilot study has been performed using intracameral triamcinolone acetonide during the congenital cataract surgery to minimize inflammation in the early postoperative period, avoiding the prolonged use of oral steroids (Fig. 19). Direct intraocular injection of steroids delivers the desired drug to its target tissue in the most direct fashion without extraocular side effects. At the end of the surgery, 0.1 ml of triamcinolone acetonide (Kenalog) is injected inside the anterior chamber, on the peripheral margin. The intraocular pressure (IOP) has been monitored systematically. In the last year two cases of transitory IOP elevation were observed (24 and 28 mmHg respectively) around two to three weeks after the surgery, controlled by IOP-lowering drops (timolol maleate 0.5%, and/or brinzolamide 1%).

POSTOPERATIVE MANAGEMENT

The residual hyperopia is corrected by spectacles adjusted according the growth and refractional changes observed in the child. The spectacles for the residual refraction should be accurate and actual, and generally they are thin and easy wearing in pseudophakic patients. The residual hyperopia can be dangerous to the visual rehabilitation if the additional refraction

for near point correction is not prescribed. In our experience, the spectacles in babies are prescribed with an additional +2.0 or +3.0D of correction to provide a near point correction. For children who have just learned walking or around one year old, bifocals or multifocals are prescribed with an additional +3.0D. (Fig. 20)

The treatment for amblyopia with patching is prescribed, using after surgery had been completed to both eyes. Occlusion therapy is indicated according to the age and amblyopia grade of the child. (Fig. 21).

The Department of Visual Stimulation is fundamental in achieving a successful visual rehabilitation, with the holistic vision of the patient's needs. A multidisciplinary team is crucial in diagnosing and treatment of them. (Fig. 22). We must, therefore, not become complacent, and should remain vigilant about potential long-term complications, especially in the infant eye. Nevertheless, early visual rehabilitation with proper refraction, spectacle prescription, and antiamblyopia therapy are necessary to ensure optimal visual outcome after pediatric cataract surgery.

BIBLIOGRAPHY

1. Argento C, Badoza D, Ugrin C. Optic capture of the AcrySof intraocular lens in pediatric cataract surgery. J Cataract Refract Surg 2001;27(10):1638-42.
2. Fan DS, Yip WW, Yu CB, Rao SK, Lam DS. Updates on the surgical management of paediatric cataract with primary intraocular lens implantation. Ann Acad Med Singapore 2006;35(8):564-70.
3. Kugelberg M, Zetterström C. Pediatric cataract surgery with or without anterior vitrectomy. J Cataract Refract Surg 2002;28(10):1770-3.
4. Lambert SR, Buckley EG, Plager DA, Medow NB, Wilson ME. Unilateral intraocular lens implantation during the first six months of life. J AAPOS. 1999;3(6):344-49.
5. Lambert SR, Lynn MJ, Reeves R, Plager DA, Buckley EG, Wilson ME. Is there a latent period for the surgical treatment of children with dense bilateral congenital cataracts? J AAPOS 2006;10(1):30-36.
6. Ledoux DM, Trivedi RH, Wilson ME Jr, Payne JF. Pediatric cataract extraction with intraocular lens implantation: visual acuity outcome when measured at age four years and older. J AAPOS 2007;11(3):218-24.
7. Lee YC, Kim HS. Clinical symptoms and visual outcome in patients with presumed congenital cataract. J Pediatr Ophthalmol Strabismus 2000;37(4):219-24.
8. McClatchey SK, Dahan E, Maselli E, Gimbel HV, Wilson ME, Lambert SR, et al. A comparison of the rate of refractive growth in pediatric aphakic and pseudophakic eyes. Ophthalmology 2000;107(1):118-22.
9. Müllner-Eidenböck A, Amon M, Moser E, Kruger A, Abela C, Schlemmer Y, et al. Morphological and functional results of AcrySof intraocular lens implantation in children: prospective randomized study of age-related surgical management. J Cataract Refract Surg 2003;29(2):285-93.

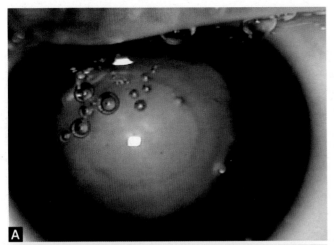

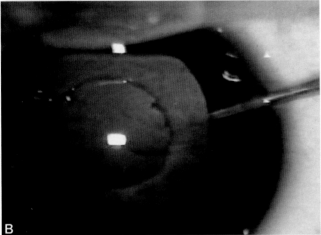

Figs 13A and B: Anterior continuous circular capsulorhexis before (A) and after (B) the lens aspiration

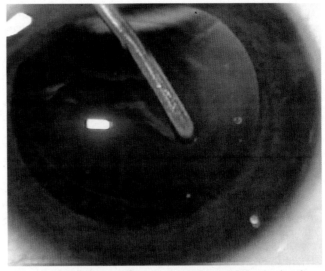

Fig. 15: The primary posterior capsulotomy performed using the radiofrequency diathermy (Easy Rhex)

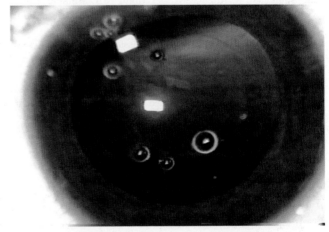

Fig. 16: Primary posterior capsulotomy

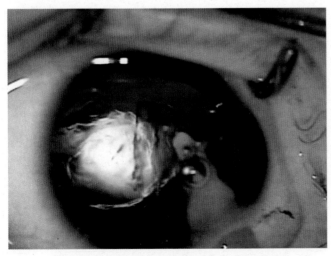

Fig. 14: Aspiration of the lens cortex and nucleus

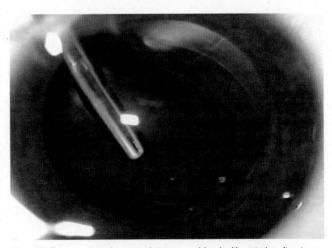

Fig. 17: Primary posterior capsulotomy combined with anterior vitrectomy

10. O'Keefe M, Fenton S, Lanigan B. Visual outcomes and complications of posterior chamber intraocular lens implantation in the first year of life. J Cataract Refract Surg 2001;27(12):2006-11.

11. Oliveira L, Carvalho M, Endriss D. Cataratas pediátricas: rehabilitación visual. In: Lorente R, Mendicute J. Cirugía del cristalino. Espanha: Sociedad Española de Oftalmología 2008;852-58.

12. Pandey SK, Wilson ME, Trivedi RH, Izak AM, Macky TA, Werner L, et al. Pediatric cataract surgery and intraocular lens implantation: Current techniques, complications, and management. Int Ophthalmol Clin 2001;41(3):175-96.

13. Ram J, Brar GS, Kaushik S, Gupta A, Gupta A. Role of posterior capsulotomy with vitrectomy and intraocular lens design and material in reducing posterior capsule opacification after pediatric cataract surgery. J Cataract Refract Surg. 2003;29(8):1579-84.

14. Shah SK, Vasavada V, Praveen MR, Vasavada AR, Trivedi RH, Dixit NV. Triamcinolone-assisted vitrectomy in pediatric cataract surgery. J Cataract Refract Surg 2009;35(2):230-2.

15. Superstein R, Archer SM, Del Monte MA. Minimal myopic shift in pseudophakic versus aphakic pediatric cataract patients. J AAPOS;2002;6(5):271-76.

16. Taylor D, Wright KW, Amaya L, Cassidy L, Nischal K, Russell-Eggitt I, et al. Should we aggressively treat unilateral congenital cataracts? Br J Ophthalmol 2001;85(9):1120-26.

17. Vasavada AR, Trivedi RH, Singh R. Necessity of vitrectomy when optic capture is performed in children older than 5 years. J Cataract Refract Surg 2001;27(8):1185-93.

18. Vasavada AR, Trivedi RH. Role of optic capture in congenital cataract and intraocular lens surgery in children. J Cataract Refract Surg 2000;26(6):824-31.

19. Ventura LO, Ventura M, Endriss D. Catarata congenital e infantil. In: Bicas HEA, Jorge AAH. Oftalmologia: fundamentos e aplicações. São Paulo: Tecmedd 2007;305-14

20. Ventura LO, Ventura M, Endriss D. Catarata infantil. In: Centurion V, Nicoli C, Villar-Kuri J. El libro del cristalino de las americas. São Paulo: Livraria e Editora Santos 2006; 695-708.

21. Ventura M, Ventura L, Endriss D. Catarata infantil: aspectos biométricos e desafios. In: Centurion V. Excelência em biometria. Rio de Janeiro: Cultura Médica 2006;157-66.

22. Ventura M. Catarata congênita. In: Rezende F. Cirurgia da catarata. Rio de Janeiro: Cultura Médica 2000;399-407.

23. Ventura M. Visual impairment due to congenital cataract. Highlights Ophthalmol 2004;32(5):17-20

24. Ventura MC, Ventura LO, Endriss D. Conduta no seguimento pós-operatório na catarata da criança. In: Verçosa IC, Tartarella MB. Catarata na criança. Fortaleza: Celigráfica 2008;245-7.

25. Ventura MC, Ventura LO, Endriss D. Implante de lentes intra-oculares na cirurgia da catarata na criança. In: Verçosa IC, Tartarella MB. Catarata na criança. Fortaleza: Celigráfica 2008;119-26.

26. Wilson ME, Pandey SK, Thakur J. Paediatric cataract blindness in the developing world: surgical techniques and intraocular lenses in the new millennium. Br J Ophthalmol 2003;87(1):14-19.

27. Wilson ME, Peterseim MW, Englert JA, Lall-Trail JK, Elliott LA. Pseudophakia and polypseudophakia in the first year of life. J AAPOS 2001;5(4):238-45.

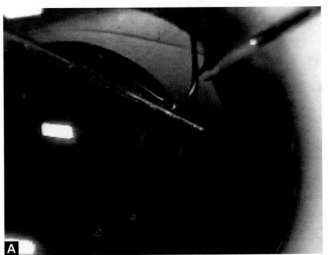

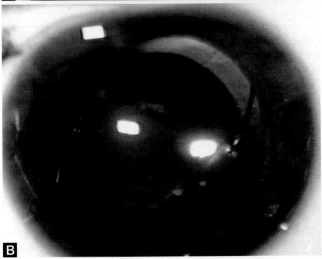

Figs 18A and B: In-the-bag IOL implantation

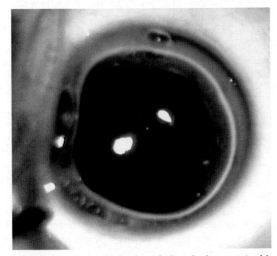

Fig. 19: Intracameral injection of triamcinolone acetonide

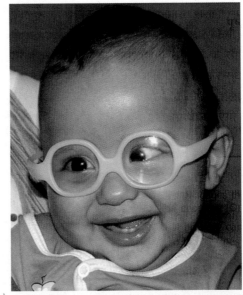

Fig. 20: Spectacles correction for the residual refraction

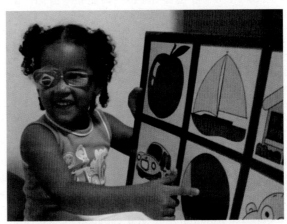

Fig. 21: Antiamblyopia therapy until 10 years of age

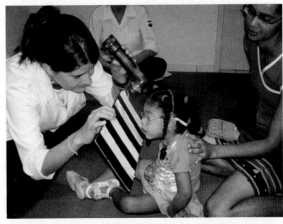

Fig. 22: Visual rehabilitation with the multidisciplinary team

Chapter 4

Bimanual Microcataract Surgery in Children

Jerome Bovet (Switzerland)

INTRODUCTION

Most of the adult cataract surgeon has to be familiar with the technique of pediatric cataract because in Europe, Africa and Asia. There are very few ophthalmologists even less pediatric ophthalmologist. If you work in an eye camp or in a Bush hospitals to do cataract surgery you will discover all kind of cataract and you will have not the possibility to say no to a children with a double white cataract.

Childhood cataract is the major preventable cause of lifelong visual impairment. In recent years technical and technological advances in adult surgery have helped pediatric cataract. Most of the surgeons agree now to implant at once as a mode of ambliopia rehabilitation.[1]

The aim of pediatric cataract surgery is to provide and maintain a clear visual axis and a focused retinal image. The long-term visual outcome is often negatively affected by the development of amblyopia secondary to the cataract itself or owing to postoperative reopacification of the ocular media.[2] One of the major challenges for pediatric cataract intraocular lens (IOL) surgery has been the adaptation of a techniques used for adult cataract—IOL surgery. The propensity for increased postoperative inflammation and capsular opacification, a refractive state that is constantly changing due to growth of the eye, a tendency to develop amblyopia are the factors that make cataract surgery in the child different from that in the adult. The management of pediatric cataracts is fare more complex than the management of cataracts in adults.[3]

The use of Bimanual microphaco[4] technique with 2 paracentesis has revolutionized cataract surgery. Most importantly it allows secure placement of the IOL within the confines of the capsular bag and limits its contact with the reactive uveal tissue. Minimal wound is also critical to the success of cataract surgery and can be achieved by the creation of a sutureless incision.

As we start doing bimanual phaco technique in 2001[8] we were surprized how easily this techniqe can be applied with very little change to pediatric cataract. This three next chapters will describe our bimanual phacotechnique apply to pediatric cataract.

I warmly recommend every surgeon to read the excellent textbook on pediatric cataract surgery by M Edward Wilson, Jr

Rupal H Trivedi and Suresh K Pandey which are the reference textbooks on the subject.[3]

HISTORY

Phacoemulsification was used in pediatric cataract surgery for the first time. In 1970 by Hiles et al and Callahan recommended phacoemulsification as a useful extension of the aspiration technique in children since the softness of the lens material can vary greatly from case to case.[2]

HISTORY BIMANUAL PHACO

To know who started the bimanual procedure we have to come back quite late the first which worked with bimanual was de Dardenne in Bonn (Germany) he has one of the first the idea to take out the cristaline of a baby with a bimanual aspiration irrigation, Brauweiller[5] come back with the technique with phaco and bimanual aspiration irrigation which is far more easier than with the monocannula. In 1982, Steven P Shearing[6] started to do phacoemulsification bimanual with a sleeveless tip.

Amar Agrawal[7] restarted the technique of phakonit which means phaco with a needle inside the hole. The reason the technique started this time that we found new lens wich can be inserted under an incision of 1.7 mm

Pediatric cataract can be removed through a relatively small wound as the lens has no hard nuclei.That is why we propose to applicate the bimanual microphaco technique which is the last and the best technique for adult cataract to children with certain modifications which is necessary to fit to children.[9]

BIMANUAL MICROPHACOEMULSIFICATION TECHNIQUE

We first measure the white to white distance to secure that we will have enough room to place a soft adult hydrophilic acrylic lens inside the bag at the end of the proceduren.[3] (Fig. 1)

We use exactly the same Instruments for adult or pediatric Bimanual Microphaco.[10] (Fig. 2) : probe sleveless 0.9 mm tip, bimanual irrigation-aspiration tip, shooter, capsulorhexis forceps, paracentesis 19G and 20G, we reserve for all children a bimanual vitrector with any vacuum pump machine to do an anterior vitrectomy.

20

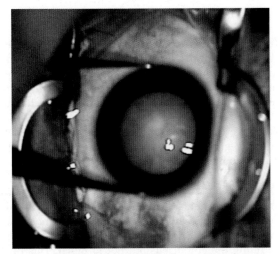

Fig. 1: Measuring the white to white

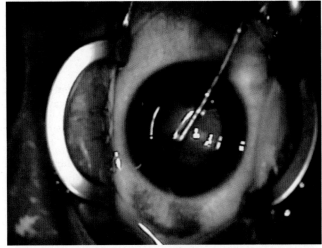

Fig. 4: Dye the anterior capsule with trypan blue

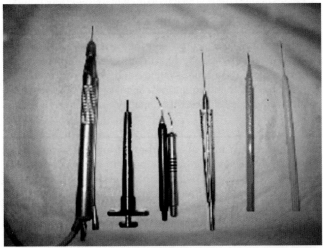

Fig. 2: Instruments

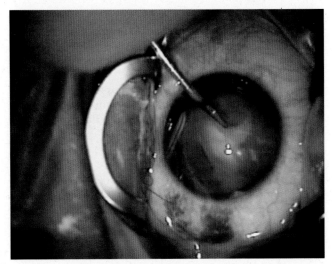

Fig. 5: Rupture of the anterior capsule

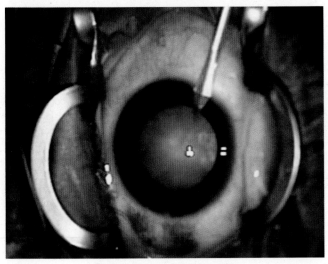

Fig. 3: First paracentesis 19G

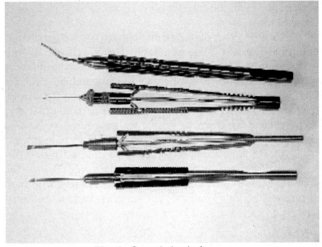

Fig. 6: Capsulorhexis forceps

ANESTHESIA

The technique we general use for a right eye is under general anesthesia.

Paracentesis[11] (Fig. 3)

We started for a right eye by 2 paracentesis at 10 and 2 O'clock create a 20 gauge respectively a 19 G opening. We always control the width of the incision.

Dye of the Capsule[12-14] (Fig. 4)

Injection of a buble of air and just after injection of trypan blue after 60 sec the excessive dye is washed out with the viscoelatic.

Viscous

Injection of high viscous acide hyaluronique, like healon GV or Healon 5.

Capsulorhexis[15]

Capsulorhexis with a double curve special 20 G forceps if the cutting force are centrifuge instead of centripet we repeat the procedure somewherelse if it is not possible we finish with a tin can opening that doesn't mean that you will change the procedure (Fig. 5).

You have to try many different forceps to find your cup of tea the most rigid, straight on used for vitrectomies are the worst, my best choice is the dobble curve first from the top (Fig. 6).

Hydrodelineation-hydrodissection

For pediatric cataract we generaly don't do any hydro-delineation because the nucleus is too soft. The hydrodissection of the cortex is more useful to detach the cortex from the capsule which is often sticky.

Phacoemulsification of the Nucleus (Fig. 7)

Bimanual microphaco technique change with the hardness of the cataract. We use most of the time very few phaco power because the pediatric cataract is very soft we aspirate most of the time the nucleus.[9]

To succed to your bimanual microphaco you have to change your fluidic system.[16] You have to change the diameter of your irrigation from 20 gauge to a 19 gauge to increase the inflow in the anterior chamber to compensate the leak and the surge the outflow has to reach 30-35 cc/min to cool down the phacotip, the paracentesis has to be 1mm and for the phaco tip of 1.2 mm. To have the same efficacity during the phacotime we have to increase the vacuum to a level of 300 mmHg of vacuum.[17,18]

Phacomachine manufacturers have devised numerous sophisticated strategies for minimizing the surge (Fig. 8). The goal has been to provide surgeons the advantages with high vacuum without the danger.[19] The simpliest and most efficacy

to rich this target is to increase the flow inside the eye in increasing the lumen of the irrigating tip.

To prevent a surge the surgeon has to verify every session that the inflow is always superior has the outflow. For examples, if you regulate your outflow to 35 cc/min and you have a 60 cc/min of inflow you will never have a surge even you have a vacuum of 500 mm Hg that the secret of the 19 G technique[20,21] (Fig. 9).

You have to play with the pedal like with the pedal of a piano not to give to much and to longer phacopower if you don't want to burn your cornea.

EPINUCLEUS REMOVAL IF EXIST

As progressively the soft nucleus is removed the posterior capsule is exposed to the phaco tip and the chamber stability becomes crucial. The vacuum has to be lower during the phase of aspirating the epinucleus but not to much. This phase is facilitated by a bimanual microphaco technique. The irrigating tip passes behind the epinucleus lo lift it in the anterior chamber.

IRRIGATION–ASPIRATION THE CORTEX

During this phase the vacuum has to be lower and the ultrasound switch off. We change the phacoemulsification probe by the irrigation-aspiration Duet systeme and we try to polish the anterior, posterior and equatorial capsule as much as we can to avoid a rapid posterior capsular opacity.

LENS

Only a few lens[22] can be injected through an incision less than 2 mm for this purpose we have to put end to end the catridge and the corneal incision (Fig. 10), then we have to shoot the lens like suppository inside the anterior chamber, we use most of the time the Acrismart 36 or 48 because of is stability and is accuracy with our biometry. The lens acrismart from Acritec is a acrylic hydrophilic-coated hydrophobic platelet lens This lens has a very good reaction and the placement inside the bag is optimal[23,24] (Fig. 10).

CONCLUSION

The difference with a conventional phaco is the sleeveless tip, the diameter of the bimanual irrigation-aspiration and the injector with a new catridge which permit to inject the lens without going inside the anterior chamber with the cartridge.

With pediatric cataract the 19G bimanual Phacotechnique allowed the surgeon to switch from the phacoemulsification probe to the vitrector probe without changing any parameter and avoiding any surge of the anterior chamber which is one difficulties when we have to do an anterior vitrectomy or posterior vitrector capsulectomy.

The examples below give you an idea of what settings are being used at the beginning of the changing technique from coaxial to bimanual microphaco (Fig. 11).

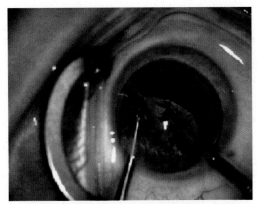

Fig. 7: Bimanual Microphaco

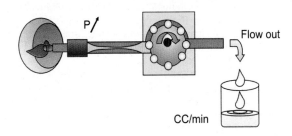

Fig. 8: Vacuum with a Peristaltique pump

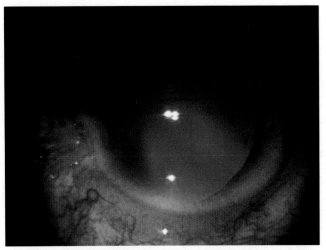

Fig .10: Injection a lens on a 1.7 mm incision

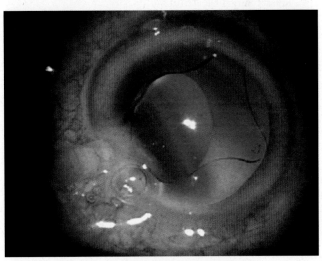

Fig. 11A: Insertion of an Acri Smart 36 A the cartridge stay outside

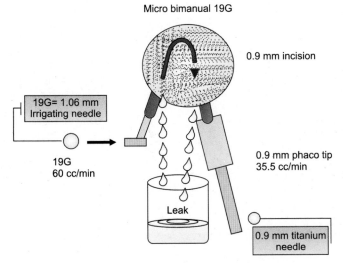

Fig. 9: Inflow-Outflow=Leak

Type of machine	Amo Gemini	Amo Gemini	Amo Gemini
Technique	Phaco chop Bimanual	Phaco chop Bimanual	Phaco chop Bimanual
Stage	Sculpting	Chopping	Epinucleus
Inflow cc/min	60.0	60.0	60.0
Real Bottle height cmH₂O	55	55	55
Pressure mm Hg inside the eye	34.5	34.5	34.5
Outflow cc/min	36.5	36.5	36.5
Vacuum mm Hg	100	300	200
Ultrasound % Linear,no pulse,no burst	30%	30%	30%

Fig. 11B: Setting bimanual Microphaco

23

REFERENCES

1. Wilson ME Jr,Bartholomev LR,Trivedi RH. Pediatric cataract surgery and intraocular lens implantation: practice styles and preferences of the 2001 ASCRS and AAPOS memberships. J Cataract Refract Surg 2003;29: 1811-20.

2. Wilson ME,Pandey SK, Werner L,et al. Pediatric cataract surgery:current techniques, complications and management.In Agarwal S,Argawal A, Sachdev MS,Metha KR, Fine IH, Argawal A (Eds). Phacoemulsification Laser Cataract Surgery and Foldable IOls.New DeIhi, India: Jaypee Brothers Medical 2000;369-88

3. Wilson ME, Jr. Trivedi RH, Pandey SK Pediatric Cataract Surgery Techniques, Complications, and Management Philadelphia, USA Lippincott WilliamsandWilkins, 2005.

4. A.Garg, Fine D, Chang K, Metha J, Bovet L, P Vejarano SK, Pandey C Metha. Mastering the art of Bimanual Microincision Phaco New Dehli Ed Jaypee Brothers Medical Publishers Ltd 2005.

5. Bimanual irrigation/aspiration. Brauweiler P. J Cataract Refract Surg 1996; 22:1013-6.

6. Sharing SP, Releya RL, Loiza A, Shearing RL. Routine phacoemulsification through a one-millimeter non sutured incision Cataract 1985;2:6-10.

7. Agarwal A, Agarwal A, Agarwal S, Narang P, Narang S. Phakonit: Phacoemulsification through a 0.9 mm corneal incision J Cataract Refract Surg 2001; 27:1548-52.

8. J Bovet, O Achard, JM Baumgartner, A Chiou, C de Courten, P Rabineau. 0.9 mm Incision Bimanual Phaco and IOL Insertion Through a 1,7 mm Incision. Symposium on cataract,IOL and refractive surgery abst ASCRS-ASOA San Francisco April 12-16,2003.

9. Scheie HG. Aspiration of congenital or soft cataracts:A new technique. A J Ophthalmol 1960;50:1048-56.

10. J Bovet, O Achard, JM Baumgartner, A Chiou, C de Courten, P Rabineau. Bimanual Phaco Trick and Track ASCRS-ASOA Film San Diego May 1-5 2004.

11. J Bovet 19 G Bimanual MicroPhaco ASCRS-ASOA abstract 2006;March 17-22.

12. Dye-Enhanced Pediatric Cataract Surgery Horiguchi M, Myake K, Otha I, Ito Staining of the lens capsule for circular continuous capsulorhexis in eyes with white cataract. Arch Ophthalmol 1998;116:535-37.

13. Melles GRJ, Waard PWT, Pameyer JH, Beekhuis.WH Tripan blue capsule staining in cataract surgery. J Cataract Refract Surg 1999;24:7-9.

14. Chang DF.Capsule staining and mature cataracts:a comparaison of indocianine green and trypan blue dyes Br J Ophthalmol (video report),July 2000.

15. Gimbel HV, Neuhann T. Development, advantage and methods oft the contiuous circular capsulorhexis technique. J Cataract Refract Surg 1990;16:31-37.

16. BS Seibel. Phacodynamics.Mastering the tools and techniques of phacoemulsification Surgery (Eds). Slack Incorporated 2005.

17. A Garg, I Fine, D Chang, IG Pallikaris, DF Chang, H Tsuneoka, J Bovet (Eds). Innovative techniques in Ophthalmology, New Dehli Jaypee Brothers Medical Publishers Ltd, 2006.

18. Jeng BH, Huang D. Anterior chamber stability during bimanual irrigation and aspiration J Cataract Refrac Surg 2001; 27:1670-78.

19. Vejarano L F, Tello A, Vejarano A. Phakonit: Incisions and use of a pressurized inflow system. J Cataract Refrac Surg 2004;30:939.

20. Barret G. Maxi-flow phaco needle. ASCRS-ASOA Film festival first place 1995.

21. Blumenthal M, Assia EI,Chen V, Avni I. Using an anterior chamber maintainer to control intraocular pressure during phacoemulsification. J Cataract Refract Surg 1994;20:93-96.

22. Tsuneoka H, Hayama A, Takahama M. Ultrasmall-incision bimanual phacoemulsification and AcrySof SA30AL implantation through a 2.2 mm incision. J Cataract Refrac Surg 2003;29:1070-76.

23. Agarwal A, Agarwal S, Agarwal A. Phakonit with an AcriTec IOL. J Cataract Refrac Surg 2003;29:854-55.

24. Wilson ME.Intraocular lens implantation:Has it become the standard of care for children?(Editorial). Ophthalmology 1996;103:1719-20.

Chapter 5

The 3-in-1 Simplified Approach for ECCE, MSICS and Phacoemulsification

Kadil Jojo Jr. Sinolinding (Philippines)

INTRODUCTION

Aside from the minimal and manageable surgery-related complications, the prime objectives in modern cataract surgery include excellent unaided visual acuity and shorter recovery time. This can be achieved by a good preoperative evaluation and preparation, a surgical technique with minimized intra-operative manipulation, and a simple post-operative require-ment. While good pre-surgical selection of patients is important in achieving targeted results, the quality of unaided postoperative vision on the other hand, is inversely related to the size of corneal incision— the smaller the better. This becomes the main topic of discussion.

The transition from intracapsular to extracapsular cataract surgery has opened the surgical arena flooded with outstanding modifications from experts and innovators around the world bringing in modern approaches and tools aimed at a common purpose— to extract the cataractous lens safely, quickly, and effectively. These include the implantation of intraocular lenses (IOLs), and cataract management utilizing either the highly technical mechanical phacoemulsification or the simpler manual small incision cataract extraction. Both phacoemulsification and manual small incision surgery enjoy the benefit of a sutureless procedure compared to the traditional extracapsular cataract extraction (ECCE) resulting to a better visual results, shorter recovery time, an expected much improved quality of life, and the dramatic acceptance of the treatment in a wide spectrum of cataract management in most surgical conditions, either ideal or not. For many years, ECCE with IOL has been the primary choice in the management of cataract. Its inherent delayed visual improvement, wound and suture related complications, including its unreliable wound integrity during healing period has led surgeons to improve existing technique paving the way to more efficient and reliable phacoemulsification and MSICS.

In manual small incision cataract surgery (MSICS), nucleus extraction is done through a 4 to 8 mm diameter incision depending on the method and intraocular lens used. Common among all techniques is the construction of a self-sealing sclero-corneal tunnel that functions like a one way valve that generally requires no suturing but provides a watertight stable wound. In the end, achieving a cost-effective, and highly predictable surgical outcome is one of the prominent advantages the MSICS offers.

Nucleus extraction in MSICS can be achieved through:
1. Hydroexpression technique. This technique uses hydrostatic pressures in the anterior chamber to aid nucleus delivery either using an irrigating vectis popularized by Dr. Natchiar of Aravind Hospital Systems or an anterior chamber maintainer connected to an IV line with a specific bottle height as popularized in the Dr. Blumenthal's Mini-Nuc technique. Dr. Ruit's Tilganga Eye Center technique utilizes modified I and A cannulae in the extraction of cataract. This technique is highly recommended for softer cataracts but dense ones can easily be managed by enlarging the wound and the tunnel.
2. Fish Hook Technique popularized by Dr. Hennig, using bent gauge 30 needle introduced and engaged in the posterior face of the nucleus. Because of the non-visualization of the hook while behind a dense cataract, many surgeons are having second thoughts despite its relative ease, effectiveness, and simplicity.
3. Hook-Sandwich Technique uses a specially designed hook engaged on top and a lens loop sandwiching the nucleus as a double protection approach to preserve the integrity of the posterior capsule while keeping the endothelium from damage during nucleus delivery. This was introduced by Dr. Sinolinding few years back. Because of the visibility of instruments used and the predictability of lens extraction, this has received wide acceptance among Filipino Ophthalmologists.
4. Phaco-Sandwich Technique is the original version of two instrument nucleus extraction introduced by Dr. Fry in 1985 using a lens loop and a Sinskey hook. Because of its limitation to hold hard cataracts in tight sclerocorneal tunnel, modi-fications were introduced then. Still, many surgeons are using this technique.

5. Manual Phacofragmentation
   a. "Phaco non-phaco technique" was introduced by Drs. Wirilayappa, Kongsap, and Samporn. This technique requires much dexterity and skills. The nucleus is pre-chopped intracamerally into small fragments before being delivered piece by piece through a 4 mm corneoscleral incision or through a modified tube (phaco-drainage technique). Foldable IOLs are used in this method.
   b. Phacofracture technique using bi-sector, tri-sector, wire loop, and other devices designed to split the nucleus into pieces before extraction. Phacofracture of lens in the tunnel is also used by other surgeons.
6. And many more techniques and modifications are used that I missed to mention.

Some basic questions in our choice of cataract surgery technique include:
- Adaptability to all types of cataracts?
- Scientifically proven to be effective: evidence based results?
- Learning curve among new learners?
- Acceptable and manageable complications?
- Capital outlay and available instrumentation?
- Cost effectiveness especially to patients?

What explains the low acceptance of the MSICS technique among many surgeons are due to limited exposure and confidence among "mentors" in training hospitals, wrongly perceived higher complication rate and difficult learning curve, limited support and scarcity teaching materials in many institutions, and minimal support from funding (Ophthalmic) companies.

Despite little support, the MSICS advocates managed to come up with modifications and studies supported by facts and figures making it time-tested technique with good if not excellent results through the years. Recently in many developing countries, more and more cataracts are managed this way that offers comparable results with the highly technical and expensive mechanical phacoemulsification in terms of safety, visual rehabilitation, applicability in all surgical center conditions and most importantly, its affordable cost.

In as much as manufacturers and surgeons would want to be perfect, no one can achieve either 100% phacoemulsification or 100% MSICS as we avoid the unreliability of visual result of the conventional ECCE or the ICCE, mostly depending on the judgment and comfort of the surgeon. In most developing countries around the globe, a white cataract is not unusual. In the Philippines alone, of the almost 4 million visually impaired affecting one or both eyes prevalence in 2002, about 41% is due to cataract. And many are mature upon diagnosis. Poverty undeniably, is claimed to be one of the reasons why people shun from early treatment. So, despite satisfactory results have been reported and published by phaco advocates regarding white cataract, mechanical phacoemulsification is still far from being an ideal method in the management of cataract considering its cost and maintenance.

The purpose of this surgical approach is to simplify the process of final technique selection on the management of cataract in all surgical conditions offering the surgeon a wide variety of choices, making him comfortable with the problem. The assumption is that the surgeon must be comfortable at any time using any of the acceptable standard techniques of cataract surgery: ECCE, MSICS, and Phacoemulsification.

WHY LEARN SIMPLIFIED 3-IN-1 TECHNIQUE?

- *Adaptation to actual capability of surgical centers.* As all eye surgeons are expected to know the three techniques, not all hospitals have state-of-the-art equipments that include phacoemuslification machine. While most paying patients are managed in adequately equipped medical centers promoted and supported by its manufacturers, a great number are still managed in modified set-up but still coming up with comparable results in terms of ease of surgery and visual outcomes.

- *Promote versatility and flexibility of the technique in unusual cases.* When dealing with soft cataracts, the choice will be easier. When patient had preference on a specific technique as requested, you are faced with a double challenge- to remove the cataract the way our patient wanted it. And if faced with dense brunescent super hard cataract, dislocated, posterior polar, pseudoexfoliation, post-uveitic, or any unusual types of cataracts, you will start making the wisest choice of approach with minimal preparation.

- *Easy conversion during unwanted situations.* No surgeon can achieve a "100% phaco" even manufacturers designed the newer machines with more outstanding features. On the other hand, MSICS cannot guarantee the same as well. Many factors have to be considered: machine failure, power failure, and even surgeon failure. Learning the 3-in-1 bails out the surgeon during surgical difficulties. It does not guarantee a 100% success rate, but assures us of a better outcome. Problems arise even in a seemingly easy and innocent looking case. And complications should not be a bigger problem than not knowing how to deal with it.

- *Inherent limitations of each technique.* Despite their "almost 100% phaco" claim, in many instances there are "shifts" done before the onset of surgery, or worse during surgery when reality of surgical limitations and surgeons comfort zones become apparent. While phaco technique offers the benefit of using a foldable lens through a 2-3 mm bloodless incision, cataract in many parts of the world are becoming "phaco-challenge" that makes the relatively safe procedure a bit risky and uncertain. This is true with hard cataracts. MSICS on the other hand becomes the preferred choice. However, patients on anti-coagulant/ thrombolytic medications are best managed with the bloodless phacoemulsification approach.

- *Achieve the confidence of a total cataract surgeon.* Easy conversion and flexibility of the surgeon towards difficult cases and unusual situations offers an advantage of a "Total Cataract Surgeon". It simply explains the capability of the surgeon to finish the task with optimal result regardless of the situation and problem.

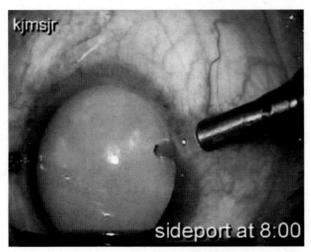

Fig. 1: Corneal sideport at 8:00

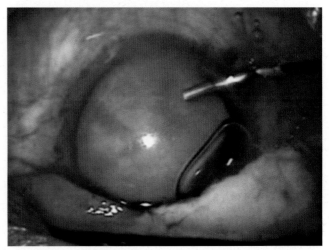

Fig. 4: Viscoelastic gel into the anterior chamber (AC)

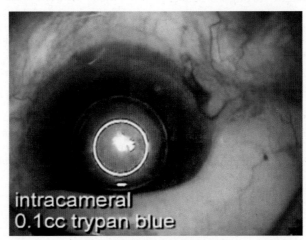

Fig. 2: Intracameral trypan blue

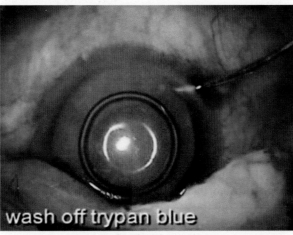

Fig. 3: Washing off trypan blue

Advantages of the 3-in-1 Approach

- All grades, all types of cataracts
- All types of IOLs
- All set-up of surgical centers (eye camp to medical centers)
- All-time all-situation, ideal for outreach or in-reach ophthalmic expeditions
- All-flexible cost of surgery
- Acceptable, minimal, and predictable complications.

Patient Preparation Includes

- Nitroglycerin patch 1/2 hour prior to surgery for >40
- Use 5% povidone iodine eye drops pre-op
- Keep BP ≤ 130/80
- Keep pupil maximally dilated
- O_2 inhalation during surgery
- Put up ear shield for fluid drips
- Make eye sheet and eye towel light but adequate, and good smelling
- Keep in touch with the patient through a relaxed conversation
- Give anxiolytic drugs (to selected patients).

The 3-in-1 Technique Precautions

- Fat, short neck patients
- Small eyes with shallow chamber
- Tight inter-palpebral fissure
- Small, non-, or poorly-dilating pupil
- High IOP
- Pseudoexfoliates at AC, weak zonules
- Cataracts: Posterior sub-capsular/polar, Inflammatory type
- Hypertensives
- Under aspirin or anticoagulant maintenance
- Patients prostate medication
- Anxious patients.

Pre-surgical Reminders

- Prepare all instruments (basic and others) in one tray
- Prepare Phaco Machine (if available)
- Use only sharp knives to decrease tissue damage
- Adequate anesthesia.

MSICS (HOOK SANDWICH), PHACOEMULSIFICATION, AND THE ECCE TECHNIQUES: THE 3-IN-1 SIMPLIFIED APPROACH (THE SINOLINDING APPROACH)

I. Planning and Evaluation

I need to emphasize that often neglected little things may save our day if we mind them ahead.

1. Patient Selection

Although some techniques of MSICS work better in specific type and grade of cataract, the Hook Sandwich Technique encompasses all the barriers even on cases that requires extreme care and holds more risks.

1a. *Type of cataract:* All types, all grades. The harder the nucleus, the hook works better but soft cataract can be managed easily as well.

1b. *Patient preparation:* A good medical history, including allergies must be considered. Pre-op antibiotic eye drops is recommended. My choice is Tobramycin 4 x a day for at least 3 days prior to surgery.

Aspirin and other anti-coagulant medications must be discontinued 2 weeks prior to surgery. Choice of surgery must be planned out well if such medications cannot be stopped.

Consider sedation to anxious patients. Constant communication and assurance to patient allays apprehension better.

Maintain blood pressure below 140/80 prior to surgery. Hypertension may lead to hyphema and unpleasant sub-conjunctival hemorrhage.

Use light but adequate drapes. Cloth made of cotton that smells good is recommended. Make sure the patient is comfortable with the drape on by asking prior to surgery.

Use improvised ear shield to seal off fluid from entering into the external auditory meatus. Some patients make unnecessary quick head turns as water drips during irrigation and aspiration.

Oxygen inhalation set at minimal level, preferable 2-3 L/min.

Nitroglycerin patch should be in place 1 hour prior to surgery among >40 years old patients or among those with heart problems. It must immediately be removed after the surgery to minimize adverse reactions such as headache and flushing to some susceptible patients.

II. Anesthesia

1. *Topical Sub Tenon Intracameral (TSI) Anesthesia is my Preferred Choice. (Table 1)* The TSI avoids the unwanted complications related to infiltration and inhalation anesthesia. Although it may have certain precautions among severely anxious and "terrified" patients towards surgery, generally, more than 95% of my patients are comfortable under TSI.
2. Retrobulbar/peribulbar
3. GA: Inhalation or IV

III. Surgical Procedure

A. *Instruments used for MSICS Hook Sandwich Technique:* Lid retractor, SRB forcep and needle holder with silk 4-0 (for retro/peribulbar/ general anesthesia), Westcott scissor, Cautery spear or wet field bipolar, Caliper, Knives (angled Crescent knife and 3.0 slit keratome) , Blade holder with blade #15, Wilder type lens loop, Lens dialer/ manipulator, "Sinolinding" Nucleus Hook, I & A Simcoe cannula, Angled 11 mm lens forcep, .12 tissue forceps.

Standby instruments: Vannas scissor, Corneal scissor, Needle holder

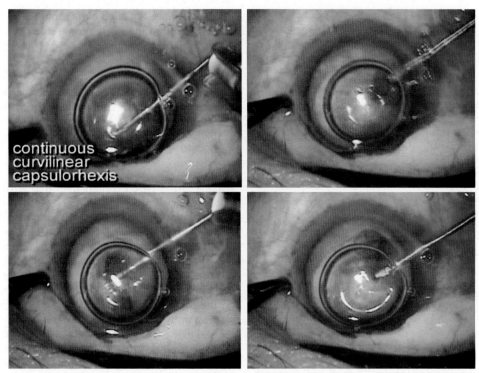

Fig. 5: Starting in the center, a continuous curvilinear capsulorhexis (CCC) is completed

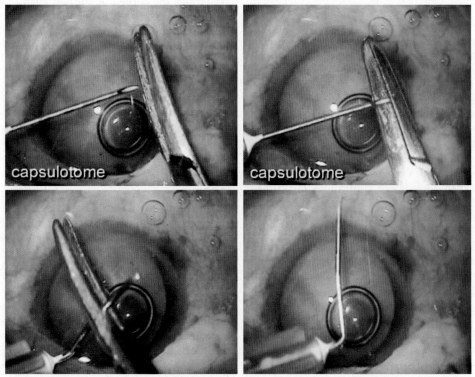

Fig. 6: The four easy steps how to prepare a capsulotome using a gauge 26 needle

Table 1: Various types of anesthesia	
Anesthesia	
TSI anesthesia	*Retro/peribulbar anesthesia*
• Topical drops initially with Propacaine 1% then may use Lidocaine 2% into the conjunctiva as maintenance • Sub Tenon injection at incision site with 3 ml premixed lidocaine 2% + 1:10000 epinephrine solution (dental anesthetic solution) • Intracameral injection with .1ml, .8% Lidocaine preservative-free solution (mix 2ml preservative-free lidocaine 2% and 3 ml BSS)	• Infiltration block with 2.5 cc (2% Lidocaine + .5% isobaric Bupivacaine solution) + hyaluronidase

B. *Additional Instrument for Phacoemulsification*: Chopper, preferably by Dr. Nagahara

The Technique

1. Initial Phase (the crossroad)

This phase is the most important part in the 3-in-1 approach. You can freely convert from one contemplated technique to another during this stage.

After an adequate anesthesia, a clear cornea side port (paracentesis) at 8:00 (another at 2:00 for Phaco) is created (Fig. 1).

Through the side port, a commercially available tryphan blue may be used to stain anterior capsule surface especially when dealing with white cataracts. During the process, an air is introduced first creating a bubble inside the eye that protects the endothelium from staining. The dye is thoroughly washed off using BSS after about 15 seconds. (Figs 2-3)

Adequate amount of hydroxymethylcellulose (viscoelastic gel) is introduced to deepen the anterior chamber. It also displaces the air bubble (Fig. 4).

A capsulotome made from a bent gauge 26 needle attached to a water-filled tuberculin syringe is inserted through the primary side port to complete a continuous curvilinear capsulorrhexis (Fig. 5).

Care must be observed not to overfill the AC. This avoids the build-up of too much intra-ocular pressure that may unnecessarily injure the endothelium and the Descemet's membrane. After CCC, hydrodissection/ hydrodelineation is done to separate the nucleus from the cortex or the capsule using the same BSS filled capsulotome syringe (Fig. 6)

After this stage, you may choose your final technique of cataract surgery.

Hint

In dealing with entumescent cataract, nick the anterior capsule to displace liquefied cortex into the AC. Introduced air will

further displace liquefied cortex into the periphery and seep outside through the capsulotome side port making the CCC easier to manage.

Hint

A superior rectus bridle suture is necessary if you chose to do the surgery under retrobulbar/peribubar/or general anesthesia.

2. Incision Phase (Figs 7-13)

MSICS

After a fornix based conjunctival flap with single temporal relaxing incision is completed, a selective and conservative hemostasis of superficial blood vessels using either a heat cautery or wet field bipolar to avoid shrinking the sclera. Using a caliper, a 5-8 mm length initial frowning scleral incision (depending on the estimated size of the lens nucleus and IOL to be used) with the apex of the frown at least 1 mm below the limbus, either at superior, superotemporal, or temporal is preferred, depending on the preference of the surgeon. Using a crescent knife and starting in the middle, keep the blade parallel with the sclero-corneal plane, insinuated in between scleral tissues until 2 mm past the limbus. Tunnel is extended towards the peripheral limbus in a straight line forming a "V" shaped tunnel. A keratome is then insinuated in the tunnel following the initial wound, careful enough not to make another surgical plane. By tilting the tip of keratome downward, a corneal "dimple" becomes visible and a gentle forward movement of the knife penetrates the cornea. A sudden gush of viscoelastic gel is apparent once cornea is penetrated. The internal wound is extended from one end to the other following the internal corneal line. The tunnel is now shaped like a funnel with a much wider internal opening than the outer.

Phaco

After a clear cornea main side port (paracentesis) at 8:00, a second side port at 2:00 is done. The former is for the capsulotome and the irrigating-aspirating cannulae while cleaning the main subincision wound area from cortical materials while the latter is for the second instrument during phacoemulsification (Fig. 14).

ECCE

After an adequate fornix based peritomy with a temporal relaxing incision, cauterization of superficial blood vessels follows. A standard ECCE approach then follows (Fig. 15).

3. Lens Delivery Phase (Figs 16-18)

MSICS

Two blunt instruments is used, the first is engaged lifting the nucleus edge towards outside the capsular bag while the other instrument holds the nucleus under it to avoid sinking back into the bag. An adequate amount of viscoelastic gel introduced into the AC and beneath the lens nucleus helps push it outside the capsular bag into the anterior chamber at the same time

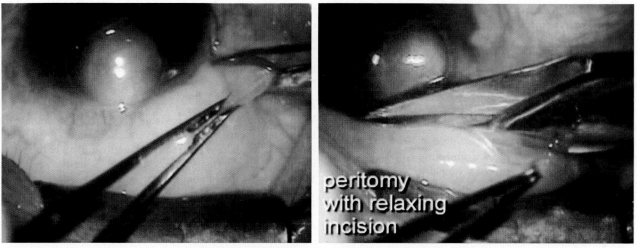

Fig. 7: Fornix based peritomy with relaxing incision

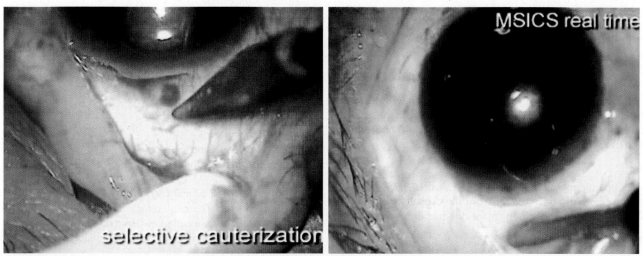

Fig. 8: Selective and conservative diathermy using heat cautery or wet field bipolar

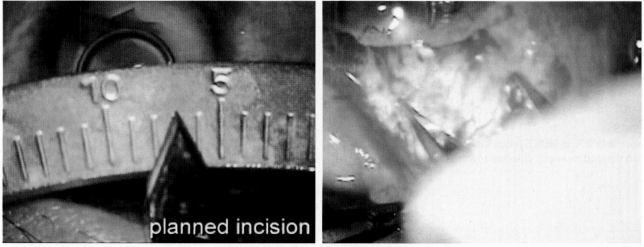

Fig. 9: Planned width of scleral incision measured with caliper

protects endothelium from trauma while lens nucleus is prolapsed using the cartwheel maneuver (make sure not to put so much tension enough to break the zonules). Complete prolapse of lens nucleus is achieved as it floats freely into the anterior chamber. With the lens loop inserted between the nucleus and the posterior capsule, the "Sinolinding" hook is placed on top of the lens 1 mm beyond the center (without touching the endothelium). After slight pressure exerted by the two instruments sandwiching the lens nucleus, a gentle traction engages the tip of the hook with the nucleus while the lens loop holds the lens nucleus from below until completely extracted through the sclerocorneal tunnel.

Care must be observed not to trap the iris during the process of extraction to avoid iridodialysis.

Hint

To avoid splitting the nucleus into small chunks, insert the hook until the tip is 1 mm beyond middle portion of the nucleus before tilting the handle upright. This maneuver engages the sharp tip of the hook right in the middle of the nucleus where it is most resistant to breakage.

Hint

When nucleus gets fractured and stuck in the tunnel, remove fractured fragment. Gently push back the remaining nucleus into the AC after injecting viscoelastic gel between the nucleus and endothelium. Reposition the nucleus with its fractured side parallel to the tunnel.

Hint

Inject copious amount of viscoelastic gel into the "space" between the posterior surface of the lens and the capsule- iris plane to push the posterior capsule-iris plane down as the nucleus floats.

Hint

During extraction under the TSI anesthesia, ask the patient to look down as you gently pull the hook and loop towards you. It acts like as a counter force.

Phaco

Using a keratome, an initial incision is done before creating a 3-plane 2-3 mm wound. A phaco tip is then inserted while a second instrument (preferably nagahara chopper) is used to assist during the procedure (Fig. 19).

4. IOL Insertion

MSICS

Insertion of IOL in MSICS follows the standard ECCE technique. With the leading haptic directed towards the capsular bag, lens is secured and pushed slowly through the tunnel until the IOL optic is halfway in the bag. The trailing haptic is then insinuated inside the bag. IOL is positioned properly by gentle manipulation until the desired position is achieved. Simcoe cannula is used to aspirate remaining VEGs inside the AC and under the lens (Fig. 20).

Phaco

With injector loaded with foldable IOL, carefully insinuate the tip through the main paracentesis and slowly inject the IOL into the AC. Lens dialer is used to manipulate until all of the IOL is inside the capsular bag. Simcoe cannula clears the remaining VEG in the AC and under the lens (Fig. 21).

IV. The Result: (Figs 22A to C, 23)

MSICS (Hook Sandwich) (Figs 22 A to C)

V. Complications

a. *During paracentesis*
>Too large/ tight side port causes leakage and difficulty of inserting instruments, respectively.

b. During capsulotomy/capsulorrhexis
>Too small/ too wide capsulorrhexis capsulotomy
>Extension of Capsulorrhexis
>Posterior capsular tear

c. During wound construction
>Hyphema
>Astigmatism
>Button hole incision
>Premature corneal entry
>Iridodialysis
>Wound leak for large incision
>Difficulty of lens extraction for small incision

d. During anterior dislocation of lens nucleus
>Rupture of lens zonules causing lens dislocation
>Injury to the endothelium
>Injury to the iris

e. During nucleus Extraction
>Descemet's membrane separation
>Injury to the endothelium by the hook
>Posterior capsule tear caused by the lens loop
>Corneal edema at incision site
>Iridodialysis

f. During Aspiration of cortical materials
>Retained cortex specially at subincision area
>Tear at posterior capsule

g. During lens implantation
>Decentered or tilted IOL
>Dropped IOL

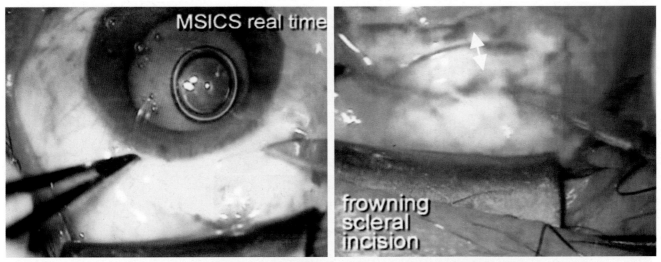

Fig. 10: Initial scleral incision using blade #15. The apex of the frown should be at least 1 mm from the limbus. Tunnel length is at least 3 mm to avoid wound leakage and control post-op astigmatism

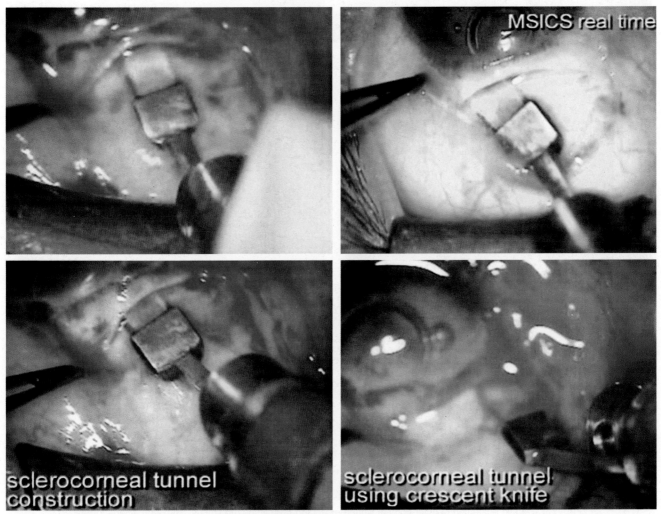

Fig. 11: Sclerocorneal tunnel with crescent knife

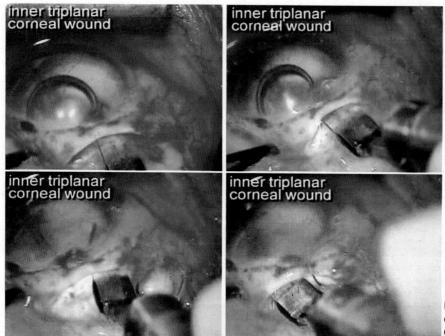

Fig. 12: Straight inner corneal wound extending from limbus to opposite limbus creating a funnel shaped sclera-corneal tunnel

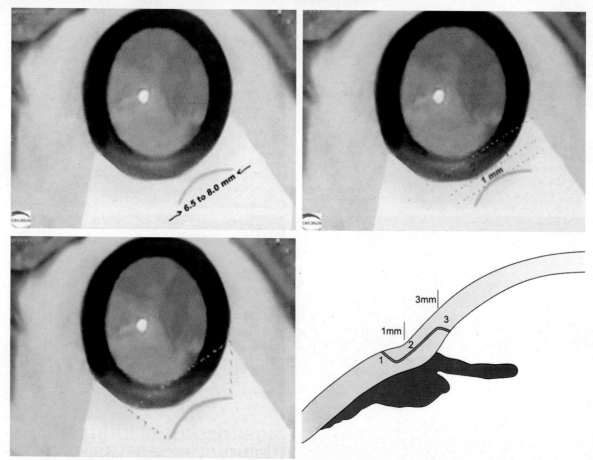

Fig. 13: Graphic illustration of inner corneal wound extending from limbus to limbus. Tri-planar sclera-corneal tunnel length is at least 3 mm: 1 mm sclera and 2 mm clear cornea

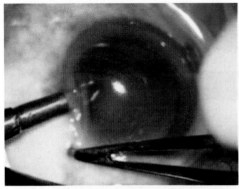

Fig. 14: Second corneal side port at 2:00

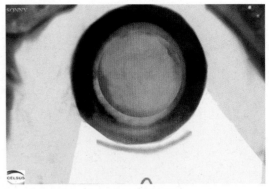

Fig. 15: Standard ECCE approach

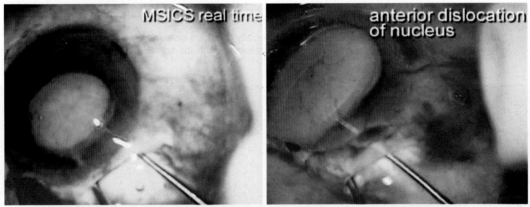

Fig. 16: Dislocation of lens nucleus into the AC using "cartwheel" technique

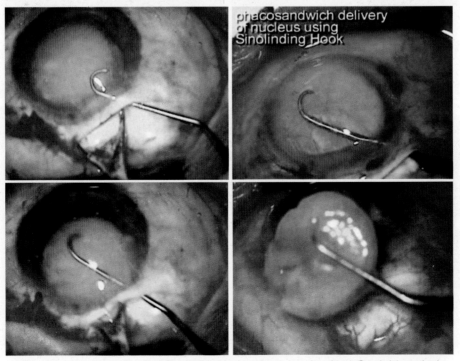

Fig. 17: Lens extraction using Sinolinding Hook and lens loop in a Hook Sandwich method

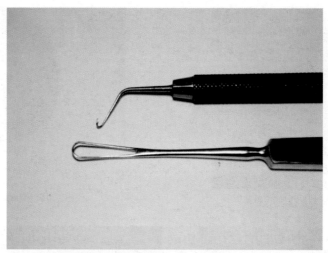

Fig. 18: Sinolinding hook is a specially designed instrument with a
45 degrees curved tip in reference with the handle

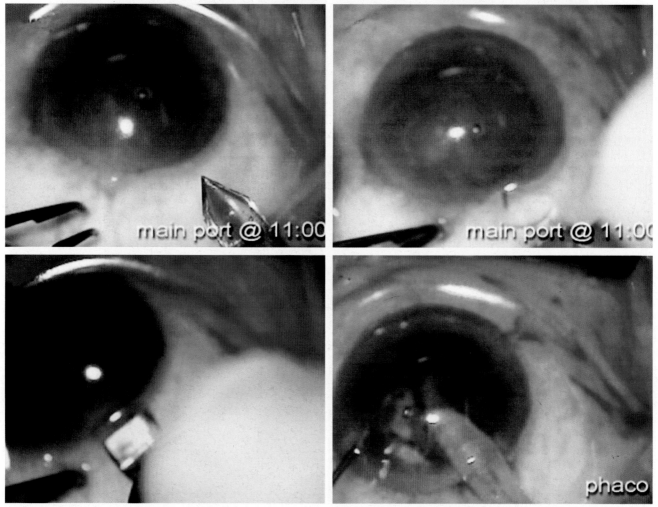

Fig. 19: Main paracentesis with a 3.0 keratome and phacoemulsification

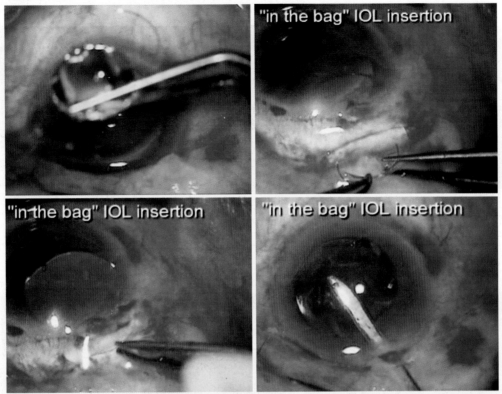

Fig. 20: Steps of insertion using a rigid type of IOL

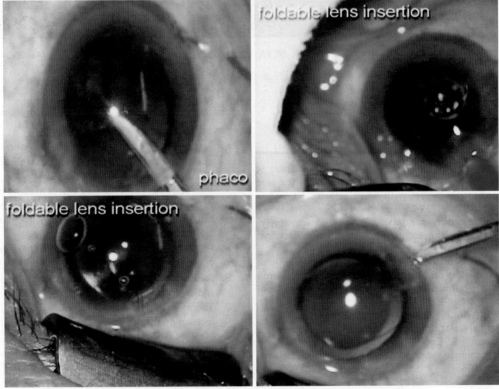

Fig. 21: The final stage of IOL insertion in phacoemulsification

Pre-op   1 day Post-op   7 days, Post-op

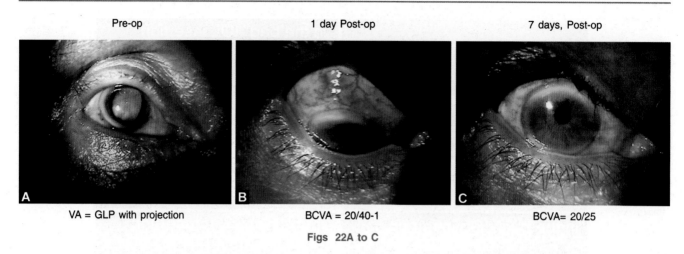

VA = GLP with projection   BCVA = 20/40-1   BCVA= 20/25

Figs 22A to C

Pre-op   1 day Post-op   7 days, Post-op

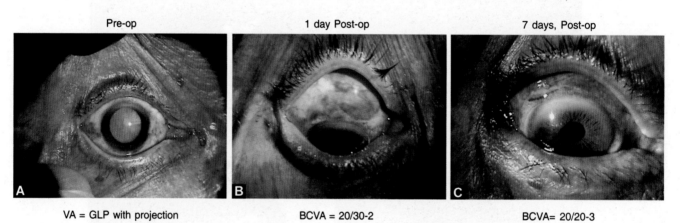

VA = GLP with projection   BCVA = 20/30-2   BCVA= 20/20-3

Figs 23A to C

BIBLIOGRAPHY

1. Jacob S, Agarwal A, Agarwal A, Agarwal S, Chowdhary S, Chowdhary R, et al . Trypan blue as an adjunct for safe phacoemulsification in eyes with white cataract. J Cataract Refract Surg 2002;28:1819-25.
2. Kansas P. Phacofracture. In: Rozakis GW, ed. Cataract surgery-alternative small incision techniques. New Jersey: Slack Inc, 1990:45-70.
3. Kothari K, Jain SS, Shah NJ. Anterior capsular staining with Trypan blue for Capsulorhexis in mature and hypermature cataracts. A preliminary study. Indian J Ophthalmol 2001;49:177-80.
4. Lam, DS, Tano, Y, Ritch, R, Rao, SK. Cataract IV, Sutureless Large Incision Manual Cataract Extraction (SLIMCE), 2008.
5. Malik Krishan PS, Goel R. Nucleus management with Blumenthal technique - anterior chamber maintainer. Indian J Ophthalmol 2008.
6. Natchiar G. Manual small incision cataract surgery - An alternative technique to instrumental phacoemulsification. Madurai: Aravind Publications; 2004.
7. Ruit S, Tabin GC, Nissman SA, et al. Low cost high volume extracapsular cataract extraction with posterior chamber intraocular lens implantation in Nepal. Ophthalmology 1999; 106:1887-92.
8. Santos EO, et al. Philippine National Survey on Blindness. 2004:6-9.
9. Srinivasan A. Nucleus management with irrigating vectis. Indian J Ophthalmology, 2008.
10. Thomas R, Kuriakose T, George R. Towards achieving small-incision cataract surgery 99.8% of the time. Indian J Ophthalmol 2000;48:145
11. Thylefors B, Negrel AD, Pararajasegram R, et al. Global data on blindness. Bull World Health Organ 1996;74:319-24.

Chapter 6

Dynamics of the Capsulorhexis

Roberto Pinelli (Italy)

When planning an extracapsular removal of the cataract, an opening of the anterior capsule has to be made in order to evacuate the opaque substance of the lens. The residual capsular tissue, the "capsular bag" can then host the artificial lens sequestrating it from the other ocular structures and giving it the best support for centration and stabilization. An intact capsular bag is more easily obtained by creating an anterior continuous curvilinear capsulorhexis (CCC) as described by Drs. Howard Gimbel and Thomas Neuhann.

The circular opening behave as a sphincter distributing the traction or dilating forces over all the circumference thus exhibiting a much higher resistance compared to an opening with a jagged margin.

A regular margin is best obtained using a continuous tear. The direction of the tear is determined by the interaction of forces exerted by
* The surgical maneuver
* The elastic properties of the capsular tissue
* The zonular attachments

APPLYING A FORCE ON A THIN SHEET OF ELASTIC TISSUE

A tractional force applied on an elastic tissue *in the same direction of the elastic fibers* causes a deformation of the tissue. The amount of deformation is proportional to the **stress** that is the amount of force divided by the cross-sectional area where the force is being applied. The change in length of an elastic strip of material divided by its original length is called **strain**. With increasing levels of stress, the strain will increase up to the elastic limit of the tissue, than beyond it causing **permanent** deformation, than further on, up to the point of breaking.

Just before the breaking point, a smaller amount of stress will be needed to cause the same amount of strain.

If one wanted to tear apart a piece of elastic fabric, he could exert a traction on the two sides of the strip of material increasing the applied force until reaching the breaking point. The rupture will happen in an uncontrolled manner, starting in an unpredictable point of less resistance and the tear will unpredictably progresses even after the traction is no longer exerted because the force stored into the elastic fibers will continue to exert stress. If a more controlled rupture is wanted,

it is better to start with creating a place of less resistance, like a small cut, in the desired location and then exert small amounts of traction making the line of rupture to progress in a controlled manner without allowing the elastic fibers to collect more than the energy just required to continue the tear. The direction of ripping will follow the rule of vectorial summation of direction and strength of the two forces (Figs 1A and 1B).

If the same traction is exerted perpendicularly to the surface of the same thin sheet of fabric, with the points of application of traction opposite to the direction of resistance, the effect will be of shearing and the tissue will behave as a stiff substance, like a piece of paper. The breaking point is always located among the points of application of the two forces: traction and resistance (Fig. 2).

RIPPING AND SHEARING

After creating a flap in the central portion of the capsule, the capsulorhexis can be continued in two ways:

Ripping

The flap is grasped with a forceps or engaged with the point of a curved needle very close to the origin of the tear. The pulling force is exerted mostly with a direction towards the center of the capsule, but changes of direction of the progression of the tear are easily and quickly done by small changes of the direction of the pulling force (Figs 1A and B).

Remember: Before the pulling is able to make the tear progresses, elastic resistance of both the capsular tissue and the zonula has to be overcome. The effect of pulling will always be displacement followed by ripping. The amount of displacement is proportional to the elasticity so that it will be larger in a young capsule compared with an old or diseased capsule. The progression of the tear will happen along with recovery of the stretched tissue and such a return movement has to be considered when planning the direction of pulling. A continuous pull toward the center of the capsule will result in a tear that extends to the periphery of the capsule, toward the zonular attachments. The tear has to be directed through continuous pull-release-pull movements changing direction of pulling according to the direction of the tear (Figs 3A and B).

Shearing

The flap is folded over the intact capsule. Pulling the flap very close to the tear, most of the force is directed pointing upward while the adherence of the capsule to the cortical material and the overall stability of the capsular bag exerts counterforce in the opposite direction. The result is a tear that progresses in a very safe manner because almost independent from the elastic forces that exert their maximum effect tangentially while the breaking effect results from forces exerted perpendicularly to the tissue. The pure shearing movement, perpendicular to the tissue, has good "steering capability", but if the movement is continued without changing the point on application of traction, the fold will gradually start to "unfold" transforming a shearing movement in a ripping movement (Figs 4A and B) so that it is safer to release the flap and regrasp it close to the tear almost every 60 degrees.

The shearing movement is safer, but the steering action is slow so that when the tear is close to the zonular attachments a ripping technique will more efficiently redirect the tear.

Dealing with the Capsule

The capsule is an elastic envelope subjected to forces coming from:
- Anterior chamber pressure
- Lens substance pressure
- Vitreous pressure
- Zonular traction

The elastic module of the capsule changes with age, being stiffer in an old patient and very elastic in a child.

Pressurizing the anterior chamber before starting the capsulorhexis is of paramount importance because it relaxes the zonular attachments on the anterior capsule (tightening those on the posterior capsule) decreasing an important counterforce able to direct the tear peripherally. On the contrary, an increased vitreous pressure tightens the anterior zonula.

A swollen lens substance (such as in an hypermature cataract) increases the tension of the capsule and increases the vectorial force directed towards the periphery.

A zonular insufficiency will make the capsulorhexis more difficult changing the ripping action in a displacement effect.

All these tissue components have to be taken in account when doing the capsulorhexis: adjusting the external forces (refilling the chamber or releasing pressure on the globe) or modifying the surgical strategy.

DYNAMICS OF THE CAPSULORHEXIS

Approach A

Many techniques of capsulorhexis are available nowadays, and most of them are very personal. The main characteristics of the different techniques are changing proportionally with the experience of the surgeon.

A common approach is to begin the capsulorhexis from the center of the capsule (point A) with a viscoelastic syringe using the needle carefully (Fig. 5).

Once created a flap from point A to point B, we can continue the maneuver with the same needle, injecting viscoelastic if needed in order to see the flap better and its integrity, and perform capsulorhexis with the visco-syringe in a clockwise direction.

The same maneuver can be performed with the capsulorhexis forceps.

In order to better control the diameter and the regularity of the capsulorhexis it is better to stop the maneuver at every quadrant (from 9 h to 12 h, from 12 h to 3 h, etc.) (Fig. 5).

Approach B

The same approach can be performed in an anti-clockwise direction. This decision is up to the surgeon, and mainly depends on his attitude (left-handed or right-handed surgeon) and in its dynamics shows no difference compared to the approach A (Fig. 6).

SMALL CAPSULORHEXIS

In case of small capsulorhexis, a careful approach can fix this problem considering the forces involved in the dynamics of this technique.

A small capsulorhexis enlargement can be performed prior to the phacoemulsification (should be) or after the insertion of the IOL in the bag (in this case, the clear red reflex through the IOL can help in clarity).

Starting from point A (Fig. 7) for the incision, it should be easier to manage the forces involved to create a new flap. Moreover, it would be also easier to perform and to manage this new flap to the diameter requested.

We consider this tangential approach safer and the most dynamically correct.

Viscoelastic injection under the small capsulorhexis can help during this maneuver.

Also in this case, the direction (clockwise or anti-clockwise) can be chosen by the surgeon depending on his personal attitude.

BIBLIOGRAPHY

1. Agarwal S, Agarwal A, Agarwal A, Phacoemulsification Third edition, Slack Inc, 2005.
2. Gimbel HV, Divide and conquer. Phacoemulsification. Video journal of ophthalmology 800-822-3100.
3. Seibel B. Phacadynamic. Mastering the tools and the techniques of phacoemulsifications surgery, Slack Inc, 2005.

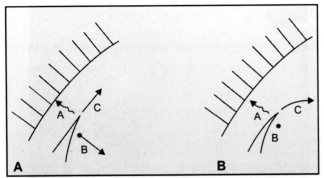

Figs 1A and B: (A) Swinging arrow A represents elastic resistance opposed by the capsular tissue plus elastic zonular traction. Arrow B is the pulling force. The effect is the direction of tear progression C resulting by two forces counteracting in the same line (B) When the pulling force is exerted in a direction forming an angle different from 180° from the direction of resistance, the direction of the tear progression will tend to intersect that angle

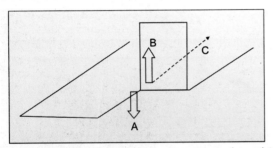

Fig. 2: B represents the shearing force, A represents the resistance. The breaking point lies in between the two forces and moves ahead in a very predictable and linear way

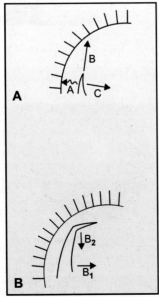

Figs 3A and B: (A) If the pulling force continues to be active in the same direction, the tear will progresses towards the zonula (B) If a change of direction of the tear is wanted, traction has to be stopped and restarted in a new point with a new direction of pulling

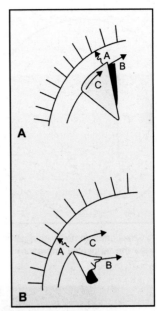

Figs 4A and B: (A) A pure shearing motion (B) A mixed shear and rip technique used to change direction of tear progression

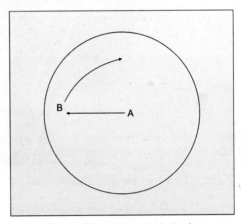

Fig. 5: Clockwise capsulorhexis

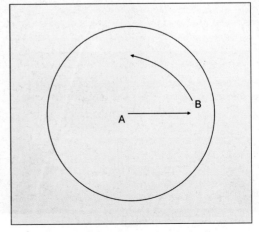

Fig. 6: Anti-clockwise capsulorhexis

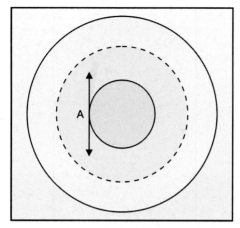

Fig. 7: Small capsulorhexis enlargement
(see the tangential approach)

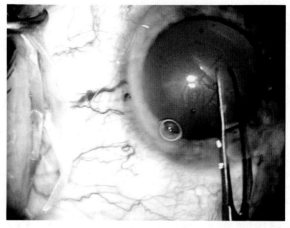

Fig. 10

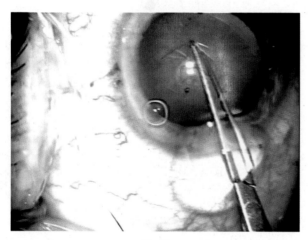

Fig. 8

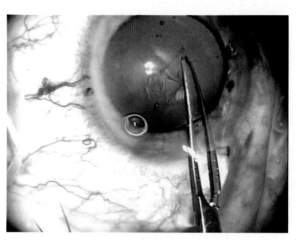

Fig. 11

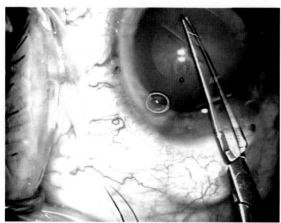

Fig. 9

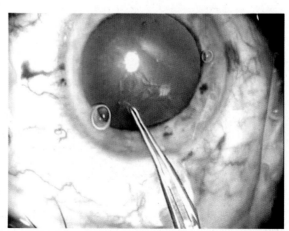

Fig. 12

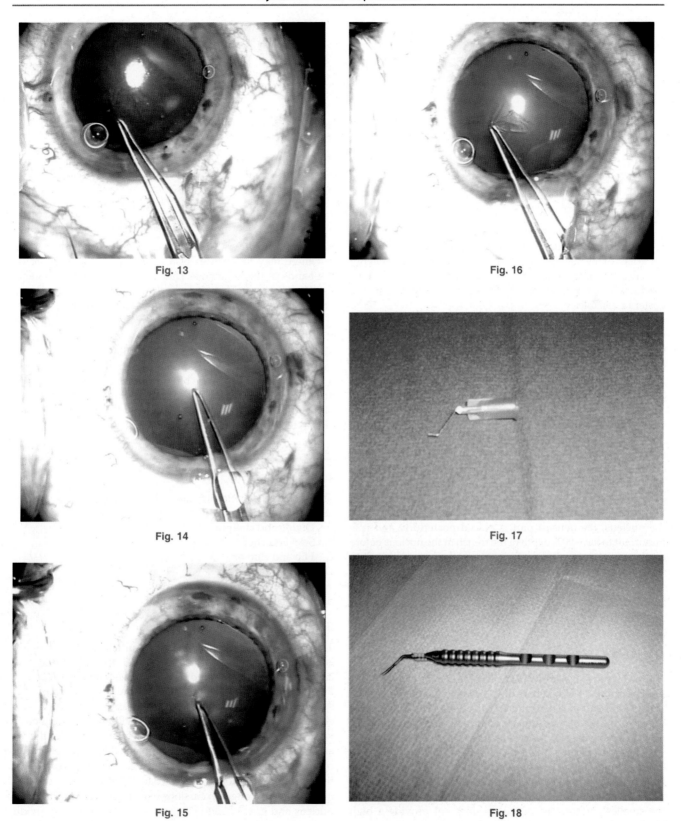

Fig. 13

Fig. 16

Fig. 14

Fig. 17

Fig. 15

Fig. 18

Figs 8 to 18: Various steps of capsulorhexis being performed by the author

Chapter 7

Dynamics of Nucleus Emulsification

AK Grover, Shaloo Bageja (India)

The aim of phacoemulsification is to emulsify the central core of the lens or the nucleus using minimum possible phaco energy and surgical maneuvers producing the least possible trauma to the intraocular structures viz the cornea, the iris and the posterior capsule.

To accomplish a successful procedure the surgeon should be well versed with anatomy of the nucleus, instruments and the dynamics of the emulsification process in order to perform the surgery safely and quickly.

APPLIED ANATOMY

The lens is divided into four parts from the surgeon's point of view - central core, epinucleus, cortex and capsule (Fig. 1).

As age advances the peripheral cortical fibers are pushed centrally and with decrease in water content, the density of the central nucleus increases. As nucleus progresses from softness to hardness there is color change from transparent to white or greenish yellow, yellow, amber brown and then black. Epinucleus also undergoes sclerosis. With increase in density of the nucleus, the densest part is placed posteriorly and it is important to have 90% depth of the trench in the nucleus before cracking is attempted as the fibers are leathery and difficult to separate.

INSTRUMENTS

1. Phaco tip
2. Chopper

Phaco Tips

Various types of tips are available like the standard, microflow, Kelman and the Kelman flare tip. Angulation of the tip may be 15°, 30°, 45° and 0°. The 0 and 15° tips have greater occlusion capacity, the 45° one has greater cutting capacity while the 30° tip is a compromise of the two features.

The *standard tip* is the most commonly used tip. It has a 0.9 mm inner and 1.1 mm outer diameter. The *microflow tip* has an internal diameter ranging from 0.45 to 0.6 mm. It is usually recommended for soft to moderate hard cataracts as the smaller surface area of the tip does not provide a high holding power. It is not recommended for the hard cataracts.

Kelman tip with downward angulation is ideal for hard cataracts but there may be chances of a posterior capsule rupture in the hands of the beginners. They should change to a regular tip after the trenching. *Kelman flared tip* has a wider distal area, transmits more power and is used for harder cataracts.

Choppers/Sinskey Hook

The Sinskey hook or chopper is a valuable second instrument for phacoemulsification. It consists of a handle, horizontal and a vertical part. They can be blunt or sharp tipped choppers or an elongated sinskey. It is used for stabilizing the globe, rotation of the nucleus, splitting and chopping of the nucleus and also aids in feeding the nuclear fragments into the tips.

NUCLEUS EMULSIFICATION

Techniques

The nucleus emulsification can be performed adopting various techniques
A. Divide and conquer
B. Stop and chop
C. Flip and chip or
D. Direct chop.

However, all these techniques, involve some basic phacodynamics which is dealt with here.

Basic Dynamics of Nucleus Phacoemulsification

The emulsification of nucleus requires ultrasonic power which is produced by the piezoelectric crystal in the hand piece. It is created by the interaction of the frequency and stroke length. Frequency is defined as the speed of the tip. It vibrates at a specific frequency when it is excited by an electrical field. The electrical energy creates an ultrasonic vibration of frequency varying from 28,000 to 60,000 Hz which is transmitted to the tip as longitudinal vibration. The mechanical energy generated contributes to emulsification of the nucleus. Phaco power implies the extent of excursion of the phaco tip. Most machines operate in 2-4 crystals. Longer excursions means greater impact on the nucleus and greater energy generation. All machines provide 0-100% power and the required power is chosen from the panel.

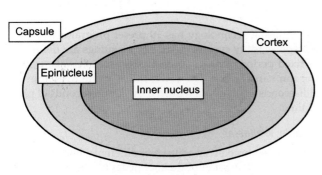

Fig. 1: Surgical anatomy of the crystalline lens

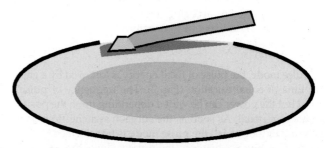

Fig. 4: Hyperpulse mode with a duty cycle of 33% phaco on time

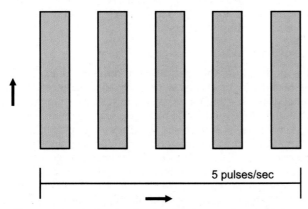

Fig. 2: Pulse mode, showing 5 pulses/sec, each pulse being 100 msec in duration

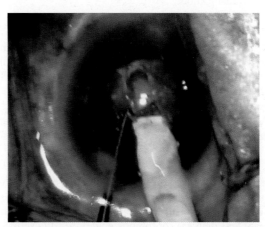

Fig. 5: Shaving action of the probe, the trench is kept short of the capsulorhexis margin

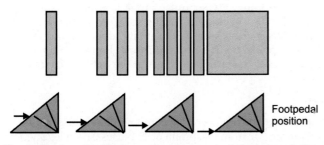

Fig. 3: Burst mode. Maximum preset power is delivered each time. Frequency of the burst varies depending upon the position of the foot pedal. On full pedal depression, the power delivery becomes continuous

Fig. 6: A photograph of the trench created in the nucleus. The trench is short of the capsulorhexis margin

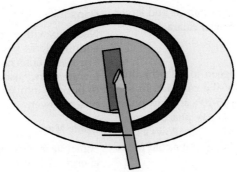

Fig. 7: Trench is behind widened by tilting the tip of the probe with bevel facing towards the center

Power Modulations in Phacoemulsification

The phaco surgeons should be aware of all the power modulations, utilizing these as one is able to emulsify hard cataract using low energy without causing any damage to endothelial cells and iris.

Phaco machine has been provided with two different modes i.e *surgeon mode* and *panel mode*. In *surgeon mode*, the delivery of power is varied from zero to maximum set power depending on the position of the foot pedal. While in panel mode, the maximum power is delivered as soon as the surgeon presses the foot pedal. The surgeon mode is usually preferred by the phaco surgeons as power can be varied according to the density of the nucleus in the part being emulsified, as we are aware the nucleus is not homogenous in density.

Pulse Phaco

In pulse mode, the pulse of fixed energy is followed by a gap of off time of equal duration (Fig. 2). The frequency of pulse is fixed but the power can be varied depending upon the position of the foot pedal. As soon as the surgeon switches to extreme position of foot pedal, the pulse mode is transformed to linear mode. The interval between the pulses allows the vacuum to build up and a good hold is achieved. Different machines have different set of pulses. As low as 2-6 pulses are adequate for nucleus emulsification.

Duty Cycle

It is the percentage of time phaco is on to total phaco time. In standard pulse mode, there is duty cycle of 50% i.e 5 pulses/second meant that each pulse interval is 200 msec, of which 100 msec is phaco on time while 100 msec is phaco offtime. With availability of newer software, the duty can be further reduced to 33% or 25%. Once chosen pulses/sec and duty cycle remain constant as set on the panel regardless of the foot pedal position.

Burst Mode

In the burst mode maximum preset power is delivered at intervals, varied according to the foot pedal position. The frequency of phaco bursts increases with depression of footpedal and delivers continuous energy at full excursion of the foot pedal (Fig. 3).

Variations of Burst Duration

Use shorter duration of 25 msec for softer cataracts and larger duration of 50 msec or even more for harder cataracts.

Hyperpulse Mode

This power modulation allows the surgeon to vary the duty cycles depending upon the density of the cataract. In soft cataract, one can have low duty cycle of 15-20% and low phaco energy such as 30%. While in harder cataracts, phacoenergy is increased to 50% with duty cycle of 25-33%. This allows a large cooling time after each pulse of power, making it a cold phaco (Fig. 4).

Whitestar

The whitestar technology has 10 preset programs regarding hyperpulse/duty cycle settings. These settings are defined by the fixed period of phaco on and phaco off intervals, which a surgeon can choose. The lowest duty cycle available is 4 milliseconds of phaco-on followed by 24 milliseconds of phaco off time.

Variable Whitestar

In this mode, surgeon can adjust four different whitestar settings through the depression of the foot pedal in position 3. At the beginning of footposition 3, one can get lower duty cycle settings but as the foot pedal is depressed, one can shift to higher duty cycles mode. This allows the surgeon a bimodal linear increase in phaco power and duty cycle and thus enhancing the phaco power and cutting when needed.

Occlusion Mode

This mode allows the application of different phaco settings before and after tip occlusion. On occlusion, one should have a higher duty cycle, higher power and lower aspiration flow rate. When the probe is occluded by the nuclear fragment, vacuum rises beyond the prefixed settings, the phaco power automatically rises for greater cutting efficiency and the flow rate decreases. This avoids the postocclusion surge. Once the occlusion is cleared, the settings return to their original levels.

The surgeon can utilize the various power modulations at different steps of surgery in achieving successful surgery. Continuous mode with phaco energy of 50-60% with low vacuum settings is used for sculpting. Microbursts with high vacuum provides strong occlusion which can also be used for direct chopping. Hyper pulse mode is used for quadrant removal with a settings of 30-50 pulses/sec with a 33% duty cycle. This increases the followability, due to rapid cycling between phaco on and phaco off time. Repulsive forces are reduced and chattering of pieces in the anterior chamber is avoided.

Infiniti

In this mode the number of maximum pulses has increased to 100 pulses/sec from maximum of 15 pulses/sec in legacy. The surgeon can also preset dutycycle from 5% to 95%, earlier being fixed at 50%. This change gives the surgeon complete control over the phaco-on and phaco-off time.

Neosonix

Neosonix with Advantec (Legacy, Alcon surgical) provides the additional low frequency oscillatory energy to the ultrasound. The oscillations can be varied upto 2 degrees at 120 HZ. The low frequency oscillations can be used alone at low frequency to burrow into the nuclear fragment or in combination with phaco power.

Sonic Mode

Sonic (Staar wave, Staar surgical) uses sonic rather than ultrasonic energy. It fragments the nucleus without generating heat. Its

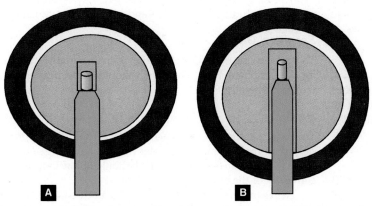

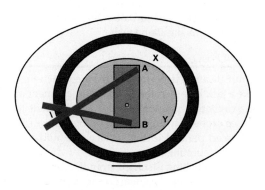

Figs. 8A and B: (A) Inadequate width of the trench as sleeve just fits into trench, (B) Showing an adequate width of the trench

Fig. 9: At position X, the force required for dialing is less as the distance from the axis of rotation is more as compared to the position Y

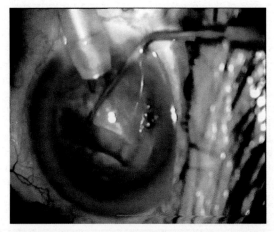

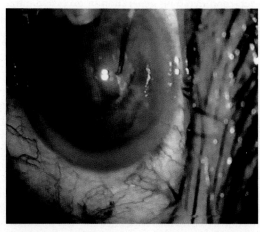

Fig. 10A: Rotating the nucleus by placing the dialer in the trench

Fig. 10B: Sculpting is continued after rotation to complete the trench

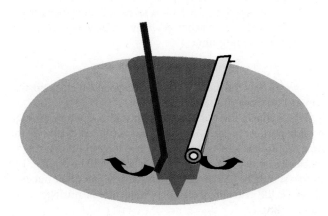

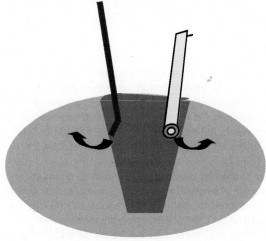

Fig. 11A: Correct placement of two instruments at the bottom of the trench and forces are applied in opposite direction

Fig. 11B: Incorrect superficial placement of instruments

47

frequency varies from 40 to 400 Hz in sonic range. The sonic phaco probe and tip can be utilized for sonic and ultrasonic mode. The surgeon can alternate between the two modes or can use them simultaneously.

TRENCHING

Emulsification is performed by the phaco tip which operates like a jack hammer, the to and fro movement of the tip and by the cavitation phenomenon. It is important to introduce the phaco probe at an angle to sculpt the surface of the nucleus. If it is placed parallel to the surface it would vibrate to and fro without sculpting.

The trenching is started from the center of the nucleus and movement is made towards the capsulorhexis margin. The forward movement consisting of shaving action, should be kept short of the capsulorhexis margin, thus avoiding injury to iris (Figs 5 and 6). The tip should not be buried more than half the width of the tip to avoid occlusion of the tip. The phaco power is adjusted to achieve a smooth sculpting without pushing the nucleus and avoiding generation of excessive intraocular energy. The power should not be too less as it may push the nucleus and exert stress on the zonules.

The power is determined by:
1. The density of the nucleus
2. Amount of tip engaged
3. Linear velocity of the tip

The phaco is kept in a linear mode during trenching for better control as the nucleus is not homogenous and has a variable density. The nucleus is less dense in the periphery and therefore the power requirement is low initially. It is increased in the central part of nucleus depressing the foot pedal and as the center of the nucleus is passed the foot pedal is raised to decrease the delivery of power. On the return, there should be no power or aspiration. The phaco surgeons should use low magnification as it provides wider field of view and allows him to assess the nuclear movements while sculpting and them to assess the depth and width of the trench. As he goes deeper, the surgeon can go beyond the capsulorhexis margin due to the available protective layer of epinucleus.

Width of the Groove

The width of the trench should be approximately two tip diameter. The width can vary according to the density of the nucleus. A wide groove in soft cataract is not required as the second instrument will not have much support to facilitate nucleus rotation. On the other hand, a hard cataract will require a wider trench. Initially a central groove is made and the trench is then widened by tilting the tip with bevel facing towards the center (Fig. 7).

One should be cautious to maintain an adequate width of the groove posteriorly even if it is adequate anteriorly. Sometimes even though the sleeve may fit into the trench, it may be pushing the nucleus, applying stress on the zonules. It may in such a situation, be necessary to widen the groove posteriorly to avoid stress on the zonules (Figs 8A and 8B). If the trench is not widened and the surgeon tries to push the tip

by increasing the ultrasound power there may be unfavorable outcomes including zonular tears and posterior capsule rupture.

Peripheral Groove

The golden ring of hydrodelineation is an important landmark for the peripheral limit. The trench should be deeper centrally than peripherally.

Depth

The required depth of the trench will vary depending upon the density of the nucleus. The harder cataract have large nucleus and will requires a deep trench which should follow the posterior convexity of the nucleus.

The required depth of trench can be assessed according to the following factors:
1. *Preoperative assessment:* Depending on the density of the nucleus.
2. *Intraoperative:*
   a. Thin epinucleus suggests large nucleus.
   b. *Size of the delineation ring:* Large ring indicates large nucleus
   c. Golden ring formation indicates a softer nucleus with small central core.

It is important for a surgeon to assess the depth of trench which can be done by:

Red reflex: The red reflex is visible peripherally in the moderate density nucleus but the reflex gets brighter as the thickness of the nucleus is reduced by sculpting.

Parallax technique: It is especially used for posterior cortical or subcapsular cataract. On moving the nucleus from side to side the movements of the posterior opacities relative to the base of the groove is assessed. The opacities will move less as trench is deepened.

NUCLEUS ROTATION

The trench is widened and deepened with multiple strokes. The nucleus can be rotated single handedly or bimanually to make the sub incisional nucleus accessible for further trenching.

The rotation of the nucleus is based on the principles of torque. The rotation is achieved if the lever arm is long and force applied is minimum.

$$\text{Torque} = \text{Force} \times \text{Lever arm}$$

As we know the initial groove is longer at 6 o'clock postion than at 12 o'clock position.

Fig. 9 shows the nucleus rotation with a spatula through the side port. At point X, if the nucleus is rotated clockwise the force required is less as the lever arm is long but if one rotates anticlockwise at point Y, the required force will be double. The spatula should be placed against the hardest part of the nucleus, otherwise the instrument may penetrate into the nucleus rather than rotating it.

After 180° rotation, trench is enlarged at 6 o'clock position. The sculpting is started superficially and continuing the shaving action, a trench of uniform depth is achieved (Figs 10A and B).

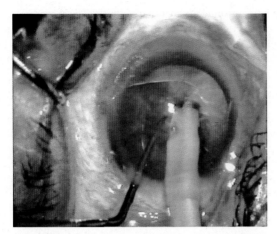

Fig. 12A: Splitting of the nucleus into two halves using the phaco probe and the dialer

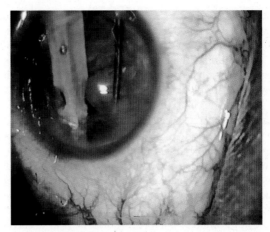

Fig. 12B: If splitting is incomplete, it is necessary to continue splitting in the peripheral part of the trench

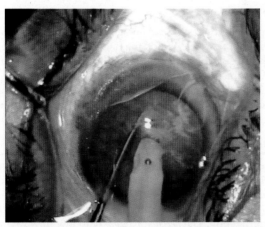

Fig. 13A: Direct chopping of the nucleus. The phaco probe is embedded in the nucleus using a burst of energy and a high vacuum

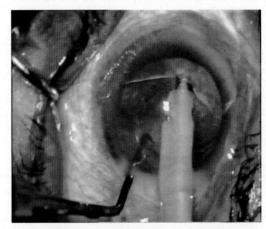

Fig. 13B: Chopping being performed, with a sideward movement splitting the nucleus into two halves

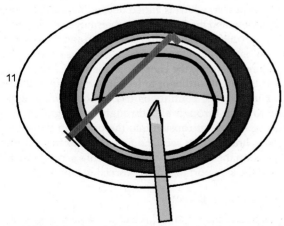

Fig. 14A: Peripheral chopping. Placement of chopper underneath the capsulorhexis margin outer to the periphery of the nucleus

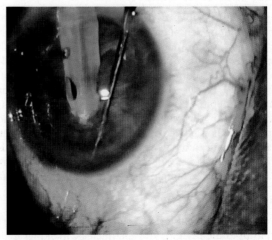

Fig. 14B: Peripheral chopping of the nuclear half

NUCLEUS ROTATION WITH PHACO TIP

The phaco tip is embedded into the nucleus with a short burst of phaco and once the vacuum seal is obtained, phaco tip is used to manipulate the nucleus. It is important to ensure that the bevel of the tip is completely embedded into the nucleus to achieve a vacuum seal.

NUCLEUS CRACKING

After achieving an adequate depth trench, the nucleus needs to be split into two halves. One should apply forces in an appropriate direction to avoid stress on the zonules. The splitting of the nucleus will depend upon its density, the distance between the points where forces are to be applied and the depth of the groove.

The application of the forces should be near to each other, in order to prevent unnecessary stress on the nucleus (Figs 11A and B). The two instruments either chopper or Sinskey hook and phaco probe should be kept near the bottom of the trench and should be close. The force applied is in the opposite directions so that center of the nucleus depresses backward and the peripheral part lifts upward. If the movement of the nucleus is not such it indicates that either the trench is superficial or the placement of the nucleus is not proper.

If splitting is incomplete, it is necessary to split in the periphery or complete it after rotating the nucleus (Figs 12A and B). In harder leathery nucleus of brown and black cataracts it is necessary to split at multiple points in order to get a complete separation.

CHOPPING

It is a technique where the nucleus is divided into smaller pieces with a chopper or sinskey hook. Chopping may be used for direct chopping of the entire nucleus or it may be used for chopping of the halves or quadrants or smaller pieces of the nucleus. Chopping can be done using a central, peripheral or a modified peripheral approach.

DIRECT CHOP OF NUCLEUS

The principle for application of forces are same. The phaco tip is embedded in the denset part of the nucleus, creating a vacuum seal by high vacuum and higher power settings, thus stabilizing the nucleus. The burst/panel mode is preferred. It is then lifted, the chopper is introduced peripheral to the phaco probe in line with it (Fig. 13A). The chopper must be directed posteriorly at a sufficient depth, towards the center of the globe. It is then moved towards the phaco probe. The phaco probe and the chopper are then moved in the opposite directions, splitting the nucleus into two halves (Fig. 13B). This technique is not preferred in the softer cataracts as the probe can go through and through. This technique uses less phaco energy and is faster.

Peripheral Chop

The chopper is introduced horizontally under the capsulorhexis margin upto the periphery of the nucleus, avoiding injury to rhexis margin (Fig. 14A). The nucleus half is positioned horizontally and is engaged by the phaco probe giving a burst of energy in the center of the piece (Fig. 14B). Once the vacuum

is built up, the nucleus is drawn centrally. The chopper is rotated vertically, engages the nucleus in the periphery in the line of the phaco probe and is pulled towards the phaco probe. When it reaches near the tip it is moved sideways, splitting the nucleus from the periphery to its center.

Central Chop

The central chop involves splitting of the fibers rather than cutting. It can be performed either by a Sinskey hook or a sharp chopper. The probe is embedded in the nucleus, vacuum hold is created and the chopper is placed just peripheral to the phaco probe and to the left to it (Fig. 15A). The chopping is performed by a posterior pressure with the chopper, at the same time pulling the chopper sideways or by pulling them both in the opposite directions (Figs 15B and C).

If the chopper is not placed properly, there will be a rotation of the nucleus.

Modified Peripheral Chop

This approach utilizes the advantages of both the central and peripheral approach. It avoids the negotiation of the chopper below the capsulorhexis margin. Once the phaco probe is buried into the fragment, vacuum builts up. The peripheral chop is performed by pulling the nucleus out of the rhexis margin and then doing a chop (Fig. 16). It is extremely useful in hard leathery cataracts.

REMOVAL OF NUCLEUS FRAGMENTS

Once each half of the nucleus is split into two or more fragments, each is held radially with a phacoprobe and moved centrally for its removal (Fig. 17).

The two systems of phaco machine—*Peristaltic and Venturi* behave differently. The *peristaltic pump* with low flow rate will have a weak attraction for the quadrant which can be increased moderately by increasing the flow rate while the *venturi pump* has a stronger attraction.

The phaco tip should be embedded in the quadrant using the phaco power, which is varied depending upon the density of the nucleus and the foot switch is then moved back to position 2. Occlusion allows the vacuum to build up and thus the nuclear fragment is moved centrally. Phaco power is used to remove the fragments, using the chopper in the other hand to divide nuclear fragment further or to feed it into the tip of the probe.

Sometimes the continuous use of power may allow the probe to pass through and through the fragment, risking engaging the iris or capsule into the probe. In these case the surgeon should bring back the foot pedal to irrigation mode and position the fragment with the help of a second instrument through the side port and then proceed to emulsify it.

Subincisional Quadrant

The beginners may find it difficult to rotate a fragment at 12 o'clock position to 6 o'clock position. Viscoelastics is injected from the side port underneath the capsulorhexis margin at 12 o'clock position which pushes the fragment forward making it easy for the fragment to be engaged.

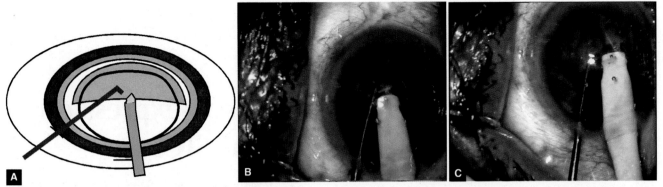

Figs 15A to C: (A) Placement of chopper in the center of the nuclear fragment to the left of the phaco probe which engages the nuclear fragment, (B) The position of the chopper after the nucleus is engaged. A backward pressure is applied by the chopper, (C) The two instruments move sideways to split the nucleus half

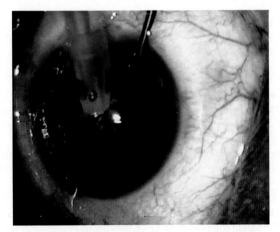

Fig. 16: Modified peripheral chop with the nuclear fragment brought to the center

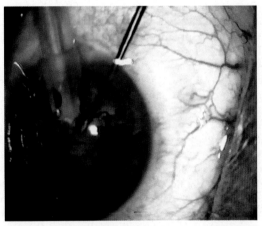

Fig. 17: Each fragment is held radially and brought to center and emulsified

BIBLIOGRAPHY

1. Badoza D., Mendy JF, Ganly M. Phacoemulsification using the burst mode.J Cataract Refract Surg 2003; 29:1101-1105 © 2003.
2. Fine IH, Packer M, Hoffman RS. Power modulations in new phacoemulsification technology: improved outcomes. J Cataract Refract Surg 2004;30(5):1014-9.
3. Lal H, Sethi A. Manual of Phaco techniques. Text and Atlas.First edition. CBS Publishers 2002.
4. Mele B, Rosa. QuickChop Phacoemulsification: Technique and Tips. Techniques in Ophthalmology 2004 March;2(1):1-4.
5. Seibel B.S. Mastering the Tools and Techniques of Phaco-emulsification Surgery, Third edition. Slack incorporated 1999;98.
6. Steinert RF. Phaco Chop. Ophthalmic surgery: Principles and Practice. (183-191) Philadelphia: WB Saunders, 2003.

Chapter 8

Nucleus Management by Visco-expression Technique in Manual SICS

Vaijayanti Deodhar, Ranjit S Dhaliwal (India)

OUR SURGICAL TECHNIQUE IS AS FOLLOWS

We perform our surgeries under topical, local, peribulbar or sub-Tenon anesthesia.

We use a superior rectus bridle suture, whenever we contemplate a superior, a superonasal or a superotemporal approach. In temporal approach we do not require a rectus bridle suture. An eye speculum is inserted in all cases.

A fornix based conjunctival flap is made and the epiciliary vessels are cauterized with a bipolar cautery (Figs 1 to 3).

We do not make any stab side port. The sclero-corneal tunnel is made as follows:

Start with a scratch frown incision (5.5 to 6 mm) with a blade fragment, a lamellar tunnel section blade or a crescent knife. The center of the groove on the sclera, i.e. the external incision is kept 1-1.5 mm from the limbus (Fig. 4).

The tunnel is dissected, starting from the 6 mm groove, using a crescent knife until the blade is 2 mm inside the clear cornea. The tunnel is fan shaped so that the internal incision is about 20% wider than the external incision. Scleral side pockets are also made with the crescent knife (Fig. 5).

A 3.2 mm keratome is then used to enter the anterior chamber (Fig. 6).

After this Trypan blue is injected into the anterior chamber, under an air bubble. The air bubble protects the endothelium from being stained with the dye. The Trypan blue is then washed out of the eye with balance salt solution leaving the anterior capsule of the mature cataract stained blue.

The anterior chamber is then reformed with the viscoelastic (Fig. 7).

A 26-gauge needle fashioned into an irrigating cystotome is used to create the continuous curvilinear capsulorhexis (Fig. 8).

In case of a swollen white cataract, the rhexis is deliberately kept very small in the beginning as the rhexis edge tends to go towards the periphery. When the capsulorhexis is nearly complete, the corneal end of the tunnel is extended on either side with the keratome or the crescent knife (Fig. 9). The anterior chamber is maintained with the viscoelastic throughout this procedure. The Utrata forces are used to complete the rhexis, making it wider at the same time.

A forceful hydrodissection makes the nucleus tilt up on one side (Fig. 10). If the nucleus is very hard and rigid, it is not flipped upside down, but is instead, gently cart-wheeled out of the capsular bag by dialling, using the bi-manual technique (Fig. 11). A smaller or a softer nucleus flipped upside down and brought gently into the anterior chamber (Fig. 12). Hydrodelineation is performed with the viscoelastic cannula in the anterior chamber itself in the case of a soft cataract (Fig. 13).

A curved cannula is then insinuated under the nucleus and viscoelastic injected beyond the inferior margin of the nucleus. All the while the posterior lip of the tunnel is gently depressed with the same cannula to make the tunnel open up and allow the nucleus to be slowly and smoothly expressed out of the eye (Figs 14 and 15). Similarly any epinucleus remaining in the anterior chamber is also expressed out with the help of the viscoelastic (Fig. 16).

A J-shaped cannula is inserted at the 12 o'clock position to remove the sub incisional cortex (Figs 17 and 18). A Simcoe irrigation/aspiration cannula is then used to aspirate rest of the cortex. The posterior capsule is polished with the Simcoe cannula itself.

A 5.25 mm posterior chamber IOL is implanted through the tunnel into the capsular bag using curved lens holding forceps. If necessary it can be dialled and centered (Fig. 19).

Viscoelastic is aspirated with the Simcoe cannula and the anterior chamber is formed with the balanced salt solution (Fig. 20).

The conjunctival flap is replaced with an iris repositor or a cotton bud, to cover the external tunnel opening (Fig. 21). It is then sealed at one end with the help of a bi-polar cautery (Fig. 22).

Postoperatively we always give a subconjunctival injection of gentamycin and dexamethasone.

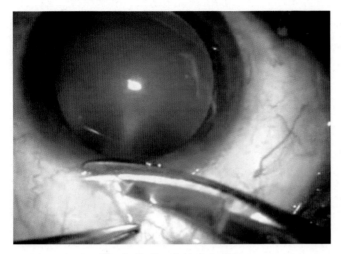

Fig. 1: Conjunctival dissection

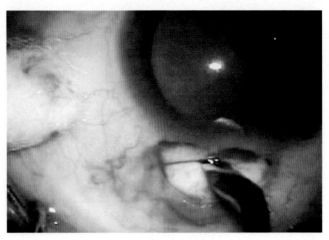

Fig. 4: Frown incision

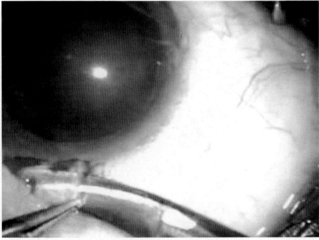

Fig. 2: Dissection of Tenon's capsule

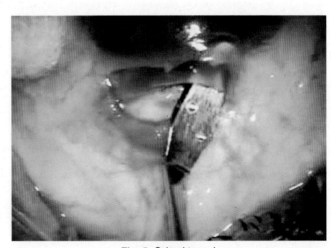

Fig. 5: Scleral tunnel

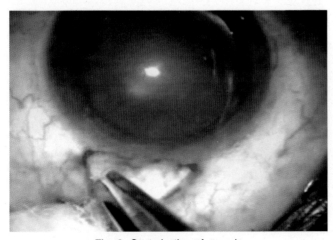

Fig. 3: Cauterization of vessels

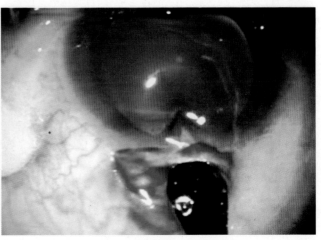

Fig. 6: AC entry by keratome

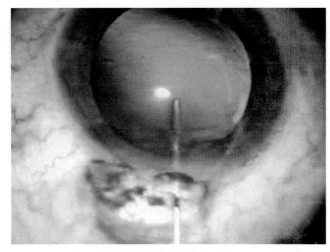

Fig. 7: Viscoelastic in AC

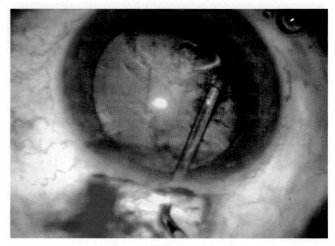

Fig. 10: Hydrodissection

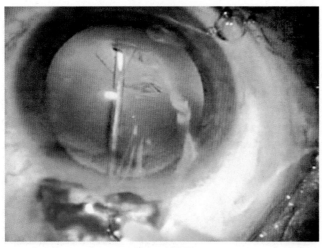

Fig. 8: "CCC"

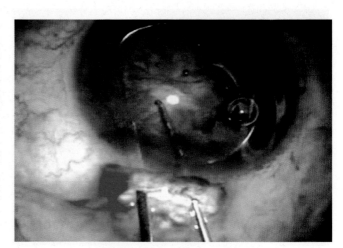

Fig. 11: Dialing of the nucleus

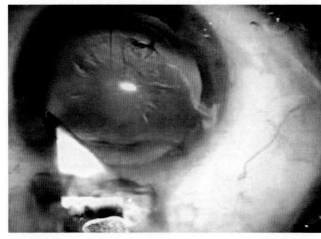

Fig. 9: Internal incision completed

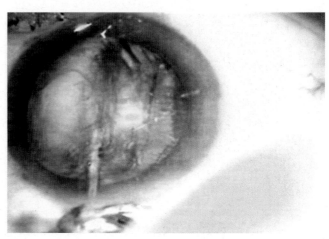

Fig. 12: Tumbling of the nucleus

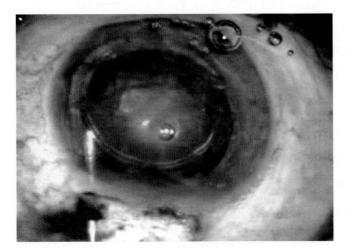

Fig. 13: Hydro-delineation in AC

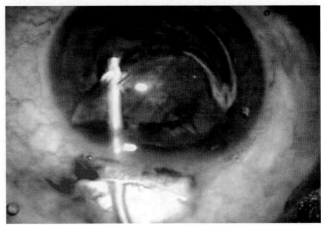

Fig. 16: Visco-expression of epinucleus

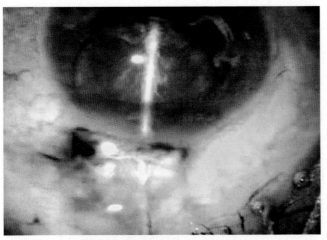

Fig. 14: Visco-expression of the nucleus

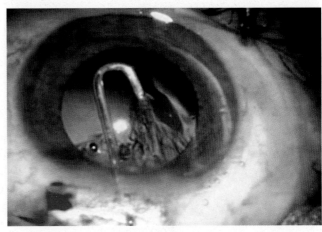

Fig. 17: Removal of sub-incisional cortex with J cannula

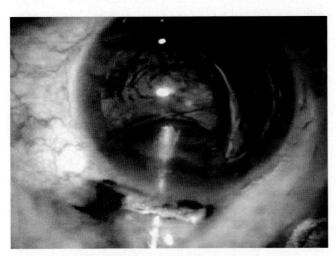

Fig. 15: Visco-expression - continued

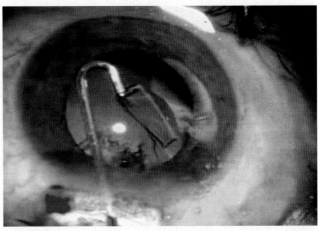

Fig. 18: Removal of sub-incisional cortex with J cannula - continued

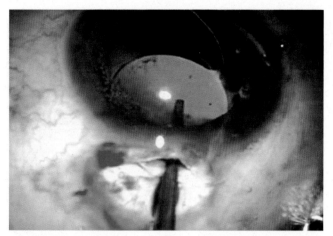

Fig. 19: Implantation of IOL

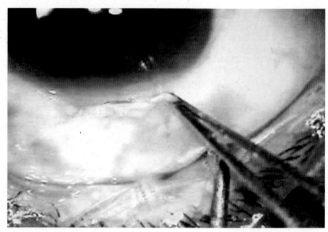

Fig. 21: Reposition of conjunctival flap

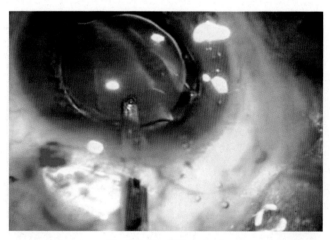

Fig. 20: I/A of Viscoelastic

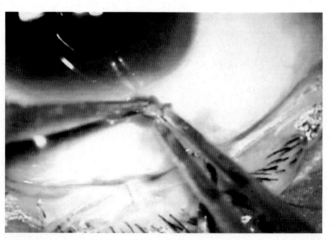

Fig. 22: Conjunctival flap cautery

THE ADVANTAGES WITH THIS TECHNIQUE ARE

1. No side ports are required and so the surgery is less traumatic.
2. The endothelium and the posterior capsule is protected during all the procedures because of the viscoelastic, which acts like a third invisible hand for the surgeon.
3. Posterior capsule rupture is rare because no instrument is inserted deep in the posterior chamber before the delivery of the nucleus.

In the initial cases we encountered complications like endothelial folds, striate keratitis, mild corneal edema, hyphema, posterior capsule rupture with vitreous in the anterior chamber, exudates in anterior chamber, raised post operative intra ocular pressure, in addition to a corneal ulcer in one case.

But now complications are far and few.

This technique has a smoother and easier learning curve; rather I would say there is NO learning curve for a surgeon who is already performing ECCE and implant surgery.

The final results with manual small incision cataract surgery with visco-expression of the nucleus and epinucleus are arguably the same as with phaco surgery.

DO'S AND DON'TS OF THE PROCEDURE

1. In addition to the use of digital massage, super pinky or balanced weight after local anesthesia, pre-operatively the patient is given Acetazolamide tablet 250 mg orally, to induce hypotension of the eyeball. Nucleus delivery by the visco-expression technique in SICS requires a hypotensive eyeball.
2. The tunnel should be made of adequate length, so that the nucleus may engage easily.
3. The nucleus should be minified in the bag or in the anterior chamber by hydrodelineation, so as to make the visco-expression of the nucleus easy.
4. As the viscoelastic is being injected with the curved cannula into the anterior chamber, beyond the nucleus, the posterior scleral lip of the tunnel is gently pressed with the same cannula. This facilitates the smooth visco-expression of the nucleus.

Chapter 9

Phaco Chopping for All Cataract Conditions

Rohit Om Parkash (India)

Chopping is the preferred technique for nucleus management. It has a longer learning curve than divide and conquer. In the chopping technique the real use and advantage of the two handed technique is employed. The chopping has becomes simple because the nucleus splits readily with the chopper because of the natural cleavage planes.

The phaco chop technique has evolved because of the following reasons:

1. There is decreased phaco time.
2. The use of high vacuum during chopping has enhanced the nuclear control.
3. The anti surge mechanisms have given a stable environment in the post occlusion phase.
4. The different choppers for different grades of cataracts have made chopping techniques more acceptable.
5. The use of different shopping techniques has also been gratifying for the Phaco surgeon.
6. The Torsional Emulsification has also helped.

CHOPPING OF GRADE 1 TO 3 SCLEROSED NUCLEI

Safe zone phacoemulsification using direct chop is the preferred technique. In this technique, no instrument is taken beyond the safe zone.

In the softer nuclei of this category, a long blunt chopper is used whereas in harder cataracts a long pointed chopper is used. The power and fluidics are also titrated depending upon the grading of the nuclei of this category.

The basic technique is the same. The ultrasonic tip penetrates the nucleus superior to the 3 o'clock 9 o'clock line. The ultrasonic energy is used to reach the core of the nucleus in its thickest part. The high vacuum in foot position 2 after the total occlusion helps in firmly holding the nucleus (Fig. 1). The tip of the chopper is embedded fully in the nucleus just inside the opposite inferior CCC margin (Fig. 2). The chopper is then moved towards the point where the ultrasonic tip is firmly holding the nucleus (Fig. 3). The moment it reaches near the ultrasonic tip (which is firmly holding the nucleus) the two instruments are moved apart in lateral and medial directions (Fig. 4). The nuclear pieces get chopped into two.

At this stage, a few things have to be borne in mind. Lateral separation usually chops the nuclear pieces (Fig. 5). If incomplete separation occurs then the separation by chopper can be tried at different places.

In the harder nuclei, additional slight pulling of the nuclear piece held with ultrasonic tip and pushing of the nuclear piece with the chopper before separating also helps to achieve total chopping into two. The nucleus is rotated and the process repeated. The first piece is usually difficult to remove. The nucleus is further rotated and the process is repeated.

BLACK CATARACT PHACOEMULSIFICATION

In Black Cataracts, the morphological details are different and there is poor visualization (Fig. 6). These Cataracts are difficult to chop and divide. They are difficult to emulsify. The excessive energy production causes more wound site thermal injury. There is higher incidence of Posterior Capsule rupture with complications. There is greater insult to Corneal Endothelium. The zonules are occasionally weak. The chamber stability with high fluidics is very important.

In Black Cataracts, high-end machine come into play because it takes care of Heat and Surge.

OZiL in Black Cataracts is a very good option. The issue of WSTI is not there. One can use tighter or otherwise routinely sized incisions. The stable chamber settings along with high fluidics further enhance the surgical results.

Adequately sized, 5.5 mm, intact CCC is a very important step in the Black Cataract Phacoemulsification. A large sized CCC is mandatory to facilitate safe and easier manipulation. Decreasing the contact between Nucleus and Anterior Capsule decreases the stress on the zonules. The size of the rhexis should be 5.5 mm.

When starting with phacoemulsification move with a definite strategy. Bevel down Sculpting is done to focus Cavitation energy into nucleus. Never push the Nucleus. (Fig. 7) A small crater is created.

A long pointed chopper is used. In our technique, the chopping is done in Safe Zone. No instrument is taken beyond the CCC edge. The chopper is long and pointed. If the chopper is not pointed or in conditions the harder nucleus does not allow deeper penetration of the chopper then the chopping motion is repeated in the same place 2-3 times to allow the chopper to penetrate deep enough before separation forces are applied.

Once the separation is to be started a few things have to be borne in mind. The posterior plate is leathery and difficult to separate. The separation, if done, has to be total.

There are a few clicks, which have to be borne in mind for achieving total separation of leathery nuclear fibers.

One has to be absolutely sure that the nucleus piece is firmly held with the Ultrasonic tip embedded in the deeper harder part of the Nucleus. The total separation is achieved by using the chopper at different planes. Chopping in different places further facilitates the total separation (Fig. 8). Sometimes separating in different directions helps. A complete separation is the key in Black Cataract Emulsification.

Chop into smaller pieces. Do not emulsify and eat up the nuclear piece. Leave them so that they act as a cushion when last piece is being separated.

The size of the pieces is also important. The harder the Nucleus the smaller the pieces should be. The smaller piece should be removed first. Larger pieces cause more turbulence. Subsequently, the nuclear pieces are easily emulsified.

What to do if initial total separation is not possible?

The brittle, leathery and sticky nuclear fibers are very difficult to separate fully in the initial stages of chopping. Continue to chop sequentially through 360 Degrees. This will give a central core and partially chopped nuclear pieces. With high vacuum lift the central core and emulsify. Now attack the nuclear pieces and separate them fully before phacoaspirating.

ENDOTHELIAL PROTECTION

Endothelial Protection is a major issue in Rocky hard Cataracts. Multiple measures have to be used to take care of the Endothelium:

- Soft shell technique of Viscoelastic substances usage in black Cataracts.
- The liberal multiple injections of visco- dispersive or Visco-adaptive at various steps help in protecting the Endothelium.
- The nuclear pieces are chopped into smaller pieces and then Emulsified. This creates lesser turbulence.
- The emulsification is carried at deeper plane.
- Stable chamber settings with appropriate incision size but not at the cost of WSTI
- Torsional Emulsification is a definite step forward in having clearer corneas.

Machine Parameters

The concept for machine parameters is based on:
-High vacuum and flow rate to allow the Nucleus to remain in contact with the tip to ensure ultrasound to be more effective.
- Cold energy modulations to have minimal WSTI
- The combination of Fluidics, energy modulations and chamber stability working with perfect balance

The final titration of machine parameters depend on the machine you are using. It is advisable to use Hyperpulse while sculpting. While chopping, the Vacuum and flow rate have to be higher. The Burst energy delivery is done. The combination of Fluidics, energy modulations and chamber stability has to work with perfect balance.

In rocky hard Cataracts, while using Torsional Emulsification, one can use the option of pressing the foot pedal fully in position 3. If one feels that the Emulsification is still difficult then a combination of torsional and traditional longitudinal is used to avoid occlusion of the handpiece tip. The problem may be caused by a large sheared-off piece obstructing the tip. The short repulsive effect of longitudinal ultrasound helps reposition the quadrant and facilitate the quadrant to be tumbled and emulsified without being lollipopped.

A programmed Torsional handpiece with a combination of 80% torsional oscillation and 20% traditional ultrasound is used for such hard Cataracts. In other words, 80 msec is used for torsional and 20 msec for traditional.

Torsional Emulsification and Hard Cataracts

In harder Cataracts, the Torsional Emulsification finds special usage because of the following reasons:
1. The wound site thermal injury (WSTI) is minimal.
2. Tighter incisions are not a problem because of minimal WSTI. Consequently, one can work in harder cataracts with stable anterior chamber settings. The advantages of stable chamber settings make it easier to work in such harder cataracts.
3. Turbulence is less because of absence of repulsion. This results in clearer corneas.
4. One can work at deeper level, which further helps in having clearer corneas.
5. Sculpting, if done, is easier, faster and more efficient with torsional ultrasound.
6. The inherent surge preventing measures in Infiniti further enhance the stable chamber settings making the Black cataract management more predictable.

Phacotips Preference

The phaco tip of choice is Kelman ABS 30 degree/45 degree Tip. This tip has the following advantages:
- Deep sculpting is facilitated
- Hard nuclei cutting is particularly enhanced
- Emulsifies 4+ nuclei at lower power levels because of increased cavitations
- Specially angled to enhance aspiration of peripheral lenticular material
- In Torsional Emulsification, 45-degree Kelman tip works a bit easier than the 30-degree tip because a 45-degree angled tip makes the quadrants tumble more easily than a 30-degree one.

Role of Fluidics

The fluidics of a machine plays a very important role in hard cataracts. A good non-compliant fluidics lets you safely go as high as 600 mm of Hg with high flow rates of 48-50 cc/min. In addition, the dynamic rise time feature in machines lets you achieve higher flow rates when the occlusion is there. Each machine has its own limitations of vacuum, which the surgeon needs to titrate. In other words, the safety has not to be compromised in machines, which do not have comparable

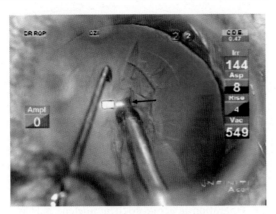

Fig. 1: Ultrasonic tip holding firmly the deeper part of the nucleus with high fluidics

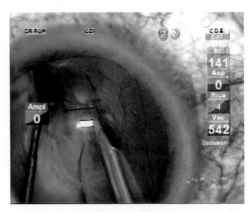

Fig. 4: Chopper tip and ultrasonic tip moving in opposite direction to achieve a division

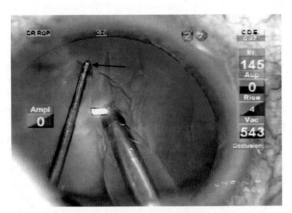

Fig. 2: Tip of the chopper embedded full thickness in the nucleus

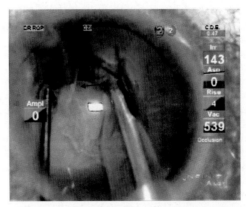

Fig. 5: Lateral separation to achieve a total division

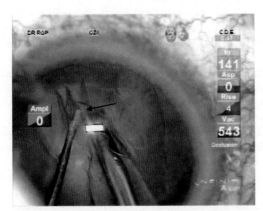

Fig. 3: Chopper tip, fully embedded in the nucleus, moving towards ultrasonic tip

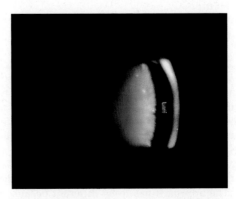

Fig. 6: Black Cataract on slit-lamp biomicroscopy

excellent fluidics. The key lies in managing fluidics successfully by maintaining stable chamber throughout the procedure.

Excellent fluidics is a boon in these rocky hard cataracts. In these Cataracts, a good followability allows the tip to remain in contact with the nuclear material thus allowing the Ultrasound to be more effective. The surge preventing measures with excellent fluidics vindicate the importance of higher end machines to successfully conquer the hardest of cataracts.

Use of Cold Infusion Solutions

The use of freezing infusion solutions is ideal where the use of U/S energy is high. It keeps the phaco tip cooler, prevents corneal burns and is said to be endothelial safe.

Predisposing Factors for Posterior Capsule Rupture in Black Cataracts Emulsification

1. Smaller Capsulorhexis
2. Peripheral Extension of CCC
3. Squirting sudden large amount of fluid for Hydrodissection
4. Tightening of the eye with fluid trapped while doing hydrodissection and trying to decompress the eye by pushing behind
5. Rotating using force with two handed technique.
6. Pushing while sculpting
7. Unsuccessful Continuous Separating force at the same point without using different places, directions or planes
8. Pulling rigid large nuclear pieces after unsuccessful chopping
9. Pointed nuclear pieces hitting the Posterior Capsule
10. Irrigation and Aspiration
11. Unstable chamber settings.

Indications for Converting Back

The success in managing Black Cataracts lies in avoiding corneal injury and maintaining the integrity of Posterior Capsule. A catastrophe can be avoided by converting. Converting back is an armamentarium which holds true for both evolving and experienced phacosurgeons. There are certain difficult situations, which can be managed as explained earlier. However, there are phaco situations wherein one needs to convert back to Extra capsular. These conditions are:
1. Extension of CCC
2. Failure to separate completely the sticky and leathery nuclear fibers while chopping or dividing.

SOFT CATARACT MANAGEMENT

Cataracts with no nuclear sclerosis or minimal nuclear sclerosis require tuning of the technique for chopping. This is a relative grey area in the chopping techniques. These cataracts are the most difficult to chop. It is easier to chop something hard like tree. However, it is difficult to chop softer like jelly. All that can be achieved is partial segmentation.

The hydrodelineation is not done if chopping has to be done. Soft cataract chopping has to be managed with a different approach. The approach has to be different because of the following reasons:

- There is no hard nuclear core
- There is difficulty in fixing the nucleus with the ultrasonic tip because power and vacuum aspirate the nucleus. This makes it difficult to impale the nucleus.
- It is difficult to chop a soft nucleus fully into two pieces.

Soft cataracts chopping require specific settings. The power has to be Zero. The vacuum and flow rate have to be dramatically reduced. The nuclear core has to be held with a non impaling technique. The foot pedal is at foot position Zero in the deeper part of the nucleus. The blunt chopper is taken beneath the anterior capsulorhexis almost to the equator. The Phaco tip and the Chopper are then moved towards each other. The moment they reach close to each other they are separated. A partial separation is achieved. The nucleus is rotated 180 degrees and the process is repeated. The procedure, if required, can be repeated at 90 degrees to the first two chopping efforts. This helps in achieving four partially chopped pieces.

At this stage the vacuum and flow rate is increased. If required, some power is also incorporated in the settings. The nuclear pieces are then aspirated using high vacuum and special vertical splitting technique. In this technique, the high vacuum and flow rate combination is used to hold and pull the partially segmented quarter/half. The chopper, in the meantime, holds the adjacent quarter/half back. The simultaneous pulling by ultrasonic tip and holding back of the adjacent nuclear piece facilitates total separation by vertical splitting. The Nucleus piece is then eaten up by using high fluidics. The process is repeated in the other quarters till the whole nucleus is removed.

The ultrasonic Energy, if required, has to be minimally used. The Torsional Emulsification helps in soft cataracts to hold the thin and soft nuclear rim. The absence of repulsion and efficient working at lower parameters has a double edged advantage in Soft Cataracts.

In Torsional Emulsification, holding of a soft and thin plate of Nucleus can be efficiently managed. In these soft Cataracts, there is a need to hold the soft nuclear piece with accurate fluidics and energy delivery. This becomes possible with OZiL while using lower machine parameters. The absence of repulsion makes the embedding and holding of a thin and softer plate of Nucleus piece easily possible.

In contrast in longitudinal Phaco, the delivery of energy associated with repulsion requires a somewhat thicker and harder nucleus plate to fully embed and hold the nucleus piece.

SMALL PUPIL

In small pupils, pupillary dilating measures are used. The pupil dilating measures take care of the problems associated with small pupil. However, postsurgically there is irregular atonic pupil. This type of pupil is associated with glare and photophobia. There is poor adaptation to light changes. Patients, at times, do complain of some loss of depth of focus.

Therefore, the surgeon has to be very discreet in using pupillary dilating measures. A perfect balance has to be created wherein the pupillary dilating measures should be used where they are absolutely mandatory. To achieve this surgeon should learn small pupil phacoemulsification without dilating aids.

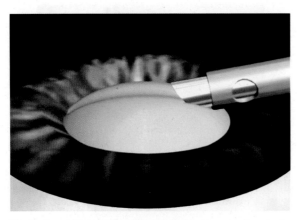

Fig. 7: Bevel down helps early on to create a small crater by focusing energy

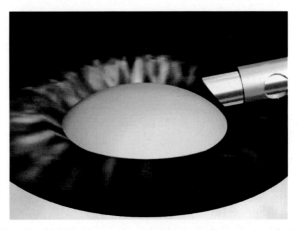

Fig. 10: Start bevel down to create space and to prevent miosis

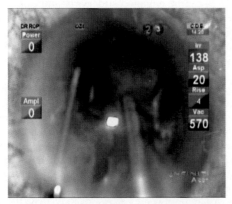

Fig. 8: Total separation being shown. Chopping at different planes, different places and different directions facilitate total separation

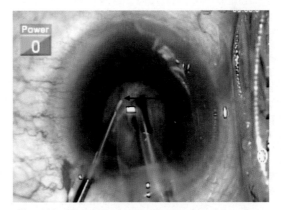

Fig. 11A: Site of burying the chopper into the nucleus

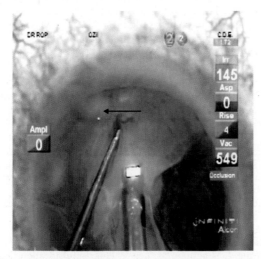

Fig. 9: Practicing small pupil safe zone phacoemulsification in an otherwise dilated pupil

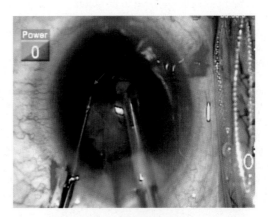

Fig. 11B: Direction of chopper-diagonal which is parallel to pupillary margin

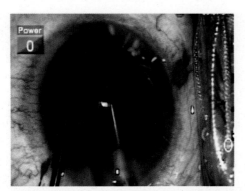

Fig. 11C: Chopper moves at a deeper plane that there is no transmission

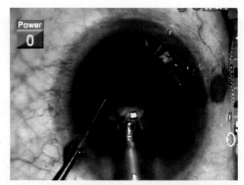

Fig. 11D: The small size of the nuclear piece helps avoid hitting the iris while nucleus piece is being pulled out

Practicing Small Pupil Phacoemulsification

The technique for phacoemulsification has to be technique of lateral separation using safe zone phacoemulsification. In this technique, the surgeon has to learn doing nucleus emulsification by not taking any instrument beyond the safe zone{beyond the CCC edge}.Those surgeons who take the chopper much beyond the CCC edge will experience that the small pupil further comes down because of traumatic miosis.

The Safe Zone Phacoemulsification has to be practiced in the dilated pupil before we really shift on to this technique in small pupil phacoemulsification (Fig. 9). Once we learn this technique, one is able to do away with moving the instruments beyond the CCC edge. Learning this technique makes you know, how not to move the instruments beyond the CCC edge. This is just like learning to practice strokes in sports with shadow practice.

Key Factors

The successful technique for small pupil Phacoemulsification without dilating aids has to revolve around some basic fundamentals:

The machine parameters have to be decreased to avoid turbulence and inadvertent aspirating of the iris tissue
• The chamber settings have to be stable
• Appropriate usage of viscoelastic usage
• All the instruments have to keep away from the pupillary margin/iris to avoid the coming down of the iris
• The nucleus pieces should not hit the iris/pupillary margin
A Viscocohesive is used before starting with Phacoemulsification. It viscodilates the pupil and creates a space. Start with bevel down initially. Sculpt a well in the central nucleus with a few passes to create a space. This helps to work under the dome of viscocohesive which at the same time maintains pupillary dilation. If the bevel is turned up at this vacuum level, the overlying viscocohesive can be engaged superiorly and pupil dilatation can be lost. Bevel up later on. There are two ways how nucleus emulsification can be done.

Chopping

Start with bevel down initially. Sculpt a well in the central nucleus with a few passes to create a space. This helps to work under

the dome of viscocohesive which maintains pupillary dilation (Fig. 10).

If the bevel is turned up at this vacuum level, the overlying viscocohesive can be engaged superiorly and pupil dilatation can be lost. Bevel up later on. Create a deep well in the centre without going beyond the 3 o'clock 9 o'clock line.

In softer Cataracts one can embed the phacotip in the inferior wall of the well using low vacuum, flow rate and minimal ultrasonic power. Torsional Emulsification is a big advantage. There is absence of repulsion makes embedding even easier into the softer wall without aspirating the nucleus. Chopping is done. Non Impaling technique can also be used to chop the nucleus.

In moderately harder and harder cataracts embed the phacotip in the inferior wall of the well and chop the nucleus. (Fig. 11A) Safe Zone Phacoemulsification with lateral separation is done. Rotate the nucleus and continue with chopping. A few important key points have to be kept in mind while chopping:

a. Do diagonal separation so that one is parallel to the pupil (Fig. 11B).
b. Chop at a slightly deeper plane so that you keep away from the iris and you do not hit the iris (Fig. 11C).
c. The pieces you make should be smaller ones because if you take out a larger piece, you can end up with making the iris come down (Fig. 11D).
d. The pupil is small and there is decreased visibility. One can leave behind a small nuclear piece.

To avoid this one should emulsify and remove the nucleus pieces sequentially starting from one end and going to the other end.

BIBLIOGRAPHY

1. Ashok Garg, I Howard Fine. Mastering the techniques of "advanced phaco surgery". Jaypee Brothers Medical Publishers, New Delhi, 2007.
2. Koch PS, Katzen LE. Stop and Chop Phacoemulsification. J Cataract Refract Surg 1994;20:565-70.
3. Sachdev M, Dada T. A practical guide to emulsification. Jaypee Brothers Medical Publishers, New Delhi, 2002.
4. Wong T, Hingorani M, Lee V. Phacoemulsification time and power requirements in phaco chop and divide and conquer nucleofractis techniques. J Cataract Refract Surg 2000;26 (9):1374-8.

Chapter 10

Quick Chop Express for Suprahard Cataract

Mohan Rajan, Sujatha Mohan, Priye Suman Rastogi (India)

INTRODUCTION

While Ultrasound Phacoemulsification can be performed on the majority of cataracts without a hitch, rock hard brunescent cataracts have always remained a challenge even for an experienced an deligent surgeon.

In our cataract population in India, suprahard cataracts (Grade IV and above) are common. Suprahard cataract are virtually all nucleus and have little or no cortical buffering material. The lens fibers of brunescent cataract are extremely tenacious and cohesive. These lens fibers being leathery resist division and makes in the bag Phacoemulsification difficult and hazardous. The surgeons may need to advocate special technique and unique instrumentation to severe the adhesions of the nuclear lens fiber completely; failure to do so results in increased risk for capsular bag distortions. Hard cataract also demands more ultrasound time and energy thus , resulting in irreparable damage to the endothelium.

SUPRAHARD CATARACTS A CHALLENGE FOR A SURGEON, WHY ?

1. Large nucleus which is difficult to crack because of leathery attachment
2. Thin posterior capsule
3. Poor or No cortical cushion
4. Inc incidence of Corneal Edema and Post-op Corneal decompensation
5. Inc incidence of Posterior Capsular Rent/Nucleus drop.

To facilitate manipulation of suprahard nuclei and to shorten the use of ultrasound energy author presents a technique called as *Quick Chop Combo Technique* using Author designed *Mohan Rajan's Super Combo Chopper* (Fig. 1). This newly designed chopper has a very sharp distal tip which cracks the posterior nuclear plate of rock hard leathery brown cataract (grade IV and above) in a single stroke.

Unique Features

1. The length of the chopper is around 1.75 mm-2 mm, which allows the chopper to penetrate into the posterior nuclear plate of Hard Brown Cataract.
2. The tip of the chopper is very sharp which enables the surgeon to crack the posterior nuclear plate in one stroke.
3. Though the chopper is very sharp it does not do any damage to the posterior capsule provided the anterior chamber is maintained deep.
4. The ability of the Super Combo Chopper to penetrate the endonucleus enables the surgeon to tackle such cataracts using very low phaco energy and high aspiration flow rate. As a result the corneas are much clearer in the 1st postoperative day.

QUICK CHOP COMBO TECHNIQUE FOR SUPRAHARD CATARACTS

Surgical Procedure

After Peribulbar anesthesia, 2.8 mm valved temporal clear corneal tunnel is created. The anterior chamber is filled with a high density viscoelastic. Using a 26-G bent cystotome/Uttata's forceps 5-5.5 mm Continuous Curvilinear Capsulorhexis is made in the anterior capsule. Hydrodissection is performed using a 24 G cannula ensuring free nucleus rotation.

Different Phaco machines are used with different parameters. While using Alcon Infinity Parameters are : Phaco power of 60%, Vacuum of 100 mm of Hg and aspiration flow rate of 25 ml/min. In Ozil technology: vacuum of 400 mm of Hg is used, Aspiration Flow Rate of 40 ml/min. While using Bausch and Lomb Millennium with Custom Control Software and Stellaris machine 20% power is used with vacuum of 300 mm of Hg – 450 mm of Hg. while using Hyperpulse technology parameters are not very much different Duty cycle of 33% is chosen , phaco power of 20% and vacuum of 300 mm of Hg – 450 mm of Hg. Surgeon first aspirate the central epinucleus with phacotip (Fig. 2).

Partial thickness trench is created sufficient to impale the phacotip in to the central nucleus. This results in sufficient vacuum seal to grip the central nucleus. By immobilizing the central nucleus against the incoming super combo chopper, the distal vertical tip of the super combo chopper is depressed posteriorly directed towards the optic nerve producing the crack (Fig. 3).

Simultaneously, the surgeon generates adequate shearing force to fracture the nuclear material full depth in single stroke. The shearing force generated by the super combo chopper extends the crack and tears the leathery fibers in to two nuclear fragments completely (Fig. 4).

The Combo Chopper is placed anterior to Phaco tip. The chopper remains with in the area of capsulorhexis. Impalling the phacotip and the chopper at a different site along the same trench producing smaller nuclear fragments (Fig. 5).

The remaining nuclear hemi section is rotated by 180 degrees and brought in to the capsular bag. Similar quick chop with super combo chopper is performed producing multiple nuclear fragments (Fig. 6).

Throughout the procedure , it is crucial to maintain the anterior chamber deep with high density viscoelastic. Using high vacuum and high aspiration flow rate surgeon elevates each small fragment out of the bag and consume it in the central space. Once the first heminucleus is evacuated there is enough room to rotate the second and emulsify using the same (Fig. 7).

ADVANTAGES OF QUICK CHOP COMBO TECHNIQUE

1. Elimination of lens sculpting that otherwise demands great phaco time and energy.
2. In chopping, the stress placed on the zonules is greatly reduced, as surgeon is immobilizing the phacotip, and the incoming mechanical force of the chopper is directed centripetally inwards, towards the phacotip rather than outward towards the capsule.
3. High vacuum is invaluable for quick chop combo with brunescent nuclei. Most phaco machines now offer burst mode which in a hard cataract, avoids the coring away of material around the tip that occurs with the continuous mode. This improves the purchase and much better vacuum seal around the tip so that piece does not dislodge easily (Figs 8 to 11).

MERITS OF QUICK CHOP COMBO TECHNIQUE

1. Helps to emulsify hard nuclei
2. Reduces the amount of phaco time
3. Reduces the amount of phaco energy
4. Reduces surgical time
5. Reduces endothelial damage and there by better postoperative rehablitation.

However this technique has limitations and steep learning curve. It requires dexterity of non-dominant hand to perform the critical maneuvers. If the surgeon has not placed the phaco and chopper tips deep enough, chop may not succeed. The thicker and denser the endonucleus, deeper the chopper tip must pass. The tendency to elevate the chopper tip during the chop arises from the fear of rupturing the posterior capsule. Instead of dividing the nucleus this may clearly crack the superficial surface.

FEW TIPS FOR THE BEGINNERS

1. Proper placement of chopper and phacotip.
2. Stabilization of the nucleus with high vacuum seal.
3. Keeping the chopper tip deeply buried in the nucleus during the actual chop.
4. Proper orientation of the chopper shaft at the limbus.

HYPERPULSE TECHNOLOGY FOR SUPRAHARD CATARACT

Term Hyperpulse is coined by David Chang. it is a variation of pulse mode of phacoemulsification in which energy is given in the form of very short pulses. In this modality of energy delivery, linear control of energy or phaco power is preserved and also allows the choice of shorter duty cycle.

Duty cycle =

$$\frac{\text{Time for which energy is delivered (on time)}}{\substack{\text{Time which energy is delivered + Time} \\ \text{for which energy is not delivered (off time)}}} \times 100$$

Cycle time = On time + Off time

In a regular phaco once the foot pedal is depressed to stage 3 energy is given continuously with/with out any break and increases linearly. In case of Pulse mode energy is given in Pulses of 10-15 pulses/sec with a break of off time in between, after every bout of energy given (on time).

Shorter the duty cycle less is the phaco energy used and more is the off period. In hyperpulse technology ultrasound energy is given in very short pulses (80-100 pulses/second).These rapid short pulses are thought to produce relatively more transient cavitations that increases ultrasonic efficiency of emulsification. More off time as compared to on time gives time for phaco probe to cool down and hence less

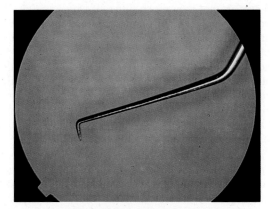

Fig. 1: Mohan Rajan's super combo chopper for quick chop combo technique

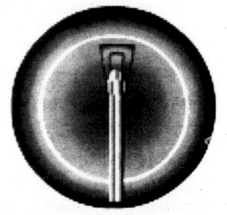

Fig. 2: Aspiration of central epinucleus with phacotip

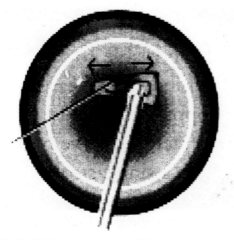

Fig. 3: Vertical chop produced by combo chopper

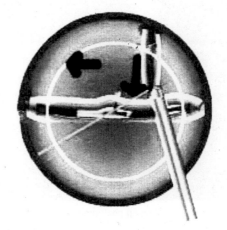

Fig. 4: Vertical chop extended by combo chopper

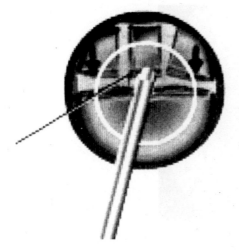

Fig. 5: Nucleus divided into small nuclear fragments

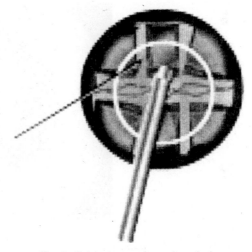

Fig. 6: Quick chop performed producing multiple nuclear fragments

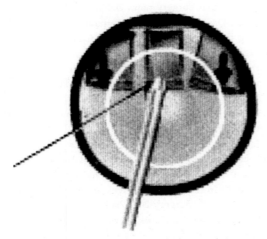

Fig. 7: Quick chop performed the second hemi nucleus

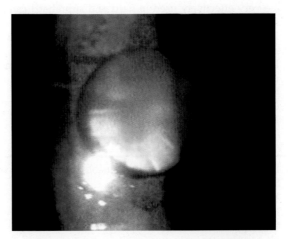

Fig. 8: Pre-op photograph of grade IV cataract

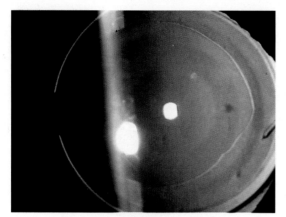

Fig. 9: Post-op photograph on day 1

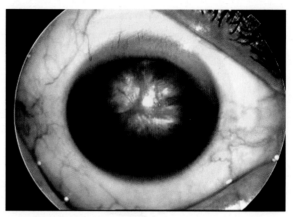

Fig. 10: Pre-op photograph of grade IV cataract

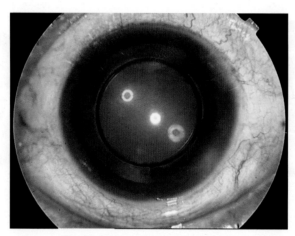

Fig. 11: Post-op photograph on day 1

complications like corneal burns. it also facilitates improved follow ability with less chattering of nucleus and more thermal protection. Hence also known as *Cold Phaco*. This technology can be very effectively used in hard and suprahard cataracts which require higher energy and more surgery time.

Hence Hyperpulse Technology in hard and Suprahard cataracts leads to:
1. Less postoperative complications due to less phaco energy used
2. Minimal endothelial cell count loss
3. Clearer corneas on day 1 postoperatively
4. Early visual rehabilitation.

CAVEATS

1. Bausch and Lomb Millennium (Custom Control Software).
2. Super Combo Chopper.
3. Vertical Chopping Technique.
4. High Molecular Weight Viscoelastic (e.g. Viscoat)
5. Hyperpulse Technology (Cold Phaco).

BIBLIOGRAPHY

1. Agarwal Amar. Hard Brown cataract can be managed using phaco. Ocular surgery news 2000;11(4).
2. Badoza Daniel Mendy, Julio Fernadez. Phacoemulsification using the burst mode. Journal of Cataract and Refractive Surgery June 2003;29:6.
3. Erbium Laser phaco requires longer time but less energy for moderately hard cataract. Binder, Stefanie Petrou – Euro Times 2003;8:2.
4. Harddril, Marilyn. Avoid heat build up in extraction of tough nucleus, Eye World 2003;8:6.
5. Mahatme, Vikas. Woodcutter technique splits hard nuclei effectively. Ocular Surgery News 2001;12:11.
6. Miyata, Toshiyukai, et al. Efficacy and safety of the soft shell technique in cases with hard lens nucleus. Journal of Cataract and Refractive Surgery 2002;28(9).
7. Vanathi M, Vajpayee, Rasik B, et al. Crater and Chop technique for phacoemulsification of hard cataract. Journal of Cataract and Refractive Surgery 2001;27(5).

Chapter 11

Chopping in Hard Cataracts—Burst Phaco

GL Arun Kumar, S Sivagnanam (India)

INTRODUCTION

The invention of phacoemulsification by Charles D.Kelman modernized cataract surgery to a more refined procedure. The usage of ultrasound energy for emulsification of the nucleus through a small incision was indeed a great invention. Ultrasound energy is heat energy which when used in excess or used incorrectly can cause thermal damage to the Cornea as well as to the ocular tissues. Recent modulations in the ultrasound modes reduces the ON TIME and increases the OFF TIME thus reducing the thermal damage.

Chopping Involves Two Main Criterias

1. The surgeon should be already trained in Stop and chop technique with more confidence of handling the chopping maneuver with the left hand (Fig. 1).
2. The Phaco machine Figs 2 and 3 used for the direct chop surgical procedure should be provided with the burst and high rates of micropulsed ultrasound modes for effective and short duration emulsification of even a hard cataract.

Different Chopping Techniques

There are different ways of chopping a hard cataract like Horizontal Chop,Vertical Chop or Karate Chop.

Horizontal chop involves the movement of the chopper tip and phaco needle tip in parallel direction to each other after embedding and piercing for atleast 2 mm separation of the nucleus substance for a perfect crack in the posterior plate of the nucleus. Figs 4, 5 and 6 show how a burst phaco mode works with the number of Bursts indication in the Phaco machine display along with the Burst time, Micropulse time and transition movement of the footpedal from step 2 to 3 for the application of the Burst U/S to embed the phaco needle tip and straight horizontal chop movement to be performed by moving the two instruments apart once the posterior plate is cracked.

Vertical Chop

Vertical chop involves the movement of the chopper tip and phaco needle tip in vertical direction to each other after embedding and piercing for atleast 2 mm separation of the nucleus substance for obtaining a crack vertically across the Y sutures.While doing so the surgeon must be very careful and observe the bottom of the Chopper tip so that it does go deep into the nucleus mass as it is very dangerous and it might sometimes even touch the Posterior Capsule.

Karate Chop

Karate chop involves the opposite direction movement of the chopper tip and phaco needle tip to each other in a horizontal plane or vertical plane according to the surgeon's preference during the chopping stroke in order to separate the nucleus completely.

Before attempting to any chopping procedure the surgeon has to be careful on the movement of the sharp chopper tip which has to pierce the Hard Nuclear girdle to accomplish a perfect cut across the Y sutures running across the nucleus mass. If the chopper tip is not sharp enough to cut the hard nuclei then it will exert mechanical force thereby pushing the nucleus away from the phaco needle tip inspite of holding with a high vacuum setting.

The vacuum of the order of 140 to 160 mm Hg should be appropriate for any grade of nucleus when a 20G phaco needle tip with 0.8 mm ID and 0.9 mm OD is used and during the embedding procedure the surgeon should see to it that the phaco needle tip projection outside the sleeve should be atleast 2 mm refer Fig. 7 and should embed atleast 1.5 mm to 2 mm into the depth of the nucleus substance in order to obtain perfect hold and leverage during the chopping stroke in any of the above mentioned three types of chopping methods.

To accomplish all the above mentioned steps the surgeon has to be conversant enough in using the Burst phaco mode available in the newer phaco machines, which provides high amplitude ultrasound energy level for a very short duration of ON time in order to completely embed into the nucleus substance with ease. Before applying Phaco Burst the surgeon should take care that the phaco needle tip is a new or sparingly used one or it is sharp enough refer Fig. 8 so that it will not waste unnecessary Ultrasound energy for incomplete partial embedding action.

The burst phaco mode is available in the Galaxy Cold Phaco Machine, Shift Portable Cold Phaco Machine Figs 9 and 10, Interface Cold Phaco from Appasamy Associates, Chennai,

India provides 100% phaco power whenever the surgeon's footpedal transition occurs from step 2 to step 3 in the downward direction for a very short duration as shown in the waveform picture the burst U/S, regular pulsed U/S and Micropulsed U/S can be applied in succession. This mode should be used only in hard cataracts grade III to grade V nucleus sclerosis.This phaco burst can be applied till the surgeon accomplishes complete embedding of the phaco needle tip in order to obtain a perfect hold of the entire nucleus mass for a direct chop technique. Once direct chops are complete the the BURST mode can be put OFF.

After downsizing the nucleus by four or five chops the chopped nuclear fragments can be removed in succession one by one by using the linear Microplused ultrasound energy with higher pulse rate available in the galaxy and shift phaco machines with 25 micropulses/second and 40 micropulses/second available in the interface phaco machines refer Figs 12A and B. Phaco power preset for these modes can be anywhere between 40 to 60% refer Figs 12A and B. At this juncture the surgeon should linearly increase the micropulse phaco power further down from the foot pedal detent 3 in order to obtain perfect and effective emulsification process without any chattering of hard nuclear pieces. During this procedure the surgeon should also downsize the chopped pie shaped pieces into smaller fragments for faster emulsification with the micropulse ultrasound.Use of these two modes effectively will drastically reduce the total ultrasound time utilized for the manipulation and emulsification of hard cataracts. If the surgeon's preference is regular pulsed U/S the same can be applied with a Pulse rate of 6 to 8 pulses/sec for the fragments emulsification but with a low phaco power of the order of 30 to 50% preset as the U/S wave duty cycle in this mode is 50% refer Figs 11A and B.

To study the wound temperature variations of these burst and micropulsed ultrasound modes a thermal study analysis was performed to study the heat generated during the emulsification of the cataract during regular phaco surgeries and bimanual phaco surgeries with different ultrasound modes like the Continuous,Pulse,Micropulse and Burst.

This thermal study was done during regular co-axial phaco and bimanual phaco surgeries on human eyes. The rise in the phaco tip temperature was analyzed using a highly sensitive infra-red camera "FLIR". The camera was placed at a distance of 1 feet from patients eye to be operated.This camera provides real time thermal still as well as video images which were later on processed in detail to study the rise in temperature during the different steps of the phaco surgery like nucleus sculpting and emulsification with different ultrasound modes. This study was performed with the Galaxy Cold Phaco Peristaltic and Venturi Phaco-emulsification Systems.

With the *continuous and pulse ultrasound modes* the rise in the phaco tip temperature was between 40 to 49 degrees centigrade for a 60 to 70% ultrasound power refer Fig. 13A. With the burst and micropulse Cold Phaco (with a reduced ON TIME and a long OFF TIME) ultrasound modes the temperature rise never exceeded 38 degree centigrade for 100% refer Figs 13B and 13C. The past studies in different countries with different phaco machines have proved that corneal wound burn occurs at or above 45 degrees centigrade.

This analysis clearly shows that the *Burst Mode and the Micropulse Cold Phaco* Mode with a reduced on time and a long of time is safe to be used in any grade of cataract as the phaco tip temperature never exceeds 38 degree centigrade in phaco and bimanual phaco surgeries. This study compares the different ultrasound modes whereas most of the previous studies done throughout the World compared between different ultrasound machines.

CONCLUSION

The advantages of the Burst Mode are:
- Decreases the amount of ultrasound energy delivered to ocular tissues.
- Very effective in chopping cataracts of nucleus sclerosis grade III to grade V in phaco and bimanual phaco surgeries.
- Decreases the amount of endothelial cell loss.
- Clearer corneas and better visual acuity on the first post-operative day.
- Very minimal wound temperature induced at the phaco needle.

Besides making a satisfied patient, the use of these ultrasound modes evolves a more Confident Surgeon

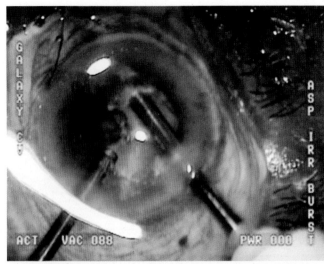

Fig. 1: Left hand manipulation is very important for a perfect chopping stroke

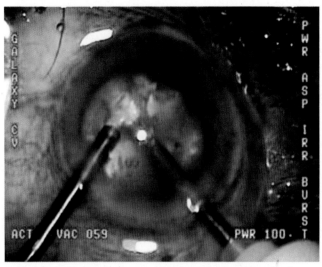

Fig. 4: 100% Burst power applied for a short on time duration

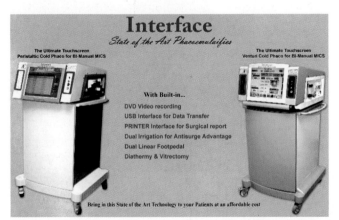

Fig. 2: Appasamy's interface touchscreen phaco machines provided with single burst phaco mode and 30/40 Micropulses per second Cold phaco mode for faster emulsification of nuclear fragments

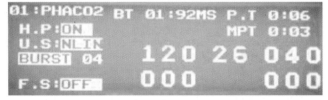

Fig. 5: Counter in the display indicates number of bursts applied and U/S time

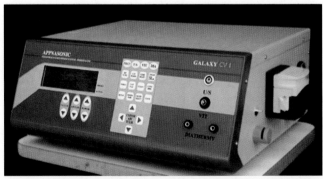

Fig. 3: Appasamy's galaxy phaco machine with burst phaco mode in succession with 25 micropulses

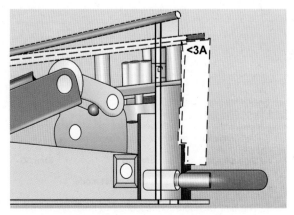

Fig. 6: Burst applied in foot transition between 2 and 3

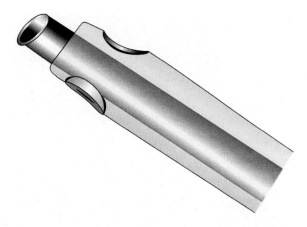

Fig. 7: The 20 G phaco needle tip projection outside the infusion sleeve should be atleast 1.5 to 2 mm in order to completely embed into the nucleus mass for a direct chop

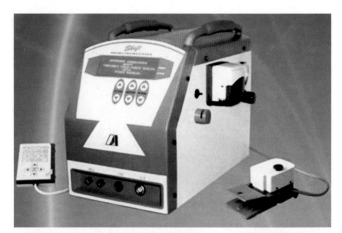

Fig. 10: Shift portable cold phaco

Fig. 8: New or sparingly used phaco needle is always preferred for the direct phaco chop technique with the burst U/S mode inorder to use effective U/S energy level

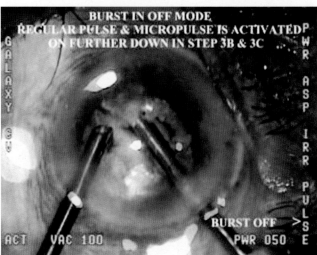

Fig. 11A: Chopped fragments are further removed with regular pulsed U/S power in step 3B

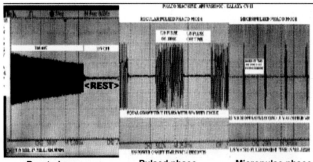

Burst phaco   Pulsed phaco   Micropulse phaco

U/S wave form pattern in burst mode phaco

Step 3A   Step 3B   Step 3C

Footpedal activation in burst mode

Fig. 9: The first waveform corresponds to burst u/s 3A then the regular pulse U/S 3B followed by 3C Micropulsed U/S power

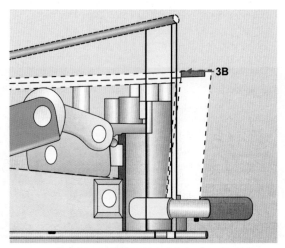

Fig. 11B: Footpedal position for regular pulsed U/S in step 3B

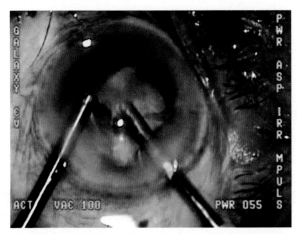

Fig. 12A: Chopped fragments are further removed with regular pulsed U/S power in step 3B

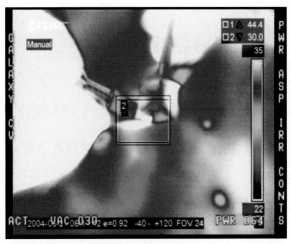

Fig. 13A: Thermal image captured with a IR thermal camera during the application of the continuous U/S mode during the bi-manual phacoemulsification surgery

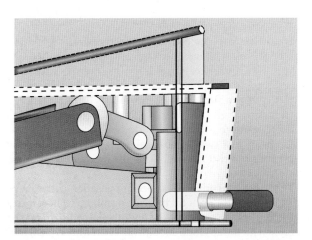

Fig. 12B: Footpedal position for regular pulsed U/S in step 3C

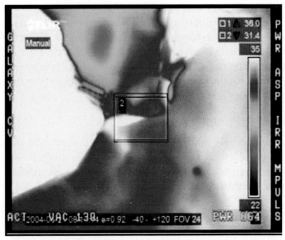

Fig. 13B: Thermal image captured with micropulse U/S

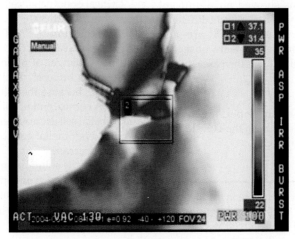

Fig. 13C: Thermal image captured with burst U/S mode

Chapter 12

Phacoemulsification Surgery Procedure and IOL-Implantation without Using Viscoelastics

Bojan Pajic, Brigitte Pajic-Eggspüehler (Switzerland)

ABSTRACT

Background

Today modern cataract surgery prefer the phacoemulsification technique with implantation of a IOL in the bag. Viscoelastics are one of the main requirements during surgery. Nevertheless it is possible to implant a foldable IOL after phacoemulsification without using viscoelastics. The aim of the study is to investigate surgery without viscoelastics regarding surgery technique, complications and endothelial cell loss.

Methods

In a prospective, randomizing and masked study 126 patients were enrolled. Parameters studied were surgery safety, preoperative and postoperative IOP, corneal endothelial cell changes with and without viscoelastics.

Results

In the BSS group at one months postoperatively a mean endothelial cell loss of 106±226 cells/mm² (corresponding 4.5%) and in the Healon group of 122±207 cells/mm² (corresponding 5.3%) were find out. Data analysis showed no significant difference between the groups. Likewise no significant difference was seen regarding cell size, cell shape and IOP pre- and postoperatively. A significant correlation were observed between patient age and endothelial cell loss increase.

Conclusions

The phacoemulsification technique can be performed with viscoelastics or continuous AC irrigation with the same level of safety regarding endothelial cell damage.

INTRODUCTION

The mean endothelial cell number at birth state in the literature differ very much between 3500-4000 cells/mm² [15,39] und 6000-7500 cells/mm².[1,5,44,66,71] The initial endothelial cell loss is above-average high, but during life the curve flattens.[67,77] From the 2 age the mean annual endothelial cell decrease around 0.5-1.0%.[45] Murphy et al.[53] calculate a mean endothelial cell reduction between the 20 and 80 years in mean 0.52% a year. In adulthood the average endothelial cell number is estimated to be 1400-2500 cells/mm².[12,15,39,44,57]

Following aspects could lead intraoperative to further endothelial cell damage: mechanically and toxically damage as liquid turbulence whirl lens fragments, ultrasound energy during the phacoemulsification, direct instrument contact, IOL implantation, keratoplasty, pharmacological affection.

Postoperative a cause of endothelial cell loss could be inflammation, IOP peaks, chronically contact damage. The most often cause for endothel cell loss are mechanically traumas during the surgery.[37,71,72]

The functional endothelial decompensation correlate poor with the absolute endothelial cell number.[39] Therefore the morphological analysis, it is said endothelial cell size and shape integrate with the absolute endothelial cell number, has a higher sensitivity regarding the evaluation of the endothelial cell damages.[40,49,60,65,71]

Critical endothelial cell number are stated very different in the literature with 300-500 cells/mm² [1,34,52,73], 500 cells/mm² [44], 400-700 cells/mm² [15,39], 500-700 cells/mm² [54] and <1000 cells/mm².[75] As soon as the critical endothelial cell number is beyond than it is a danger of permanent stroma edema [11,39,70] or of a keratopathia bullosa[6]. The endothelial cell number decreases during life, because the cell loss can not be compensated with mitosis. A corneal endothelial dystrophy and degeneration cause a endothelial cell decrease respectively glaucoma or uveitis could favor an endothelial cell loss. All this factors lead to corneal function decrease.[39]

Viscoelastic solutions are used in modern cataract surgery for ever as a space maintainer during IOL implantation and as prevention of corneal endothelial cell loss.

The aim is to analyze a safe cataract surgery method without viscoelastica investigating corneal endothelial cell pattern and IOP.

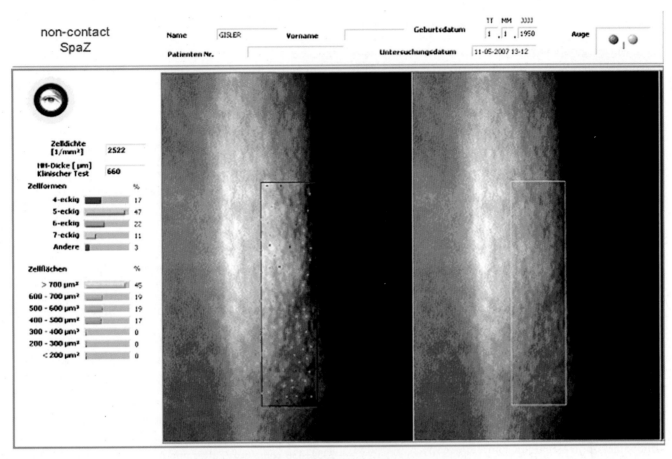

Fig. 1: Endothelial cell image with cell count and analysis

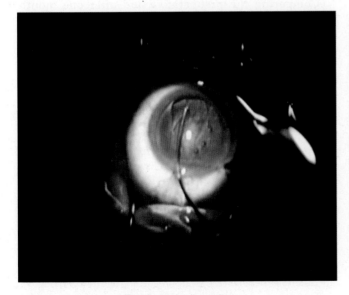

Fig. 2: Hydrodissection

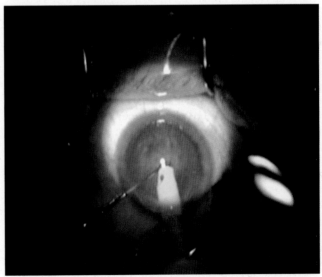

Fig. 3: Phacoemulsification with chop and stop technique

PATIENTS AND METHODS

In a prospective, randomized, masked study during 12 months 126 patient in 2 groups were carried out. Each patient was agree with the study and give us a permit to perform it. In the Healon group there were 62 and in the BSS group 64 patients. Patients were excluded with glaucoma[4], uveitis, pseudoexfoliation, where a postoperative inflammation and fibrinous reaction is more frequently[74], with diabetes mellitus type I, malignant tumors, endothelial dystrophy and cornea guttata.[13,74]

In the Healon respectively BSS group 45 respectively 47 patients were analyzed for the study. In each group there was a follow-up loose of 17 patients, because they did not come for the postoperative examination or death.

Overall the surgery was done in the Healon- respectively BSS group 23 (51.1%) respectively 22 (46.8%) on the left eye and 22 (48.9 %) respectively 25 (53.2 %) on the right eye. Mean age of patients in the Healon group was 71.2 years (range: 40.6-91 years) and 71.2 years (range: 43.6-87.6 years) in BSS group. In the Healon group, 30 patients (32.6%) were female, 15 patients (16.3%) male and in the BSS group, 29 patients (31.5%) were female, 18 patients (19.6%) male.

In all patients, preoperative evaluations included manifest refraction, best-spectacle-corrected visual acuity (BSCVA), intraocular pressure (IOP), corneal endothelial cell number, corneal radius and slit-lamp examination of the anterior and posterior segment. Additional the IOP was measured 6 hours after surgery. Patients were evaluated preoperatively and 1 day, 1 week and 1 months after surgery.

Noncontact Corneal Endothelium Microscopy

For corneal endothelium cell number and pattern investigation the noncontact corneal endothelium microscopy (Noncontact Slit Lamp Device, Rhine-Tec, Krefeld, Germany) was used.

Endothelium cells were counted at area of 860 μm x 650 μm. Counting frame is positioned manually with evaluation of cells divided by left and lower edge. Cell shape specification are done in percent of evaluated cells; based on cell shape of quadrangular, pentagonal, hexagonal, heptagonal and other cells. Cell area specification are stated in percent of evaluated cells; based on cell size, divided into cells bigger than 700 μm², 600–700 μm², 500–600 μm², 400–500 μm², 300–400 μm², 200–300 μm², smaller than 200 μm². Qualitative endothelial changes (polymegatismus und pleomorphismus) were assess with a image analyses procedure. The analyzed endothelial cell number is defined with CD (Zellen/mm²). The mean endothelial cell size is described with AVE (unity: μm²), the standard deviation with SD. The number of analyzed cells is apparent with the parameter NUM. The variation coefficient CV is received by division of the cell size standard deviation with the mean endothelial cell size. For obtaining size in percent, the coefficient have to be multiply with 100 (SD/AVE x 100). The percentage of hexagonal cells is defined with 6A. The hexagonal cell (apex) percentage and the average dispersion of endothelial cell size (area) were imaged by a diagram (Fig. 1).

Surgery Method with BSS

The anesthesia is done subconjunctival and parabulbar with Xylocain 2% and Carbostesin 0.5%. Two paracentesis were put at 10 and 2. The chamber anterior is maintained with the irrigation terminal during performing a circular capsulorhexis with a 25 G needle. A clear corneal approach with a width of 2.8 mm is done at 11h with consecutive hydrodissection (Fig. 2). The lenticular nucleus is removed by phacoemulsification (Fig. 3) and the cortex by bimanual irrigation/aspiration (I/A) system (Fig. 4). A acrylic IOL (type PhysIOL 65 C/N) is implanted by an injector in the chamber posterior in the bag during irrigation (Fig. 5A, B). IOL center with the aspiration unit (Fig. 6 A, B, and 7). Application of 0.25 ml Carbachol (Miostat®) and 1 mg Cefuroxim (Zinacef®) is done in the chamber anterior.

Surgery Method with Healon®

In this group a circular capsulorhexis is performed under the protection of Healon with a 25 G needle. The IOL was implanted by Healon in the bag with a consecutive bimanual aspiration of Healon with an irrigation/aspiration (I/A) system.

Results

There was no statistical significant difference between the BSS and Healon group preoperative regarding endothelial cell number, age and gender.

Corneal Endothelial Cell Number and Shape

At BSS group mean endothelial cell number was preoperative 2334±436 cells/mm², after one day postoperative 2250±472 cells/mm², after one week postoperative 2211±485 cells/mm² and after one month postoperative 2228 ±471 cells/mm².

Comparing the preoperative and after one month postoperative values at BSS group, than an endothelial cell loss was detected of 106.2 ±226 cells/mm², what corresponds a loss of 4.5% (Fig. 8).

At Healon group the mean endothelial cell number was preoperative 2307±427 cells/mm², after one day postoperative 2243±435 cells/mm², after one week postoperative 2195±452 cells/mm² and after one month postoperative 2185±389 cells/mm².

Comparing the preoperative and after one month postoperative values at the Healon group, than an endothelial cell loss was detected of 122.2±207 cells/mm², what corresponds a loss of 5.3% (Fig. 8).

Regarding the corneal endothelial cell number loss there is no significant difference between the BSS and Healon group at day one (p=0.61), at week one (p=0.84) and at month one (p=0.72) postoperative.

Preoperative patient age was in BSS group at 71.213±9.7 years and in the Healon group at 71.210±10.6 years. There is no significant difference between the groups regarding age (p=0.99) (Fig. 9).

There is no statistical significant correlation (p=0.059) between preoperative corneal endothelial cell number and age.

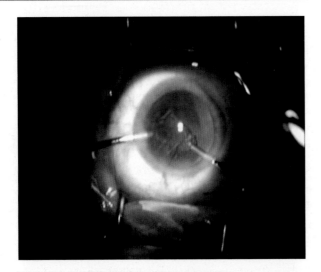

Fig. 4: Irrigation / Aspiration

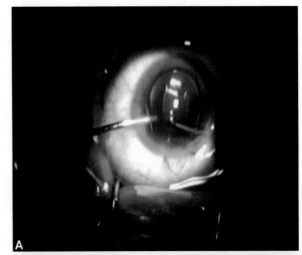

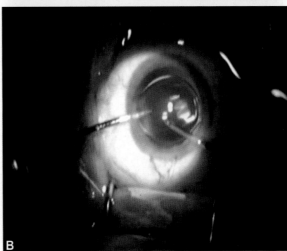

Figs 6A and B: Corneal endothelial cell loss 1 month postoperative

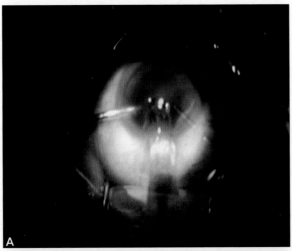

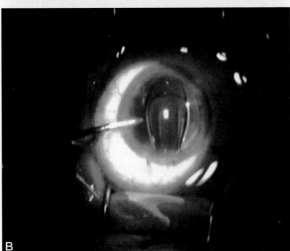

Figs 5A and B: Acrylic IOL (type (Phys IOL 65C/N) implantation by an injector in the bag during irrigation

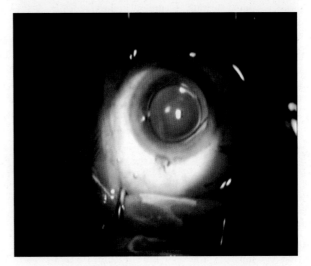

Fig. 7: Age distribution with mean, standard deviation and range values

There is a significant correlation between age and endothelial cell loss at day 1 (p=0.04), at week 1 (p=0.003) and at months 1 (p=0.049) postoperative. The higher the age, the higher is the endothelial cell loss after cataract surgery.

Preoperative mean average cell area (AVE) is in BSS group 457.7 ± 252 µm² (range 170.1 to 942.6 µm²) and in Healon group 452.3 ± 126 µm² (range 158.2 to 933.9 µm²). Coefficient of variation (CV) is in BSS group at 34.7±5.9 with a percent of hexagonal cells (6A) of 60.4%. Coefficient of variation (CV) is in Healon group at 34.9 ±5.1 with a percent of hexagonal cells (6A) of 58.8% (Table 1).

Table 1: Preoperative endothelial cell area pattern and shape					
	AVE	SD	MAX	MIN	CV	6A
BSS-group	457.7 µm²	±252 µm²	942.6 µm²	170.1 µm²	34.7 ±5.9	60.4%
Healon-group	452.3 µm²	±126 µm²	933.9 µm²	158.2 µm²	34.9 ±5.1	58.8%

1 day postoperative mean average cell area (AVE) is in BSS group 481.8 ± 211 µm² (range 170.0 to 1014.0 µm²) and in Healon group 467.0 ± 116 µm² (range 150.0 to 962.3 µm²). Coefficient of variation (CV) is in BSS group at 36.7 ±6.0 with a percent of hexagonal cells (6A) of 57.9%. Coefficient of variation (CV) is in Healon group at 35.5 ±5.2 with a percent of hexagonal cells (6A) of 57.1% (Table 2).

Table 2: 1 day postoperative endothelial cell area pattern and shape					
	AVE	SD	MAX	MIN	CV	6A
BSS-group	481.8 µm²	±211 µm²	1014.0 µm²	170.0 µm²	36.7 ±6.0	57.9%
Healon-group	467.0 µm²	±116 µm²	962.3 µm²	150.0 µm²	35.5 ±5.2	57.1%

1 week postoperative mean average cell area (AVE) is in BSS group 504.9 ±274 µm² (range 173.6 to 1036.5 µm²) and in Healon group 490.7 ±179 µm² (range 163.1 to 1012.6 µm²). Coefficient of variation (CV) is in BSS group at 36.5 ±5.7 with a percent of hexagonal cells (6A) of 57.2%. Coefficient of variation (CV) is in Healon group at 36.3 ±6.3 with a percent of hexagonal cells (6A) of 56.7% (Table 3).

Table 3: 1 week postoperative endothelial cell area pattern and shape					
	AVE	SD	MAX	MIN	CV	6A
BSS-group	504.9 µm²	±274 µm²	1036.5 µm²	173.6 µm²	36.5 ±5.7	57.2%
Healon-group	490.7 µm²	±179 µm²	1012.6 µm²	163.1 µm²	36.3 ±6.3	56.7%

1 month postoperative mean average cell area (AVE) is in BSS group 495.8 ±248 µm² (range 177.7 to 994.0 µm²) and in Healon group 476.8 ± 123 µm² (range 152.8 to 989.4 µm²). Coefficient of variation (CV) is in the BSS group at 36.5±7.9 with a percent of hexagonal cells (6A) of 56.6%. Coefficient of variation (CV) is in Healon group at 36.9 ±5.6 with a percent of hexagonal cells (6A) of 55.6% (Table 4).

Table 4: 1 month postoperative endothelial cell area pattern and shape					
	AVE	SD	MAX	MIN	CV	6A
BSS-group	495.8 µm²	± 248 µm²	994.0 µm²	177.7 µm²	36.5 ±7.9	56.6%
Healon-group	476.8 µm²	± 123 µm²	989.4 µm²	152.8 µm²	36.9 ±5.6	55.6%

There is a decrease of hexagonal cells 1 months postoperative comparing with the preoperative values of 3.5% in the BSS group and 3.2% in the Healon group. The difference between the groups is not statistical significant (p=0.05). There is an increase of CV factor comparing to the preoperative values of 1.7 in the BSS group and 2.0 in the Healon group. The difference between the groups is not statistical significant (p=0.8).

Intraocular Pressure

Preoperative mean intraocular pressure in BSS group respectively Healon group was 15.2±3.8 mm Hg (range 6.0 to 24.0 mm Hg) respectively 13.9 ± 2.7 mm Hg (range 7.0 to 19.0 mm Hg). The difference between groups is not statistical significant (p=0.054) (Fig. 10).

6 hours postoperative intraocular pressure increases 6 hours postoperative in BSS group around 1.8 mm Hg and in Healon group around 1.3 mm Hg. The mean IOP is in BSS group at 17.1 ±6.9 mmHg (range 10.0 - 37.0 mm Hg) and in Healon group at 15.2 ± 5.4 mm Hg (range 8.0 - 39.0 mm Hg). IOP peak could be seen in BSS group in 9 cases and in the Healon group in 5 cases (Figs 11 and 12).

The difference between the groups is not statistical significant (p=0.66).

1 day postoperative intraocular pressure decreases again 1 day postoperative. The mean IOP is in BSS group at 12.1 ±3.5 mm Hg (range 5.0 -22.0 mm Hg) and in Healon group at 11.3 ±3.1 mm Hg (range 5.0 -19.0 mm Hg). Difference between the groups is not statistical significant (p=0.47).

1 week postoperative mean IOP is in BSS group at 13.6 ±3.3 mmHg (range 6.0-21.0 mmHg) and in Healon group at 12.6 ±2.5 mmHg (range 6.0-17.0 mmHg). The difference between groups is not statistical significant (p=0.68).

1 month postoperative mean IOP is in BSS group at 13.2 ± 3.0 mmHg (range 5.0 - 19.0 mmHg) and in the Healon group at 13.2 ± 2.6 mmHg (range 7.0 - 20.0 mmHg). The difference between the groups is not statistical significant (p=0.09) (Fig. 10, Table 5).

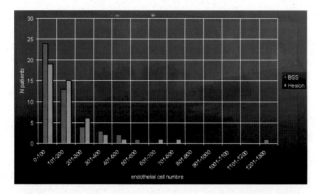

Fig. 8: Corneal endothelial cell loss 1 month postoperative

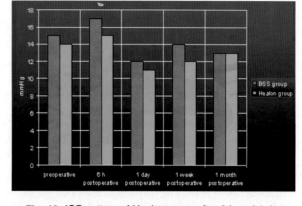

Fig. 10: IOP pattern of Healon group after 6 h and 1 day postoperative

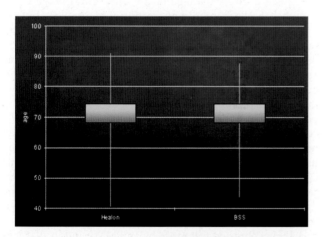

Fig. 9: Age distribution with mean, standard deviation and range values

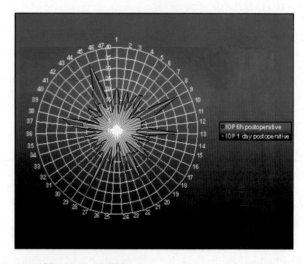

Fig. 11: IOP pattern of BSS group after 6 h and 1 day postoperative

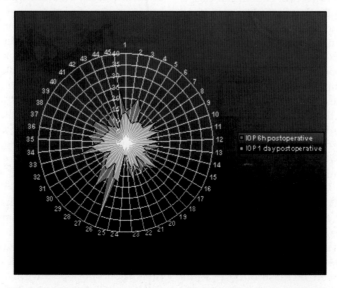

Fig. 12: IOP pattern of Healon group after 6 h and 1 day postoperative

	1 day	6h	1 day	1 week	1 month
	preoperative		postoperative		
BSS-group	15.2 ±3.8 mm Hg	17.1 ±6.9 mm Hg	12.1 ±3.5 mm Hg	13.6 ±3.3 mm Hg	13.2 ±3.0 mm Hg
Healon-group	13.9 ±2.7 mm Hg	15.2 ±5.4 mm Hg	11.3 ± 3.1 mm Hg	12.6 ± 2.5 mm Hg	13.2 ± 2.6 mm Hg

Table 5: IOP pattern

Refraction Values and Visual Acuity

Mean preoperative spherical correction is in BSS group at -1.1±3.7D mm Hg with cylinder values of 0.8±0.6D and axis of 69.9±64° and in Healon group at –2.1±3.8D with cylinder values of 0.7±0.7D and axis of 66±50.8°.

1 month postoperative the mean spherical correction is in BSS group at –1.2±1.2D mm Hg with cylinder values of –0.1±0.9 D and axis of 67.4±58.2° and in Healon group at –1.6±1.2D with cylinder values of –0.1±1.1D and axis of 57±57.1°.

Mean best corrected visual acuity increases in BSS group from 0.33±0.17 preoperative to 0.77±0.24, 1 months postoperative and in Healon group from 0.31±0.17 preoperative to 0.77±0.22 1 months postoperative.

DISCUSSION

The cataract surgery has to be performed as careful as possible regarding the endothelial cell layer. In the past the indication for a perforated keratoplasty[8,45,63] was a keratopathia bullosa after traumatic cataract surgery.

The corneal endothelial cells are after birth substantial amitotic and decrease during life.[73,76] After postoperative trauma corneal endothelium heals by magnification and migration of endothelial cells contemporary absolute cell density decreases. The barrier and pump function of corneal endothelial cells is affected therefore depending on the data in the literature if cell density decreases under a critical number of 300 to 700 cells/mm^2 [1,15,34,39,44,52,54,73] than the cornea leads to a decompensation with epithelial and stroma edema.

We observe 1 month postoperative after cataract surgery that there is a significant endothelial cell loss in both, BSS and Healon groups, whereas there is no significant difference between the groups. 1 month postoperative the mean endothelial cell loss was in the BSS group 4.5% (106.2 ± 226 cells/mm^2) and in the Healon group 5.3 % (122.2 ± 207 cells/mm^2). Our results are favorable comparing with the values declared in the literatures of endothelial cell loss between 3.8 and 11.8%.[19,21,22,32,40]

The corneal endothelial cell density must not obligate correlate with endothelial cell function. The morphometric analysis of cell size (Polymegathismus) and cell shape (Pleomorphismus) seems to be a more sensitive indicator.[49,50,62] 1 month after cataract surgery we stated in the BSS- respectively Healon group a endothelial cell increase of 38.1±4 μm^2 respectively 24.5 ±3 μm^2 contemporary a decrease of hexagonal cells (Pleomorphismus) around 3.5% respectively 3.2% and

coefficient of variation of cell size (Polymegatismus) around 1.8% respectively 2% (not significant between the groups). 1 month after cataract surgery with Healon Koch et al.[40] find out a decrease of hexagonal cells around 2.6% and coefficient of variation around 2.7%, what is comparable with our results.

We find out a significant difference between patient age and a endothelial cell decrease, it is said the older the patient is, the higher is the endothelial cell loss. A possible explanation could be that older patients have harder lens nucleus with a consecutive longer phacoemulsification time.[29,72] Dick et al.[21] favor this theory the findings that there is a correlation between phacoemulsification time and corneal endothelial cell loss, it is said the longer the phacoemulsification time is the more is a endothelial cell loss.

Regarding the endothelial cell loss is not only the surgery technique, clear corneal versus extracapsular extraction[17,21,31], cleaner rest on the phacoemulsification tip[9], phacoemulsification energy as a direct damage of the ultrasound wave to the endothelial cells or indirect by creating of free radicals, but also the choice of irrigation solutions for the chamber anterior. In comparison to the physiological liquid of the chamber anterior BSS does not contain glucose as energy source, no glutathione as protection again oxidants and free radicals, instead of bicarbonate there is citrate acetate buffer. Thus it could be shown that after a prolongate BSS stream a significant increase of polymegatismus und pleomorphismus with a decrease of endothelial cells can be seen.[2,25] It is a little bit difficult to compare our study with those from the literature because all of them used different baseline parameters, drugs and treatments. Glasser et al.[27] describe that with BSS+ irrigation solution he safe 7.3% more endothelial cells than with BSS irrigation solution, though he used in his study an extracapsular cataract surgery technique. In an experimental study was shown that in a corneal endothelial abrasion test made by an PMMA intraocular lens, 48.1±4.8 % was damaged of endothelial cells using BSS versus 10.1±1.7% using Natriumhyaluronate 1%.[46] Specific natrium-hyaluronate receptors were identified at the corneal endothelium.[23,30,47,48,55] Thus natrium hyaluronate may protect corneal endothelium during an IOL implantation.

In our study we did not found a difference between the BSS and Healon group. For achieving this result it was important to have an enough deep chamber anterior, a careful implantation of a posterior chamber IOL through 3 mm aperture without touching the corneal endothelium.

The postoperative IOP peak after using viscoelastica is explained with a viscosity depended increasing trabecular outflow resistance by obstruction of the aqueous drainage system.[33,46] Accordingly IOP peaks up to 67 mm Hg were described using Healon.[3,7,14,16,33,43,46,58] Most often the IOP peaks are seen within the first 12 hours postoperative. Despite of viscoelastica elimination a transitory IOP increase can not be prevent for all cases. So an intraoperative application of Carbachol can be recommended.[27] In contrast to an other study[64] a transitory IOP peak over 20 mm Hg was seen in 9 cases 6 hours postoperative in the BSS group, which normalized at the 1. postoperative day (Fig. 11). The reason may be a small quantity of methyl cellulose as lubricating agent in injector.

Overall we stated in the BSS group after a transitory IOP peak around 1.9±3.9 mm Hg after 6 hours an IOP decrease at the 1. postoperative day of 3.1±0.3 mm Hg and at 1 postoperative month of 3±0.8 mm Hg. In the Healon group only 5 cases had 6 hours postoperative IOP peak over 20 mm Hg, which normalized at the 1. postoperative day (Fig. 12). In the Healon group was seen a transitory IOP peak of 1.3±5.2 mm Hg after 6 hours an IOP decrease at the 1. postoperative day of 2.6±3.2 mm Hg and at 1 postoperative month of 0.7±0.1 mm Hg. This good results are explained by good remove of Healon and the application of Carbachol at the end of surgery. It is important to remove viscoelastic solution even behind the IOL. The visual acuity pattern pre-and postoperative was analogous in both groups. Regarding complications we detected only some IOP peaks and there was no significant differences between the groups.

CONCLUSION

Regarding the complications and corneal endothelium cell pattern after cataract surgery we showed that there is not difference using Healon or only BSS, it is said that both methods are safe if applied properly.

REFERENCES

1. Alvarado JA. Pathogenesis of Chandler's syndrome, essential iris atrophy and the Cogan-Reese syndrome II. Invest Ophthalmol Vis Sci 1986; 27: 873-82.
2. Araie M. Barrier function of corneal endothelium and the intraocular irrigating solutions. Arch Ophthalmol. 1986; 104: 435.
3. Assia EI, Apple DJ, Lim ES, Morgan RC, Tsai JC. Removal of viscoelastic materials after experimental cataract surgery in vitro. J Cataract Refract Surg 1992;18:3-6.
4. Axenfeld Th. Lehrbuch der Augenheilkunde von Axenfeld. Hrsg von Pau; Stuttgart, Jena, New York: G Fischer 1992; 13. Auflage.
5. Bahn CF. Postnatal develoment of corneal endothelium. Invest Ophthalmol Vis Sci 1986; 27: 44-51.
6. Bates AK, Cheng H. Bullous keratopathy: A study of endothelial cell morphology in patients undergoing cataract surgery. Br J Ophthalmol 1988; 72: 409-12.
7. Binkhorst CD. Inflammation and intraocular pressure after the use of Healon in intraocular lens surgery. Am Intra Ocular Implant Soc J 1980; 6:340-41.
8. Brady SE, Rapuano CJ, Arentsen JJ. Clinical indications for and procedures associated with penetrating keratoplasty. Am J Ophthalmol 1989;108:118.
9. Breebart AC, Nuyts RMMA, Pels E. Toxic endothelial cell destruction of the cornea after routine extracapsular cataract surgery. Arch Ophthalmol 1990; 108:1121.
10. Bourne WM, Enoch JM. Some optical principles of the clinical specular microscope. Invest-Ophthalmol 1976; 15(1): 29-32.
11. Bourne WM, Kaufman HE. Specular microscopy of human corneal endothelium in vivo. Am J Ophthalmol 1976; 81(3): 319-23.
12. Bourne WM, Kaufman HE. Endothelial damage associated with intraocular lenses. Am J Ophthalmol 1976; 81(4): 482-85.
13. Bourne WM, Nelson LR, Hodge DO. Central corneal endothelial cell changes over a ten-year period. Invest Ophthalmol Vis Sci 1997;38(3):779-82.
14. Cherfan GM, Rich WJ, Wright G. Raised intraocular pressure and other problems with sodium hyaluronate and cataract surgery. Trans Ophthalmol Soc UK 1983;103: 277-79.
15. Collins JF. Augenheilkunde von Collins. Hrsg Augustin AJ; Berlin, Heidelberg, New York: Springer 1997.
16. Cochener B, Jacq PL, Colin J. Capsule contraction after continuous curvilinear capsulorhexis: Poly (methyl-methacrylate) versus silicone intraocular lenses. J Cataract Refract Surg 1999;25:1362-69.
17. Cozean CHJr, Waltman SR. The effects of posterior chamber phacoemulsification and secondary Kelman anterior chamber lens implantation on the corneal endothelium. J Am Intraocul Implant Soc 1981; 7:237.
18. Craig MT, Olson RJ, Mamalis N, Olson RJ. Air bubble endothelial damage during phacoemulsification in human eye bank eyes. J Cataract Refract Surg 1990;16(5):597-602.
19. Diaz D, del Castillo Sanchez JMB, Castillo A, Sayagnes O, Moriche M. Endothelial damage with cataract surgery techniques. J Cataract Refract Surg 1998;24:951-55.
20. Dick B, Schwenn O, Pfeiffer N. Einteilung der viskoelastischen Substanzen für die Ophthalmochirurgie. Der Ophthalmologe 1999;96:193-211.
21. Dick HB, Kohnen T, Jacobi FK, Jacobi KW. Long-term endothelial cell loss following phacoemulsification through a temporal clear corneal incision. J Cataract Refract Surg 1996;22: 63-71.
22. Faulkner GD. Endothelial cell loss after phacoemulsification and insertion of silicone lens implants. J Cataract Refract Surg 1987;13:649-52.
23. Forsberg N, Von Malmborg A, Madsen K, Rolfsen W, Gustafson S. Receptors for hyaluronan on corneal endothelial cells. Exp Eye Res 1994;59:689-96.
24. Galin MA, Lin LL, Fetherolf E, Obstbaum SA, Sugar A. Time analysis of corneal endothelial cell density after cataract extraction. Am J Ophthalmol 1979;88:93-96.
25. Glasser DB, Matsuda M, Ellis JG. Effects of intracular irrigating solutions on the corneal endothelium after in vivo anterior chamber irrigation. Am J Ophthalmol 1985; 99:321.
26. Glasser DB, Katz HR, Boyd JE. Protective effects of viscous solutions in phacoemulsification and traumatic lens implantation. Arch Ophthalmol 1989;107:1047-51.
27. Glasser DB, Edelhauser HF. Toxicity of surgical solutions. International Ophthalmol Clinics 1989; 29:179-87.
28. Glasser DB, Osborn DC, Nordeen JF, Min YI. Endothelial protection and viscoelastic retention during phacoemulsification and intraocular lens implantation. Arch Ophthalmol 1991;109:1438-40.
29. Graether JM, Davison JA, Harris GW. A comparison of the effects of phacoemulsification and nucleus expression on endothelial cell density. J Am Introcul Implant Soc 1983; 9:420.
30. Härfstrand A, Molander N, Stenevi U, Apple D, Schenholm M, Madsen K. Evidence of hyaluronic acid and hyaluronic acid binding sites on human corneal endothelium. J Cataract Refract Surg 1992;18:265-69.
31. Hayashi K, Nakao F, Hayashi F. Corneal endothelial cell loss after phacoemulsification using nuclear cracking procedures. J Cataract Refract Surg 1994;20:44.
32. Hayashi K, Hayashi H, Nakao F, Hayashi F. Corneal endothelial cell loss in phacoemulsification surgery with silicone intraocular lens implantation. J Cataract Refract Surg 1996;22:743-47.
33. Hessemer V, Dick B. Viskoelastische Substanzen in der Kataraktchirurgie. Grundlagen und aktuelle Uebersicht. Klin Mbl Augenheilk 1996;209:55-61.

34. Hoffer KJ. Vertical endothelial cell disparity. Am J Ophthalmol 1979;87(3):344-49.

35. Hogan MJ, Alvarado JL, Weddell JS. In histology of the human eye; Philadelphia: WB Saunders 1971;102-03.

36. Holmberg AS, Philipson BT. Sodium Hyaluronate in cataract surgery. I. Report on the use of Healon in two different types of intracapsular cataract surgery. Ophthalmology 1984;91(1):45-52.

37. Holmberg AS, Philipson BT. Sodium hyaluronate in cataract surgery. I. Report on the use of Healon in extracapsular cataract surgery using phacoemulsification. Ophthalmology 1984;91(1):53-59.

38. Kaufman E, Katz JI. Endothelial damage from intraocular lens insertion. Invest Ophthalmol. 1976;15(12):996-1000.

39. Kaufman HE, Barron BA, McDonald MB. The Cornea. Edited by Kaufman HE, Barron BA, McDonald MB; Butterworth-Heinemann 1997; 2nd edn.

40. Koch DD, Liu JF, Glasser DB, Merin LM, Haft E. A comparison of corneal endothelial changes after use of Healon or Viscoat during phacoemulsification. Am J Ophthalmol 1993;115:188-201.

41. Kreyszig E. Statistische Methoden und ihre Anwendungen. Hrsg von Kreyszig E; Vandenhoeck und Ruprecht 1991; 7 Auflage.

42. Laing RA, Neubauer L, Oak SS, Kayne HL, Leibowitz M. Evidence for mitosis in the adult corneal endothlium. Ophthalmology 1984; 91:1129-1134.

43. Liesegang TJ. Viscoelastic substances in ophthalmology. 1990;34(4):268-93.

44. Liesegang TJ. The response of the corneal endothelium to intraocular surgery. Refractive & Corneal-Surg 1991;7:81-86.

45. Lindquist TD, McGlothan JS, Rotkis WM. Indications for penetrating keratoplasty. Cornea 1991;10:210.

46. MacRae SM, Edelhauser HF, Hyndiuk RA, Burd EM, Schultz RO. The effects of sodium hyaluronate, chondroitin sulfate, and methylcellulose on the corneal endothelium and intraocular pressure. Am J Ophthalmol. 1983; 95(3): 332-341

47. Madsen K, Stenevi U, Aplle DJ, Härfstrand A. Histochemical and receptor binding studies of hyaluronic acid and hyluronic acid binding sites on corneal endothelium. Ophthalmic Practice 1989a; 7:92-97.

48. Madsen K, Schenholm M, Jahnke G, Tengblad A. Hyaluronate binding to intact corneas abd cultured endothelial cells. Invest Ophthalmol Vis Sci 1989b;30:2132-37.

49. Matsuda M, Suda T, Manabe R. Serial alterations in endothelial cell shape and pattern after intraocular surgery. Am J Ophthalmol 1984; 98:313-19.

50. Matsuda M, Miyake K, Inaba M. Long-term corneal endothelial changes after intraocular lens implantation. Am J Ophthalmol. 1988;105:248.

51. Miller D, Stegmann R. The use of Healon in intraocular lens implantation. Int Ophthalmol Clin 1982;22(2):177-87.

52. Mishima S. Clinical investigations on the corneal endothelium. Am J Ophthalmol 1982; 93:1-29.

53. Murphy C, Alvarado J, Juster R. Prenatal and postnatal cellularity of the human corneal endothelium. Inv Ophthalmol Vis Sci 1984; 25:312-22.

54. Naumann GOH. Pathologie des Auges von Naumann, Hrsg von Doerr, Seifert; Berlin, Heidelberg, New York: Springer 1997,Bd 12/I, 2. Auflage

55. Nguyen LK, Yee RW, Sigler SC, Ye HS. Use of in virto models of bovine corneal endothelial cells to determine the relative toxicity of viscoelastic agents. J Cataract Refract Surg 1992;18:7-13.

56. Noden DM. Periocular mesenchyme: Neural crest and mesodermal interactions. In: Tasman W, Jaeger EA (Eds): Biomedical foundations of ophthalmology, Vol 1, Philadelphia 1989, Lippincott

57. Nucci P. Normal endothelial cell density range in childhood. Arch Ophthalmol 1990;108:247-248.

58. Pape G, Balazs EA. The use of sodium hyaluronate (Healon) in human anterior segment surgery. Ophthalmology 1980;87:699-705.

59. Polack FM. Healon (Na Hyaluronate). A review of the literature. Cornea 1986;5(2):81-93.

60. Rao GN, Shaw EL, Arthur EJ, Aquavella JV. Endothelial cell morphology and corneal deturgescence. Ann Ophthalmol 1979; 885-99.

61. Rao GN, Lohman LE, Aquavella JV. Cell size-shape relationships in corneal endothelium. Invest Ophthalmol Vis Sci 1982; 22: 271-74.

62. Rao GN, Aquavella JV, Goldberg SH, Berk SL. Pseudophakie bullous keratopathy: relationship to preoperative corneal endothelial status. Ophthalmology 1984;91:1135.

63. Robin JB, Gindi JJ, Koh K. An update of the indications for penetrating keratoplasty. Arch Ophthalmol 1986;104:87.

64. Schipper I, Lechner A, Senn P. Intraokulardruck nach Phakoemulsifikation mit Implantation einer Silicon-Plattenhaptik-Intraokularlinse ohne Viscoelastica. Klin Monatsbl Augenheilkd 2000 Feb;216(2):96-8.

65. Schultz RO, Matsuda M, Yee RW, Edelhauser HF, Schultz KJ. Corneal endothelial changes in type I and type II diabetes mellitus. Am J Ophthalmol 1984; 98(4):402-410.

66. Speedwell L. The infant corneal endothelium. Arch Ophthalmol 1988; 106:771-75.

67. Sturrock GD, Sherrard ES, Rice NSC. Specular microscopy of the corneal endothelium. Br J Ophtahlmol 1978;62:809-814.

68. Sugar J, Mitchelson J, Kraff M. The effect of phacoemulsification on corneal endothelial cell density. Arch Ophthalmol 1978; 96:446-48.

69. Sugar J, Mitchelson J, Kraff M. Endothelial trauma and cell loss from intraocular lens insertion. Arch Ophthalmol 1978; 96:449-450.

70. Svedbergh B, Bill A. Scanning electron microscopic studies of the corneal endothelium in man and monkeys. Acta Ophthalmol 1972; 50:321-35.

71. Tuft SJ, Coster DJ. The corneal endothelium. Eye 1990;4: 389-424.

72. Waltman SR, Cozean CH. The effect of phacoemulsification on the corneal endothelium. Ophthalmic Surg 1979; 10:31-33.

73. Waring GO 3rd, Bourn WM, Edelhauser HF, Kenyon KR. The corneal endothelium: normal and pathologic structure and function. Ophthalmology 1982; 89:531.

74. Wirbelauer Ch, Anders N, Pham DT, Wollensak J. Corneal endothelial cell changes in pseudoexfoliation syndrome after cataract surgery. Arch Ophthalmol 1998;116:145-49.

75. Wilson RS, Roper-Hall MJ. Effect of age on the endothelial cell count in the normal eye. Br J Ophthalmol 1982;66:513-15.

76. Yee RW, Geroski DH, Matsuda M, Champeau EJ, Meyer LA, Edelhauser HF. Correlation of corneal endothelial pump site density, barrier function, and morphology in wound repair. Invest Ophthalmol Vis Sci 1985; 26(9):1191-201.

Chapter 13

Prechop with Two 25 G Cannulas and Micro-Biaxial Cataract Technique (No Irrigating Chopper Microphakonit)

Arturo Pérez-Arteaga (Mexico)

INTRODUCTION

The objective of this technique is not to use prechop forceps, non-irrigating or irrigating choppers and so to learn how to perform the mechanical fragmentation of the cataract with two 25 G cannulas previous to start phacoemulsification (Fig. 1). It helps to decrease the possible damage to the capsular bag and the zonulae.

INSTRUMENTATION

The instrumentation is very simple; it uses only the knifes, the micro-capsulorhexis forceps, an irrigating cannula, a phaco tip, an aspirating cannula and two 25 G viscoelastic cannulas with their syringes, for the entire lens extraction procedure.

The use of biaxial techniques is preferable, nevertheless is not mandatory; in all the cases that the surgeon has two incisions (paracentesis-kind or phaco incisions) where the possibility to introduce two viscoelastic cannulas exist, the technique is possible by complete (Fig. 2). Maybe is preferable to perform the technique under a biaxial approach because the incisions are smaller (700 micron in cases of micro-biaxial or microphakonit techniques) and the advantage of an almost closed chamber without leakage improves the mechanical forces for nuclear fracture of the nucleus, and helps to protect the capsular bag and the endothelial cells (Fig. 2).

SURGICAL TECHNIQUE

The main goal in of this technique is to perform a mechanical fragmentation of the cataract outside the capsular bag, utilizing only the viscoelastic cannulas, avoiding the transmission of the mechanical forces to the capsular bag and zonula, but also far away from the endothelial cells of the cornea. It is a mechanical fracture of the nucleus at the iris plane in a bimanual fashion (Fig. 1).

The steps to perform this surgical technique are as follows:

1. A wide capsulorhexis is performed in order to facilitate the luxation of the nucleus outside the capsular bag (Figs 2 and 3).

2. After the hydrodissection a rotation of the nucleus is performed (Fig. 4) developing a "hemiluxation" of the nucleus, taking outside the capsular bag only one pole of the lens. This technique was described as "the lens salute technique" by Dr. Keiki Mehta from Mumbai India (Fig. 5).

3. Once the nucleus is in lens salute position, the surgeon introduces the viscoelastic cannula through the non-dominant hand corneal incision and place viscoelastic between the rear part of the nucleus and the capsular bag, just to protect it from some eventual damage (Fig. 6). Then the cannula is maintained just below the hemiluxated nucleus, with the non dominating hand.

4. Then, the surgeon introduces another viscoelastic cannula through the corneal incision for the dominant hand. It is helpful for the vectorial forces, if this incision is placed somewhere between 120 to 180 degrees away from the non-dominant hand incision (at the opposite meridian). The surgeon introduces viscoelastic material between the nucleus and the corneal endothelium, with the objective to protect intraocular structures and finally place this cannula at the front of the lens in the central portion (Fig. 7).

5. Once the surgeon reaches this position, the work is to capture the nucleus between both instruments. Beware to maintain the cannulas at the iris plane, enough far away from the cornea and from the capsular bag (Fig. 8).

6. Then, with the anterior chamber wide open (full of visco) and with minimum leakage (micro-incisional techniques), the surgeon applies gentle pressure between the two instruments with the nucleus in the middle (Fig. 9); this maneuver produces the first "crack" and then the nucleus is divided in two halves with a prechop technique, outside the capsular bag with the force of only two 25 G cannulas (Fig. 10).

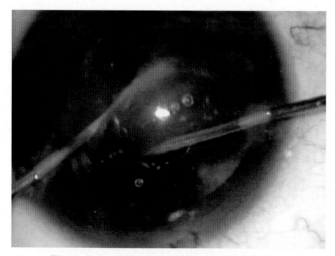

Fig. 1: Bimanual mechanical fracture of the nucleus

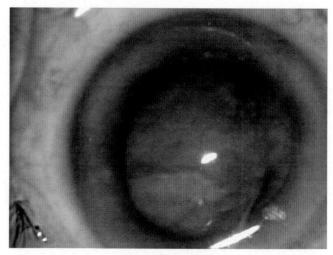

Fig. 4: Hydrosurgery

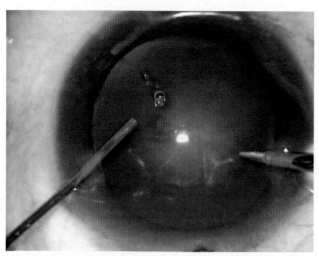

Fig. 2: Wide capsulorhexis being performed

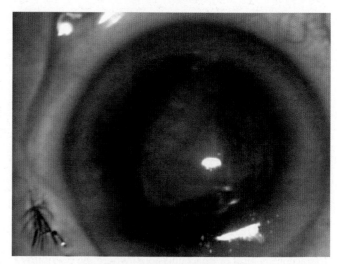

Fig. 5: Nucleus in lens salute position

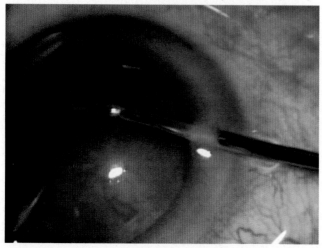

Fig. 3: Creation of wide capsulorhexis

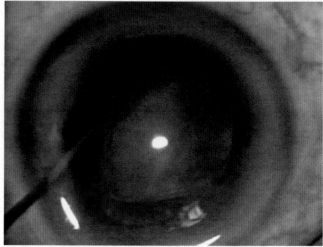

Fig. 6: Introduction of viscoelastic cannula

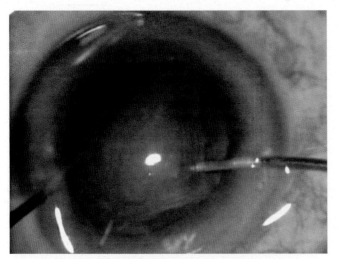

Fig. 7: Placing the cannula at the front of the lens
in the central position

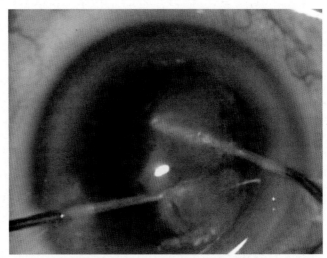

Fig. 10: Nucleus divided into two halves

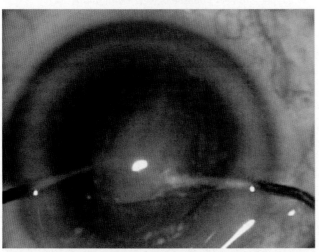

Fig. 8: Cannula in the Iris plane far away
from corneal and capsular bag

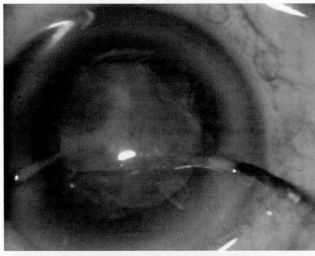

Fig. 11: Nucleus divided into various pieces

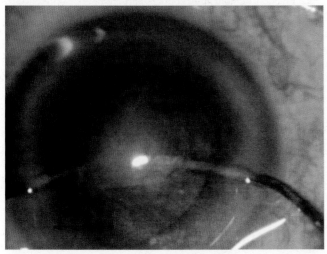

Fig. 9: Surgeon applies gentle pressure between two instruments
with the nucleus in the middle

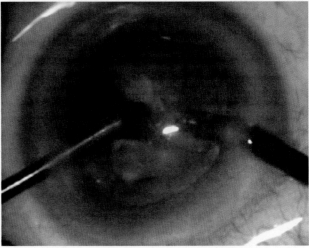

Fig. 12: Phacoemulsification being performed

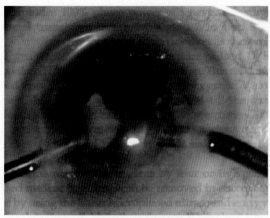

Fig. 13: Phaco of last nuclear piece

7. When possible, more nuclear fragmentations can be made in the same fashion; the surgeon is able to obtain 3, 4 or more nuclear pieces according the applied forces and the advance of the learning curve. As in all the prechop techniques, as much as more pieces are obtained, less ultrasonic time and power will be needed (Fig. 11).

8. Once the nuclear pieces are obtained, the surgeon starts the phacoemulsification process, utilizing intermittent modulation modalities of ultrasonic power, and no more choppers are needed, just a second instrument (preferable an irrigating cannula) to serve as a help for the phacoemulsification (Fig. 12). The surgeon must remember at this time that current phacoemulsification techniques are phacofragmentation techniques, followed by phacoaspiration assisted by ultrasound managed with intermittent power modulations (Fig. 13).

CONCLUSION

We strongly believe that this technique is the latest and master evolution of the bimanual surgery. It combines the Bimanual Irrigation/Aspiration concepts, the art of the Phakonit, the latest evolution of Microphakonit and the "state-of-the-art" of the prechop concepts without any prechopper device, without irrigating chopper and with out stress over the zonula and posterior capsule. Future will tell...
The main advantages of this technique that we find are:
1. It keeps the anterior chamber wide open during the entire procedure.
2. There is no stress over the zonula

3. There is not need of a sharp instrument inside the eye.
4. There is not need to switch many instruments during the entire surgery; when the nuclear fragmentation has been done with the cannulas, there is only a switch to the phaco tip and the aspiration cannula.
5. There´s less incision edema because there is not "inside and out" of many instruments.
6. Less time consuming, situation that can lead benefit for the patient.
7. There is less cost in the use of the viscoelastic cannulas for prechop, in comparison to expensive prechoppers (irrigating and no irrigating) or forceps.

BIBLIOGRAPHY

1. Agarwal A, Agarwal S, Agarwal A. Phakonit : lens removal through a 0.9 mm incision. (letter) J Cataract Refract Surg 2001;27:1531-32.
2. Arturo Perez-Arteaga. Step by Step to Biaxial Lens Surgery. Jaypee Brothers Publishers, New Delhi, India, 2008.
3. Ashok Garg. Biaxial Pre-chop without choppers; chapter by Arturo Pèrez-Arteaga in "Pre-chop techniques". Textbook by Jaypee Publishers, India, 2008.
4. Ashok Garg. Mastering the Phacodynamics (Tools, Technology and Innovations). Chapter 12. Dynamics of Capsulorhexis. Roberto Pinelli, P. Fazio.2007, Jaypee Brothers Medical Publishers. India.
5. Aravind Haripriya, Srinivasan Aravind, Kavitha Vadi, Govindappa Natchiar. Bimanual microphaco for posterior polar cataracts. Journal of Cataract % refractive Surgery June 2006;32(6):914-17.
6. Jorge Alió, José Luis Rodríguez-Prats, Ahmed Galal, Mohamed Ramzy. Outcomes of microincision cataract surgery versus coaxial phacoemulsification. Ophthalmology November 2005:112 (11):1997-2003.
7. Kawai K, Suzuki T, Hayakawa K. The 23 gauge capsulorhexis forceps having a cystotome function. Tokai J Exp Clin Med Apr 2005;30(1):11-3.
8. Packer M., Hoffmann R., Fine H. Refractive lens surgery. Ophthalmology Clinics of North America March 2006; 19(1):77-88.
9. Prechop without pre-choppers and choppers; conference by Arturo Pèrez-Arteaga Chop Techniques Symposium. World Ophtghalmology Congress, at Hong Kong, China, 2008. Chief Instructor, Prof. Ashok Garg.
10. Sabine Kurz, Frank Krummenauer, Pia Gabriel, N. Pfeiffer, H. Burkhard Dick. Biaxial Microincision versus Coaxial Small-Incision Clear Cornea Cataract Surgery. Ophthalmology October 2006;113(10):1818-26.
11. Tsuneoka H, Takuya S, Takahashi Y. Feasibility of ultrasound cataract surgery with a 1.4 mm incision. J Cataract Refract Surg 2001;27:934-40.

Chapter 14

Biaxial Phacoaspiration with 700 micron Technology

Arturo Pérez-Arteaga (Mexico)

INTRODUCTION

In this chapter we will describe how to perform a complete lens extraction avoiding by complete the use of ultrasonic energy and using only vacuum and infusion as the forces to apply inside the eye to complete the entire surgery, with 700 micron technology (Fig. 1).

This technique is useful for many kind of lens extraction procedures with the feature that the nucleus can be soft enough, like congenital cataract, posterior subcapsular cataract, traumatic cataract, posterior polar cataract, intumescent cataract, milky cataract, clear lens extraction and refractive lensectomy procedures between others (Fig. 2). In these cases the surgeon can avoid any kind of ultrasonic power (linear or torsional) and some other technologies for lens fragmentation (e.g. Aqualase, Photolysis), performing so the entire lens extraction using only aspiration of the lens material; irrigating force and vacuum force.

WHY IN BIAXIAL AND NOT IN COAXIAL

There are important differences of biaxial phacoaspiration versus coaxial or micro coaxial phacoaspiration (Fig. 3):

1. We are working in a complete closed environment. No surge at all is occurring.
2. As the irrigation force goes inside there is only one way to go outside, the aspirating cannula; there is not leakage, it means the followability concept.
3. The use of forced infusion and vacuum as operating tools decrease the amount of movements performed by the surgeon inside the eye.
4. Less amount of irrigation is in use in comparison with coaxial and micro coaxial. Even less with 700 micron instrumentation; a complete biaxial phacoaspiration procedure can be performed with this technology utilizing no more than 40 to 50 cc of BSS.
5. Access to all meridians. No problem with subincisional, epinuclear or cortical material, as in coaxial technology.

SURGICAL TECHNIQUE

1. When using smaller diameters -like the 700 micron technology- forced infusion is mandatory (Fig. 1).
2. Be aware of your parameters; if using 700 micron cannulas apply between 90 to 120 cm H_2O of infusion and 400 mm Hg of vacuum. Change your parameters according your skills, instrumentation and learning curve (Fig. 4).
3. Perform your two incisions with the proper knife taking care of the wound architecture. A closed environment is mandatory for the correct work of the "invisible hydrodynamic forces".
4. Perform biaxial microcapsulorhexis (Fig. 5).
5. Perform hydrodissection and hydrodelineation in a bimanual mode; then you are able to feel the real softness of the nucleus and you can help your self to decide if it is a good case for biaxial phacoaspiration (Fig. 6).
6. If the nucleus is too soft it withdraw outside the capsular bag in an easy way and then you are ready to start to aspirate (Fig. 7).
7. If the nucleus is a little harder you might need some biaxial prechop approach. Perform prechop maneuvers with two viscoelastic cannulas (25gauge); one entering the eye through each incision. Better to perform at the iris plane in "lens salute" position. There is no case to perform the prechop maneuvers inside the capsular bag if you can avoid risks with this maneuver (Fig. 8).
8. Once the nucleus has been divided in multiple pieces you are ready to start phacoaspiration (Fig. 9).
9. Enter first the irrigating cannula and then press the foot pedal to start irrigation. If the incisions were made in the correct mode, even your cannula is inside the eye with the irrigation on, a balance of pressures will occur and no leakage at all will happen (Fig. 10).
10. Keeping the irrigation on, introduce the aspiration cannula; the intraocular pressure acts as a counterforce and you can introduce it easily (Fig. 11).
11. Start with a small cleanup of the cortex. Once you can see the nuclear pieces you have fragmented, go for them. So you are sure you are keeping the cushion of the epinuclear material behind it (Fig. 12).
12. Once you are able to see the epinuclear material, go to aspirate it, first at the opposite side of your aspirating cannula and then the rest (Fig. 13).

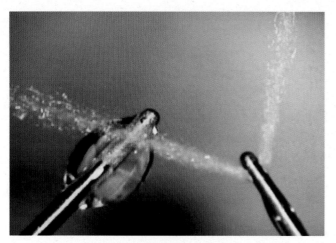

Fig. 1: The 700 micron irrigation-aspiration system

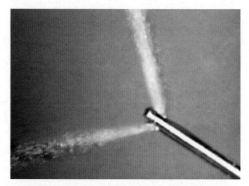

Fig. 4: Forced infusion through a 0.7 double ended cannula

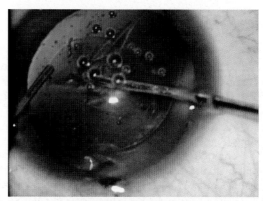

Fig. 5: Biaxial approach to perform capsulorhexis through two 700 micron incisions

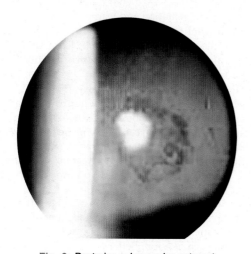

Fig. 2: Posterior subcapsular cataract

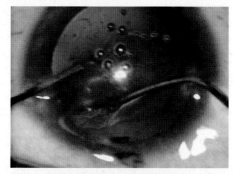

Fig. 6: Biaxial hydrosurgery in a soft nucleus

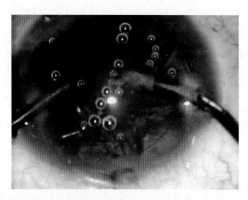

Fig. 3: Advantages of biaxial irrigation-aspiration

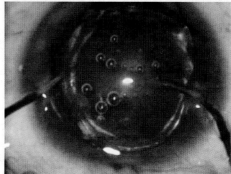

Fig. 7: Hydro-expulsion of the soft nucleus

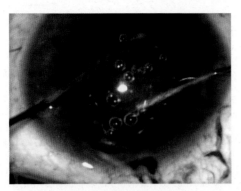

Fig. 8: Biaxial prechop with 25G cannulas in a soft nucleus

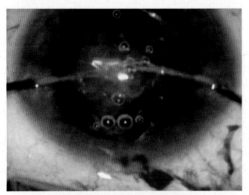

Fig. 9: Nucleus fragmented

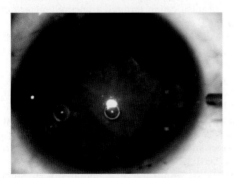

Fig. 10: A 22 gauge irrigating cannula is inside the eye and no
leakage is present

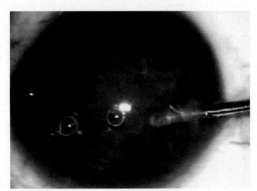

Fig. 11: Both cannulas have been introduced to the anterior chamber

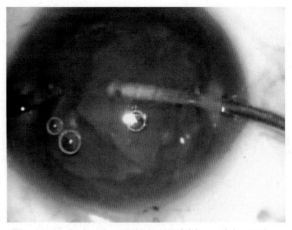

Fig. 12: Aspirating the cortical material front of the nucleus

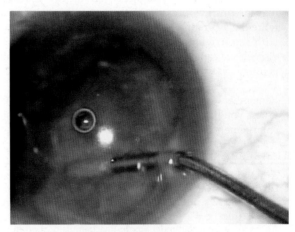

Fig. 13: Aspirating the nucleus

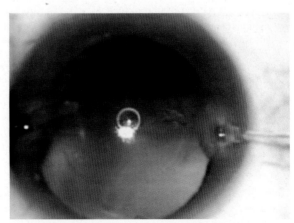

Fig. 14: Keeping the positive IOP with the irrigation

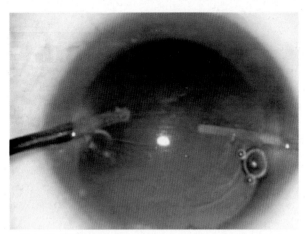

Fig. 15: Distending the anterior chamber with viscoelastic

13. Finish your phacoaspiration process by cleaning the cortical material with the same biaxial approach (Fig. 3).

14. Do not withdraw both cannulas from the eye; remember that the positive pressure is the key in biaxial surgery; retire the aspirating cannula with the irrigation on, keep with the irrigation on while switching and enter the viscoelastic cannula (Fig. 14). Once the anterior chamber is full of visco you can retire the irrigating cannula (Fig. 15).

15. Remember to perform a third incision to implant the IOL, unless you have a kind of IOL that doesn´t need incision enlargement.

BIBLIOGRAPHY

1. Aravind Haripriya, Srinivasan Aravind, Kavitha Vadi, Govindappa Natchiar. Bimanual microphaco for posterior polar cataracts. Journal of Cataract % refractive Surgery 2006;32(6):914-17.

2. Abhay Vasavada, Raminder Singh. Phacoemulsification in eyes with posterior polar cataracts. Journal of Cataract and Refractive Surgery 1999;25(2):238-45.

3. Agarwal A, Agarwal S, Agarwal A. Phakonit : lens removal through a 0.9 mm incision. (letter) J Cataract Refract Surg 2001;27:1531-32.

4. Cavallini GM, Lugli N, Campi L, et al. Surgically induced astigmatism after manual extracapsular cataract extraction or after phacoemulsification procedure. Eur J Ophthalmol 1996; 6:257-63.

5. Chee SP, Ti SE, Sivakumar M, Tan DT. Postoperative inflammation: extracapsular cataract extraction versus phacoemulsification. J Cataract Refract Surg 1999; 25:1280-5.

6. David Plager. Pediatric Cataract Surgery, Techniques Complications, and Management. American Journal of Ophthalmology 2005;140(4):778.

7. Francis PJ, Morris RJ. Post-operative iris prolapse following phacoemulsification and extracapsular cataract surgery.Eye 1997;11(Pt 1):87-90.

8. Girard LJ. Ultrasonic fragmentation for cataract extraction and cataract complications. Adv Ophthalmol 1978.

9. Jagat Ram, Gagandeep S Brar, Sushmita Kaushik, Amit Gupta, Amod Gupta. Role of posterior capsulotomy with vitrectomy and intraocular lens design and material in reducing posterior capsule opacification after pediatric cataract surgery. Journal of Cataract and Refractive Surgery 2003;29(8):1579-84.

10. Linebarger EJ, Hardten DR, Shah GK, Lindstrom RL. Phacoemulsification and modern cataract surgery . Surv Ophthalmol 1999; 44:123-47.

11. Luis Fernández-Vega, José F. Alfonso, Pedro P. Rodríguez, Robert Montés-Micó. Clear Lens extraction with Multifocal Apodized Diffractive Intraocular Lens Implantation. Ophthalmology 2007;114(8):1491-98.

12. Mark G Wood, Gregory SH Ogawa. The challenge of pediatric cataract surgery. Journal of AAPOS 2000;4(5)323.

13. Minassian DC, Rosen P, Dart JK, et al. Extracapsular cataract extraction compared with small incision surgery by phacoemulsification: a randomized trial. Br J Ophthalmol 2001; 85:822-9.

14. Refractive Lens Surgery. Mark Packer, I. Howard Fine, Richard S. Hoffman. Ophthalmology Clinics of North America 2006;19(1):77-88.

15. Shearing SP, Relyea RL, Loaiza A, Shearing RL. Routine phacoemulsification through a one-millimeter non- sutured incision. Cataract 1985; 2(2):6-11.

16. Sleeveless bimanual phaco with Millennium system delivers less thermal energy to the eye. Ocular Surgery News US. Edition April 1, 2003. Rosa Braga-Mele.

17. Trivedi, ME Wilson, RL Golub. Incidence and risk factors for glaucoma after pediatric cataract surgery with and without intraocular lens implantation, 23 August 2006 RH. American Journal of Ophthalmology 2006;142(4):714-15.

18. Tsuneoka H, Takuya S, Takahashi Y. Feasibility of ultrasound cataract surgery with a 1.4 mm incision. J Cataract Refract Surg 2001;27:934-40.

19. Watson A, Sunderraj P. Comparison of small-incision phacoemulsification with standard extracapsular cataract surgery: post-operative astigmatism and visual recovery. Eye 1992 6 (Pt 6):626-9.

20. Wilson ME, Bartholomew LR, TrivediRH. Pediatric cataract surgery and intraocular lens implan-tation: Practice styles and preferences of the 2001 ASCRS and AAPOS memberships. J Cataract Refract Surg 2003;29(9):1811-20.

Chapter 15

Avoiding and Solving the Incomplete Capsulorhexis Cases with Biaxial Techniques

Arturo Pérez-Arteaga (Mexico)

INTRODUCTION

To deal with an incomplete capsulorhexis is a situation affecting every surgeon. Terrible complications can occur if an appropiate management is not done, like vitreous loss, nuclear and epinuclear fragments dislocated to the vitreous, a complete luxation of the nucleus to the vitreous cavity and problems in intraocular lens (IOL) placement that can go from descentration until a complete dislocation. The good management of it will avoid the surgeon to deal with truly complications.

The biaxial approach has many advantages in comparison with the coaxial approach, not only during the routine performance of the microcapsulorhexis, but evenmore, during the management of the surgical complications.

In this chapter we will describe the different degrees of "incomplete capsulorhexis" that can occur and the way to solve them in a biaxial approach and finaly we will be describing some particular variations to the phacoemulsification approach that must be put in practice in these particular cases, pointing the advantages of biaxial phaco over the coaxial style.

Avoiding Complications while Constructing the Microcapsulorhexis

The advantages of perform the capsulorhexis with a Biaxial approach through micro-incisions are as follows (Fig. 1):
1. The incisions are smaller so the anterior chamber remains wide open.
2. The microcapsulorhexis forceps has not the "opening movement" at the incision site.
3. The non-dominant hand is holding the eye through the another incision.
4. It is helpful if the instrument in the non-dominant hand is a viscoelastic cannula, because the surgeon can inject visco.
5. The surgeon can have two angles of attack while performing capsulorhexis.

Now we will describe step by step how to avoid an incomplete capsulorhexis, while performing capsular surgery. Please notice that we are not going to talk about other possible surgical maneuvers and/or devices (e.g. capsular rings, capsular staining).

a. Initial Capsule Puncture. The anterior chamber must be completely full of viscoelastic material; if low IOP exist, a tear can run easily to the periphery. The initial puncture is the correct moment to obtain information regarding the capsule, the zonula and the hardness of the cataract (Fig. 2).

b. "To cut the capsule" micro-biaxial capsulectomy is the technique of choice. It avoids the transmission of forces to the capsular bag and the zonula. Insert a micro-scissors with your dominating hand through the phaco incision, and cut the capsule as much as you can advance in a CCC mode (Fig. 3).

c. Pulling towards your meridian of forceps insertion: if you pull, instead of push, you can control the eye movements with the no dominating hand, holding the eye at the opposite meridian (Fig. 1).

d. Pulling a new capsular tear to the opposite side (Fig. 4.)

e. Performing a new puncture to start in another place (Fig. 5.).

f. Microcapsulectomy to re-direct capsulorhexis (Fig. 6). Because you are working in a biaxial approach you have the facility to use micro-scissors any time you want to give a new direction to the new flap (Fig. 7).

g. Multiple capsulectomies. If you find still some difficulty in controlling the anterior capsule and the possibility of some peripheral tear exist, you can use the micro-scissors to cut the capsule by complete in a round fashion.

h. Multiple capsular punctures or capsular relaxing incisions as the final option, when everything has failed.

Avoiding Complications during Biaxial Phaco with an Incomplete Capsulorhexis

Some years ago, Prof. Keiki Mehta from Mumbai, India, described what he called, "The Lens Salute Technique", that consists in a hemi-luxation of the nucleus to the iris plane, during the hydrodissection and hydrodelineation (Fig. 8). It helps to decrease the transmission of forces to the capsular bag and to the zonula.

The steps to follow to obtain advantage of this technique are:

a. Performing gentle hydrodissection (Fig. 9). The maneuvers of hydrodissection and hydrodelamination should be very similar to those cases of posterior polar cataracts.

b. Searching for an easy "Lens Salute Position" (Fig. 10). The key factor to control your phacoemulsification procedure is to work at the iris plane. You can place your irrigating cannula (or irrigating chopper) behind the nucleus (Fig. 11.), helping with this maneuver to separate planes with the irrigation.

b.1: Perform the "Lens Salute Technique" during the hydroprocedures (Fig. 10.) avoiding rotation of the nucleus during hydrosurgery. The final position that the nucleus reaches with this maneuver is a "tilt" position, (Fig. 8).

b.2: Also it is possible"to pull the nucleus with vacuum" (Fig. 12). Start the irrigation and embded the phaco needle with a small amount of ultrasonic power inside the center of the nucleus (Fig. 13B) and pull the unit phaco needle-nucleus outside the capsular bag, in a maneuver (Fig. 12). Once your irrigating device is behind the nucleus, keep holding it with vacuum, do not miss it, and simply move your irrigating device to cut the nucleus (Fig. 13A)–sustained with vacuum at the iris plane- from the rear to the front; you will obtain a nice division in two halves at the iris plane (Fig. 14).

c. Biaxial I/A. After switching instrumentation, Biaxial I/A is performed in the usual fashion.

d. Biaxial anterior vitrectomy if needed. If you have not ready your vitrector, or if you want to have a complete visualization of the intraocular structures without a hurry, before withdraw the irrigating device, switch from your aspirating cannula to a viscoelastic syringe using your dominant hand, and inject visco before retiring the irrigating cannula. Once you are sure that the eye has been filled by compete and you have enough positive pressure, stop irrigation and retire the irrigating cannula.

CONCLUSIONS

Many advantages have been observed when performing biaxial lens surgery in cases of complicated capsular management. These advantages can be noticed since the first maneuvers when you start to feel the capsular tissue and the maneuvers that can be performed in order to avoid entering to a more complicated case. But furthermore, these advantages go along the case during the management of the chop maneuvers, phacoemulsification, I/A and biaxial anterior vitrectomy when needed. It is completely true that MICS is not a matter of incision size, is a matter of management of new tools, new maneuvers, new forces, new fluidics inside the eye, that helps the surgeon to decrease the possible complications of cataract surgery, but

furthermore, of great value in solving complex and challenging cases like the presented in this chapter.

BIBLIOGRAPHY

1. Ahmed Sallam, Hooman Sherafat. Intraocular lens implantation in cases with anterior capsule tears extending to the posterior capsule. Journal of Cataract & Refractive Surgery. June 2007 (Vol. 33, Issue 6, Pages 938-939).

2. Anterior lens capsule management in pediatric cataract surgery.Wilson ME. Trans Am Ophthalmol Soc. 2004 (Vol. 102, Pages 391-422).

3. Arturo Perez-Arteaga. Step by Step to Biaxial Lens Surgery. Jaypee Brothers Medical Publishers, New Delhi, India, 2008.

4. Assia EI, Apple DJ, Barden A, Tsai JC, Castaneda VE, Hoggatt JS. An experimental study comparing various anterior capsulectomy techniques. Arch Ophthalmol. May 1991 (Vol. 109, Issue 5, Pages 642-7).

5. Assia EI, Apple DJ, Tsai JC, Morgan RC. Mechanism of radial tear formation after anterior capsulectomy. Ophthalmology, 1991; 98: 432-37.

6. Capsule Staining as an Adjunt to Cataract Surgery: A report from the American Academy of Ophthalmology.Deborah S. Jacobs, Terry A. Cox, Michael D. Wagoner, Reginald G. Ariyasu, Carol L. Karp. Ophthal-mology..April 2006 (Vol. 113, Issue 4, Pages 707-13.

7. D Wasserman, DJ Apple, VE Castaneda, JC Tsai, RC Morgan, EI Assia. Anterior capsular tears and loop fixation of posterior chamber intraocular lenses. Ophthalmology 1 April 1991 (Vol. 98, Issue 4, Pages 425-431).

8. Effect of Optic Material and Haptic Design on Anterior Capsule Opacification and Capsulorhexis Contraction.Stefan Sacu, Rupert Menapace, Oliver Findl. American Journal of Ophthalmology.March 2006 (Vol. 141, Issue 3, Pages 488-93.

9. Fate of anterior capsular tears during cataract surgery. Marques FF, Marques DM, Osher RH, Osher JM. Journal of Cataract & Refractive Surgery 2006 (Vol. 32, Issue 10, Pages 1638-42).

10. Fishkind WJ. Intraoperative management of capsular tears in phacoemulsification and intraocular lens implantation. Discussion paper by Gimbel HV, Sun R. Ferensowics M. Ophthalmology. 2001;108;2190-92.

11. Gimbel HV, Sun R, Ferensowicz M, Anderson Penno E, Kamal A. Intraoperative management of posterior capsule tears in phacoemulsification and intraocular lens implantation. Ophthalmology. Dec 2001 (Vol. 108, Issue 12, Pages 2186-9; discussion 2190-2).

12. Gimbel HV, Teuhann T. Development, advantages and methods of continuous curvilinear capsulorhexis technique. Journal of Cataract & refractive Surgery. 1990; 16: 31-37.

13. Hamada S, Low S, Walters BC, Nischal KK. Five-year experience of the 2.incision push-pull technique for anterior and posterior capsulorhexis in pediatric cataract surgery. Ophthalmology.Aug 2006 (Vol. 113, Issue 8, Pages 1309-14).

14. Hettlich HJ, El-Hifnawi ES. Scanning electron microssopy studies of he human lens after capsulorhexis. Ophthalmologe 1997;(Vol. 94, Issue 4, Pages 300-2).

15. Intraoperative Floppy Iris Syndrome. Mahiul M.K. Muqit, Mitch J. Menage. Ophthalmology.October 2006 (Vol. 113, Issue 10, Pages 1885-86.

16. Kawai K, Suzuki T, Hayakawa K. Tokai. The 23 gauge capsulorhexis forceps having a cystotome function. J Exp Clin Med. Apr 2005 (Vol. 30, Issue 1, Pages 11-3).

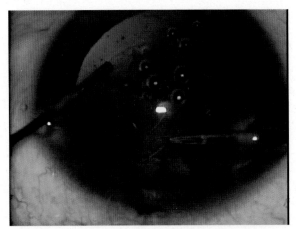

Fig. 1: Advantages of capsulorhexis performance in a biaxial fashion

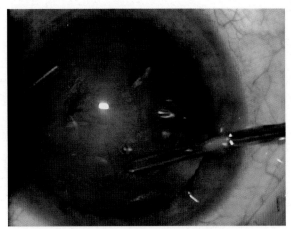

Fig. 4: Performing CCC in the opposite direction

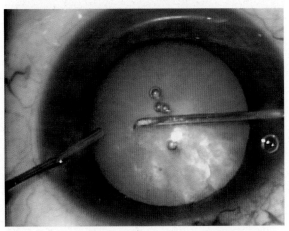

Fig. 2: Initial capsular puncture in a biaxial approach

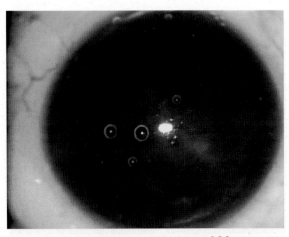

Fig. 5: Two differents points of start CCC were done in the anterior capsule

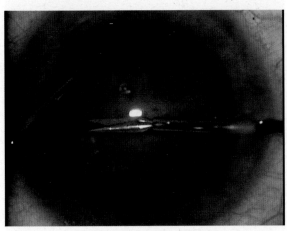

Fig. 3: Biaxial capsulectomy

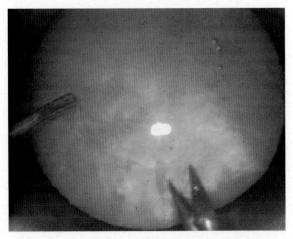

Fig. 6: Using micro-scissors to save the rhexis

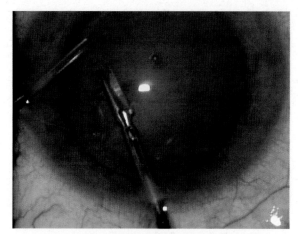

Fig. 7: Micro-scissors entering at a new angle to give direction to the capsular tear

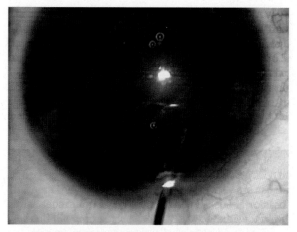

Fig. 10: Placing the nucleus in lens salute position

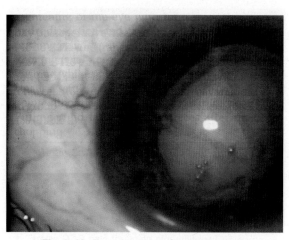

Fig. 8: Nucleus placed in lens salute position

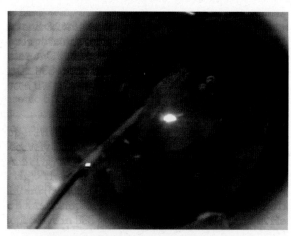

Fig. 11: Hydrodissection behind the nucleus

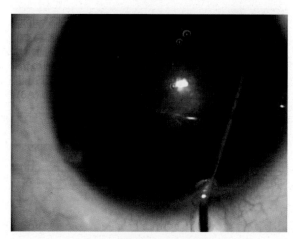

Fig. 9: Gentle hydrosurgery

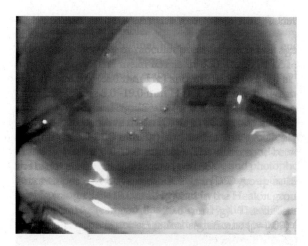

Fig. 12: Pulling the nucleus with vacuum

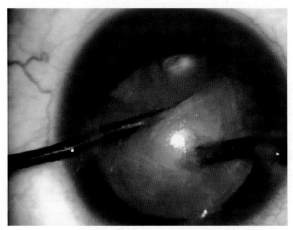

Fig. 13A: Biaxial prechop with vacuum

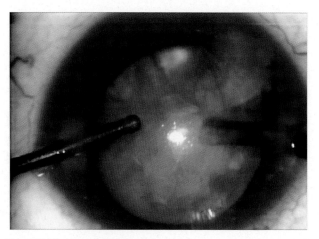

Fig. 13B: Small amount of US power to penetrate the nucleus with the phaco needle

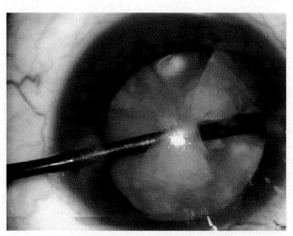

Fig. 14: Biaxial prechop completed

17. Kawai K. Comparison of 23 gauge and 25 gauge anterior capsulotomy forceps. Tokai J Exp Clin Med. Sep 2004 (Vol. 29, Issue 3, Pages 105-10).

18. Kwartz J. Implantation of foldable intraocular lenses in the presence of anterior capsular tears. Eye.1996 (Vol. 10 (Pt 4), Pages 529-30)

19. Mastering the Phacodynamics (Tools, Technology and Innovations). Ashok Garg. Chapter 12. Dinamics of Capsulorhexis. Roberto Pinelli, P. Fazio.2007, Jaypee Brothers Medical Publishers. India.

20. Navneet Brar, Sandra Lora Cremers. Assesing surgery skills. Ophthalmology. August 2007 (Vol. 114, Issue 8, Pages 1587-87).

21. Oner FH, Durak I, Soylev M, Ergin M. Long term results of various anterior capsulotomies and radial tears on intraocular lens centration. Ophthalmic Surg Lasers (Vol. 32, Issue 2, Pages 118-23).

22. Outcomes of Microincision Cataract Surgery versus Coaxial Phacoemulsification. Jorge Alió, José Luis Rodríguez-Prats, Ahmed Galal, Mohamed Ramzy. Ophthalmology. November 2005 (Vol. 112, Issue 11, Pages 1997-2003.

23. Packer M, Hoffmann R, Fine H. Refractive lens surgery. Ophthalmology Clinics of North America. March 2006 (Vol. 19, Issue 1, Pages 77-88).

24. Reply: Intraocular lens implantation in cases with anterior capsule tears extending to the posterior capsule. Osher RH. Journal of Cataract & Refractive Surgery. Jun 2007 (Vol. 33, Issue 6, Pages 939-40).

25. Sabine Kurz, Frank Krummenauer, Pia Gabriel, N. Pfeiffer, H. Burkhard Dick. Biaxial microincision versus coaxial small-incision clear cornea cataract surgery. Ophthalmology. October 2006 (Vol. 113, Issue 10, Pages 1818-1826.

26. Sallam A, Sherafat H. Intraocular lens implantation in cases with anterior capsule tears extending to he posterior capsule. Journal of Cataract & Refractive Surgery. Jun 2007 (Vol. 33, Issue 6, Pages 938-9; author reply 939.40)

27. Vajpayee RB, Sharma N, Dada T, Gupta V, Kumar A, Dada VK. Management of posterior capsule tears. Surv Ophthalmol.(Vol. 45, Issue 6, Pages 473-88).

28. VE Castaneda, UF Legler, JC Tsai, JP Hoggatt, EI Assia, C Hogan, DJ Apple. Posterior continuos curvilinear capsulorhexis. An experimental study with clinical applications. Ophthalmology.1 January 1992 (Vol. 99, Issue 1, Pages 45-50).

Chapter 16

How to Perform Biaxial MICS Step by Step ?

Gilles Lesieur (France)

- Microincision cataract surgery (MICS) with biaxial approach is not yet widely adopted.
- This technique can offer less traumatism and less complications with a faster visual recovery for the patient.
- A new phacoemulsification system brings an optimization of fluidics during microincision cataract surgery.
- A wireless pedal, with blue tooth technology, optimises the space used in the operating room.

This phaco system comprises 3 others elements:
- The computer is based on an algorithm used in both aviation and also in food processing industries. It allows regulation of vacuum settings 250 times per second.
- The VFM module for vacuum fluidic module including a vacuum new cassette, pinch valves and vacuum sensor.
- The compressor module with the new vacuum pump and the compressor.
- The main goal is to preserve a good fluidic balance that is a positive pressure in the eye.
- BSS infusion provides irrigation flow.
- Aspiration through phaco needle provides aspiration flow.
- The wireless Bluetooth pedal controls the user interface. The bottle height setting is programmed in the computer via the screen interface provoking irrigation flow to the eye.
- In the same way, the vacuum setting is programmed on the computer via a screen interface and then information is transferred to the couple "pump & servo valve".
- The major improvement is the new vacuum pump. Its role is to generate a depression inside the cassette and therefore aspiration flow.
- The vacuum can reach a maximum of 600 mm Hg and vacuum rise speed can be adjusted according to surgeon preference.
- A vacuum sensor measures 250 times per second the supplied real value. Algorithm will analyse these datas. This active feedback loop is able to adjust in real time the exact vacuum value expected by surgeon.
- And finally, the compressor creates a reserve of air available at any time during the surgery. Its main role is to activate pneumatic pinch used to control aspiration, irrigation, venting, reflux and the vitrectomy cutter.
- The venting is an automatic procedure that creates some positive pressure inside the aspiration tubing to avoid surge effect.
- The reflux is the same process but it is voluntary activated by the surgeon with the pedal.
- During a test with a flexible balloon fixed on aspiration tubing, we can simulate the strong aspiration flow provoked by occlusion break. At that precise moment, venting role is crucial because it will automatically compensate in a way to keep fluidic balance and so anterior chamber stable.
- This test also shows that tubing must have low compliance power to avoid distension under internal pressure.
- Moreover, a flow reducer of 10 cm has been associated to the aspiration tubing. Internal diameter between the entry and the exit is reduced by 50%. Big nucleus fragments are retained by the filter. BSS can pass through without any resistance.
- With this new technology, aspiration tubing cannot be clogged. This also avoids instability of anterior chamber.
- This phacoemulsification system has an overboost function. It allows to use higher vacuum settings when necessary at any time during the surgery.
- Chop technique is then easier thanks to a better nucleus gripping ability.
- From the side view, we can judge the excellent efficiency in term of mobilization and followability of crystalline lens fragments as well as perfect anterior chamber stability especially with high vacuum levels.
- In my daily practice, I work with a high vacuum setting of 420 mm Hg and 500 mm Hg with overboost for chop phase. On the inverse way, ultrasound power is very low: only 15%
- Others elements also have a key role in fluidics. Lot of care must be taken with incisions. They must be performed with an appropriately shaped knife (MicroCut PhysIOL) to preserve the wound architecture. Introducing the phaco probe vertically will avoid descemetic and stromal tears.

- The instruments, such as the irrigating chopper must provide an irrigation flow sufficient enough to also vary according to bottle height.
- As we can notice, with a 20G irrigation cannula (Lesieur Hydrochopper Katena) and a different bottle height, we obtain the following irrigation flow:
  - 80 cm-38 cc/mn
  - 90 cm-42 cc/mn
  - 100 cm-44 cc/mn
  - 110 cm-48 cc/mn
  - 120 cm-50 cc/mn
  - 130 cm-52 cc/mn
  - 140 cm-56 cc/mn
- The first goal of all these technical evolutions is to improve our surgical results.
- Indeed, even if various publications proved the negative role of the high amount of ultrasound emission, what about too much irrigation flow washing endothelial cells.

- We realize a study about 100 patients undergoing biaxial cataract surgery.
- Average ECC Preop 2328 cc/mm^2
- Average ECC Postop 2182 cc/ mm^2
- 6.28% endothelial cells loss
- Preop pachymetry and at 1 day and 1 month
- Pachy Preop 518 µm
- Pachy D1 557µm average edema 8.3%
- EPT meaning effective phaco time
- Average EPT 0.8s
- And BSS quantity
- BSS volume average 26,96 cc
- 12 moderate corneal edemas postoperative (including 30% Guttata cornea) resolved following days. The most important endothelial cell loss concerned a case where EPT was over 1s and BSS volume > 50 cc.
- The right phaco machine settings will allow you to obtain efficiency, stability and precision in any simplicity for the safety and faster visual recovery of your patients.

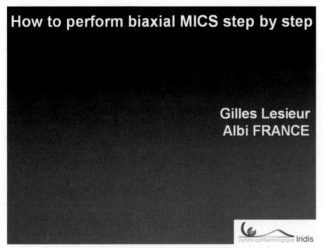

Fig. 1: How to perform biaxial MICS step by step

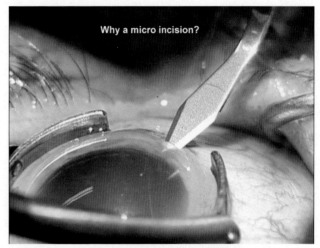

Fig. 2: Why a micro incision?

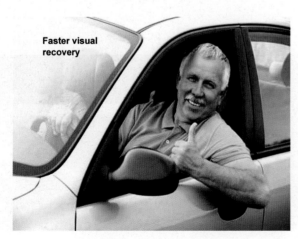

Fig. 3: Faster visual recovery

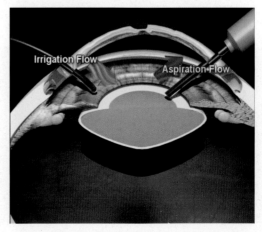

Fig. 4: Goal of biaxial: to preserve positive pressure inside the eye

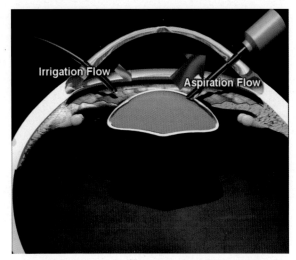

Fig. 5: Too much aspiration = capsular bag rising

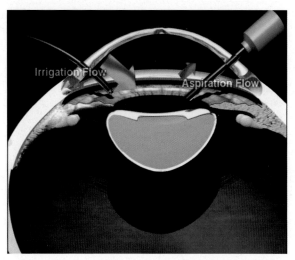

Fig. 6: Too much irrigation = capsular bag pushed down

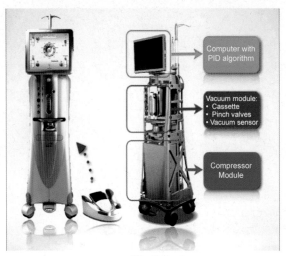

Fig. 7

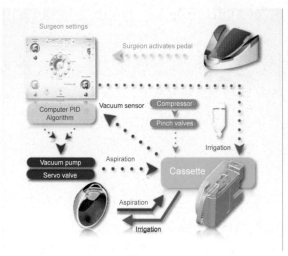

Fig. 8

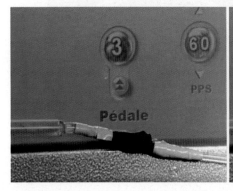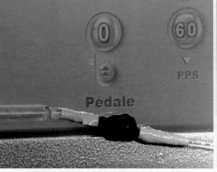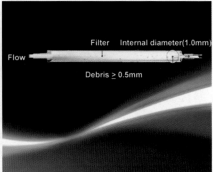

Fig. 9: Anterior chamber stability

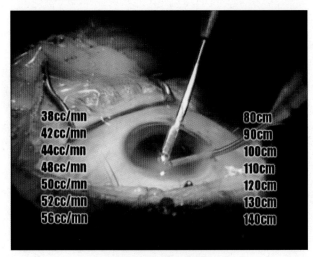

Fig. 10: Infusion height

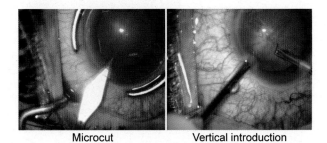

Microcut   Vertical introduction

Fig. 11: Surgery incision

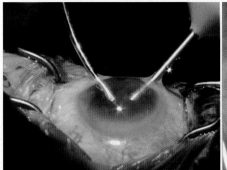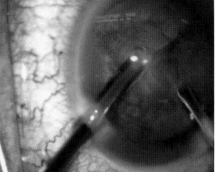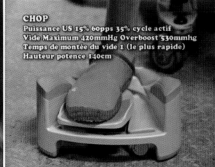

Fig. 12: Surgery

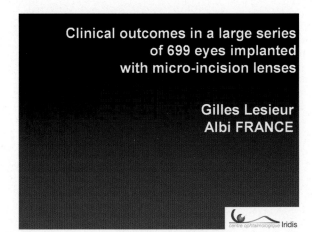

Fig. 13: Clinical outcomes in a large series of 699 eyes implanted
with micro-incision lenses

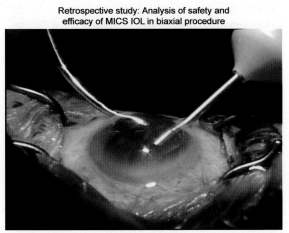

Fig. 14: Purpose

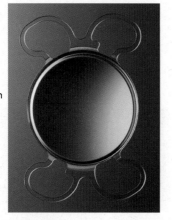

Modern standard
• 25% hydrophilic acrylic
• Optical zone: 6.15mm
• Total diameter: 10.75 mm
• 360° Square edge
• Haptic thickness: 300 μm
• Features at 1-7 o'clock
• +10 to + 30 by 0.5D
• IOlmaster 118.9

Fig. 15: MicroSlim

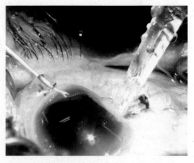

• Medicel injector 1.8 mm
• 450 pateints: 262 F 188 M
• 656 eyes: 315 OD 341 OS
• Mean age: 70.52 years (3895)
• Mean preop VA: 5.28/10
• Postop Va: 8087/10(ARMD
  included)
• Mean SE: 0.052(-2.45 to +1.96)
• Mean follow-up: 248.44 days
  (8-609)

Fig. 16: MicroSlim

• Same desing and material as Microslim
• Blue - light filtration: Blue Tech ® (0.05% polymerized yellow
  chromophore) balancing photo - protection and quality of vision

• Macular edema 0.30%
  - 1 with ERM 6/10 - Final VA 8/10
  - 1 normal macula 6/10 - Fianal VA 10/10
• Yag capsulotomy 1.22%
  - 8/656 implantations
  - Time to Yag: 10 month (127 to 465 days)
  - Preop VA: 95/10 (8 to 10/10)

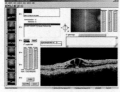

Fig. 17: MicroSlim

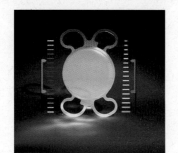

Fig. 18: Micro Ay

• Same design and material as MicroSlim
• Aspheric optic moderate level of negative SA (-0.11μ) to
  preserve the natural positive balance of the eye for
  providing depth of field and contrast sensitivity

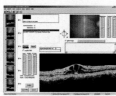

Fig. 19: Micro Ay

• Same design and material as MicroSlim
• More compressible
• Thickness reduction:2.25%

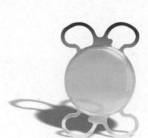

Fig. 20: Micro Ay

- Medicel Injector 1.8
- 36 patients: 16 F 20 OS
- 43 eyes: 23 OD 20 M
- Mean age: 75.54 years (42-95)
- Mean power:21.62D (18-23.5)
- Mean preop VA:4.93/10
- Postop VA: 87/10 (ARMD inculded)
- Mean follow - up: 55.25 days (8-89)

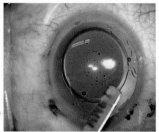

Fig. 21: Micro Ay

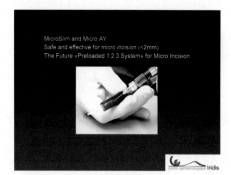

Fig. 22

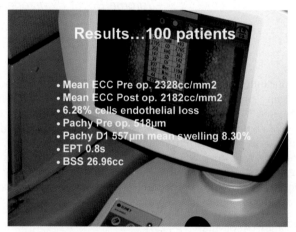

Fig. 23

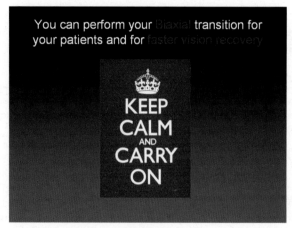

Fig. 24

Chapter 17

BiMICS versus CoMICS Our Actual Technique (Bimanual Micro-Cataract Surgery versus Coaxial Micro-Cataract Surgery)

Jerome Bovet (Switzerland)

INTRODUCTION

These two surgical techniques are not in conflict, but result from the common goal to better control and reduce the induced astigmatism during cataract surgery[12] (Fig. 1).

The 3 mm [4,14] incision has already become obsolete, just as the 12 mm and thereafter the 6 mm incisions did.

The reduction of the size of cataract incisions will self establish itself by reducing induced astigmatism thus bringing it better under the control[9] of the surgeon. It opens the road to refractive lens surgery (as an application of bioptics to cataract surgery) with the association of phacoemulsification and IOL with LASIK during presbysurgery.

HISTORICAL BACKGROUND

Biaxial and coaxial microincision cataract surgery are complementary as Olson[16] says and are likely to dominate lens surgical techniques in the very near future.

BiMICS (FIG. 2)

Introduction

BiMICS,[6,13] (Bimanual Micro Incision Cataract Surgery) is a surgical technique performed through two micro incisions, one for irrigation and the other one for aspiration, of a reduced size, usually under 1 mm.

Material (Fig. 3)

The material for BiMICS presents only slight changes in regards to conventional phaco. However particular attention will have to be paid to the microphacodynamics, as well as to the incisions, which have to be chosen and tested meticulously.

Microphacodynamics[3,5,8] (Fig. 4)

The incoming flow should be superior to the outgoing flow and with regards to the law of Poiseuille it is possible to increase significantly the flow without modifying notably the intraocular pressure by using only slightly increased internal tubing diameter.

The choice of the irrigation instrument is very important in order to adapt the fluidic dynamics: the internal diameter of the irrigation tube must be of a superior gauge than the gauge of the internal diameter of the aspiration tube, in order to compensate for fluid losses, diminish intraocular pressure and to avoid instabilities of the anterior chamber.

Irrigation- Aspiration[10] (Fig. 5)

In bimanual phaco, if you use an aspiration instrument with an internal diameter of 20 G, you should use an irrigation instrument with an internal diameter of 19G.[5] If you use an aspiration instrument with an internal diameter of 21 G,[16, 17] then you will use with advantage an irrigation instrument with an internal diameter of 20 G.

This compensates for surge and to reduce intraocular pressure as well.

Actually the instruments for irrigation and aspiration DUET MST for Micro Surgical Technology (MST) offer the optimal relationship between the internal and external diameters of these instruments.

If you use the BIMIC technique you have to use the irrigator manipulator with the irrigation at the head of the instrument to avoid a surge when you go back with the manipulator.

Phacotips

The phacotips usually are equipped with an external diameter of 21 G (0.9 mm); it is important to control the internal diameter in order to avoid surge. The tip is straight with a 30¡ bevel.

Capsulorhexis (Fig. 6)

The needle is the simplest way to create a capsulorhexis through a micro incision; it is easily done under the protection of a

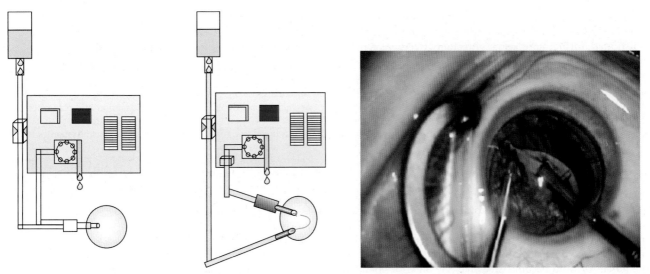

Fig. 1: Set up CoMICS versus BiMICS

Fig. 2: BiMICS technique

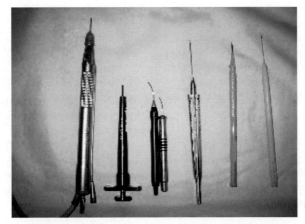

Fig. 3: Material for the bimanual phaco technique

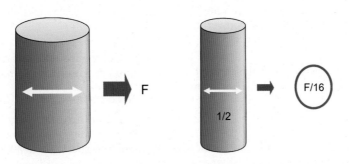

Fig. 4: Law from Poiseuille-Hagen relationship between flow and diameter

viscoelastic gel like methylcellulose, which has a reduced cost. The micro instrument for capsulorhexis is quite a bit more sophisticated; furthermore, using vitrectomy tweezers is not a simple task either.

Capsulorhexis tweezers should have a smaller diameter than the incision, the bytes being able to open without a movement of the body of the instrument; also, it should have a double curvature, in order to allow picking up the edges of the rhexis in vicinity to the corneal incision. Capsulorhexis tweezers from Zeiss Jena[15] fulfill these requirements.

Blades

The straight blades allow a cleaner incision than the triangular blades. There are multiple trapezoidal sizes of blades from allowing to perform the desired incision; it is effectively important to remember that the tolerance of variation in incision sizes is much more sensitive with BiMICS. If the incision is too large, losses of fluid become excessive, the anterior chamber presents instabilities, and recurrent iris herniation may be encountered. If the incision is too small, not infrequently corneal burns and Descemet folds may occur.

The Phaco Machines

Starting with the newest generation phaco machines will considerably simplify the transition to microincision cataract surgery. The recent phaco machines should allow sufficient aspiration flow rate, since the smaller the diameter, the greater the aspiration flow rate to be applied to obtain adequate suction.

Another advantage of last generation phaco machines is to facilitate the control of heat production by the phaco tip at the level of the incision.

Phaco Pumps

The newer phaco pumps associate a peristaltic to a venture pump. They allow for more adaptability to start with, and more efficacies in the presence of hard nuclei. They are also equipped with systems, which enable a considerably better stabilization of the anterior chamber.

Ultrasound Power Delivery

The most recent machines have notably reduced thermal energy due to power modulation that includes pulses and bursts with microsecond duration. However, even with the old phaco machines, it is possible to reduce the thermal energy using the foot pedal during short interval reducing the phacopowertime.

Implant insertion[11] (Fig. 7)

Rather than widening one of the microincision which most of time induce a Seidel. We make a third incision between them to inject the lens.

Astigmatism

This technique allows a total neutralization of induced astigmatism, the microincisions leaving the original astigmatism unchanged if needed.

Table 1: Advantages/disadvantages of BiMICS	
Advantages BiMICS	Disadvantages BiMICS
• Two micro incisions down to 0.9 mm in width	• Steep learning curve
• Injection of an IOL through an incision below 2.2 mm wide	• Precise setting of the parameters for irrigation and aspiration flow mandatory
• No induced astigmatism, which allows a precise control of astigmatism	• Sensitive phacodynamics
• Separated irrigation flow allowing minimum turbulence during aspiration	• Specific instrumentation required
• Most appropriate technique for small pupils or in the case of a floppy iris syndrome	

Table 1A: Advantages/disadvantages of BiMICS	
Advantages BiMICS	Disadvantages BiMICS
• New instruments	• Possible to adjust the incision for the astigmatism
• Change the phacotips	
• Change the parameters	• Injection of the lens through 1.5 mm
• Surge if we don't use the right parameters	• Easy to work to 0,9 mm
• Wound not stable and burn	

Coaxial Microincision Cataract Surgery[12,15,18]

CoMICS surgical technique was developed after BiMICS surgical technique to avoid the learning curve and the difficulties encounter with the BiMICS technique.

CoMICS was the perfect choice for the injection of a lens at 2.2 mm incision width without changing much of your conventionnal phacotechnique.

At that size they have no risk of inducing anterior instability, as well as corneal heating.

CoMICS surgery do not need to change all your instruments set and it is cheaper.

Capsulorhexis

Most of the fine capsulorhexis tweezers can be used through a 2.2 mm incision. Below that size, it becomes necessary to use a capsulorhexis tweezers with distal activation.

Phacotips

2 sizes of phacotips with external diameter sizes of 0.9 to 1.1 mm are used, with an angulation of 30° or 45°.

The Phaco Machines (Fig. 11)

The level of the irrigation bottle should be between 80 cm and 100 cm. The flow of aspiration used is 25 cc/minute. The aspiration pressure is set at 400 mm Hg. It is imperative to set the irrigation bottle sufficiently high in order to avoid corneal burns by the phacotip.

BiMiCS 20G
1.2 mm
incision

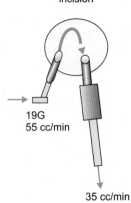

20G
35 cc/min

35 cc/min

Irrigating needle
20G = 0.88 mm
titanium phacotip
0.9 mm

BiMiCS 19G
1.2 mm
incision

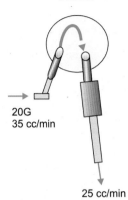

19G
55 cc/min

35 cc/min

Irrigating needle
19G = 1.06 mm
titanium phacotip
0.9 mm

Microphaconit
0.9 mm
incision

20G
35 cc/min

25 cc/min

Irrigating needle
20G = 0.88 mm
titanium phacotip
0.7 mm

Fig. 5: Microphacodynamics BiMICS

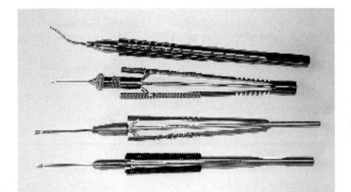

Fig. 6: Capsulorhexis forceps

• 1 Paracentesis for irrigation
• 1 Paracentesis for Phacoemulsification
• 1 incision for injection the lens

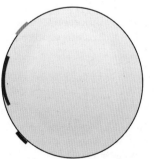

Fig. 8: BiMICS incision

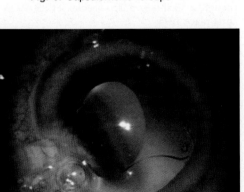

Fig. 7: Insertion of an Acri Smart 36 A
the cartridge stay outside

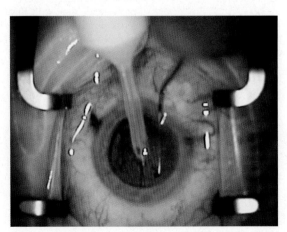

Fig. 9: CoMICS technique

103

The Pumps

It is easier to use a machine combining peristaltic and venturi pumps.

Ultrasound Delivery

Any phaco machine can be used with CoMICS.

Irrigation- Aspiration

The aspiration instrument should be replaced by a 2.2 mm diameter instrument when using a bimanual irrigation aspiration system to maintain water tightness so that the anterior chamber remains stable.

Incision-assisted Implantation (Fig.12)

Most IOLs can be injected through a 2.2 mm incision by applying the injector directly against the incision with a certain pressure and then ejecting with force the plate or monobloc IOL into the tunnel and the anterior chamber.

CONCLUSION

The BiMICS and CoMICS techniques are two complimentary methods of practical phacoemulsification practised nowadays by surgeons. As we have already seen, each method has its advantages and its disadvantages. We will outline here the most important differences that enable a surgeon to choose between one method and another.

It is easier to pass from the classic emulsification technique to the CoMICS technique as one only needs to change the

parameters of the machine being used. The learning curve in the CoMICS technique is simpler than that used in the BiMICS technique. Bad management in the handling of the inlet and outlet of the BiMICS technique can lead to instability in the anterior chamber.

The BiMICS method allows a wider margin for maneuver in management of the inlet and outlet as well as in the handling of the instruments. Any complications experienced during the operation are easier to manage using the BiMICS technique.

These two differences can help the surgeon to choose one surgical technique over another.

If we now consider the technical results for the patient, it is important to note the two following points:

The current method of incision by the CoMICS, with a minimum length of 1.6 mm, cannot be reduced due to the inlet and outlet. The incision is the same for phacoemulsification as for the injection as it is difficult to position it more precisely in the periphery – this can lead to astigmatism.

The BiMICS method allows reduction of the irrigation inlet and outlet up to 0.7 mm. The incision for the implant injection can be carried out in the second stage. This allows the incision to be the exact size of the implant. It also allows a more precise positioning of the incision in relation to the patient's pre-operative astigmatism.

The toric implants already present an important improvement and the only real technique for fine correction of astigmatism.

BiMICS will be, therefore, the method of the future for allowing neutrality of astigmatism.

This means to say that it is the better possibility for implanting aspheric or multifocal lenses.

Table 2: Advantages/disadvantages of CoMICS	
Advantages CoMICS	*Disadvantages CoMICS*
• No learning curve	• The incision's width is limited to 1.6 mm, because of the phacodynamics
• Increased water tightness of the incision	• Management of posterior capsular rupture is more problematic than with BiMICS
• The setting for the phacomachine is comparable to the 3 mm incision technique	• Small pupils are more delicate to deal with than with BiMICS
• IOLs and injectors are well-adapted to a 2.2 mm incision	

Table 2A: Advantages/disadvantages of CoMICS	
Advantages CoMICS	*Disadvantages CoMICS*
• Nothing to change • Change the phacotips • Change the parameters • Easy to work to 2.2 mm • Easy to inject a lens to a 2.2 mm	• Not possible to adjust the incision for the astigmatism • Not possible to go below 1.6 mm without any surge

REFERENCES

1. Agarwal A, Agarwal A, Agarwal S, Narang P, Narang S. Phakonit: phacoemulsification through a 0.9 mm corneal incision. J Cataract Refract Surg 2001;27:1548-52.
2. Agarwal A, Agarwal S, Agarwal A. Phakonit with an AcriTec IOL. J Cataract Refract Surg 2003;29:854-55.
3. Barret G. Maxi-flow phaco needle ASCRS-ASOA Film festival first place 1995.
4. Bovet J J, Baumgartner JM, Bruckner JC, Ilic V, Paccolat F, Maroni O, Bovet F. Chirurgie de la cataracte en topique intracamŽrulaire. Abstract SSO-SOG.sept 1997.
5. Bovet J. 19 G Bimanual MicroPhaco ASCRS-ASOA abstract March 17-22, 2006.
6. Bovet J. Achard O, Baumgartner JM. Chiou A. de Courten, C Rabineau P. Bimanual Phaco Trick and Track ASCRS-ASOA Film San Diego.
7. Bovet J, Achard O, Baumgartner JM. Chiou A de Courten, C Rabineau P. 0.9 mm Incision Bimanual Phaco and IOL Insertion Through a 1,7 mm Incision. Symposium on cataract,IOL and refractive surgery abst ASCRS-ASOA San Francisco April 12-16, 2003.
8. Bovet J. Phacodynamics: Bimanual microphaco, in Mastering the phacodynamics (Tools, Technology and Innovations) Ashok Garg, I Howard Fine, Jorge L Alio, David F ChangŽ, Keiki R Mahta, JŽr™me J Bovet, Hiroshi Tsuneoka, Cyres K Mehta Jaypee Brothers, 2007.

- 2 Paracentesis 20G for injection, phacochops manipulation irrigation aspiration
- 1 Incision for phacoemulsification and injection the lens

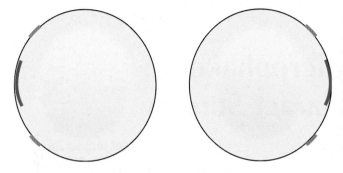

Fig. 10: CoMICS incision

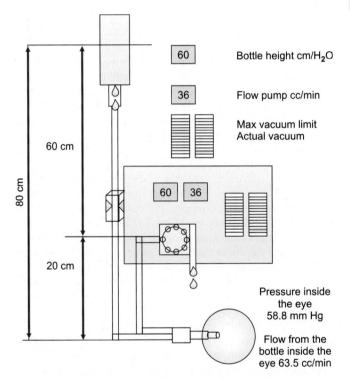

Fig. 11: Real pressure and flow inside the eye coaxial phaco

60 — Bottle height cm/H$_2$O

36 — Flow pump cc/min

Max vacuum limit
Actual vacuum

60 cm

80 cm

60 36

20 cm

Pressure inside the eye 58.8 mm Hg

Flow from the bottle inside the eye 63.5 cc/min

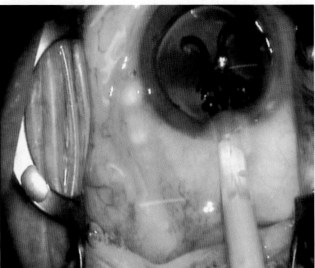

Fig. 12: IOL insertion on a 2.2 mm incision CoMICS technique

9. Bovet J. Break the Phaco Barrier. in Mastering the Phacodynamics (Tools, Technology and Innovations) Ashok Garg, I Howard Fine, Jorge L Alio, David F Chang, Keiki R Mehta, JŽr™me J Bovet, Hiroshi Tsuneoka, Cyres K Mehta Jaypee Brothers, 2007.

10. Brauweiler P. Bimanual irrigation/aspiration. J Cataract Refract Surg 1996;22:1013-16.

11. Dogru M, Honda R, Omoto M, Fujishima H, Yagi Y, Tsubota K. Early visual results with the rollable ThinOptX intraocular lens. J Cataract Refract Surg 2004;30:558-65.

12. Cavallini GM, Campi C, Masini C, Pelloni S, Pupino A. Bimanual microphacoemulsification versus coaxial miniphacoemulsification: Prospective study. J Cataract Refract Surg 2007;33:387-92.

13. Garg A. Fine I. Chang D. Mehta K. Bovet J. Vejarano LP, Pandey SK, Mehta C. In mastering the art of bimanual microincision phaco Ed Jaypee Brothers Medical Publishers Ltd 2005.

14. Kelman CD. Phacoemulsification and aspiration: A new technique of cataract extraction. Am J Ophthal 1967; 64: 23

15. Buratto L, Werner L, Zanini M, Apple DJ. Phacoemulsification: (Principles and Techniques, Second Edition Eds Slack Incorporated 2003.

16. Olson RJ. Clinical experience with 21 gauge manual microphacoemulsification using sovereign WhiteStar technology in eyes with dense cataract. J Cataract Refract Surg 2004;30:168-72.

17. Sharing SP, Releya RL, Loiza A, Shearing RL. Routine phacoemulsification through a one-millimeter non sutured incision. Cataract 1985;2:6-10.

18. Tsuneoka H, Shiba T, Takahashi Y. Feasibility of ultrasound cataract surgery with a 1.4 mm incision. J Cataract Refract Surg 2001;27:934-40.

19. Wong V. WY Lai, TYY Lee, GKY Lam, PTH. Lam DSC. Safety and Efficacy of Micro-Incisional Cataract Surgery with Bimanual Phacoemulsification for White Mature Cataract Ophthalmologica 2007;221:24-28.

Chapter 18

Advances in Microphakonit: 700 micron Cataract Surgery

Amar Agarwal, Athiya Agarwal,
Sunita Agarwal, Ashok Garg (India)

HISTORY

On August 15th 1998 the authors (Amar Agarwal) performed 1 mm cataract surgery by a technique called PHAKONIT[1-13] (Phako being done with a Needle Incision Technology). Dr. Jorge Alio (Spain) coined the term MICS or Microincision cataract surgery[14] for all surgeries including laser cataract surgery and Phakonit. Dr. Randall Olson (USA) first used a 0.8 mm phaco needle and a 21 gauge irrigating chopper and called it Microphaco.[15-18]

On May 21st 2005, for the first time a 0.7 mm phaco needle tip with a 0.7 mm irrigating chopper was used by the authors (Am A) to remove cataracts through the smallest incision possible as of now. This is called Microphakonit.

MICROPHAKONIT (0.7 MM) NEEDLE TIP

When we wanted to go for a 0.7 mm phaco needle the point which we wondered was whether the needle would be able to hold the energy of the ultrasound. We gave this problem to Larry Laks from MST, USA to work on. He then made this special 0.7 mm phaco needle (Fig. 1). As you will understand if we go smaller from a 0.9 mm phaco needle to a 0.7 mm phaco needle the speed of the surgery would go down. This is because the amount of aspiration flow rate would be less.

It was decided to solve this problem by working on the wall of the 0.7 mm phaco needle. There is a standard wall thickness for all phaco tips. If we say the outer diameter is a constant, the resultant inner diameter is an area of the outer diameter minus the area of the wall.

The inner diameter will regulate the flow rate/ perceived efficiency (which can be good or bad, depending on how you look at it). In order to increase the allowed aspiration flow rate from what a standard 0.7 mm tip would be, MST (Larry Laks) had the walls made thinner, thus increasing the inner diameter. This would allow a case to go, speed wise, closer to what a 0.9 mm tip would go (not exactly the same, but closer). With the gas forced infusion it would work very well. Finally we decided to go for a 30 degree tip to make it even better.

MICROPHAKONIT (0.7 MM) IRRIGATING CHOPPER

In Figure 2 you will notice two designs of 20 gauge (0.9 mm) irrigating choppers which we designed. On the left is the Agarwal irrigating chopper made by the MST (Microsurgical Technology) company. This is incorporated in the Duet system. The irrigating chopper on the right is made by Geuder, Germany. Notice in the right figure the opening for the fluid is end opening, whereas the one on the left has two openings in the side. Depending on the convenience of the surgeon, the surgeon can decide which design of irrigating chopper they would like to use. There are advantages and disadvantages of both types of irrigating choppers. The end opening chopper has an advantage of more fluid coming out of the chopper. The disadvantage is that there is a gush of fluid which might push the nuclear pieces away. The advantage of the side opening irrigating chopper is that there is good control as the nuclear pieces are not pushed away but the disadvantage is that the amount of fluid coming out of it is much less. That is why if one is using the side opening irrigating chopper one should use an air pump or gas forced infusion.

The MST in their irrigating chopper increased flow by removing the flow restrictions incorporated in other irrigating choppers as a bi-product of their attachment method. They also had control of incisional outflow by having all the instruments to be of one size and created a matching knife of the proper size and geometry.

When we decided to go smaller to using a 0.7 mm irrigating chopper (Fig. 3) we decided to go for an end-opening irrigating chopper. The reason is as the bore of the irrigating chopper was smaller the amount of fluid coming out of it would be less and so an end-opening chopper would maintain the fluidics better. With gas forced infusion we thought we would be able to balance the entry and exit of fluid into the anterior chamber and that is what happened.

We measured the amount of fluid coming out of the various irrigating choppers with and without an air pump (Table 1). We also measured the values using the simple aquarium air pump

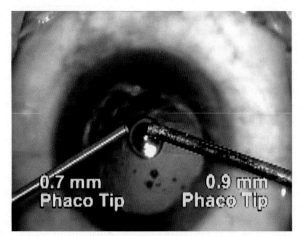

Fig. 1: 0.7 mm phaco tip (microphakonit) as compared to a 0.9 mm phaco tip (phakonit)

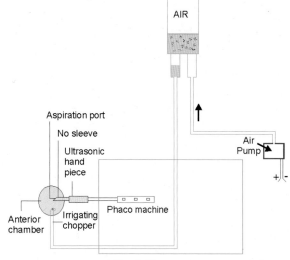

Fig. 4: Air pump

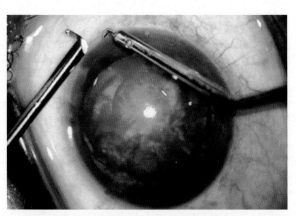

Fig. 2: Two designs of Agarwal irrigating choppers. The one on the left has an end opening for fluid (microsurgical technology). The one on the right has two openings on the sides (Geuder –Germany).

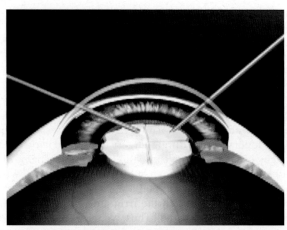

Fig. 5: Illustration showing normal anterior chamber when case is started. Air pump is not used

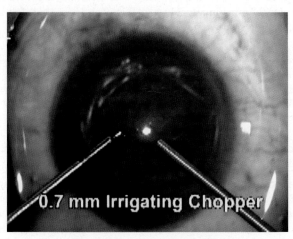

Fig. 3: 0.7 mm irrigating chopper

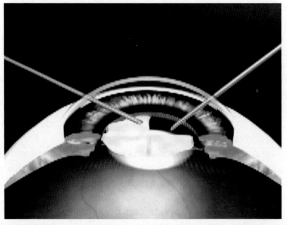

Fig. 6: Illustration showing surge and chamber collapse when nucleus is being removed. Air pump is not used. Note the chamber depth has come down. When we use the air pump this problem does not occur

Irrigating chopper	Without gas forced infusion	With gas forced infusion using the accurus machine at 50 mm Hg	With gas forced infusion using the accurus machine at 75 mm Hg	With gas forced infusion using the accurus machine at 100 mm Hg	Air pump with regulator at low	Air pump with regulator at high
0.9 mm side opening	25	36	42	48	37	51
0.9 mm end opening	34	51	57	65	52	68
0.7 mm end opening	27	39	44	51	41	54

Table 1: Fluid exiting from various irrigating choppers (values in ml/minute)

(external gas forced infusion) and the accurus machine giving internal gas forced infusion.

The microphakonit irrigating chopper which we have designed is basically a sharp chopper which has a sharp cutting edge and helps in karate chopping or quick chopping. It can chop any type of cataract.

AIR PUMP AND GAS FORCED INFUSION

The main problem in phakonit we had was the destabilization of the anterior chamber during surgery. We solved it to a certain extent by using an 18-gauge irrigating chopper. Then one of us (S.A.) suggested the use of an antichamber collapser,[19] which injects air into the infusion bottle (Fig. 4). This pushes more fluid into the eye through the irrigating chopper and also prevents surge (Figs 5 and 6). Thus, we were able to use a 20/21 gauge irrigating chopper as well as solve the problem of destabilization of the anterior chamber during surgery. Now with a 22 gauge (0.7 mm) irrigating chopper it is extremely essential that gas forced infusion be used in the surgery. This is also called external gas forced infusion.

When the surgeon uses the air pump contained in the same phaco machine, it is called internal gas forced infusion (IFI). To solve the problem of infection we use a millipore filter connected to the machine. The advantages of the Internal Forced Infusion over the External are:

1. The surgeon doesn't have to incorporate an external air pump to the surgical system to obtain the advantages of the forced infusion.
2. The surgeon can control all the parameters (forced infusion rate, ultrasonic power modulations and vacuum settings) in the same panel of the surgical system he or she is working with.
3. The forced infusion rate can be actively and digitally controlled during the surgery, adjusting the parameters to the conditions and/or the surgical steps of each individual case.

When we decided to use the 0.7 mm MST Duet set we decided to use the internal gas forced infusion of the accurus machine to measure the pressure of air exactly. This is from Alcon. The advantage by this was that we could regulate the amount of air entering into the infusion bottle and thus titrate the system in such a way that there is no surge or collapse of the anterior chamber. When we are using a 0.7 mm irrigating chopper the problem is that the amount of fluid entering the eye is not enough. To solve this problem gas forced infusion is a must.

The anterior vented gas forced infusion system (AVGFI) of the accurus surgical system helps in the performance of phakonit. This was started by Arturo Pérez-Arteaga from Mexico. The AVGFI is a system incorporated in the Accurus machine that creates a positive infusion pressure inside the eye. It consists of an air pump and a regulator which are inside the machine; then the air is pushed inside the bottle of intraocular solution, and so the fluid is actively pushed inside the eye without raising or lowering the bottle. The control of the air pump is digitally integrated in the Accurus panel. We preset the infusion pump at 100 mm Hg when we are operating microphakonit.

As you will notice in Table 1 if we use the air pump at high it is equal to using the accurus machine at about 100 mm Hg pressure and if we use the air pump at low it is equal to using the accurus machine at 50 mm Hg pressure. Some air pumps come with such a regulator so that one can have more air coming out of them. The regulator has a switch for low and high pressure. The cost of the air pump is about US $ 2 to US $ 10/- depending on the country. This can be got from an aquarium shop. If one uses an air pump one can connect a millipore filter to it to prevent any infection. Alternatively one can use a gas forced internal infusion system using the accurus machine. In such a case preset the pump at 100 mm Hg.

BIMANUAL 0.7 MM IRRIGATION ASPIRATION SYSTEM

Bimanual irrigation/aspiration is done with the bimanual irrigation/aspiration instruments. These instruments are also designed by Microsurgical Technology (USA). The previous set we used was the 0.9 mm set. Now with microphakonit we use the new 0.7 mm bimanual I/A set (Figs 7 and 8) so that after the nucleus removal we need not enlarge the incision.

DUET HANDLES

All these instruments of the 0.7 mm set fit onto the handles of the Duet system. So if a surgeon has already got the handles and is using it for phakonit they need to get only the tips and can use the same handles for microphakonit.

TECHNIQUE

Incision

The incision is made with a keratome. This can be done using a sapphire knife or a stainless steel knife. One should be careful when one is making the incision so that the incision is a bit long as one would be using gas forced infusion in microphakonit. Before making the incision, a needle with viscoelastic is taken

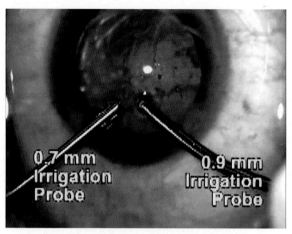

Fig. 7: 0.7 mm irrigation probe used for bimanual i/a compared to the 0.9 mm irrigation probe

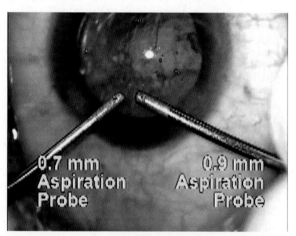

Fig. 8: 0.7 mm aspiration probe used for bimanual I/A compared to the 0.9 mm aspiration probe

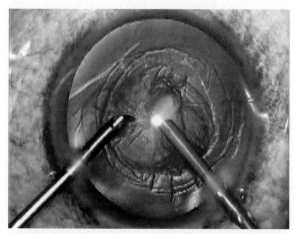

Fig. 9: Microphakonit started. 0.7 mm irrigating chopper and 0.7 mm phako tip without the sleeve inside the eye. All instruments are made by MST, USA. the assistant continuously irrigates the phaco probe area from outside to prevent corneal burns

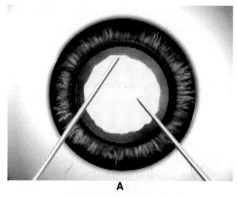

A

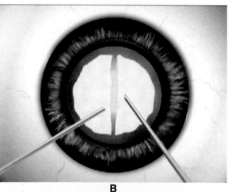

B

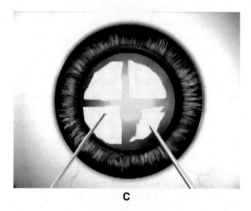

C

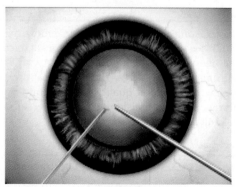

D

Figs 10A to D: Illustration showing the nucleus removal

109

and pierced in the eye in the area where the side port has to be made . The viscoelastic is then injected inside the eye. This will distend the eye so that the clear corneal incision can be made easily. Make one clear corneal incision between the lateral rectus and inferior rectus and the other between the lateral rectus and superior rectus. This way one is able to control the movements of the eye during surgery.

Rhexis

The rhexis is then performed of about 5-6 mm. This is done with a needle . In the left hand a straight rod is held to stabilize the eye. This is the Globe stabilization rod. The advantage of this is that the movements of the eye can get controlled if one is working without any anesthesia or under topical anesthesia.

Hydrodissection

Hydrodissection is performed and the fluid wave passing under the nucleus checked. Check for rotation of the nucleus. The advantage of microphakonit is that one can do hydrodissection from both incisions so that even the subincisional areas can get easily hydrodissected. The problem is as there is not much escape of fluid one should be careful in hydrodissection as if too much fluid is passed into the eye one can get a complication.

Microphakonit

The 22 (0.7 mm) Gauge irrigating chopper connected to the infusion line of the phaco machine is introduced with foot pedal on position 1. The phaco probe is connected to the aspiration line and the 0.7 mm phaco tip without an infusion sleeve is introduced through the clear corneal incision (Fig. 9). Using the phaco tip with moderate ultrasound power, the center of the nucleus is directly embedded starting from the superior edge of rhexis with the phaco probe directed obliquely downwards towards the vitreous. The settings at this stage are 50% phaco power, flow rate 24 ml/min and 110 mm Hg vacuum. Using the karate chop technique the nucleus is chopped (Figs 10A to D). Thus the whole nucleus is removed (Fig. 11). Cortical wash-up is then done with the bimanual irrigation aspiration (0.7 mm set) technique (Figs 12 and 13). During this whole procedure of microphakonit gas forced infusion is used.

SUMMARY

With microphakonit a 0.7 mm set is used to remove the cataract. At present this is the smallest one can use for cataract surgery. With time one would be able to go smaller with better and better instruments and devices. The problem at present is the IOL. We have to get good quality IOL's going through sub 1mm cataract surgical incisions so that the real benefit of microphakonit can be given to the patient.

REFERENCES

1. Agarwal A, Agarwal S, Agarwal AT. No anesthesia Cataract surgery; In: Agarwal et al. Textbook Phacoemulsification, Laser cataract surgery and foldable IOL's, First edition; Jaypee , India 1998; 144-54.
2. Pandey S, Wener L, Agarwal A, Agarwal S, Agarwal AT, Apple D. No anesthesia Cataract surgery. J Cataract and Refractive Surgery; 2001;28:1710.
3. Agarwal A, Agarwal S, Agarwal AT. Phakonit: A new technique of removing cataracts through a 0.9 mm incision; In Agarwal et al. Textbook Phacoemulsification, Laser cataract surgery and foldable IOL's, First edition; Jaypee, India, 1998; 139-43.
4. Agarwal A, Agarwal S, Agarwal AT. Phakonit and laser phakonit: Lens surgery through a 0.9 mm incision; In Agarwal et als textbook Phacoemulsification, Laser cataract surgery and foldable IOL's, Second edition; Jaypee, India 2000;204-16.
5. Agarwal A, Agarwal S, Agarwal AT. Phakonit; In: Agarwal et al. Textbook Phacoemulsification, Laser cataract surgery and foldable IOL's, Third edition; Jaypee , India, 2003; 317-29.
6. Agarwal A, Agarwal S, Agarwal AT. Phakonit and laser phakonit; In Boyd/Agarwal et als textbook Lasik and Beyond Lasik, Higlights of Ophthalmology, Panama, 2000; 463-68.
7. Agarwal A, Agarwal S, Agarwal AT. Phakonit and laser phakonit- Cataract surgery through a 0.9 mm incision; In Boyd/Agarwal et als textbook Phako, Phakonit and Laser Phako, Higlights of Ophthalmology, Panama 2000; 327-34.
8. Agarwal A, Agarwal S, Agarwal AT. The Phakonit Thinoptx IOL; In Agarwals textbook Presbyopia, Slack, USA, 2002;187-94.
9. Agarwal A, Agarwal S, Agarwal AT. Antichamber collapser. J Cataract and Refractive Surgery 2002;28:1085.
10. Pandey S, Wener L, Agarwal A, Agarwal S, Agarwal AT, Hoyos J. Phakonit: Cataract removal through a sub 1.0 mm incision with implantation of the Thinoptx rollable IOL. J Cataract and Refractive Surgery 2002;28:1710.
11. Agarwal A, Agarwal S, Agarwal AT. Phakonit: phaco-emulsification through a 0.9 mm incision. J Cataract and Refractive Surgery 2001;27:1548-52.
12. Agarwal A, Agarwal S, Agarwal AT. Phakonit with an acritec IOL. J Cataract and Refractive Surgery 2003;29: 854-55.
13. Agarwal S, Agarwal A, Agarwal AT. Phakonit with Acritec IOL; Highlights of ophthalmology, 2000.
14. Jorge Alio. What does MICS require in Alios textbook MICS; Highlights of Ophthalmology 2004;1-4.
15. Soscia W, Howard JG, Olson RJ. Microphacoemulsification with Whitestar. A wound-temperature study. J Cataract and Refractive Surgery 2002;28:1044-46.
16. Soscia W, Howard JG, Olson RJ. Bimanual phacoemulsification through two stab incisions. A wound-temperature study. J Cataract and Refractive Surgery 2002;28;1039-43.
17. Randall Olson. Microphaco chop in David Changs textbook on Phaco Chop; Slack, USA 2004;227-37.
18. David Chang. Bimanual phaco chop in David Changs textbook on Phaco Chop; Slack, USA 2004;239-50.
19. Agarwal A. Air pump in Agarwal's textbook on Bimanual phaco: Mastering the phakonit/MICS technique; Slack, USA 2005.

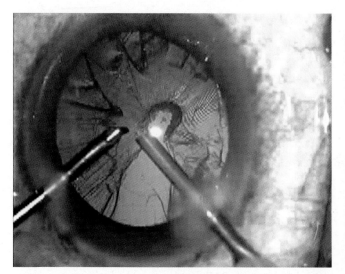

Fig. 11: Microphakonit completed. The nucleus has been removed

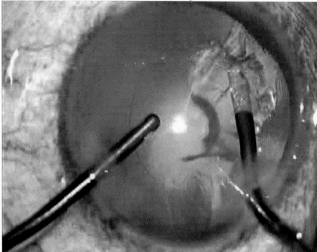

Fig. 12: Bimanual irrigation aspiration started with the 0.7 mm set

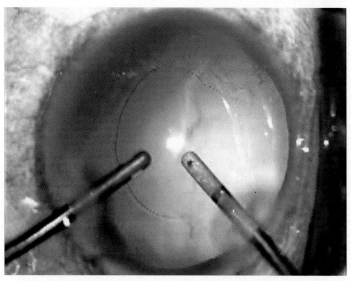

Fig. 13: Bimanual irrigation aspiration completed

Chapter 19

Microincision Coaxial Phaco is the Everyday Phacoemulsification

Simonetta Morselli, Antonio Toso (Italy)

INTRODUCTION

Microincision coaxial phacoemulsification could be the every day phacoemulsification.[1]

The technique is the same of the standard phaco technique that we are normally able to do every day for cataract surgery. For microcoaxial phaco (MICS) we want to describe around 2 mm incision cataract surgery. Between 1.8 and 2.2 mm incision is possible to perform cataract surgery with dedicated phaco machine. We don't need dedicated instruments, with normal capsulorhexis forceps we are able to do capsulorhexis through 2.2 mm incision. A lot of single piece hydrophilic acrylic IOLs are able to insert through 2.2 mm with viscoject injector.[2] With this technique we induce very low postoperative astigmatism.[3]

PHACO MACHINE AND TECHNIQUE

Coaxial microincision will soon be the everyday standard in cataract surgery, according to us.

The technique is similar to what we have been traditionally doing in cataract surgery. The change that really matters is the phaco machine and the US setting.

There are now new machines with the capability of producing a high vacuum and, consequently, a fast removal of the nucleus fragments in safe conditions.

We have a special experience with [Bausch & Lomb] Stellaris. Created specifically for MICS, this system is exceptionally fast and safe. I experience everyday how quickly the nucleus fragments are removed while the chamber remains perfectly stable. This machine, give us the opportunity to set the ultrasound in a two different sub mode. Burst and micropulse. Only changing the duration and the duty cycle of the ultrasound we are able to adapt the power at any type of cataract. Even with very hard cataract we are able to remove the pieces with not more than 10% US power. Our parameters with Stellaris machine are:

Sub mode 1 used for "normal 2+/3+ cataract:
- Dual foot pedal system
- 10 % US linear
- Pulse mode 80 Pulse per second
- 35 % duty cycle (Fig. 1).

Sub mode 2 used for 3+/4+ cataract:
- Dual foot pedal system
- 10% US linear
- Fix burst 160 millisec. duration
- 320 millisec Intervals of pulse duration (Fig. 2).

Sub mode 3 for 5+ /6+ cataract:
- Dual foot pedal system
- 10 % fix US
- Multiple burst 40 millisecond burst duration
- 60 % duty cycle (Fig. 3).

With these multiple regulation we are able to use all parameters during surgery. For example, if we want to remove the final little pieces that are floating into the anterior chamber we can use the sub model number 1. If we want to chop the nucleus at the beginning of the surgery we probably use the sub mode 3.

Our machine setting is studied to have the opportunities to change during the surgery the sub mode system only turning the foot pedal on the left during surgery. We are using dual foot pedal system. The ultrasound power is obtained turning the foot pedal on the right and the vacuum is obtain depressing the foot pedal. With this system we don't need any type of pre-set mode on the machine. The surgeon could adapt the sub mode at every moment during surgery.

VERY HARD CATARACT REMOVAL

With this system we are able to remove very hard cataract with MICS and with very low trauma for the eye structures. The most important thing is to know very well the possibilities that your machine offer to You to obtain high efficacy with less trauma for the patient (Fig. 4).

Another pearl to manage hard cataracts that we suggest is the use of various ophthalmic viscosurgical devices (OVDs) and chop-technique.

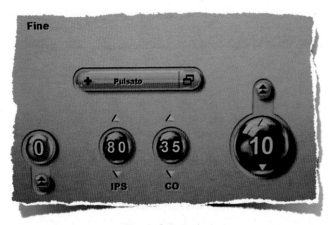

Fig. 1: Sub mode 1

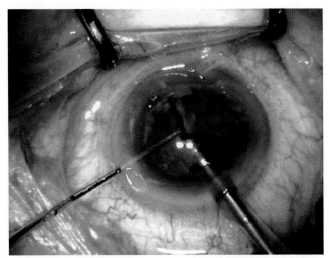

Fig. 4: MICS with very hard cataract

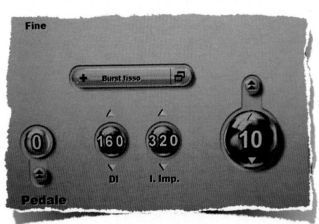

Fig. 2: Sub mode 2

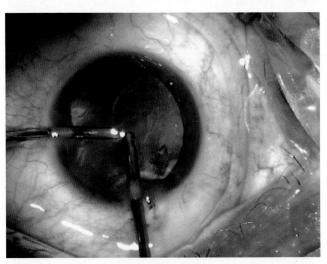

Fig. 5: Vitreous loss

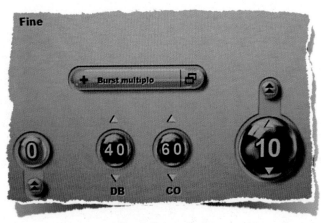

Fig. 3: Sub mode 3

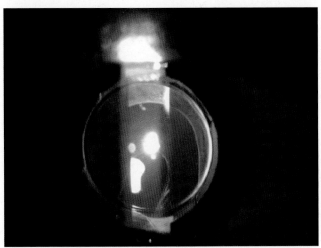

Fig. 6: MI60 in the capsular bag after 6 months

We like to use a brand new viscoelastic substance which contains sodium hyaluronate 2% and with molecular weight of 2,3 mil. dalton, giving it dispersive properties with a medium viscosity. This type of OVD provides a good anterior chamber stability, a safe adhesion to the corneal endothelium and a good protection of inner structures of the eye. This OVD gives to the surgeon the option to perform a large and controlled capsulorhexis. Unlike others dispersive OVDs, this OVD doesn't keep adhesion of the cataract fragments to the posterior corneal surface. For these reasons this OVD gives a better quality of vision during phacoemulsification.

When we remove hard cataract we performed a large capsulorhexis (6-6.5 mm) to move the nucleus out of the capsular bag into the anterior chamber during hydrodissection. This technique provides a safe chop fracture of the nucleus. The chopper is positioned at the equatorial edge of the nucleus without the risk to damage the capsular bag, even in case of PEX or zonular weakness. A little amount of OVD is injected over the capsular bag under the nucleus. The nuclear fracture is obtained by chopper, stopping the nucleus with bevel down phaco tip into the center of the nucleus. The phaco tip is inserted in the center as deep as possible. The sleeve must be retracted to obtain almost 1.8-2 mm of available tip to stop the center of the nucleus. After the first cracking, the nucleus is divided in other small slices and it is emulsified with the manipulator to avoid the capsular bag damage. During these maneuvers the anterior chamber viscoelastic refilling is mandatory, to protect the endothelium and to have a more stabilization of the nucleus.

IN CASE OF COMPLICATIONS

The microcoaxial incision cataract surgery could be the every day phacoemulsification technique even when complications occurred. In case of posterior capsule rupture, anterior vitrectomy could be performed with and without infusion. 2 mm incision is enough to mange minor complications that occurred during cataract surgery, bi-manual irrigation and aspiration with very low bottle level is and advantage during complication with vitreous loss (Fig. 5). When a complication with vitreous loss happened 1.8-2 mm incision cataract surgery is enough to manage anterior segment surgery complications with vitreous loss. MI60 IOL implantation is possible through 2 mm incision even if there is a hole in the posterior capsule. This IOL stabilized the capsular bag with four loops and the IOL remain centered into the capsular bag after 3 months (Fig. 6).

REFERENCES

1. Thomas R, Navin S, Parikh R. Learning microincision surgery without the learning curve. Indian J Ophthalmol 2008;56(2):135-7.
2. Alió y Sanz JL. Micro incision cataract surgery time has arrived. Arch Soc Esp Oftalmol 2003;78(2):65-6. Spanish.
3. Masket S, Wang L, Belani S. Induced astigmatism with 2.2- and 3.0-mm coaxial phacoemulsification incisions. J Refract Surg 2009;25(1):21-4.

Chapter 20

Advances in Fluid Dynamics of Micro-coaxial Incision Surgery

Simonetta Morselli, Roberto Bellucci (Italy)

The fluid dynamics control the environment of cataract surgery and consists of five fundamental elements:

- The size of the sleeve
- The size of the needle
- The irrigation line
- The aspiration line
- The dynamics of the pump
- The Leakage of fluid from the incision.

PHACO SLEEVE

Mini-incision coaxial phaco surgery is defined as conventional phacoemulsification taking place through a 2-2.5 mm incision. The side-port incision is performed in the usual manner, as preferred by the surgeon. The claimed advantages of this surgical procedure are the match of small incisions with minimal modifications in the usual techniques and instruments.

The standard phaco sleeve/needle cannot be used through a sub-2.5 mm incision. It can enter the eye, but several unwanted complications occur. The incision borders can be damaged, and the incision can be stretched and enlarged by phaco tip insertion. The standard phaco tip fits tight in small incisions, and movements are greatly limited. The standard soft sleeve is compressed against the phaco needle, thus limiting irrigation with reduced anterior chamber stability and increased thermal damage (Fig. 1A). In addition, the sleeve softness and compression allow the phaco needle to move forward and backwards with respect to the sleeve itself, that tends to remain consistent with the incision (Fig. 1B). As phacoemulsification is a precise surgical procedure, the characters of the tip must be adapted to the incision size. The sleeve modifications are the main element of mini-incision phaco. The sleeve must be smaller than the regular, but stiffer to avoid collapse with the above mentioned consequences. The Alcon Microsmooth, the Bausch & Lomb and the Prodis::::: are examples of such reduced sleeves (Fig. 1C). They can fit a 19 G flare, a 20 G or a 21 G phaco needle, allowing almost the same irrigation as the standard sleeve around a standard 19 G needle. To increase irrigation, and to help avoiding irish touch, a third hole can be produced in the part of the tip that is kept inferior during surgery, at the cost of precise control of its position.

The rigidity of the mini sleeve avoids its compression against the phaco needle, and allows the required movements inside the anterior chamber. In addition, it allows a minimal fluid egression at both sides at incision edges. As with standard 19 G phaco, this fluid egression could help needle cooling and could prevent excessive pressure rise in the anterior chamber, but on the other side it could favour anterior chamber collapse.

NEEDLES FOR MINI-INCISION COAXIAL PHACOEMULSIFICATION

Several approaches have been developed to find the proper phacoemulsification tip for 2-2.5 mm incisions:

- The use of 19 gauge phaco needle together with a modified sleeve
- The use of 20 gauge phaco needle together with a modified sleeve
- The use of 21 gauge phaco needle together with a modified sleeve

For the 19 G approach, the flare phaco needle seems the best option (Fig. 2A). This needle has a distal tip 1.1 mm wide with 0.9 mm internal diameter, and a body 0.8 mm wide with 0.6 mm internal diameter. This tip allow additional space for irrigation through a reduced sleeve, while maintaining some of the properties of the standard 1.1 mm needle when operating inside the eye.

A 20 G needle is produced by Bausch & Lomb. This Stable flow needle has an outer diameter of 0.9 mm, and an inner diameter of 0.4 mm, that are different from the 0.9 outer-0.6 inner diameters of the needle employed for bimanual (biaxial) surgery. The Stable flow 0.4 mm inner diameter is also available for 19 G needles (Fig. 2B).

Many companies are now producing new 21 G needles, with an outer diameter of 0.8 mm and inner diameters that vary from 0.35 to 0.6 mm. (Fig. 2C) From a practical point of view, the outer diameter dimensions no longer represent the characters of the phaco needle. Therefore a labelling including both diameters should be adopted. For instance, a 0.9/0.4 mm needle is a 20 G needle with a 0.4 mm inner diameter. Alcon also provide to insert a little hole on the tip . This system is called ABS and it was crated to minimize the surge phenomenon

115

because the tip is never complete occluded during the surgery (Fig. 2D).

THE ASPIRATION LINE

We will use an example to understand better which are the differences in aspiration line between normal 19-20 G tip and micro 21 G tip. If you try to drink a liquid with a small straw you need more "aspiration force" and you need "more time" to drink the same quantity of liquid as you drink with a large straw. The same thing happen during micro-coaxial incision phacoemulsification. With a 21 G tip we need a very high vacuum from 250 to 500 mm Hg to remove emulsified cataract pieces. There are some differences if we use peristaltic or Venturi pump.

ASPIRATION FLOW RATE

All these needles with reduced inner diameters produce some modifications in the aspiration line. With vacuum control pumps, the aspiration flow is reduced – at the same vacuum settings – as compared with standard needles (Fig. 3A). With fluid control pumps, the aspiration flow could be less than indicated by the machine, especially for high settings (Fig. 3B). With both pumps, the vacuum at phaco tip without occlusion is increased as compared with larger needles, that could favor followability and holdability. Because of the reduced aspiration flow and because of the more elevated vacuum at phaco tip when no occlusion is present, the post occlusion surge is diminished. As a consequence, maintaining high irrigation levels is of minor importance.

The amount of fluid removal through a 0.35 mm to 0.6 mm inner diameter needle is much less than through a 0.9 mm inner diameter needle, when the same vacuum is applied. This reduction in aspiration flow is more evident with vacuum control pumps than with fluid control pumps, when no occlusion is present. To maintain the same amount of aspiration, additional vacuum has to be provided with vacuum control pumps and additional aspiration with fluid control pumps. This is the reason why vacuums up to 600 mm Hg are provided by newer machines, with aspiration rates up to 60 cc/min for the fluid control pumps.

IRRIGATION LINE

The irrigation line must be enough to maintain the stability of the anterior chamber during the phacoemulsification. With the regular 19–20 G we are able to use a normal soft sleeve that permit an adequate fluid irrigation of the anterior chamber of about 110 cc/min with 19 G tip and 100 cc/min with 20 G with 110 cm of height of the bottle that used for 3-3.2 mm incision.

By using a 21 G very small tip a special rigid sleeve is used to maintain a fluid irrigation about 90 cc/min that used for 2.2-2.4 mm incision with 140 cm of height of the bottle and 80 cc/min for 110 cm of height of the bottle. (Fig. 4) If not a rigid sleeve is used the small size of the incision compress the sleeve and the flow of BSS is not enough to maintain the anterior chamber

stability during the procedure. Some modern machines use special larger tubes for micro incision surgery even if the irrigation flow is related to the height of the bottle and the sleeve size.

Regardless the maximum vacuum and aspiration settings, reduced fluid removal from the anterior chamber takes place with low internal diameter phaco needles. The need for high irrigation volume is thus reduced, allowing the use of smaller sleeves with normal bottle height. The fluid balance within the anterior chamber is settled at a lower exchange rate than with standard phaco needle and sleeve. This lower fluid exchange does not lead to an increase in pressure within the anterior chamber, but can reduce the cooling effect on the phaco needle. Therefore, small incision coaxial phaco can only be performed with cold phaco techniques.

DYNAMICS OF THE PUMPS

Peristaltic Pump

Peristaltic pump is a flow control pump. Using this pump we can set the flow rate and the vacuum separately as we want and as our technique requires. With micro coaxial incision cataract surgery we must set the flow rate from 35 to 60 cc/min to remove cataract fragments. In some modern machines there is a possibility to set the flow rate in a liner mode. The vacuum will be set from 350 to 500 mm Hg to obtain an effective and quite rapid removal of emulsified cataract pieces. The correct balance of the flow rate and the vacuum could reduce the time of surgery and the surge. A suggestion is to start with 35 cc/min of flow rate and increase the value during the surgery until this value appears suitable for our technique.

Venturi Pump

Venturi pump is a vacuum control pump. We can set the maximum level of vacuum but the flow rate could not be set and increases automatically with the vacuum. We can recommend to use dual foot pedal system (when it is available) with this pump. With 21G small tip we can use 350-500 mm Hg of Vacuum. In some machines (like Millenium B&L) the value of vacuum rise could be set. We recommend to start with lower level of vacuum rise setting and increases it during the procedure if it is necessary.

MINI-COAXIAL PHACO: GRIP

The reduced vacuum at phaco distal tip as compared with larger needles involves a reduction of the gripping force. This reduction is especially evident with the Flare tip, because of the larger opening. With the 20 G and the 21 G needles the vacuum reduction does affect grip at a lesser extent, unless the inner diameter of the needle is lower than 0.5 mm. However, with these needles the use of any second instrument, chopper or manipulator, must be mechanically very precise to avoid fragment rotation because of instrument misalignment (Fig. 5). Increasing the vacuum setting can increase the gripping force up to the normally obtained levels.

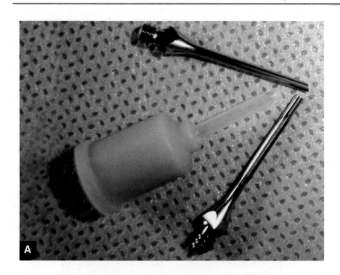

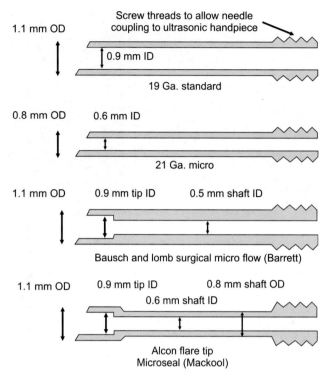

1.1 mm OD — Screw threads to allow needle coupling to ultrasonic handpiece

0.9 mm ID

19 Ga. standard

0.8 mm OD — 0.6 mm ID

21 Ga. micro

1.1 mm OD — 0.9 mm tip ID — 0.5 mm shaft ID

Bausch and lomb surgical micro flow (Barrett)

1.1 mm OD — 0.9 mm tip ID — 0.8 mm shaft OD

0.6 mm shaft ID

Alcon flare tip
Microseal (Mackool)

Fig. 2A

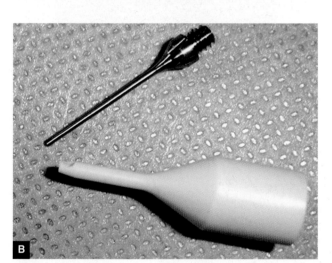

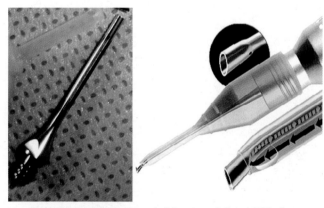

Fig. 2B: Stable flow Bausch & Lomb and flared ABS alcon

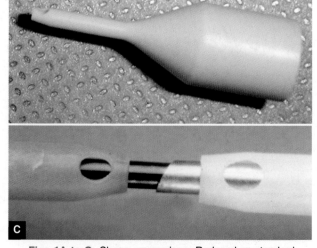

Figs 1A to C: Sleeve comparison: Reduced vs standard

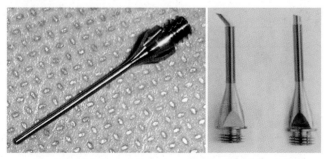

Fig. 2C: 21G Tip and Alcon flare tip microseal (Mac Kool)

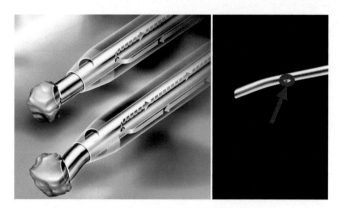

Fig. 2D: Aspiration bypass system (ABS)

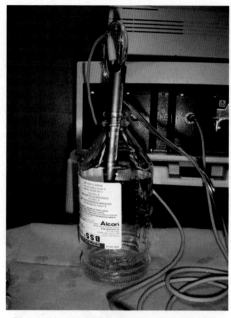

Fig. 4: How we measured the irrigation flow

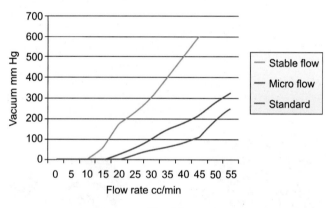

Fig. 3A

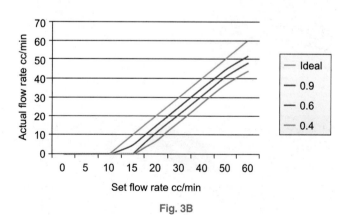

Fig. 3B

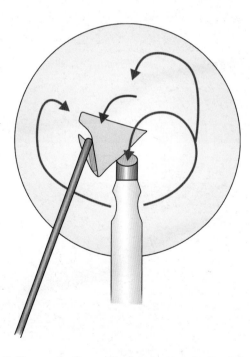

Fig. 5: The smaller the needle, the more precise has to be the second instrument movement

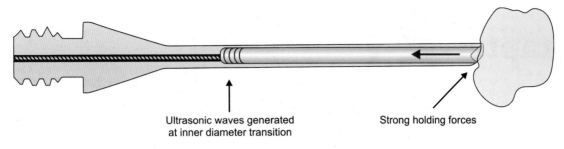

Ultrasonic waves generated
at inner diameter transition

Strong holding forces

Fig. 6

MINI-COAXIAL PHACO: FRAGMENTS REMOVAL

Because of the reduced aspiration port, fragment removal can take a longer time with mini-incision coaxial phacoemulsification. Although fragment removal is aided by the production of ultrasound at the location of the inner diameter transition inside the phaco needle (Fig. 6), the removal time could be even twice as the time requested by 1.1/0.9 mm needles, especially with hard cataracts.

MINI-COAXIAL PHACO: SURGE

The problem of SURGE is very minimized with the small tip. It is well known that the surge is a sort of extra fluid aspiration when the tip is suddenly disoccluded and one solid piece of cataract is pulled into the tip. The surge phenomenon is caused by some factors:

- The compliance of the tubes: special rigid aspiration tubes with small internal diameter are used with this technique
- Peristaltic pump suffer more than the Venturi pump: this is due to the differences between the two pumps working
- Correct settings of the machine, correct balance between flow rate and vacuum
- The size of the aspiration tip: less diameter it means less extra fluid aspiration after the occlusion and it is not related to the pump used or tubes used.

The lower fluid exchange during phacoemulsification does not produce an increase in the risk for surge. The lower aspiration rate that occurs both with Venturi and with peristaltic pump is the main reason for this reduced risk. A second reason is the higher vacuum at phaco needle distal opening. This higher vacuum as compared with standard needles helps maintaining some tube collapsing during the entire procedure, thus limiting both further collapsing during occlusion and expansion on disocclusion

BIBLIOGRAPHY

1. Barry S Seibel. Phacodinamics, mastering the tools and techniques of phacoemulsification surgery. Third edition. SLACK INC 1999.
2. Barry S Seibel: Phacodinamics, mastering the tools and techniques of phacoemulsification surgery. Fourth edition. SLACK INC 2005.
3. Buratto L, Werner L, Zanini M, Apple D. Phacoemulsification: Principle and Techniques. 2nd ed. Thorofare, NJ: SLACK INC 2003.
4. Hoffman RS, Fine IH, Packer M. New phacoemulsification technology. Curr Opin Ophthalmol 2005;16(1):38-43.
5. Packer M, Fishkind WJ, Fine IH, Seibel BS, Hoffman RS. The physics of phaco: A review. J Cataract Refract Surg 2005;31(2):424-31.
6. Weikert MP. Update on bimanual microincisional cataract surgery. Curr Opin Ophthalmol. 2006;17(1):62-7.
7. Wilbrandt HR. Comparative analysis of the fluidics of the AMO Prestige, Alcon Legacy, and Storz Premiere phacoemulsification systems. J Cataract Refract Surg 1997; 23(5):766-80.

Chapter 21

Bimanual Microphacoemulsification

GM Cavallini, C Masini, S Pelloni, L Campi (Italy)

The *bimanual microphacoemulsification* or **B-MICS** *technique*, is a product of a ceaseless technological advance, as it is a less invasive variation of traditional coaxial phacoemulsification that allows cataract extraction through incisions of 1.5 mm or smaller.

We shortly describe the surgical steps of this technique.

Although all types of **anesthesia** are compatible with bimanual phaco, local anesthesia remains the most reasonable alternative as compared to locoregional or general anesthesia in microincision cataract surgery. *Microincisions* must be created in order to prevent leakage and enable easy insertion of the instruments to be used. I usually perform two 1.4 mm trapezoidal incisions in the clear cornea at 10 o'clock and 2 o'clock (Fig. 1) with a precalibrated diamond knife (e. Janach, Como, Italy). The *capsulorhexis* can be performed, as I usually do, with cystotome 26 G needle, but it may be easier by using capsulorhexis forceps (Fig. 2), that enables perfect control of the circular cutting of the anterior capsule. A viscoelastic device combining both dispersion and cohesion agents, is particularly appropriate for bimanual microphacoemulsification. The correct capsulorhexis diameter in order to avoid surgical difficulties and complications, is between 5 mm and 6 mm. The *hydrodissection* does not require specific instruments for bimanual microphaco, as it can be used a normal 26 G cannula properly introduced through microincision, placed under the capsulorhexis and slightly lifted to create a small tent under the anterior capsule to facilitate the progression of BSS (Fig. 3). If the nucleus does not turn, the surgeon can repeat the procedure in the opposite quadrant. For *phacofracture* we need dedicated instruments for bimanual microphaco: an irrigating chopper, a 20-gauge 30-degree-angled sleeveless probe (Fig. 4), and phaco machines with ultrasound power modulation technologies, which enable discontinuous US emission and avoid thermal burns in the corneal tunnel. One of the most diffuse phaco machine, that I use, is the AMO-signature phacoemulsificator, but there are also other machines that allow the optimization of ultrasound power with different technologies.

For phacofracture we can adopt the usual techniques, but I suggest to use the "divide and conquer" or "stop and chop" technique for normal nuclei, and "vertical phaco-chop" for harder ones. Whatever is the phacofracture procedure, the great advantages of the bimanual technique over traditional coaxial phaco and mini-coaxial phaco are:

- The use of an irrigating chopper, that allows to direct the nucleus fragments towards the phaco-tip, with better followability and less turbulence in anterior chamber (AC);
- The optimization of fluidics, that allows a great AC stability;
- A greater visibility of the surgical field for the minimal size of the surgical instruments, that make this technique ideal for microphthalmos and infantile cataracts.

The *irrigation/aspiration* phase is greatly facilitated by the bimanual technique. The separated aspiration and irrigation probes are introduced through microincisions into the AC, with the aspiration probe in the dominant hand. The infusion probe in the other hand works in a continuous infusion mode, in order to avoid AC collapse, and helps to direct the cortical material towards the aspiration probe minimizing turbulence. After having performed aspiration of material on the opposite half of the entry point of the aspiration probe, the surgeon

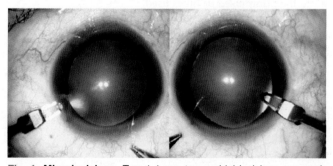

Fig. 1: Microincisions. Two 1.4 mm trapezoidal incisions are made in the clear cornea at 10 o'clock and 2 o'clock with a precalibrated diamond knife (E. Janach)

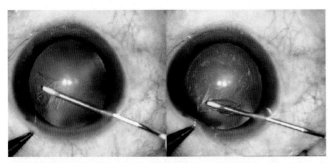

Fig. 2: Capsulorhexis (CCC). A continuous curvilinear capsulorhexis with a diameter between 5.0 mm and 6.00 mm is made with a cystotome. It may be also performed with dedicated microforceps, with "squeeze-handle" mechanism, that well fit with the microincisions and allow a safe and easy capsulorhexis phase

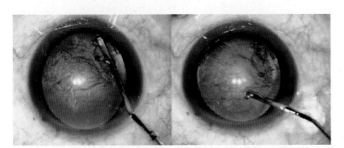

Fig. 3: Hydrodissection. This phase is performed with a 26-gauge cannula

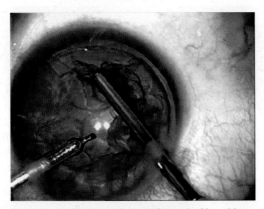

Fig. 4: Phacoemulsification. It is performed with a 20-gauge, 30-degree-angled sleeveless probe, kept with the dominant hand, and with an irrigating chopper (E. Janach) kept with the other hand and inserted through the contralateral microincision

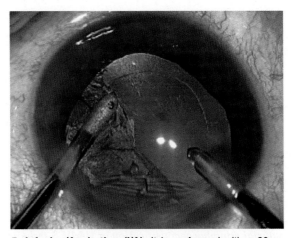

Fig. 5: Infusion/Aspiration (I/A). It is performed with a 20-gauge-probe with an oval shape section (American Medical Optics) introduced through the microincisions. Gradual suction of the cortical remnants and epinucleus is done with the aspiration probe in the dominant hand and the irrigation probe in the other, using the continuous infusion mode to avoid sudden collapse of the anterior chamber. In order to easily polish all the capsular bag, you can change the instruments from one hand to the other

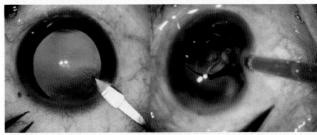

Fig. 6: IOL implant. For the implant of the IOL (Akreos MI60, Bausch & Lomb) one of the two microincisions is enlarged from 1.4 mm to 1.8 mm. Alternatively, the IOL is inserted through a third incision created at 12 o'clock, between the original two. The microincision IOLs are inserted through their own dedicated injector, and the implant is safe and easy

changes hands and keeps the aspiration probe with the other hand in order to perform aspiration of material in the other half. I usually use 20 G probes with oval section (AMO), that perfectly fit with the trapezoidal microincisions (Fig. 5).

Finally, for *IOL implantation* I usually enlarge to 1.8 mm the incision at 10 o'clock. There are now available many IOLs for microincisions that can be easily introduced in posterior chamber with a dedicated injector through the microincisions (Fig. 6). At the end of the implant I usually perform a simple *suture hydration* (Fig. 7), but it's also possible to suture the major incision with Nylon 10-0.

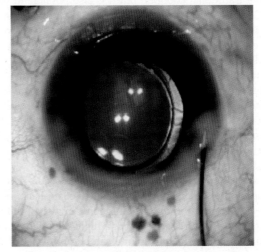

Fig. 7: Suture hydration. Surgery ends with hydration of the microincisions

121

Chapter 22

Coaxial Miniphacoemulsification

GM Cavallini, C Masini, S Pelloni, L Campi (Italy)

The *coaxial miniphacoemulsification* or **C-MICS** *technique* is another mini-invasive cataract surgery technique that some Italian surgeons proposed in 2004 (Caporossi, personal communication, 2004) as alternative to the bimanual phaco. It consists on a minimally invasive coaxial phacoemulsification technique using incisions smaller than those in traditional coaxial phacoemulsification (2.0 mm versus 2.8 mm) allowing surgeons to use the same surgical approach. So, the only difference from the traditional coaxial phaco is the use of a phaco-tip with a 21-G Ultrasleeve, that allows the insertion of the instrument through a 2.0 mm incision.

My personal technique for minicoaxial phaco is the following: after local *anesthesia*, I perform two 1.4 mm *incisions* in clear cornea at 10 o'clock and 2 o'clock with a precalibrated diamond knife (Fig. 1); then, I create a *capsulorhexis* with a cystotome 26 Gauge needle (Fig. 2). After *hydrodissection* (Fig. 3), I enlarge one of the incisions to 2.0 mm with a calibrated blade, to produce a trapezoidal 1.8- to 2-mm internal and 2.0- to 2.2-mm external incision that facilitate instrument insertion. Than, I perform *phacoemulsification* with a 20-gauge, 30-degree-angled probe with Ultrasleeve (Fig. 4). In the other hand I keep a traditional chopper, but it is also possible to use the same 20-gauge chopper as in the bimanual technique, although it is closed and not linked to the irrigating source. The ultrasound (US) energy and the fluidics control must be changed accordingly, usually by increasing the US power, bottle height, vacuum, and the flow rate. I perform *bimanual I/A* of the residual fragments with 20-gauge probes with an oval section, that can be interchanged for a complete cleaning of the capsular bag (Fig. 5). Finally, I *implant the IOL* through the 2.0 mm incision used for phacoemulsification (Fig. 6), then I finish with *suture hydration* (Fig. 7), but it's also possible to suture the major incision with Nylon 10-0.

The main advantage of C-MICS technique is the possibility of keeping the same surgical habits of coaxial phaco, with no learning curve for a traditional surgeon. Anyway, I think that this technique has already reached its highest limit in a 2.00 mm incision, while B-MICS technique can be performed through 1.4 mm incisions and it is expected to achieve the IOL insertion through a sub 1.8 mm incision.

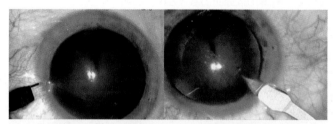

Fig. 1: Incision. Two trapezoidal incisions are made in the clear cornea: one of 1.4 mm at 10 o'clock with a precalibrated diamond knife (E. Janach), and the other of 1.8 mm at 2 o'clock by using a precalibrated steel knife

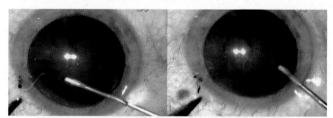

Fig. 2: Capsulorhexis (CCC). A continuous curvilinear capsulorhexis with a diameter between 5.0 mm and 6.00 mm is made with a 26 gauge needle bent twice, with a cystotome or with forceps, according to the surgeon habits

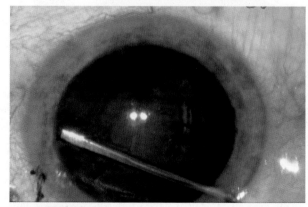

Fig. 3: Hydrodissection. This phase is performed with a 26-gauge cannula, that can be introduced both through the main incision and through the side access

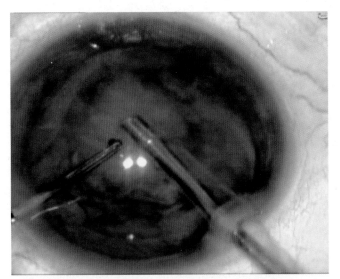

Fig. 4: **Phacoemulsification**. It is performed with a 21-gauge, 30-degree-angled probe with Ultrasleeve (Oertly), kept with the dominant hand, and with a non irrigating chopper kept with the other hand and inserted through the side access. You can use the preferred phacofracture technique, also according to the cataract hardness

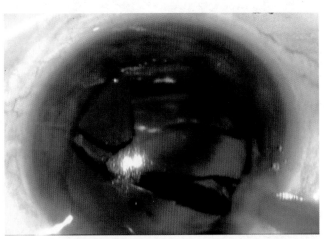

Fig. 6: **IOL implant.** For the implant we use a microincision IOL that is inserted through the main incision at 10 o'clock by using its own dedicated injector. In this case we implant a Akreos MI60 (Bausch & Lomb)

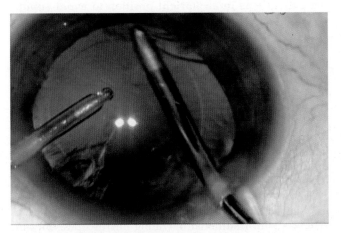

Fig. 5: **Infusion/Aspiration (I/A)**. It is performed in a bimanual way with a 21-gauge-probe with a round shape section (Bausch & Lomb) introduced through the incisions. In order to easily polish all the capsular bag, you can change the instruments from one hand to the other

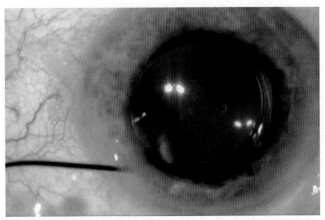

Fig. 7: **Suture hydration**. Surgery ends with hydration of the side access and of the main incision

Chapter 23

Heads Up Cataract Surgery with the True Vision 3D Visual Display System

Robert J Weinstock, Neel Desai (USA)

INTRODUCTION

Since the earliest days of intraocular surgery, the surgeon has looked through an ocular microscope to perform the delicate tasks required. Standard operating microscopes have changed little over the last many decades and have consistently suffered from limitations in function and design. As a result, many surgeons have suffered the long-term effects of this ergonomically deficient manner of operating. Inherent to its design, a surgeon must adjust the microscope to the patient's particular positioning and then adjust his shoulders, neck, and back to reach the oculars of the microscope, often yielding chronic occupational injuries. Furthermore, surgeons who use traditional operating microscopes have been unable to take advantage of many of recent advances in digital imaging and real-time operator feedback.

Recently, a few surgeons have made the transition to the digital era by freeing themselves from the ergonomic and functional confines of a standard operating microscope. By employing a cutting edge high-definition video camera and 3-dimensional display system, called True Vision, these surgeons are able to operate in a comfortable heads-up fashion with improved depth of field and unmatched ergonomics. The surgeon simply centers the digital system, which is integrated into the operating microscope, over the patient's eye and operates by wearing polarized glasses that allow 3D viewing of the projection screen without any bodily stress. Surgeons are now able to sit in an comfortable fashion with proper spinal alignment and relaxed neck and shoulder positioning. If a patient's medical condition (eg. severe kyphosis or positional apnea) requires special positioning of the bed, it would compromise the position of the operating microscope and hence the comfort of the surgeon. In such cases, the advantages of the True Vision system are magnified as the surgeon has little trouble adapting comfortably to the patient and is able to operate with consistent and safe visualization of the operating field.

The True Vision 3D system also breaks the ceiling on the traditional microscope in terms of digital on-screen applications to aid the surgeon. Traditional microscopes offered the surgeon only the view provided. Other helpful patient data, such as keratometric information, corneal topography, and lens implant information had to be kept separately on paper for review. If astigmatism correction with limbal relaxing incisions, astigmatic keratectomy, or placement of a toric lens was indicated, axis markings had to be placed at the limbus preoperatively while the patient was in an upright position to avoid supine-cyclotorsional error. The traditional operating microscope and oculars offered no additional help with these issues. Now, the applications available with the True Vision 3D system allow the digital overlay of data and markings on to the surgeon's view in real-time. For instance, a slit-lamp camera image taken with the True Vision system can be combined with preoperatively entered keratometric data to produce integrated on-screen overlays for LRI placement or lens positioning with automatic cyclotorsional registration to limbal vessels or iris-features. Thus, in the surgeon's view a perfectly on-axis mark overlies his real-time view of the eye to allow tracing of the mark to produce a precisely placed LRI or AK.

From an educational standpoint, the 3D system elevates teaching of surgical techniques to an entirely new level. Whereas with traditional operating microscopes, only the surgeon had a good stereoscopic view of the procedure while looking through the oculars, the 3D heads-up display allows everyone in the operating theatre to enjoy the surgeon's view with excellent depth-perception and clarity. Hence, for the first-time surgeons and technicians in training can fully appreciate important hands-on lessons during surgery where instrument position within the eye and depth of field are critical. In addition, surgery can be digitally recorded in this 3D format, edited, and played back for larger audiences for the purposes of teaching or discussion. Our practice, has integrated this 3D system into our series of patient education seminars on cataract surgery, that allow prospective patients to watch live cataract surgery in 3D with narration and interactive questions and answers.

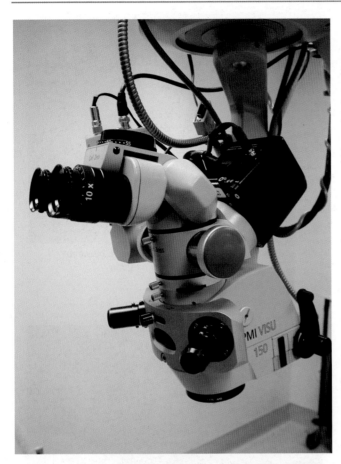

Fig. 1: The first part of the True Vision system consists of a specialized High definition 3D video camera that attaches to the surgical microscope. In this case it hooked to the backside of the oculars via a special bridge

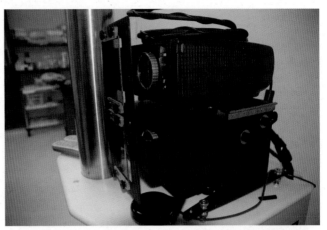

Fig. 3: The two projectors have polarizing filters in front of them. The surgeon and observers also wear polarized glasses. When the screen is viewed with the glasses on, the left eye only sees the image from one projector and the right sees the image from the other projector. The brain then fuses the two images to provide the 3D view

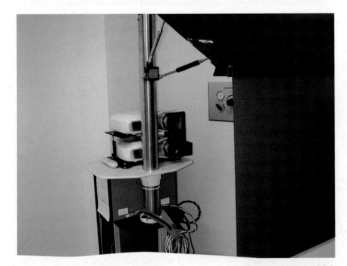

Fig. 2: The second part consists of a computer processor, two high resolution projectors, and a specialized rear projection screen

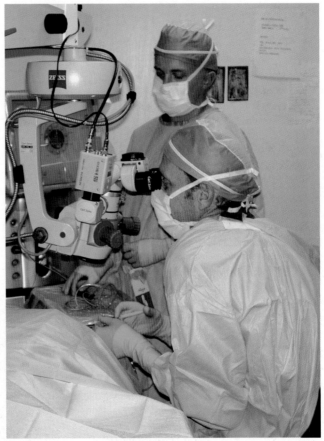

Fig. 4: One of the primary advantages of the heads up 3D view is to allow the surgeon to operate in a more comfortable ergonomic position and avoid neck and back strain. This image shows the tendency of surgeons to assume an unnatural and uncomfortable position when looking through the oculars

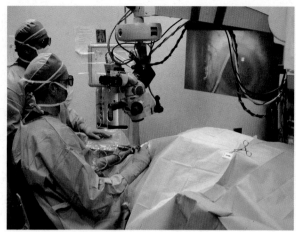

Fig. 5: This image illustrates how the surgeon can sit upright with good posture while operating. Notice that the surgical assistant is also wearing polarized glasses and viewing the case in 3D. This can aid in the efficiency of instrument passing and the assistants ability to anticipate the surgeons needs

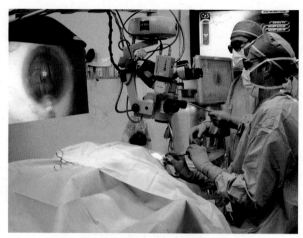

Fig. 7: Optimum screen placement is between 5-10 feet from the surgeon

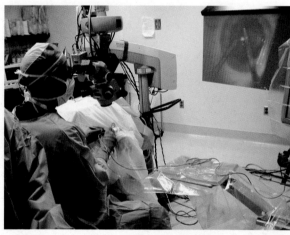

Fig. 6: Since the oculars are still attached to the scope, the surgeon can lean forward and look through them if he or she is uncomfortable with the image on the 3D display. This helps in transitioning to heads up surgery

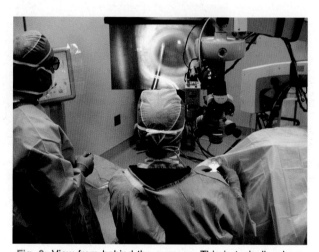

Fig. 8: View from behind the surgeon. This is typically where observers can stand to get the best 3D image

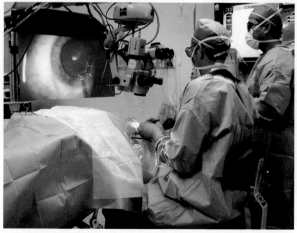

Fig. 9: Typical setup for the left eye. Notice how the screen is perpendicular to the surgeon and how he looks to the right of the microscope head to see the display

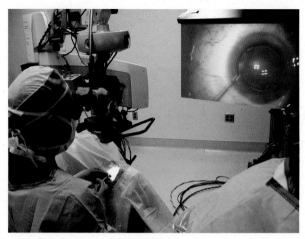

Fig. 10: The large size and magnification of the 3D system allows for a tremendous depth of field and sense of immersion in the eye for the surgeon

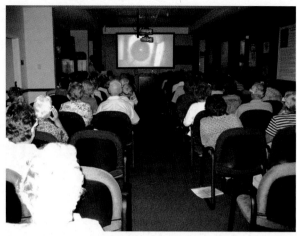

Fig. 12: The system can also be used to educate patients. In this picture patients observe live cataract surgery in 3D. The surgery is being performed in the operating room just above the auditorium they are sitting in

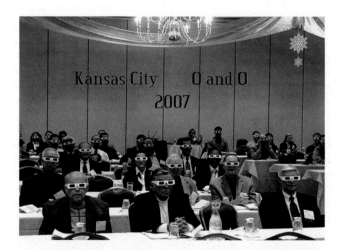

Fig. 11: Cases can be recorded in 3D format and played back to an audience for educational purposes. This slide shows a group of surgeons in Kansas City watching recorded surgical cases in 3D. Watching in 3D greatly improves the educational value

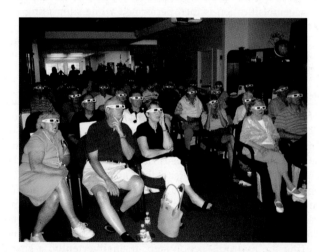

Fig. 13: Viewing the surgery in 3D lets the patients better understand the procedure and often eases their anxiety about cataract surgery

Chapter 24

Pearls of Supracapsular Surgery Using the Tilt and Tumble Technique

Elizabeth A Davis, Richard L Lindstrom (USA)

The technique of tilt and tumble is a modified form of supracapsular phacoemulsification. It uses a bimanual technique to tilt one pole of the nucleus above the anterior capsule. Phacoemulsification is then performed while supporting the lens in the iris plane with a nucleus rotator.

In the following paragraphs we will describe and illustrate this technique in enough detail to allow an ophthalmologist to perform it on their own.

INDICATIONS

The indications for the tilt and tumble phacoemulsification technique are quite broad. It can be utilized in either a large or small pupil situation. Some surgeons favor the technique with small pupils where the nucleus can be tilted up such that the equator is resting in the center of the pupil and is then carefully emulsified. It does require a larger continuous tear anterior capsulectomy of at least 5.0 mm. If a small anterior capsulectomy is created, the hydrodissection step of tilting the nucleus can be dangerous, and it is possible to rupture the posterior capsule during the hydrodissection step. If, inadvertently, a small anterior capsulectomy is created, it is probably safest to convert to an endocapsular phacoemulsification technique or enlarge the capsulorhexis. If it is not possible to tilt the nucleus with either hydrodissection or a manual technique, the surgeon should also convert to an endocapsular approach. Occasionally the entire nucleus will subluxate into the anterior chamber. In this setting if the cornea is healthy, the anterior chamber deep, and the nucleus soft, then the phacoemulsification can be completed in the anterior chamber supporting the nucleus away from the corneal endothelium. The nucleus can also be pushed back inferiorly over the capsular bag to allow the iris plane tilt and tumble technique to be completed.

In patients with severely compromised endothelium, such as Fuchs' dystrophy or previous keratoplasty patients with a low endothelial cell count, endocapsular phacoemulsification is preferred to reduce endothelial cell loss. In a normal eye, corneal clarity on the first day postoperatively is excellent. Nevertheless, the tilting and tumbling maneuvers do increase the chance of endothelial cell contact of lens material compared to an endocapsular phacoemulsification. Therefore, the endocapsular technique should not be employed in eyes with borderline corneas or shallow anterior chambers.

PREOPERATIVE PREPARATION

The patient enters the anesthesia induction or preoperative area and Tetracaine drops are placed in both eyes. The placement of these drops increases the patient comfort during the placement of the multiple dilating and preoperative medications, decreases blepharospasm and also increases the corneal penetration of the drops to follow.

The eye is dilated with 2.5% neosynephrine and 1% cyclopentolate every 5 minutes for three doses. Additionally, preoperative topical antibiotic and anti-inflammatory drops are administered at the same time as the dilating drops. We favor the combination of a preoperative topical antibiotic, topical steroid and topical non-steroidal. The rationale for this is to pre-load the eye with antibiotic and non-steroidal prior to surgery. The pharmacology of these drugs and the pathophysiology of postoperative infection and inflammation support this approach. An eye that is pre-loaded with anti-inflammatories prior to the surgical insult is likely to have a much reduced postoperative inflammatory response. Both topical steroids and non-steroidals have been found to be synergistic in the reduction of postoperative inflammation. In addition, the use of perioperative antibiotics is supported in the literature as reducing the small chance of postoperative endophthalmitis. Since the patient will be sent home on the same drops utilized preoperatively, there is no additional cost.

Our usual anesthesia is topical tetracaine reinforced with intraoperative intracameral 1% non-preserved (methylparaben free) xylocaine. For patients with blepharospasm a "miniblock" O'Brien facial nerve anesthesia, utilizing 2% xylocaine with 150 units of hyaluronidase per 5 cc of xylocaine, can be quite helpful in reducing squeezing. This block lasts thirty to forty-five minutes and makes surgery easier for the patient and the surgeon. Patients are sedated prior to the block to eliminate any memory of discomfort. One way to determine when this facial nerve block might be useful is to ask the technicians to

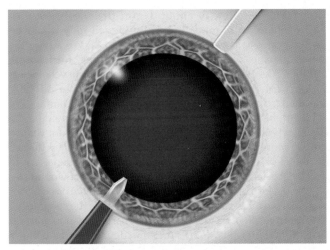

Fig. 1: Counterpuncture site of 1.0 mm is made with a diamond stab knife

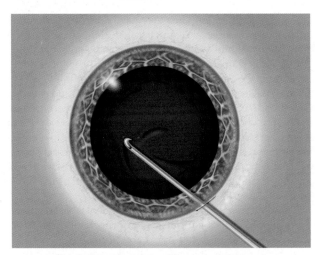

Fig. 4: A continuous curvilinear capsulotomy is made with a cystotome

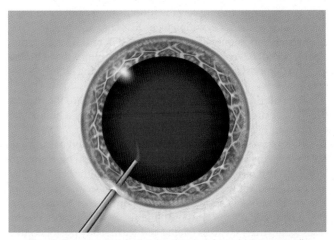

Fig. 2: Preservative-free xylocaine is injected intracamerally

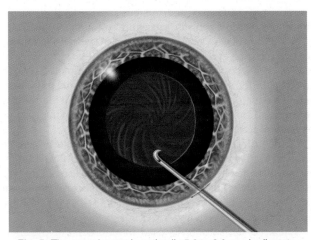

Fig. 5: The capsulotomy is optimally 5.0 to 6.0 mm in diameter

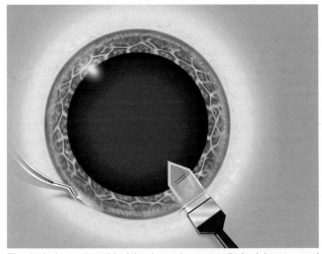

Fig. 3: A clear corneal incision is made temporally in right eyes and nasally in left eyes

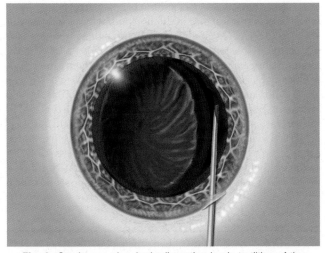

Fig. 6: Continuous slow hydrodissection leads to tilting of the nucleus out of the bag

make a note in the chart when they have difficulty performing applanation pressures or A-scan because of blepharospasm. In these patients a mini facial nerve block can be quite helpful.

In younger anxious patients and in those with difficulty cooperating, we perform a peribulbar block. Naturally, general anesthesia is used for very uncooperative patients and children. While this is controversial, in some patients where general anesthesia is chosen and a significant bilateral cataract is present, we will perform consecutive bilateral surgery completely re-prepping and starting with fresh instruments for the second eye. Again, this is a clinical decision weighing the risk to benefit ratio of operating both eyes on the same day versus the risk of two general anesthetics.

Upon entering the surgical suite the patient table is centered on pre-placed marks so that it is appropriately placed for microscope, surgeon, scrub nurse and anesthetist access. We favor a wrist rest, and the patient's head is adjusted such that a ruler placed on the forehead and cheek will be parallel to the floor. The patient's head is stabilized with tape to the head board to reduce unexpected movements, particularly if the patient falls asleep during the procedure and suddenly awakens. A second drop of tetracaine is placed in each eye. If the tetracaine is placed in each eye, blepharospasm is reduced. A periocular prep with 5% povidone-iodine solution is completed. We do not irrigate the ocular surface and fornices with povidone-iodine. Under topical anesthesia we have found that the patients note a significant burning. If a few drops leak into the eye this is certainly acceptable.

An aperture drape is helpful for topical anesthesia to increase comfort. We have noted that when the drape is tucked under the lids this often irritates the patient's eye and also reduces the malleability of the lids, decreasing exposure. Since it is important to isolate the meibomian glands and lashes a Tegaderm adhesive cut in half for the upper and lower lids may be used.

Balanced salt solution is used in all cases. For the short duration of a phacoemulsification case, BSS plus does not provide any clinically meaningful benefit. We place 0.5cc of the intracardiac non-preserved (sodium bisulfate free) epinephrine in the bottle for assistance in dilation and perhaps hemostasis. We also add 1ml (1,000 units) of heparin sulfate to reduce the possibility of postoperative fibrin. This is also a good anti-inflammatory and coating agent. At this dose there is no risk of enhancing bleeding or reducing hemostasis.

The lids are separated with a Lindstrom/Chu aspirating speculum (Rhein Medical). A final drop of tetracaine is placed in the operative eye or the surface is irrigated with the non-preserved xylocaine. We do not like to utilize more than three drops of tetracaine or other topical anesthetic as excess softening of the epithelium can occur, resulting in punctate epithelial keratitis, corneal erosion and delayed postoperative rehabilitation.

OPERATIVE PROCEDURE

The patient is asked to look down. The globe is supported with a dry Merocel sponge, and a counter puncture is performed superiorly at 12 o'clock with a diamond stab knife. (Osher/

Storz) The incision is about 1 mm in length (Fig. 1). Approximately 0.25 ml of 1% non-preserved methylparaben free xylocaine is injected into the eye (Fig. 2). We advise the patient that they will feel a "tingling" or "burning" for a second, and then "the eye will go numb". This provides a psychological support for the patient that they will now have a totally anesthetized eye and should not anticipate any discomfort. We tell them that while they will feel some touch and fluid on the eye, they will not feel anything sharp, and if they do, we can supplement the anesthesia. This injection also firms up the eye for the clear corneal incision. We do not find it necessary to inject viscoelastic prior to constructing the corneal wound.

We perform a temporal or nasal anterior limbal or posterior clear corneal incision. Care is taken not to incise the conjunctiva as this can result in ballooning during phacoemulsification and irrigation aspiration. Some surgeons define this as being a posterior clear corneal incision and others as an anterior limbal incision. The anatomical landmark is the perilimbal capillary plexus and the insertion of the conjunctiva. Since the incision is into a vascular area, long-term wound healing can be expected to be stronger than it is with a true clear corneal incision. True clear corneal incisions, such as performed in radial keratotomy, clearly do not have the wound healing capabilities that a limbal incision demonstrates where there are functioning blood vessels present.

The anterior chamber is then entered parallel to the iris at a depth of approximately 300 microns. This creates a hinge type of incision (Fig. 3).

In right eyes the incision is temporal, and in left eyes, nasal. This allows the surgeon to sit in the same position for right and left eyes. The nasal cornea is thicker, has a higher endothelial cell count and allows very good access for phacoemulsification. The nasal limbus is approximately 0.3 mm closer to the center of the cornea than the temporal limbus, and this can, in some cases where there is excess edema, reduce first day postoperative vision more than one might anticipate with a temporal incision. There also can, in some patients, be pooling of irrigating fluid. For this reason, an aspirating speculum is useful. It is also helpful to tip the head slightly to the left side. Nonetheless, in left eyes a nasal clear corneal approach is an excellent option, particularly for surgeons who find the left temporal position uncomfortable.

In some patients it may be safest to create a corneal scleral incision. Examples of these include patients who have had a previous radial keratotomy or demonstrate findings of peripheral corneal ulcerative keratitis, in some patients with very low endothelial cell counts, and any case where there is any significant peripheral pathology or thinning. The anterior limbal or posterior corneal incision described above can be made temporally, nasally, in the oblique meridian or even superiorly without induction of significant corneal edema or endothelial cell loss.

The incision, if 3 mm in length, tends to cause an induction of 0.25 ± 0.25 diopters of astigmatism. If it is placed on the steeper meridian, it can therefore be expected to reduce the astigmatism somewhere between 0 and 0.50 diopters. An incision in the 3 mm range will almost always be self sealing.

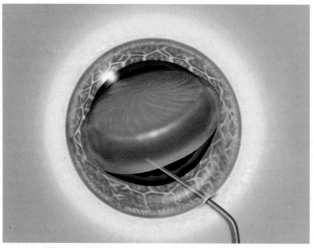

Fig. 7: The nucleus is rotated to face the incision

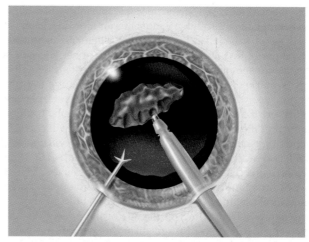

Fig. 10: Emulsification is completed in the iris plane

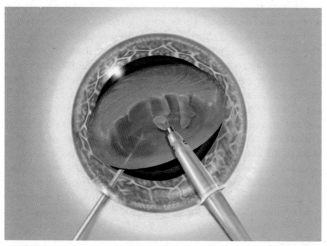

Fig. 8: The nucleus is supported during phacoemulsification with a second instrument

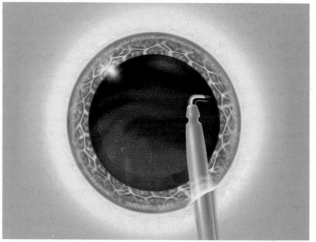

Fig. 11: Subincisional cortex is removed with a right angled tip

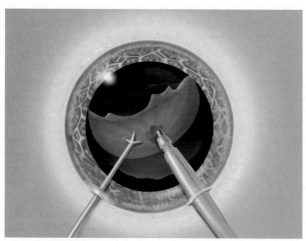

Fig. 9: The second half of the nucleus is tumbled upside down

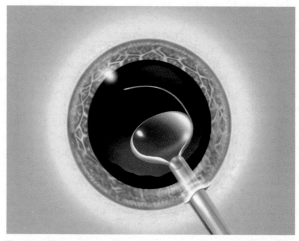

Fig. 12: The intraocular lens is inserted with an injector system

With modern injector systems most foldable intraocular lenses can be implanted through a 3 mm anterior limbal incision.

In select patients an intraoperative astigmatic keratotomy can be performed at the 7 to 8 mm optical zone. This can be done at the beginning of the operation. The patient's astigmatism axis is marked carefully using an intraoperative surgical keratometer which allows one to delineate the steeper and flatter meridian and not be concerned about globe rotation. One 2 mm incision at a 7 to 8 mm optical zone will correct 1 diopter of astigmatism and two 2 mm incisions will correct 2 diopters of astigmatism in a cataract age patient. One 3 mm incision will correct 2 diopters, and two 3 mm incision 4 diopters. One can combine a 3 and 2 mm correcting 3 diopters. Larger amounts of astigmatism can also be corrected utilizing the Arc-T nomogram. Depending on the age of the patient one can correct up to 8 diopters of astigmatism with two 90° arcs. Many surgeons have moved to a more peripheral corneal limbal arcuate incision, but we favor the 7 - 8 mm optical zone because of years of experience with this approach. There certainly is a variation in response, but there have not been any significant induced complications with this approach. The outcome goal is 1 diopter or less of astigmatism in the preoperative axis. It is preferable to under-correct rather than over-correct. The key in astigmatism surgery is "axis, axis, axis". If one is not careful in preoperative planning and the incision are placed more than 15° off axis, one is better avoiding this approach.

The anterior chamber is constituted with a viscoelastic. Our studies have not found any significant difference between one viscoelastic or another in regards to postoperative endothelial cell counts. Amvisc Plus works well and we can obtain 0.8 cc of it at a very fair price.

Next a relatively large diameter continuous tear anterior capsulectomy is fashioned (Figs 4 and 5). This can be made with a cystotome or forceps. The optimal size is 5.0 to 6.0 mm in diameter and inside the insertion of the zonules (usually at 7 millimeters). Larger is better than smaller, as there is less subcapsular epithelium and thus lower risk of capsular opacification. Additionally, a larger capsulorhexis makes for an easier cataract operation. With this technique there has not been any change in the incidence of intraocular lens decentration. With some intraocular lenses the capsule will seal down to the posterior capsule around the loops rather than be symmetrically placed over the anterior surface of the intraocular lens. These eyes do extremely well and this might be preferable to having the capsule anterior to the optic. This is also certainly a controversial position.

Hydrodissection is then performed utilizing a Pearce hydrodissection cannula on a 3cc syringe filled with BSS. Slow continuous hydrodissection is performed gently lifting the anterior capsular rim until a fluid wave is seen. At this point irrigation is continued until the nucleus tilts on one side, up and out of the capsular bag (Fig. 6). If one retracts the capsule at approximately the 7:30 o'clock position with the hydrodissection cannula, usually the nucleus will tilt superiorly. If it tilts in another position, it is simply rotated until it is facing the incision (Fig. 7).

Once the nucleus is tilted some additional viscoelastic can be injected under the nucleus pushing the iris and capsule back. Also, additional viscoelastic can be placed over the nuclear edge to protect the endothelium. The nucleus is emulsified from outside-in while supporting the nucleus in the iris plane with a second instrument, such as a Rhein Medical or Storz Lindstrom Star or Lindstrom Trident nucleus rotator (Fig. 8). Once half the nucleus is removed, the remaining one half is tumbled upside-down and approached from the opposite pole (Fig. 9). Again, it is supported in the iris plane until the emulsification is completed (Fig. 10). Alternatively the nucleus can be rotated and emulsified from the outside edge in, in a carousel or cartwheel type of technique. Finally, in some cases, the nucleus can be continuously emulsified in the iris plane if there is good followability until the entire nucleus is gone.

This a very fast and very safe technique, and as mentioned before, it is a modification of the iris plane technique taught by Richard Kratz, MD in the late 1970's and 1980's. It is basically "back to Kratz" with help from Brown and Maloney in the modern phacoemulsification, capsulorhexis, hydrodissection and viscoelastic era. Surgery times now range between four and seven minutes with this approach rather than ten to fifteen minutes for endocapsular phacoemulsification. In addition, our capsular tear rate has now gone under 1%. Therefore, we find this technique which to be easier, faster and safer. It is true that in this technique the phacoemulsification tip is closer to the iris margin and also somewhat closer to the corneal endothelium. There is, however, a significantly greater margin of error in regards to the posterior capsule. Care needs to be taken to position the nucleus away from the corneal endothelium and away from the iris margin when utilizing this approach.

If the nucleus does not tilt with simple hydrodissection, it can be tilted with viscoelastic or a second instrument such as a nuclear rotator, Graether collar button or hydrodissection cannula.

The dual function Bausch and Lomb Millennium™ is excellent for all cataract techniques including "tilt and tumble." The vacuum is set with a range of 325 to 400 mm Hg and the ultrasound power set in a pulse mode from 10 to 30%. The foot pedal is arranged such that there is surgeon control over ultrasound on the vertical or pitch motion of the foot pedal, and then on the yaw or right motion foot pedal, there will be vacuum control. This allows very efficient emulsification, and the Millennium ™ is currently our preferred machine. The microflow plus needle with a 30° angle tip works well with the Millennium.

Following completion of nuclear removal, the cortex is removed with the irrigation aspiration hand piece. We prefer a 0.3 mm tip and utilize the universal hand piece with interchangeable tips. A curvilinear tip is used for most cortex removal. Sub-incisional cortex can be aspirated with a Lindstrom right angle sand blasted tip currently manufactured by Rhein and Storz (Fig. 11). If there is significant debris or plaque on the posterior capsule, one can attempt some polishing and vacuum cleaning but not so aggressively as to risk capsular tears.

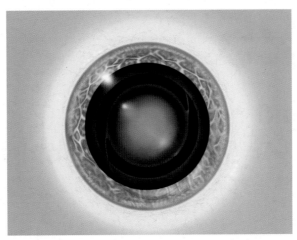

Fig. 13: The lens is centered in the capsular bag

The anterior chamber is reconstituted with viscoelastic and the intraocular lens is inserted utilizing an injector system (Figs 12-13).

Excess viscoelastic is removed with irrigation aspiration. Pushing back on the intraocular lens and slowly turn the irrigation aspiration to the right and left two or three times allows a fairly complete removal of viscoelastic under the intraocular lens.

We favor injection of a miotic and tend to prefer carbachol over miochol at this time, as it is more effective in reducing postoperative intraocular tension spikes and has a longer duration of action. It is best to dilute the carbachol 5 to 1, or one can obtain an excessively small pupil which results in dark vision for the patient at night for one to two days. The anterior chamber is then refilled through the counter-puncture and the incision is inspected. If the chamber remains well constituted and there is no spontaneous leak from the incision, wound hydration is not necessary. If there is some shallowing in the anterior chamber and a spontaneous leak, wound hydration is performed by injecting BSS peripherally into the incision and hydrating it to push the edges together. We suspect that within a few minutes these clear corneal or posterior limbal incisions seal, much as a LASIK flap will stick down, through the negative swelling pressure of the cornea and capillary action. It is important to leave the eye slightly firm at 20 mm Hg or so to reduce the side effects of hypotony and also help the internal valve incision appropriately seal.

At completion of the procedure another drop of antibiotic, steroid and non-steroidal, is placed on the eye. Additionally, one drop of an anti-hypertensive such as Betagan or Alphagan is applied to reduce postoperative intraocular tension spikes.

POSTOPERATIVE CARE

No patch is routinely utilized for the topical and intracameral approach. If a mini-block of the lids has been performed, this will wear off in thirty to forty-five minutes, and there is usually adequate lid function for a normal blink at the completion of the procedure. Patients are advised that they will have some erythropsia, meaning they will see a pink after image for the rest of the day, but usually this will resolve by the next morning. They are also told that their vision may be a little dark at night from the miotic, and not to be concerned if they wake up at night and their vision seems dimmer.

The patient is seen on the first day postoperative and then at approximately two to three weeks postoperative. At this time a refraction, slit-lamp, and fundoscopic examination is performed. If there is no inflammation, patients are seen again one year postoperative. If at three weeks there is still persistent inflammation, additional postoperative anti-inflammatory medications are recommended, and the patient is asked to return again at two to three months postoperative.

Topical antibiotic, steroid and non-steroidal, are utilized twice a day, usually requiring a 5 cc bottle and three to four weeks of therapy. Occasionally a second bottle of steroid and non-steroidal is necessary if flare and cell persist at the three week examination. There are minimal restrictions, including a request that there be no swimming and no very heavy lifting for two weeks. We consider the ideal postoperative refractive spherical equivalent for a monofocal lens to be -0.62 diopters with less than 0.50 diopters of astigmatism in the same axis as existed preoperatively. Most patients can see 20/30+ and J3+ with this type of correction. Monovision can be utilized in the appropriate settings. Good results can also be obtained accommodating or multifocal intraocular lens.

The second eye is done at 2 weeks or greater postoperatively except in rare situations. Any YAG lasers are deferred for 90 days in order to allow the blood aqueous barrier to become intact and capsular fixation to be firm.

CONCLUSION

We hope other surgeons will find this approach to cataract surgery useful. These techniques must be personalized, and every surgeon will find that slight variations in technique are required to achieve optimum results for their own individual patients in their own individual environment. Continuous efforts at incremental improvement result in meaningful advances in our ability to help the cataract patient obtain rapid, safe, visual recovery following surgery.

Chapter 25

Intrepid Microcoaxial (2.2 mm) System for Safe Phacoemulsification

Keiki R Mehta, Cyres K Mehta (India)

The Alcon has introduced a new "Intrepid" micro-coaxial technology is changing the way cataract surgery is performed with smaller, less invasive procedures without compromising on surgical techniques

Microincision Sleeve developed by Alcon permits the phacoemulsification using the standard 0.9 mm tip to be done successfully via a 2.2 mm incision. Alcon also developed an experimental "ultra" sleeve able to do it to through a 1.8 mm incision also but the flow tends to be severely restricted not allowing the full vacuum to be utilized as effectively . With the Intrepid 2.2 mm system utilizing the Alcon Infiniti, one has the ability to combines unparalleled fluidics with an unique energy delivery systems that provide you with options for efficient cataract lens removal OZil® Torsional Hand piece. This technologies deliver enhanced fluidic stability and surgical control. Torsional phaco improves efficiency and offers precise energy delivery with reduced repulsion that increases followability with an improved thermal safety profile.

The INFINITI® Vision System's revolutionary Intrepid micro-coaxial technology is changing the way cataract surgery is performed with smaller, less invasive procedures without compromising on surgical techniques.

The essential component of the Fluidic management system (FMS) is an advanced cassette which has a a low-compliance (rigid) design that increases surgical efficacy without sacrificing efficiency. Superior surge suppression and a high performance pump mechanism allow for smooth and precise fluidic sensing and adjustments in the changing ocular environment. The way this cassette works is due to the molded fluid paths and thick-wall polymer aspiration tubing decrease post-occlusion surge and increase fluidic response and accuracy. In addition an uique sensor based on a elastomer membrane allows vacuum levels up to 600 and above to help increase the effectiveness of delivered energy and decrease peristaltic pulsations.

The FMS system also has an advanced pump mechanism which has tapered rollers designed for instantaneous, smooth peristaltic response and has greater pumping capability, with forward and reverse actuation up to 100 cc per minute. Accurate alignment of the consumable and pump head enables more precise calibration and measurement and monitors vacuum pressure at an unprecedented rate.

Application of the OZil® Torsional handpiece to Microphaco technology.

The OZil® Torsional handpiece delivers side-to-side oscillating ultrasonic movement. With virtually no repulsion, it delivers a high level of followability. The unique movement of torsional phaco shears the lens material, providing decreased repulsion while improving the thermal safety profile over traditional ultrasound. Thus it is the decreased repulsion: increased followability, reduced potential for turbulence, and increased cutting efficiency which would seem to make all the difference. Interestingly the Ozil uses a lower frequency of 32kHz which thus induceslLess frictional movements and thus) reduce the risk for thermal injury significantly. Thus it permits the use of sealed incisions and continuous torsional modes increasing surgical efficiency and thus facilitates the emerging trend of micro-coaxial phaco.

Naturally using the custom power modulations provide for a choices of energy options.

Pulse and Hyperpulse. Provides access to high pulse rates with customizable on times and variable, easy-to-understand duty cycles. The customized energy modulations allow for reduced repulsion and an improved thermal safety profile when compared to continuous ultrasound.

Smart Pulse allows low energy delivery to complement and aid in traditional micropulse phaco settings below 20 ms.**Linear**

Burst adds control of energy power to the traditional burst mode – allowing increased precision, more instantaneous control and decreased repulsion based on lens densities. The customized burst off limit improves the thermal safety profile by providing modulation of ultrasound energy delivery.

The continuously variable footswitch controls optimizes control of burst delivery, burst energy level and duty cycle, enabling better occlusion.

The advantage of the thinner 2.2 mm sleeve is that I support smaller incisions by reduce shaft diameter. The soft flexible sleeve minimizes wound leakage. Made from a translucent

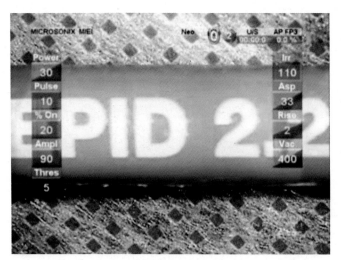

Fig. 1: The intrepid system

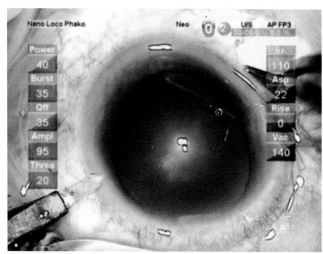

Fig. 4: 0.9 mm side port at 2 o'clock position

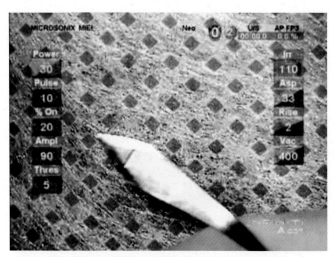

Fig. 2: Intrepid 2.2 mm blade with groove at 1.8 MM

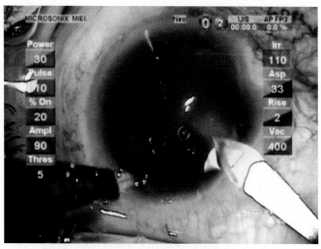

Fig. 5: Main phaco entry with special intrepid blade

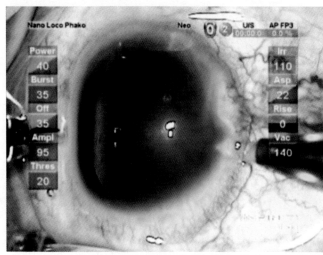

Fig. 3: 0.9 side port at 9 o'clock position

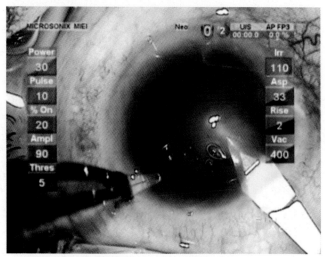

Fig. 6: Blade advanced upto groove in tunnel

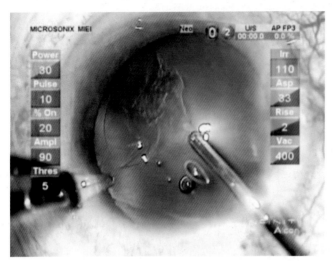

Fig. 7: Hydrodissection

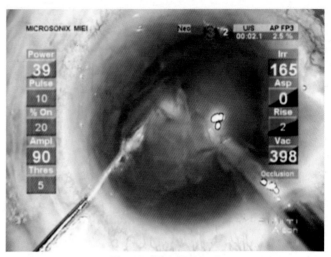

Fig. 10: Chop instituted

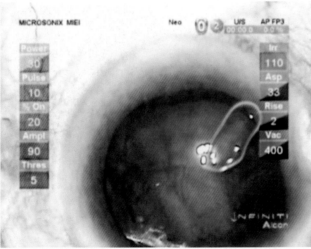

Fig. 8: Lens tipped up at 5 o'clock position (Lens Salute)

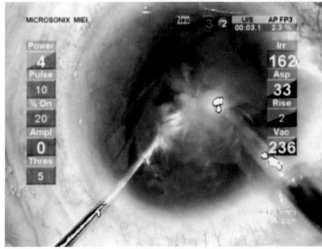

Fig. 11: Nucleus being separated

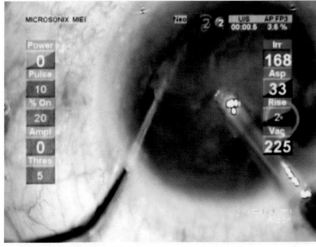

Fig. 9: Notice thin sleeve on phaco chopper supports nucleus.
Phaco advanced into nucleus

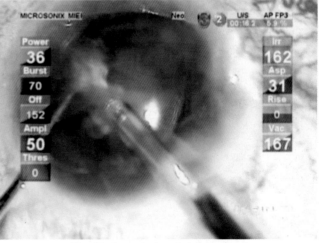

Fig. 12: Second piece being chopped

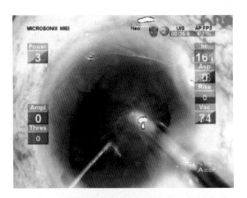

Fig. 13: Final fragment being removed

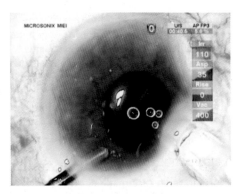

Fig. 16: Assisted delivery by invaginating injector under superior lip

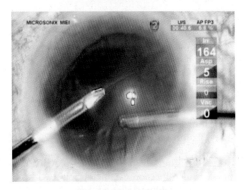

Fig. 14: Bimanual IA

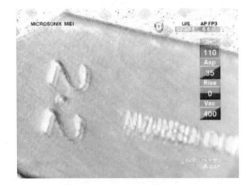

Fig. 17: 2.2 mm measuring gauge

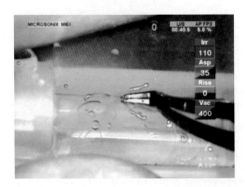

Fig. 15: Rayner lens being prepared for insertion

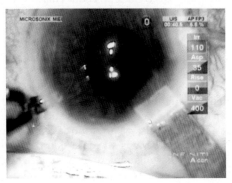

Fig. 18: Gauge just enters

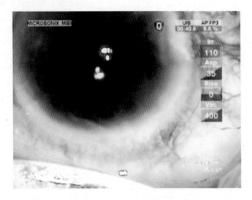

Fig. 19: Final appearance

material with very thin walls it permits a high flow, at the same time minimizing bulk and has large side openings to permit unrestricted flow. Its smooth profile, narrowing to the front permits an simple ease of insertion. It is recommended by Alcon that the Irrigation Flow show be derived from a 78 cm H_2O bottle height.

Complimenting the system is a 2.2 mm smooth entry blade with a marker at the tip indicative of 1.8 mm in case the narrower "ultra " sleeve is to be utilized.

SURGICAL TECHNIQUE

Two side ports incisions are made at 9.00 o'clock and at 1.30 o'clock. Viscoelastic is perfused in my personal preference is for Viscoat (Alcon) simply because it preserves the chamber well and at the same time protects well the endothelial cells . I have found using the 'soft shell' technique of Arshinov also useful especially in highly myopic eyes or eyes with deep chambers.

The corneal entry is done at 11.00 o'clock using the special 2.2 mm knife with the gradated tip. It slips in very smoothly leaving a good well designed tunnel.

Rhexis is done with a MST (MicroSurgical Technology) rhexis forceps which easily slips in via a 0.9 mm opening or alternatively with the Indo German rhexis forceps designed in India. The rhexis needs to be at least 6.5 mm in size. The next step of hydrodissection is done at two planes, first horizontally and then vertically, repeated if necessary till the edge of the nucleus tips forward at the 5.00 o'clock position. This in my opinion is an essential step because it immediate simplifies all the procedure which will follow.

The phaco sleeve is checked (especially if reused as the sleeve is very fragile and tears easily). The flow is evaluated (bottle at least 3 feet higher than the eye).

The blunt chopper is introduced and the phaco tip inserted. It often needs a slightly screwing motion to get the tip in smoothly in these tight incisions. A simple tip is to place a drop of viscoelastic on the incisions prior introducing the phaco tip as it lubricates it and permits an easier entry. I prefer to use either the regular phaco handpiece or more recently the OZil handpiece with a vacuum of 380, a with a burst mode with 40% power for a Grade 3 cataract. Usually after the first two chops I change to hyperpulse dropping the power. The phaco can proceeds as normal with no difficulty.

Bimanual hand pieces used to complete the I/A and an IOL can be implanted using a smooth hook to take support from the the side incision keeping the tip of the injector pressed tightly against the incision (assisted technique. It is possible to implant an Alcon IQ , or a Raynar IOL or for that matter virtually all 5.5 to 6.0 mm foldable IOL's provided the procedure is followed carefully and the tip of the injector is invaginated into the superior lip of the incision.

Results

I have used this technique in a fairly large series of cases and have now virtually adopted this technique as a routine in most cases. The results are predictable. The opening is for all practical purposes a zero astigmatic incision, the eyes are very quiet the next day and the technology is similar to the standard phaco technique so adopting it is your practice needs only little practice with the assisted implantation but otherwise it is virtually the same. Just simply be careful in implanting higher powers (+25 and above) as the bulk of the lens increases and unless you are very careful the IOL will simply open outside the eye. I have never had a phaco burn and the average surgery time for the phaco component is 38.8 seconds over the last 380 serial cases done with the OZil . The average phaco power was 12 % .

Reducing the size of the incision does not in any way compromise the length of the procedure or the endothelial cells as I have found absolutely no change.

BIBLIOGRAPHY

1. Alió J, Rodríguez-Prats JL, Galal A, Ramzy M. Outcomes of microincision cataract surgery versus coaxial phaco-emulsification. Ophthalmology 2005;112(11):1997-2003. Epub 2005 Sep 23.Comment in: Ophthalmology 2006;113(9):1687; author reply 1687.

2. Alió J, Rodríguez-Prats JL, Galal A, Ramzy M. Outcomes of microincision cataract surgery versus coaxial phaco-emulsification. Ophthalmology 2005;112(11):1997-2003. Epub 2005 Sep Comment in: Ophthalmology 2006;113(9):1687; author reply 1687.

3. Alió JL, Rodriguez-Prats JL, Vianello A, Galal A. Visual outcome of microincision cataract surgery with implantation of an Acri.Smart lens. J Cataract Refract Surg 2005;31(8): 1549-56.

4. Crema AS, Walsh A, Yamane Y, Nosé W. Comparative study of coaxial phacoemulsification and microincision cataract surgery. One-year follow-up. J Cataract Refract Surg 2007; 33(6):1014-8.

5. Kahraman G, Amon M, Franz C, Prinz A, Abela-Formanek C. Intraindividual comparison of surgical trauma after bimanual microincision and conventional small-incision coaxial phacoemulsification. J Cataract Refract Surg 2007;33(4):618-22.

6. Kurz S, Krummenauer F, Gabriel P, Pfeiffer N, Dick HB. Biaxial microincision versus coaxial small-incision clear cornea cataract surgery. Ophthalmology 2006;113 (10):1818-26.

7. Liu Y, Zeng M, Liu X, Luo L, Yuan Z, Xia Y, Zeng Y. Torsional mode versus conventional ultrasound mode phaco-emulsification: Randomized comparative clinical study. J Cataract Refract Surg 2007;33(2):287-92.

8. Mencucci R, Ponchietti C, Virgili G, Giansanti F, Menchini U. Corneal endothelial damage after cataract surgery: Microincision versus standard technique. J Cataract Refract Surg 2006;32(8):1351-4.

9. Osher RH, Injev VP. Microcoaxial phacoemulsification Part 1: laboratory studies. J Cataract Refract Surg 2007;33(3): 401-7.

10. Vasavada V, Vasavada V, Raj SM, Vasavada AR. Intra-operative performance and postoperative outcomes of microcoaxial phacoemulsification. Observational study. J Cataract Refract Surg 2007;33(6):1019-24.

11. Wilczynski M, Drobniewski I, Synder A, Omulecki W. Evaluation of early corneal endothelial cell loss in bimanual microincision cataract surgery (MICS) in comparison with standard phacoemulsification. Eur J Ophthalmol 2006; 16(6):798-803.

Chapter 26

Locomotive Cored Technique for Rapid Fast Safe Phacoemulsification

Keiki R Mehta, Cyres K Mehta (India)

Phacoemulsification is now become the simplest and the easiest way to conduct cataract surgery will any level of efficiency. For many year researchers have made many efforts to produce a technique, which would permit phacoemulsification to be done with a high level of safety and efficiency even in hard cataracts. The newer techniques have ranged from new choppers, which chop vertically horizontally or even vertically. Newer techniques of splitting the lens nucleus in a vertical and horizontal or oblique fashion have all been attempted. However none of the techniques have really been based on functional reality. One has to clearly appreciate that the maximum density of the nucleus to be removed lies in the rotund middle, and hence a technique, which would remove, or core out the center, would logically is most efficient and effective method for removal of a nucleus with total safety.

MATERIAL AND METHODS

The technique for doing locomotive phacoemulsification is fairly simple. It requires nothing much more than a blunt tipped sharp edged chopper which is 1.5 mm long and which can act as a support for the nucleus while it is being cored. The technique is essentially very simple. Following a standard tunnel incision, which is corneal based, a good rhexis is carried out. Next, hydrodissection is carried out at the horizontal and then the vertical plane, alternating till the nucleus of the lens tips out at the half way pint of the hydrodissection, namely the 10.30 position. It is then gently spun from side to side while it still stands vertical to be sure to break the adhesions.

Now viscodissection is carried out at the right quadrant at 10 o'clock. This permits the left side of the nucleus to literally come up ands stay up permitting the very easy insertion of the chopper. This phase of the nucleus, when it tips up is termed as the "Lens Salute".

THE TECHNIQUE

The phaco tip is exposed till almost 2.5 mm of the tip is exposed. Considering thickness of a normal phako microtip is 0.9 mm, three times the thickness of the needle is the approximate amount to expose. The phacoemulsification settings are now changed. In coring mode, the ultrasound power is set at 75%, aspiration rate at 12 and vacuum at 40 mm Hg. The reason for these settings is that one needs to only core the nucleus without holding the nucleus. Since the phaco tip will bury itself into the substance of the lens, U/S energy is not liberated onto the cornea.

The chopper is now introduced via the side port and allowed to support the nucleus. The phaco is now introduced via the corneal tunnel is now impacted on the surface of the nucleus so as to core out the center of the nucleus.

Nucleus is supported for from the left inner aspect utilizing the flat chopper, using the blade of the chopper and not the tip. The phacoemulsification tip is now placed in the middle or as near to the middle of the nucleus and ultrasound energy is utilized to let it sink itself into the nucleus. It is never possible to place it directly in the middle, but as much as possible is acceptable. It is important not to push the tip in, simply let the phaco energy carry it passively in. The entire procedure is based on simply coring out of the central nucleus. After the first core is made, as the phaco tip comes out of the nucleus use it to rotate the nucleus into position for the next core. Each core should be separated from the other by the thickness of the core . Place four cores in the middle of the nucleus in a symmetrical fashion at 12, 3, 6 and 9 o'clock. In very hard nucleus, it may prove necessary to core out 6-8 openings.

As a next step, It is easy to imagine that you have now converted the lens into a doughnut by coring the nucleus center out. Now one needs to only to pull the core apart so that a thin rim is left over.

The chopper, which till the present was lying flat against the surface of the nucleus, is now rotated sp that its tip is rotated towards the center of the nucleus. Using the phaco tip the nucleus is now split open. Since there are multiple cores the nucleus simply opens up easily. All this is done with the phaco in the 'core' mode.

The next step following the breaking of the rim is to change the phaco parameters. Change the ultrasound power to 40%,

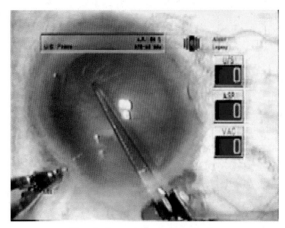

Fig. 1: A good rhexis is essential

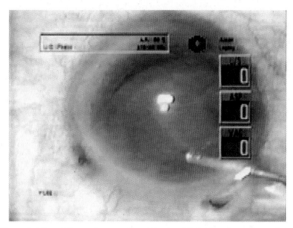

Fig. 4: Viscodissection at 12 o'clock which lifts the edge of the lens up. This technique is called as the "lens salute"

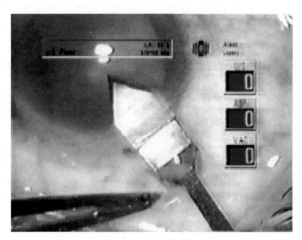

Fig. 2: Tunnel incision with a diamond knife

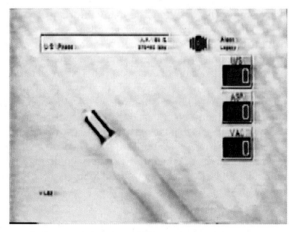

Fig. 5: Expose the needle more, almost 3.00 mm

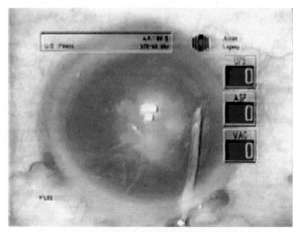

Fig. 3: Hydrodissection at two opposite points

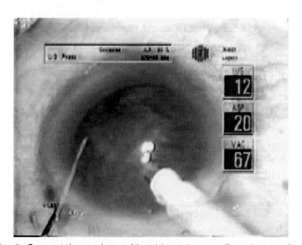

Fig. 6: Support the nucleus with a blunt chopper. Bury the needle to its hilt in the middle of the nucleus

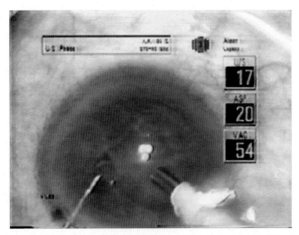

Fig. 7: Remove the needle (easy as there is no suction) and prepare to bury it again

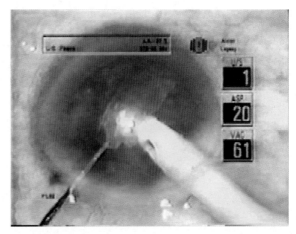

Fig. 10: Snap open the ring created by coring out of the nucleus

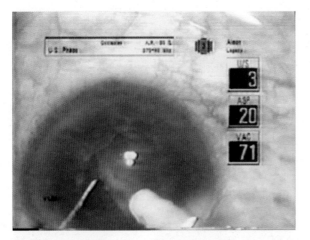

Fig. 8: Once again bury the needle upto the hilt in the nucleus

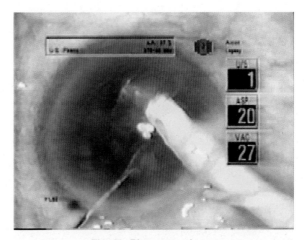

Fig. 11: Ring snapped open

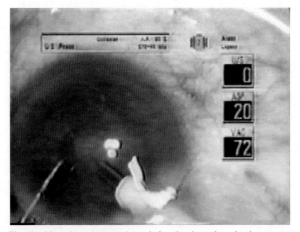

Fig. 9: After three cores, bury it for the last time in the center

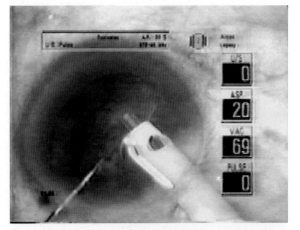

Fig. 12: Switch to pulse phaco and proceed to aspirate the ring residual in the eye

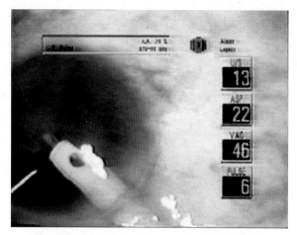

Fig. 13: Final fragments removed with final phaco

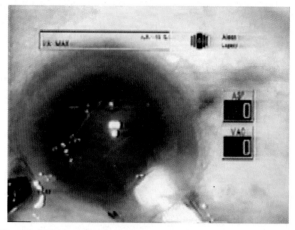

Fig. 16: Silicone lens injected into the eye with an M port injector (Storz)

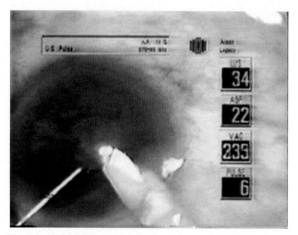

Fig. 14: Use high vacuum with low u/s power and proceed to gradually phaco off the ring of the dough nut

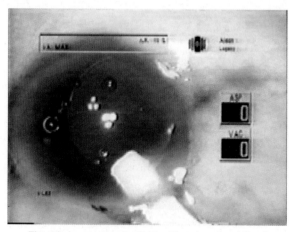

Fig. 17: Lens rotated with the M port and stabilized

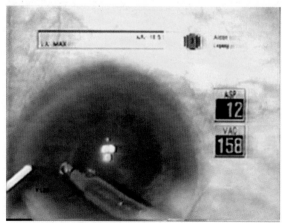

Fig. 15: I/A used to remove the cortical debris

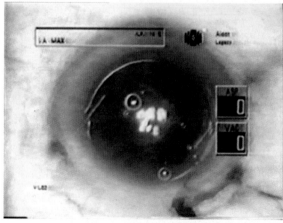

Fig. 18: Good stable positioned lens

aspiration rate to 28 and vacuum to 450 mm Hg. Place the tip of the phaco onto the edge of the rim, and utilizing the pulse phaco mode (at 5 pulses per second), simply carrousel the rim into the phaco tip. If you are using the Ozil mod with a Alcon phaco, life becomes exceedingly simple as the rims simply vanishes . Keep the Ozil mode on 80%. It is a very fast and effective technique which literally scoffs at a hard lens .

Complications of the procedure are virtually nil. Since one is never near the capsule, there can be no risk of a capsular break. Ultrasound energy used is very low and what energy is liberated is usually when the phaco tip is buried in the nucleus. Carousel ling the rim out with pulse phaco, or OziL uses minimal energy. In 600 serial cases conducted both in the rural and the urban circumstance no cases of capsular break were recorded.

SUMMARY

The Locomotors phaco technique is a very simple and effective method which is easy to learn and as easy to teach. It is applicable in the urban as well as the rural milieu. It is very effective and totally safe.

Chapter 27

Microincisional Lens Surgery

Jorge L Alió, Pawel Klonowski, Bassam El Kady (Spain)

CORE MESSAGES

- The minimization of the incision is a consequence of a natural evolution of the cataract surgery technique.
- Microincision Cataract Surgery (MICS) is the surgery performed through incisions of 1.5 mm or less.
- With MICS you can operate all grades of cataract LOCS III, even hard cataracts, subluxated lenses, post traumatic lenses, zonular laxity and congenital cataracts.
- One of the most important achievements of MICS is the reduction of the US power delivered into the eye.
- Among the major advantages of MICS is the reduction of surgical trauma resulting in a reduction of surgically induced astigmatism (SIA).
- However a major problem remains in the possibility of lens compression.
- The future belongs to the miniaturization of the tools and the wound size.
- MICS is ready to extract cataract through sub 1 mm incision.

1. INTRODUCTION: THE TRENDS TOWARDS MICROINCISION CATARACT SURGERY (MICS)

Biaxial microincision clear corneal phacoemulsification was a new method which made the corneal incision smaller. This method was described by Shearing in 1985.(35) This procedure uses separate irrigations with an irrigating chopper, sleeveless phacoemulsification tip, and also requires pulsed phacoemulsification energy.

The minimization of the incision is a consequence of a natural evolution of the cataract surgery technique in the search of excellence. When we place cataract surgery within the context of Gaussian distribution, it is clear that the standard of practice today is standard coaxial phacoemulsification (Fig. 1). Extracapsular 6 mm surgery is a procedure still in practice today, but rarely performed, hence between -2 and -2.6 standard deviation. The Gaussian curve is like a wave. It moves from ancient to new surgical techniques. Nowadays the standard coaxial technique is still the most popular type of cataract surgery in the world. The coaxial wound size is still 2.75 mm, in spite of the availability of the newest foldable intraocular lenses which can be injected through smaller incisions. Microincision Cataract Surgery (MICS) can make the incision smaller than 1.5 mm and it should be considered beyond the 2 up to the 2.6 standard deviations of our Gaussian distribution. MICS will be the standard of practice in future, and what we could call sub 1 mm MICS or micro-MICS will be the next standard.[1] MICS is the next stage in the evolution of cataract surgery.

Summary for the Clinician

- The minimization of the incision is a consequence of a natural evolution of the cataract surgery technique

2. MICS DEFINITION

In 2001, MICS was patented as a new operating method by Jorge Alio. The definition of Microincision Cataract Surgery (MICS) is the surgery performed through incisions of 1.5 mm or less. Understanding this global concept implies that it is not only about achieving a smaller incision size but also about making a global transformation of the surgical procedure towards minimal aggressiveness. In other words, a transition from conventional small incision surgery to the more developed concept of MICS.[4]

Confirmed Advantages of MICS

- Surgery
  - I/A separation
    - No leakage (tight incision and well profiled tools make wounds impermeable)[10,14,37]
    - Fluidics work as an instrument (high vacuum is the third power which can crumble the lens mass)[1,3,4]
    - Flexible surgery, assisted by fluidics (proper fluidics flow assures anterior chamber stability, profundity and separated tools allow the possibility of faster and more precise surgery)[4,5,41]
    - Intraoperative control of intraocular pressure – IOP (permanent and sufficient infusion keep the eye globe in stable condition)[4,22]
  - Smaller incision
    - New MICS irrigating hydromanipulators and the new use of fluidics leads to a reduction in the dimension of the incision.[1,3,4,5,41]

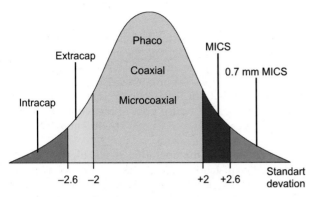

Fig. 1: Natural evolution of cataract surgery

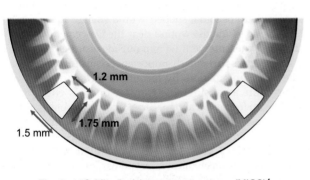

Fig. 2: 19G Microincision cataract surgery (MICS)[4]

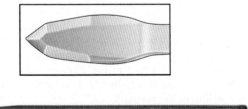

Fig. 3: Alio´s MICS metal knife (Katena Inc, Denville, NJ, USA)

Fig. 4: Alio´s MICS diamond knife (Katena Inc, Denville, NJ, USA)

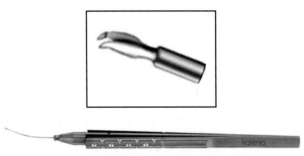

Fig. 5: Alio's MICS capsulorhexis forceps (Katena Inc, Denville, NJ, USA)

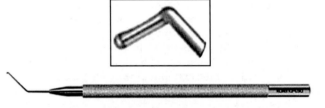

Fig. 6: Alio-Rosen Phaco Prechopper for microincision cataract surgery (Katena Inc, Denville, NJ, USA)

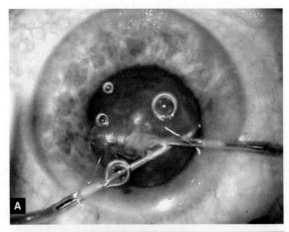
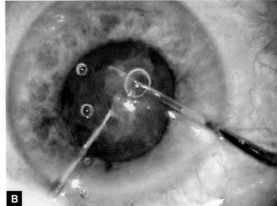
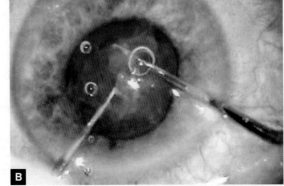

Figs 7A and B: MICS prechopping with Alio-Rosen phaco prechoppers

145

– Decreased Effective Phaco Time (EPT)
  - Prechopping, new irrigating hydromanipulators, fluidics as a tool, effective decrease time of phacoemulsification.[10,11,20,23,39]
- Patient
  – Minimal surgical induced astigmatism
    - Smaller incision means smaller astigmatism[15,30,44]
  – Minimal aberration induction
    - Minor intraoperative injury does not lead to permanent injury of the cornea.[10,14,15,17, 37,44]
  – Faster postoperative recovery
    - Safe and stable anterior chamber operating system with minimal corneal injury reduce recovery time.[10,14,20,23,26,37]
  – Excellent visual acuity
    - Fast and safe operation technique, minimal harmful influence on corneal optic property[5,6,7,15,23,37]

Ophthalmic surgeons who perform cataract surgery in the standard phacoemulsification mode will not have a problem to change the operation technique to MICS because the principle idea of the manipulation inside the eye remains unchanged. The main aim of MICS is to understand the principles.

Summary for the Clinician

- Microincision Cataract Surgery (MICS) is the surgery performed through incisions of 1.5 mm or less
- MICS advantages
  - I/A separation with fluidics work as an instrument
  - Smaller incision
  - Decreased Effective Phaco Time (EPT)
  - Minimal surgical induced astigmatism
  - Minimal aberration induction
  - Faster postoperative recovery
  - Excellent visual acuity

3. INDICATION FOR MICS SURGERY

There is no limitation to indicate a MICS cataract operation. You can operate all grades of cataract LOCS III, even hard cataracts. The subluxated lenses, posttraumatic lenses, zonular laxity and congenital cataracts can also be operated with MICS, with small doses of ultrasound. Generally MICS does not induce astigmatism. MICS is especially dedicated for "refractive cataract operation". MICS can be used for refractive cataract surgery by injecting multifocal lenses and toric lenses.[7,8]

Summary for the Clinician

- All grades of cataract LOCS III can be operated with MICS

4. OUR SURGICAL TECHNIQUE STEP BY STEP

4.1. MICS Anesthesia

After the incision, intraocular anesthesia and mydriatics are applied to the eye. We use 1% lidocaine injecting it into the anterior chamber. Pupil dilatation is achieved by intraocular tropicamide 10% and fenilefrine 10% combination.

4.2. MICS Incision

The incision optimization results from maintaining a stable anterior chamber depth, adapting the incision size to the tools used, implantation of the lens and counter stretching in the route of manipulation. The minimization of the incision is required to carry out MICS correctly. Incisions lower than 1.5 mm do not normally induce post-operative astigmatism.[5] Nowadays we use 19 G (1 / 1.1 mm) i 21 G (0.7 mm) tools to do MICS.

The first stage of the operation is making two corneal incisions with a distance of 90°-110° angle steps. To assure the reduction of existing astigmatism, a dominant incision must be made in a positive meridian of astigmatism. It led to 30% reduction in the refractive cylinder.[6] Relaxing incisions can also be made.[21, 29] Incisions should allow correct tool manipulation, be watertight and the wound should be correctly closed in the postoperative period. The shape of the wound is very important, it should be trapezoidal shaped with a smaller measurement 1.2 mm wide inside the wound near the Descemet membrane and a wider measurement 1.4 mm outside near the epithelium.

This shape is particularly important because of the necessity of the tool manipulation. By forming the wound this way it enables quite a considerable transfer of tools without any distortion, deformation and maceration. It also protects against induced post-operative astigmatism. This is essential as the structure of the wound must be protected against leakage and at the same time it provides an opportunity to work without tissue injury. The mechanical injury to tissues can lengthen the healing process and contribute to leakage, hypotony and increased risk of endophthalmitis. It is also necessary to remember that too small incisions will not allow us to correct manipulations and a too big incision will lead to the uncontrolled leakage from the wound (Fig. 2). The value of such incisions reduces the possibility of exchanging liquids between the anterior chamber and the conjunctiva sack.[9,25,28] To make the incision, we use trapezoidal knives, which allow different widths of incision from 1.2 mm at the peak to 1.4 mm at the base (Katena Inc, Denville, NJ, the USA). To achieve this target two kinds of knives can be used:

Alio´s MICS Knife (Katena Inc, Denville, NJ, the USA). Trapezoid shape 1.25 mm/1.4 mm/2.0 mm angled, double bevel (Fig. 3).

MICS Diamond Knife (Katena Inc, Denville, NJ, USA) trapezoid shaped pale 1.25 mm/1.4 mm/2.0 mm width laser etched line indicating 1.25 mm width (Fig. 4).

4.3. MICS Capsulorhexis

Correctly performed capsulorhexis is vitally important for the MICS procedure. For this we used Alio's MICS Capsulorhexis Forceps (Katena Inc, Denville, NJ, the USA). These are exquisitely delicate forceps with a 23 G diameter (Fig. 5).

They can be easily located in the wound of the cornea. The correct profile of the hilt assures the ergonomic use and normal movements inside the eye. At the end of the forceps a pointed

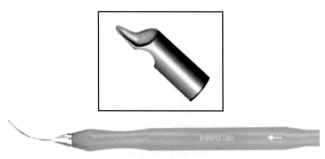

Fig. 8: Alio's original fingernail MICS irrigating hydromanipulator (Katena Inc, Denville, NJ, USA)

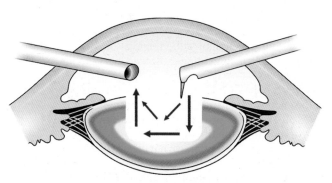

Fig. 9: Posterior irrigation helps to open the capsular bag which does not induce turbulences, elevates nucleus fragments towards the phaco tip and helps in cortex cleaning[4]

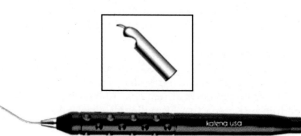

Fig. 10: Alio's MICS Irrigating Stinger (Katena Inc, Denville, NJ, USA)

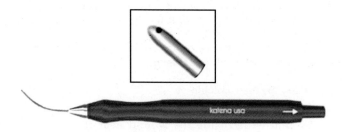

Fig. 11: Alio's MICS aspiration handpiece (Katena Inc, Denville, NJ, USA)

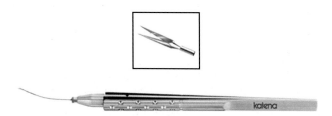

Fig. 12: Alio's MICS scissors (Katena Inc, Denville, NJ, USA)

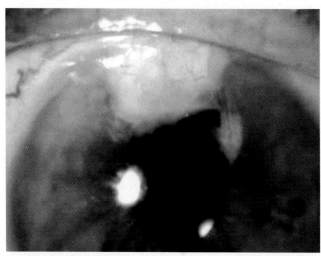

Fig. 13: Corneal burn after surgery. Personal case. This is the only corneal burn so far in our transmission period to MICS and was related to the use of high viscosity viscoelastics

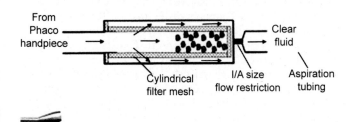

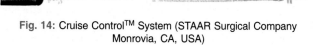

Fig. 14: Cruise Control™ System (STAAR Surgical Company Monrovia, CA, USA)

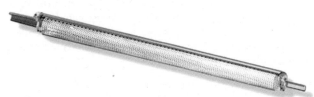

Fig. 15: Stable chamber system (Bausch & Lomb, Rochester, NY, USA)

147

hook is found. This enables a controlled puncturing of the anterior capsule of the lens. Pressure is applied on the capsule and then with a little movement a cut is made. The wide gauged shoulder forceps enable free manipulation of the torn capsule.

The next step is to pull the flap by tearing the capsule clockwise or anticlockwise. The size of the surgical wound and the diameter of the forceps prevent the possibility of the OVD leakage and flattening of the anterior chamber. The lens and the capsule are stabilized. The probability of bad tearing decreases. MICS capsulorhexis forceps allows capsulorhexis without the necessity of the help of the second tool.

4.4. MICS Hydrodissection, Hydrodelineation

The next stage of the cataract operation is the dissection of the lens from the cortex. This is important for pre-chopping as it enables the process of pre-chopping to be carried out in a safe way and does not cause complications. Hydrodissection can diminish the power of ultrasound and surgery time.[42]

In hydrodelineation, liquid is applied under the ring of the anterior capsule into the space of the lens. It enables the nuclei to be elevated and separated from the cortical masses. The maneuvers should be carried out as quickly as possible and with very little amount of liquid. If the nuclei rotation is not possible, hydrodissection maneuvers should be repeated.[34]

4.5. MICS Prechopping

After the hydrodissection of the lens a mechanical division is made. This activity is aimed to make four lens quadrants. Prechopping reduces the amount of the ultrasonic, laser or mechanical energy delivered into the anterior chamber for fragmentation. This is a very important activity in the process of the energy reduction delivered to the eye. This is made with the help of two pre-choppers - Alio-Rosen MICS prechoppers (Katena Inc, Denville, NJ, the USA) (Fig. 6).

Two prechoppers should be inserted into the capsule under the anterior capsular rim, so that they are opposite to each other. The hook of the chopper should be parallel to the anterior capsule. Next the chopper should be gently rotated along the axis of the tool. The chopper should now be situated in the lens under the anterior capsule on the perimeter (Fig. 7).

This activity should be made symmetrically by both hands. The Choppers are crossed by situating each one symmetrically opposite to the other. Next a cutting movement of the lens is made, gently crossing the prechoppers. The cut will be made from the perimeter to the center of nuclei. Internal edge prechoppers have a sharp edge which facilitates the incisions of the lens. This ambidextrous activity is important so that zonular stress does not occur. When the cut is made, two dividing hemispheres are formed. The nucleus is then rotated about 90° and then the prechopping process is repeated as described. After carrying out prechopping we have four lens quadrants in the capsular bag.

4.6. MICS Phacoemulsification and Removal Section

Having shared quadrants we can start phacoemulsification from the first quadrant. We use Alio's MICS hydromanipulator

irrigating fingernail (Katena Inc, Denville, NJ, the USA). Its end is fingernail-like shaped. This tool helps to remove rather soft cataracts. There is an irrigation hole on the bottom lower side of the tool. The hole diameter is 1 mm. It has also very thin walls to increase internal diameter of instrument. This irrigation cannula assures infusion of about 72 cc/min (Fig. 8).

An outstanding stability of the anterior chamber is assured through the infusion and directs the liquid to the lens masses at the back of the capsule, independently from high vacuum sets of the phacoemulsification machine (Fig. 9).

The strength of the stream permits the capsule to be held at a safe distance from the phacoemulsification tip and at the same time enables convenient manipulations of tools and lens masses. Additionally, this stream can clean the back capsule from the remaining cortical cells. A very fertile directed stream to the back capsule is provided with the preservation of corneal endothelial cells from mechanical and thermal damage.

The tool which allows the removal of harder cataracts is Alio´s MICS Irrigating Stinger (Katena Inc, Denville, NJ, USA) (Fig. 10).

This tool has a 19G diameter and it is equipped with a tip at the end which is angled downwards. This tool is useful to chop off segments or dividing masses of the nucleus in the phacoemulsification tip.

In the case of soft cataracts having established the pressure at 500-550 mm Hg we can only use Alio's MICS hydromanipulator irrigating fingernail. This makes it possible to divide and aspirate fragments of the cataract without using ultrasound or using ultrasound in the minimum way. In this case, a torsional phacoemulsification system can be helpful. In the case of hard cataracts, when total occlusion of the tip occurs preventing aspiration, Alio´s MICS Irrigating Stinger would be more useful. This handpiece has a narrow edge at the end which divides the masses and allows easy aspiration of the phacoemulsification tip. The fragmented elements of the hard cataracts are now easily aspirated using the high under pressure and in occasionally using ultrasound energy.

For removing cortical remains, Alio's MICS Aspiration Handpiece (Katena Inc, Denville, NJ, the USA) is a useful instrument (Fig. 11).

It has the port diameter 0.3 mm which assures the stability of the hydrodynamic of liquid within the anterior chamber.

Another auxiliary instrument - Alio's MICS scissors exist for complicated cataracts which may require cutting within the anterior chamber. It can cut delicate membranes, adhesions, to make iridotomy, and also cut the fibrosis of capsules. This tool has 23 gauge curved shaft with horizontal micro blades (Fig. 12).

Their shape allows the comfort of free manipulation in the corner parts of the anterior chamber.

Summary for the Clinician

- Incision - trapezoidal shaped with a smaller measurement 1.2 mm wide inside the wound near the Descemet membrane and a wider measurement 1.4 mm outside near the epithelium.

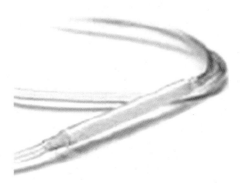

Fig. 16: Stable chamber tubing system (Bausch & Lomb, Rochester, NY, USA)

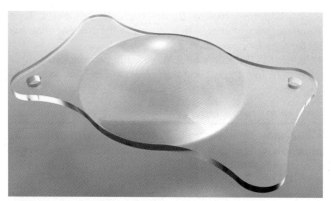

Fig. 17: AcriLisa 366D ACRITEC, Bifocal, aberration correcting, aspherical, foldable one piece lens for capsular capsule fixation and microincision (MICS)

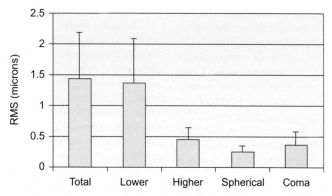

Fig. 18: RMS values and standard deviation of total, lower order, higher order, spherical- and coma-like intraocular aberrations

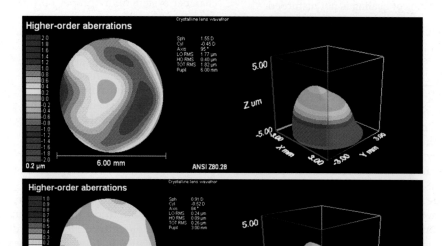

Fig. 19: Wavefront intraocular aberrations after surgery of the AcriLISA 366D at both (a) 6 mm and (b) 3 mm pupil diameters

149

- Prechopping - reduces the amount of the ultrasonic, laser or mechanical energy delivered into the anterior chamber for lens fragmentation
- Alio's MICS hydromanipulators assure an infusion of about 72 cc/min it allows the fluidics to act as a tool and to cool the phaco tip.

5. FLAT INSTRUMENTS CONCEPT

Wound integrity is one of the most important factors that may influence outcome of the surgery. The assurance of the proper amount of the fluidics in MICS requires large dimension of the tools. That is why the corneal tissue can be stressed during the operation. Mechanical tissue stress can evoke leakage, astigmatism, problems of anterior chamber stability.[9,10,14,37] The requirement of tool improvement has become most important. The new Alio's MICS flat tools were made by Katena. The irrigation and aspiration tools have rectangular cross-section. The change of the shape did not influence the fluidics parameters. The fluidics flow of these tools is correct for MICS. The leakage around the tool is absent. The tool manipulation is easy and does not cause corneal tissue stress. Vertical manipulating does not stretch the wound and the horizontal movements do not press the angle of the wound due to the trapezoidal shape. This concept of irrigation-aspiration flat tools is new way of treating the wound. The tools are adapted to the wound, but the wound does not have to be stressed by the tools. The tissue of the wound is untouched.

The self-sealing capability of the incision is mainly dependent on the construction of the wound: the angle, the width to depth ratio and multiple-plane construction of incision. The disturbance of these conditions can have an effect on the postoperative healing. The flat instruments do not affect the edges so the natural process of healing is not disturbed.

Summary for the Clinician

- MICS flat tools don't stretch the wound

6. FLUIDICS IN MICS

In order to use the additional tool the flow of liquids must be fulfilled with the following conditions:
1. Stable incision with no leakage
2. Stable anterior chamber
3. High vacuum

When the diameter of the infusion cannulas is decreased a serious problem occurs. The anterior chamber does not start to fill up with the adequate amount of liquid. An infusion cannula diameter of 21 G is not able to maintain a stable anterior chamber at aspiration and under pressure of 500-600 mm Hg. Each attempt would end with the collapse of the anterior chamber.

Getting the high inflow of liquids into the anterior chamber is possible thanks to a new generation of tools. These tools have a relatively large infusion diameter and the right profile allowing the right flow of liquid and a low level of internal resistance. These conditions do not allow the anterior chamber

to become shallow or rippling of the posterior capsule. Also, the correct amount of liquid ensures chilling of the phacoemulsification tip, and can function with highly efficient aspiration pumps.

According to laws of physics the interior diameter of the tool has a major influence on fluidic resistance, because resistance is proportional to the diameter. Therefore, one is not allowed to apply standard infusion tools from the attention to the insufficient hydrodynamics of these units. Tools assuring the flow higher than 50 cc/min are needed for doing MICS. Current aspiration pumps have a utility which considerably exceeds the flow function of standard tools. The activity of standard infusion cannulas is estimated only for 30 cc/min.

Therefore the need for creating new tools arose in order to meet MICS needs. Katena Inc (Denville, NJ, USA) took on the design and manufacture. A tool set came into existence with a very small diameter in answer to MICS requirements but at the same time with a high flow of about 72 cc/min.

Using the highly efficient pump we must allow the correct inflow of liquid into the anterior chamber. In the case of Accurus, Infinity type equipment we have the additional mechanism of pressurized inflow of fluidics -"gas forced infusion". This can allow controlling the increase in the pressure of the irrigation bottle. This mechanism pumps filtered gas into the irrigation bottle. It allows an additional increase in infusion. Highly efficient irrigation cannulas and the mechanism of gas forced infusion helps provide the comfort of working in stable anatomical conditions.

We can achieve anterior chamber stability in two ways. First, the high inflow of fluidics with proper instrument fluidics flow and forced infusion of fluidics. Secondly, reduced outflow. The diminished diameter of tools and the Cruise Control stable chamber system allow proper outflow without reducing the vacuum.

MICS can be done with different kinds of aspiration systems. However, a Venturi Pump system is most popular and recommended. It has great flexibility, fast reaction. It allows high value of under pressure and the flow as the additional important tool in breaking and removing masses of the lens. The flow can be adjusted, through the amount of vacuum and degree of occlusion of the tip. At present venturi is the most efficient system. MICS settings with different phaco-emulsification platforms are shown in Tables 1 to 3.

Avoiding Corneal Burn

At present biaxial microincision clear cornea phacoemulsification makes it possible to do the treatment practically with no temperature elevation. However, development of high temperatures and incidence of corneal burns are possible (Fig. 13). For example, they may appear when the phaco-emulsification tip is occluded for a long time with lens fragments associated with the use of highly OVD material.[40] They do not occur with the normal flow of liquids as long as the infusion liquid is circulated adequately. Flow control seems to be one of basic conditions of the entire procedure.

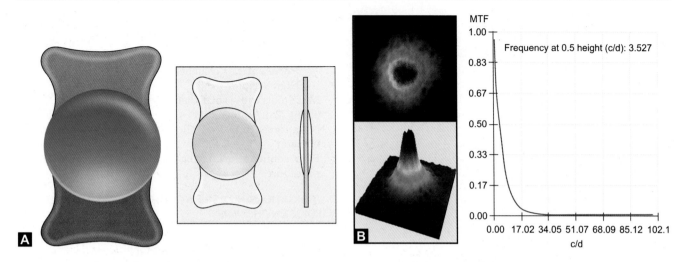

Figs 20A and B: Acri.Smart lens (a)Acri.Smart lens. (b)Optical Quality Analysis
System (OQAS) image comparison with the PSF of treated and untreated Acri.Smart IOL

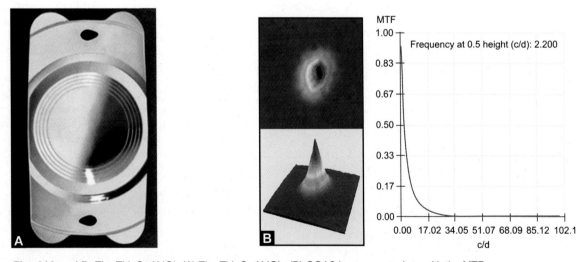

Figs 21A and B: The ThinOptX IOL (A) The ThinOptX IOL. (B) OQAS image comparison with the MTF
of treated and untreated ThinOptX IOL

Table 1: Accurus 600 Alcon settings for 19G MICS		
Quad	Phacoemulsification power	20%
	Vacuum	300 mm Hg
	Irrigation	90
	Mode burst	30 ms

Table 2: Infinity Alcon settings for 19G MICS		
Chop	Phacoemulsification power	0
	Dynamic rise	0
	Vacuum	150
	Irrigation	110
	Torsional amplitude	Limit 40
		On: 20
		Off: 40
	Aspiration rate	15
Quad	Phacoemulsification power	0
	Dynamic rise	2
	Vacuum	500
	Irrigation	110
	Torsional amplitude	Limit 80
		On: 20
		Off: 40
	Aspiration rate	30
Epi	Phacoemulsification power	0
	Vacuum	28
	Irrigation	110
	Torsional amplitude	Limit 30
		On: 20
		Off: 40
	Aspiration rate	28

Note: For 21 G MICS forced air infusion with air pump is necessary

Table 3: Millennium Bausch & Lomb settings for 19G MICS		
Sculpture	Bottle height	100 cm
	Maximum bottle infusion	40 mm Hg
	Fixed vacuum	200 mm Hg
	Fixed U/S	10%
	Duration	20 ms
	Duty cycle	60%
Quadrant	Bottle height	100 cm
	Maximum bottle infusion	40 mm Hg
	Fixed vacuum	470 mm Hg
	Fixed U/S	10%
	Duration	20 ms
	Duty cycle	60%
I/A	Bottle height	80 cm
	Maximum bottle infusion	40 mm Hg
	Maximum vacuum	550 mm Hg

Note: For 21 G MICS forced air infusion with air pump is necessary

Summary for the Clinician

- Fluidics conditions
  - Stable incision with no leakage
  - Stable anterior chamber
  - High vacuum
- MICS tools with a small diameter have a high liquid flow of about 72 cc/min.
- "Gas forced infusion" allows an additional increase in infusion
- Flow control is one of the basic conditions of the entire procedure.

7. IRRIGATION AND ASPIRATION: CREATING A BALANCED FLUIDICS ENVIRONMENT

The aspiration cannula has a smaller internal diameter than the irrigation cannula. This will cause disproportion in the resistance of the flow between infusion and aspiration and additionally will guarantee the anterior chamber stability. The aspirating cannula has a hole of about 0.3 mm diameter. However, increasing the depth of the anterior chamber causes movement of the lens diaphragm which can make the lens fragments enter the space behind the iris. Fragments can get between the iris and the anterior capsule in the space surrounding the sulcus and cannot be seen. However, occasionally the fragments can be observed in the anterior chamber several hours after the operation. Rinsing out and cleaning this space is extremely important.

The stability of the anterior chamber in the case of MICS is indisputably higher than in coaxial phacoemulsification. MICS does not cause frequent and considerable changes in the anatomical proportion of the eyeball and traction does not occur during the operation. From capsulorhexis to filling up with OVD before lens injection it is possible to maintain the anterior chamber stable.

Stable Chamber System

Cruise Control[TM] of the STAAR Surgical Company is an additional system streamlining the irrigating-aspirating system.[12] It is a device specially designed for cataracts in the bimanual microincisional phacoemulsification mode at the high vacuum settings. Cruise control has a disposable flow restrictor with a 0.3 mm internal diameter. It is fixed between the phacoemulsification handpiece and the aspiration tubing. It prevents surges during occlusion breaks at higher vacuum level. It has a mesh filter which safeguards against blocking. Lens fragments remain on the filter. The restrictor limits the flow. At the underpressure of 500 mm Hg, the anterior chamber does not become shallow (Fig.14).

A similar device is offered by Bausch & Lomb. The Stable Chamber differs in size restrictor, however the principle of action remains similar. This device can be attached to the standard phaco machine tubes. (Fig.15)

The Stellaris (Bausch & Lomb, Rochester, NY, USA) offers new tubing technology called Stable Chamber tubing system. This kit consists of tubes integrated with a micromesh filter.

The tubes have reduced diameter and the wall is much more durable. These modifications help to achieve greater power of fluidics and reduces postocclusion surge (Fig 16).

Summary for the Clinician

- Flow restrictor makes the procedure safer and it helps to achieve greater power of fluidics and it reduces postocclusion surge.

8. IS MICROINCISION CATARACT SURGERY WORTHWHILE?

8.1. Clinical Outcome

One of the most important achievements of MICS is the reduction of the US power delivered into the eye. The nucleus breaking is done by mechanical movements of tools, high volume fluidics activity and US power in cataract surgery system. The total effective US power and total ultrasound time can be diminished in MICS surgery. Alio et al indicated that the MICS surgery technique compared to standard coaxial phacoemulsification diminishes the mean incision size with statistical significance (p < 0.001), mean total phacoemulsification percent (p < 0.001) and the mean effective phacoemulsification time (p<0.001).[5] Kahraman et al show that in MICS the mean ultrasound time is statistically lower than in the coaxial group.[20] In Kurz at al the microincision group had shorter EPT and BCVA improved more rapidly than in the coaxial group.[23] Also Cavallini et al explain that microincision surgery can be less invasive, safer, resulting in less postoperative intraocular inflammation, fewer incision related complications and shorter surgical time.[11]

For the corneal endothelium; the clinical evaluations after MICS are variable. But most of them indicate that there is no difference between the coaxial and MICS group. Crema et al indicate in their microincision cataract surgery and coaxial surgery comparative study with one year follow up that central endothelial cell loss can be significant in the MICS group after 1 year. This study also shows that endothelial cell loss 6 months after surgery did not change.[13] Wilczynski et al did not find any difference in endothelial cell loss between the MICS and standard phacoemulsification group. The endothelial cell loss was similar in both groups and the difference was not statistically significant.[43] Kahraman et al confirm this in their investigation.[20] Also Mencucci et al report that the endothelial cell loss was similar in the MICS and coaxial group.[26]

8.2. Outcome of the Incision

MICS is performed using new technology, so the US tip does not need to be extensively cooled. Using rapid on-off cycles you can reduce power delivered to the tip. Donnenfeld et al. showed that increase of the temperature during bimanual phacoemulsification can be lower than temperature increase during coaxial phacoemulsification, and no wound damage was observed.[14]

Experimental models of sleeveless bimanual phacoemulsification indicate that advanced microburst or hyperpulse technology does not enhance corneal temperature over the corneal damage threshold and additionally did not pass 39.0ºC even with tip occlusion.[10] The total amount of the US power used in MICS surgery is much lower than the power which can damage the cornea.[38] The sleeveless US tip does not deform the incision and there is a sufficient flow to cool the tip during phacoemulsification so the risk of thermal burn is minimal.[41] Additionally the corneal swelling is much less significant in smaller incisions than in standard coaxial incisions.[16]

The problem with leakage after the wound stress has been described.[9] However, the integrity of the wound can be achieved using MICS tools and the new Alio's MICS flat instruments. The incision can be tight with no leakage and the tissues are not stressed. The sub 2.0 mm MICS incision has good self-sealing ability and additionally does not cause postoperative astigmatism in most cases.[5]

8.3. Astigmatism Control with MICS

Among the major advantages of MICS is the reduction of surgical trauma resulting in a reduction of surgically induced astigmatism (SIA), aberrations and improvement of the optical quality of the cornea after surgery, thus leading to improvement of visual outcome and high patient satisfaction.[3, 27]

Degraded optical quality of the cornea after incisional cataract surgery would limit the performance of the pseudophakic eye. Thus, it is important not to increase or to induce astigmatism and/or corneal aberrations after cataract surgery.[44] Even with MICS, we could achieve reduction of astigmatism and higher order corneal aberrations.[19] The optical quality of the cornea plays an important role in the recovery of the visual function after cataract surgery, and this is determined by a combination of corneal and internal aberrations generated by the IOL and those induced by the surgery. These corneal refractive changes are attributed to the location and size of the corneal incision. The smaller the incision, the lower the aberrations, the better the optical quality.[18]

We have described the improved control of surgically induced astigmatism with MICS when compared to conventional 3 mm phacoemulsification. A great advantage of MICS is the reduction of SIA and that the microincisions do not produce an increase in astigmatism.[5] The shorter the incision, the less the corneal astigmatism, as it was estimated that the magnitude of the SIA studied by vector analysis is around 0.44 and 0.88 diopters, rising as the size of the incision increases.[36, 42] This is considered important because cataract surgery today is considered more and more a refractive procedure.[5]

Also, small-incision surgery (3.5-mm incision without suture) does not systematically degrade the optical quality of the anterior corneal surface. However, it introduces changes in some aberrations, especially in non-rotationally symmetric terms such as astigmatism, coma, and trefoil.[17] Therefore, one has to expect better results and fewer changes with sub 2 mm incision (MICS).

This is supported by the finding that the corneal incision of < 2 mm had no impact on corneal curvature.[19, 30, 32] Going hand in hand with the modern concept of making cataract surgery a refractive procedure, by controlling and even decreasing astigmatism and HOA by using MICS, which is the state-of-the-art.

8.4. Corneal Aberration Control with MICS

Nowadays cataract surgery is not only removal of an opaque lens, but also it is a part of refractive surgery. The technical progress generated high standards of ophthalmic machines and tools. We can obtain precise IOL power calculation, reduce residual astigmatism and do surgery without surgically induced astigmatism (SIA). Corneal refractive surgery becomes more popular and more excellent. For this reason the lens we are using should be perfect.

Optical Quality of MICS IOL

Our experience with MICS has proved its effectiveness in stabilizing the corneal optics after surgery without degradation of the corneal optical quality.[15] Thus for a MICS IOL to fulfill this advantage, it should help to improve the control of the optical performance of the human eye. Consequently, such IOL should be aberration and scattering free, not to cause night-vision complaints such as halos and glare, with similar or even better optical outcome when compared to conventional lenses.[3]

The optical quality of the psuedophakic eye is largely affected by aberrations induced by the implanted IOL. These aberrations depend on two characteristics of the lens, thickness and surface quality, and will vary depending on the type of IOL implanted.[7]

Among the currently available MICS IOLs, only few of them have been evaluated from the optical quality point of view. Generally, obtaining optical quality and biocompatibility similar to conventional intraocular lenses in vivo.[3, 7]

For Acri.Smart IOLs (Acri-Tec GmbH, Berlin, Germany), studying the point spread function (PSF) before and after pushing the lens through the Acri.Glide cartridge (Acri-Tec GmbH, Hennigsdorf, Germany), revealed no difference between the Acri.Smart lens before and after. This was further supported by an interesting study comparing the retinal image quality after implantation of 2 MICS IOLs and a conventional IOL, by evaluating the modulation-transfer function (MTF), 0.1 and 0.5 values for Acri.Smart and ThinOptX UltraChoice 1.0 IOL (ThinOptX Inc, Abrindon, Virginia, USA) for MICS versus AcrySof conventional lens (AcrySof MA60BM, Alcon Laboratories Inc, Ft Worth, USA), with no statistical difference between all of these lenses (Table 4).[7] Also, the manufacturing company studied the MTF for the ThinOptX MICS IOL,

concluding that each stepped ring provides the same optical information to the same focal point on the retina and MTF and visual acuity, therefore providing excellent refractive design.[3] Recently, the aberration-correcting effect of ThinOptX IOL has been evaluated by comparing the spherical aberration between ThinOptX and Alcon Acry S of lens. The results demonstrated that although no statistically significant difference in the root mean square (RMS) for spherical aberration, the ThinOptX eyes showed smaller spherical aberrations being designed for negative spherical aberration.[33]

Recently we evaluated a new MICS multifocal IOL, the Acri.LISA 366D (Acritec GmbH, Hennigsdorf, Germany) (Fig. 17).[2] We analyzed objectively the intraocular optical quality in vivo of this diffractive asymmetrical light distribution multifocal IOL, the main outcomes were RMS values for intraocular aberrations, Strehl ratio and the MTF (0.5 and cut-off), by using an intraocular optical analysis model.[31] The Acritec Acri.LISA 366D showed excellent intraocular optical performance as demonstrated by good values for the intraocular optical aberrations, Strehl ratio and MTF, (Figs 18 and 19). Such an effect can be additionally explained by Acri.LISA neutral asphericity and aberration correcting profile.[2]

Finally, we can conclude that for an ideal MICS IOL it is not enough to have low optical aberrations but it must also be able to compensate for corneal aberrations (coupling of 2 optical systems), an effect which can work with MICS in stabilizing corneal optical quality. The evaluation of MTF in vivo may be the best method to study the optical quality of eyes implanted with IOLs which could be objectively measured by the Optical Quality Analysis System (OQAS, Visiometrics S.L. Tarrasa, Spain) which calculates also the PSF. Consequently, MICS IOLs perform well inside the eye, their folding and unfolding does not cause structural and functional defects, which together with neuroprocessing allows excellent IOL optical performance in vivo.[3, 5, 7]

The other study shows that UltraChoice 1.0 ThinOptX and Acri.Smart 48S MICS lenses have excellent MTF performance. In this study there was no difference between these lenses and AcrySof MA60BM lenses. This indicates that there is no difference between MICS lenses and conventional cataract lens. Small incision, folding and unfolding did not cause structural and functional defects (Figs 20 and 21).[3, 7]

IOL type	Incision size (mm)	Mean IOL power (D ± SD)	Mean after surgery defocus equivalent (D ± SD)	Mean BCVA after surgery	Mean spatial frequency (cpd) at 0.5 MTF ± SD	Mean spatial frequency (cpd) at 0.1 MTF ± SD
Alcon AcrySof MA60 BM	3.2	19.86 ± 6.21	1.13 ± 0.72	20/20	2.647 ± 0.833	8.720 ± 3.074
ThinOptX Ultra Choice 1.0	1.6–1.8	20.39 ± 1.05	0.88 ± 0.35	20/20	2.601 ± 0.986	8.814 ± 4.380
Acri. Smart 48S	1.6 - 1.8	23.25 ± 4.6	1.00 ± 0.63	20/20	3.453 ± 0.778	11.418 ± 2.574

Table 4: MTF value of Acri.Smart IOL, ThinOptX IOL and AcrySof IOL[3]

Summary for the Clinician

- MICS surgery technique compared to standard coaxial phacoemulsification:
    - diminishes the mean incision size
    - diminishes the mean effective phacoemulsification time
    - diminishes surgical time
    - diminishes postoperative intraocular inflammation
    - diminishes complications
    - diminishes surgically induced astigmatism
- With MICS, we can achieve a reduction of astigmatism and higher order corneal aberrations

9. END OF THE SURGERY

Endophthalmitis prevention is the last part of the surgery. The procedure is finished by injecting 0.1-0.2 cc of cefuroxime into the anterior chamber. Next, corneal wound hydratation should be done to close the wound and 2-3 drops of povidone iodine administrated into the conjunctival sac. The state of incisions is verified in the slit lamp after half an hour. If leakage appears, the procedure of hydratation should be repeated.

10. FUTURE OF MICS

Unfortunately, new ideas in the field of the cataract surgery are limited by technical possibilities. However a major problem remains in the possibility of lens compression. The foldable intra-ocular lenses are compressed only to 1.5 mm.of incision. MICS makes the wound smaller and it will evolve into reduction of incision, energy and eye injury. The future belongs to the miniaturization of the tools and the wound size. A minimization of the energy and manual activities must occur in the anterior chamber. The problem of energy still remains a problem to be solved. The next step could be subsonic oscillation and lasers. In the future, the laser will supply the ultrasound energy and may become standard technology of breaking nuclei of the lenses. However, it is not possible to remove hard cataracts with the help of new types of lasers at the present stage of technology. Also the ultrasound energy and laser energy connection can bring the desired effect in the future. Laser energy will make it possible to remove cataracts with incisions smaller than 0.7 mm.

Managing the flow of liquids also will change together with the development of infusion and aspirating pumps. The problem with providing large amounts of liquids by irrigation tools still occurs. The development of highly efficient fluid injectors and new liquid substances with a different viscosity will be the perfect solution.

MICS development and evolution will be necessary in the future.

REFERENCES

1. Alió JL. What is the future of cataract surgery?. Ocular Surg News 2006;17:3-4.
2. Alió JL, Elkady B, Ortiz D, Bernabeu G. Clinical Outcomes and Intraocular Optical Quality of a Diffractive Asymmetrical Light Distribution Multifocal Intraocular Lens (Acri.LISA 366D). J Cataract Refract Surg. Accepted for publication, 2007.
3. Alio JL, Rodriguez-Prats JL, Galal A. Advances in microincision cataract surgery intraocular lenses Curr Opin Ophthalmol 2006;17:80–93.
4. Alio JL, Rodriguez Prats JL, Galal A. MICS Micro-incision Cataract Surgery. Highlights of Ophthalmology International, Miami, 2004.
5. Alio JL, Rodriguez-Prats JL, Galal A, Ramzy M. Outcomes of microincision cataract surgery versus coaxial phacoemulsification. Ophthalmology 112:1997-2003.
6. Alio JL, Rodriguez-Prats JL, Vianello A, Galal A. Visual outcome of microincision cataract surgery with implantation of Acri Smart Lens J Cataract Refract Surg 2005;31:1549–56.
7. Alió JL, Schimchak P, Montés-Micó R, Galal A. Retinal image quality after microincision intraocular lens implantation. J Cataract Refract Surg 2005;31:1557-60.
8. Assaf A, El-Moatassem Kotb AM. Feasibility of bimanual microincision phacoemulsification in hard cataracts. Eye 2007;21:807-11.
9. Berdahl JP, DeStafeno JJ, Kim T. Corneal wound architecture and integrity after phacoemulsification evaluation of coaxial, microincision coaxial, and microincision bimanual techniques. J Cataract Refract Surg 2007;33: 510-15.
10. Braga-Mele R. Thermal effect of microburst and hyperpulse settings during sleeveless bimanual phacoemulsification with advanced power modulations. J Cataract Refract Surg 2006;32:639-42.
11. Cavallini GM, Campi L, Masini C, Pelloni S, Pupino A. Bimanual microphacoemulsification versus coaxial miniphacoemulsification: Prospective study. J Cataract Refract Surg 2007;33:387-92.
12. Chang DF. 400 mm Hg High-Vacuum Bimanual Phaco Attainable with the Staar Cruise Control Device J Cataract Refract Surg 2004;30:932-33.
13. Crema AS, Walsh A, Yamane Y, Nosé W. Comparative study of coaxial phacoemulsification and microincision cataract surgery. One-year follow-up. J Cataract Refract Surg 2007;33:1014-8.
14. Donnenfeld ED, Olson RJ, Solomon R, Finger PT, Biser SA, Perry HD, Doshi S. Efficacy and wound-temperature gradient of WhiteStar phacoemulsification through a 1.2 mm incision. J Cataract Refract Surg 2003;29:1097-100.
15. Elkady B, Alió JL, Ortiz D, Montalbán R. Corneal aberrations after microincision cataract surgery. J Cataract Refract Surg 2008;34:40-45.
16. Fine IH, Hoffman RS, Packer M. Profile of clear corneal cataract incisions demonstrated by ocular coherence tomography. J Cataract Refract Surg 2007;33:94-7.
17. Guirao A, Tejedor J, Artal P. Corneal aberrations before and after small-incision cataract surgery. Inves Ophthalmol Vis Sci 2004;45:4312-4319.
18. Holladay JT. Optical quality and refractive surgery. Int Ophthalmol Clin 2003;43:119-136.
19. Jiang Y, Le Q, Yang J, Lu Y. Changes in corneal astigmatism and high order aberrations after clear corneal tunnel phacoemulsification guided by corneal topography. J Refract Surg 2006;22:1083-88.
20. Kahraman G, Amon M, Franz C, Prinz A, Abela-Formanek C. Intraindividual comparison of surgical trauma after bimanual microincision and conventional small-incision coaxial phacoemulsification. J Cataract Refract Surg 2007;33(4): 618-22.

155

21. Kaufmann C, Peter J, Ooi K, Phipps S, Cooper P, Goggin M. The Queen Elizabeth Astigmatism Study Group. Limbal relaxing incisions versus on-axis incisions to reduce corneal astigmatism at the time of cataract surgery. J Cataract Refract Surg 2005;31:2261-65.

22. Khng C, Packer M, Fine IH, Hoffman RS, Moreira FB. Intraocular pressure during phacoemulsification. J Cataract Refract Surg 2006;32:301-08.

23. Kurz S, Krummenauer F, Gabriel P, Pfeiffer N, Dick HB. Biaxial microincision versus coaxial small-incision clear cornea cataract surgery. Ophthalmology 2006;113:1818-26.

24. Masket S, Tennen DG. Astigmatic stabilization of 3.0 mm temporal clear corneal cataract incisions. J Cataract Refract 1996;22:1451-55.

25. Mehran T, Behrens A, Newcomb R, Nobe M, Saedi G, McDonnell P. Acute Endophthalmitis Following Cataract Surgery and Systematic Review of the Literature. Arch Ophthalmol 2005;123:613-20.

26. Mencucci R, Ponchietti C, Virgili G, Giansanti F, Menchini U. Corneal endothelial damage after cataract surgery: Microincision versus standard technique. J Cataract Refract Surg 2006;32:1351-4.

27. Naeser K, Knudsen EB, Hansen MK. Bivariate polar value analysis of surgically induced astigmatism.J Refract Surg 2002;18:72-78.

28. Nagaki Y, Hayasaka., Kadoi C, Matsumoto the M, Yanagisawa, Watanabe K, Watanabe K, Hayasaka Y, Ikeda N, Sato, Kataoka Y, Togashi M, Abe J. Bacterial endophthalmitis after small-incision cataract surgery: Effect of incision placement and intraocular lens type Cataract Refract Surg 2003;29:20-26.

29. Nichamin L. Treating astigmatism at the time of cataract surgery. Current Opinion in Ophthalmology 2003;14: 35-38.

30. Olson RJ, Crandall AS. Prospective randomized comparison of phacoemulsification cataract surgery with a 3.2-mm vs a 5.5-mm sutureless incision. Am J Ophthalmol 1998;125: 612-620.

31. Ortiz D, Alió JL, Bernabeu G, Pongo V. Optical quality performance inside the human eye of monofocal and multifocal intraocular lenses. J Cataract Refract Surg Accepted for publication, 2007.

32. Oshika T, Tsuboi S. Astigmatic and refractive stabilization after cataract surgery. Ophthalmic Surg 1995;26:309-15.

33. Ouchi M, Kinoshita S. Aberration-correcting effect of ThinOptX IOL. Eye 2007;21.

34. Peng Q, Apple DJ, Visessook N, Werner L, Pandey SK, Escobar-Gomez M, Schoderbek R, Guindi A. Surgical prevention of posterior capsule opacification. Part 2: Enhancement of cortical cleanup by focusing on hydrodissection. J Cataract Refract Surg 2000;26:188-97.

35. Shearing SP, Relyea RL, Loaiza and, Shearing RL. Routine phacoemulsification through and they millimeter non-sutured incision. Cataract 1985;2:6-11.

36. Simsek S, Yasar T, Demirok A, Cinal A, Yilmaz OF. Effect of superior and temporal clear corneal incisions on astigmatism after sutureless phacoemulsification. J Cataract Refract Surg 1998;24:515-18.

37. Soscia W, Howard JG, Olson RJ. Bimanual phacoemulsification through 2 stab incisions. A wound-temperature study. J Cataract Refract Surg 2002;28:1039-43.

38. Soscia W, Howard JG, Olson RJ. Microphacoemulsification with WhiteStar. A wound-temperature study. J Cataract Refract Surg 2002;28:1044-6.

39. Tanaka T, Koshika S, Usui M. Cataract surgery using the bimanual phacoemulsification technique with an Accurus system and Mackool microphaco tip. J Cataract Refract Surg 2007;33:1770-74.

40. Tsuneoka H, Hayama A, Takahama M. Ultrasmall-incision bimanual phacoemulsification and AcrySof SA30AL implantation through a 2.2 mm incision J Cataract Refract Surg 2003;29:1070–76.

41. Tsuneoka H, Shiba T, Takahashi Y. Feasibility of ultrasound cataract surgery with a 1.4 mm incision. J Cataract Refract Surg 2001;27(6):934-40.

42. Vasavada AR, Singh R, Apple DJ, Trivedi RH, Pandey SK, Werner L. Effect of hydrodissection on intraoperative performance: Randomized study. J Cataract Refract Surg 2002;28:1623-28.

43. Wilczynski M, Drobniewski I, Synder A, Omulecki W. Evaluation of early corneal endothelial cell loss in bimanual microincision cataract surgery (MICS) in comparison with standard phacoemulsification. Eur J Ophthalmol 2006;16:798-803.

44. Yao K, Tang X, Ye P. Corneal astigmatism, high order aberrations, and optical quality after cataract surgery: Microincision versus small-incision. J Refract Surg 2006;22: 1079-82.

Chapter 28

A Challenging Case of IOL Power Calculation after Previous Refractive Surgery

Frank Goes (Belgium)

Since we started excimer laser surgery in 1991 we gathered clinical experience of more than 100 cataract and lens Implant surgeries in eyes that had previous refractive surgery such as—**Radial keratotomy -Excimer laser (LASIK-EpiLASIK-LASEK-PRK) - LTK –CK.**

We started Radial keratotomy in 1981and performed more than 1300 surgeries.

We started Excimer laser surgery in 1991 and have performed more than 13.000 cases until now.

We started LTK in 1998 and have performed 450 cases.

We started CK in 2005 and have experience of 40 cases.

We will analyse here a complicated case/How to determine the emmetropizing IOL power in an eye after previous RK and LASIK surgery.

PATIENT CHRIS VT/AGE 53

1. In **1988** this patient underwent **Radial keratotomy** for - 4,75 cyl -1 axis /16K1 43.25 K2 43.50 uncomplicated surgery; 8 incisions was performed.
2. **In 1999**-11 years-later she developed a progressive hyperopic shift: +4cyl -1.25 axis 70: K1 39.7 -K2 34.9-UCVA 0.1 -BSCVA 0.8
   HYPEROPIC LASIK with A Hansatome was performed; the incisions did not open during the keratotomy. Postop UCVA 0.9
3. **In 2003** she had a regression
   +3.5 CYL -2.5 AXIS 65: K1 37.2- K2 34.- AXL 25.42 mm. UCVA 0,2-BSCVA 0.7
   REDO HYPERLASIK was performed. Again the incisions did not split during the opening of the flap.
4. In 2008 October / development of cortical cataract r eye; acuity under glare 0.05.

IOL MASTER

AXL 25.5 mm.-K1 38.01 AXIS 39-K2 41.77 A1XIS 129 -ACD 3.51 mm.

Tomey Values

K1 38.1 AXIS 41 -K2 42.2 AXIS 131

DISCUSSION

We know that there are 3 kinds of errors after refractive surgery: radius error, K-index error, IOL formula error.

Since the Haigis formula is not suffering from the IOL formula error, this the best choice. After RK, there is no K-index error. To minimize a possible radius error, IOL Master keratometry has to be used which is known to measure closer to the optical axis than any other keratometer. So, prior to the hyperopic LASIK correction, IOL Master data with the Haigis formula would have been the choice.

After hyperopic LASIK, there will be no radius error, but a K-index and IOL formula error. Ignoring radius and K-index error and again using the Haigis formula , an average myopic shift in refraction of the order of 0.5 D is expected.

Thus, with the constants for the Alcon SN60WF, the following results are obtained using this rationale:

IOL = 20.0 D → Rx = + 0.1 D
IOL = 20.5 D → Rx = – 0.2 D

and we would expect a refraction a little (0.3 -0.5D) more myopic than calculated.

Also, applying paraxial thick lens ray-tracing, Prof. Haigis obtained an emmetropizing IOL power of 20.5 D for emmetropia.

Dr Warren Hill also advised to use the Haigis L formula after hyperopic LASIK.

Calculation outcomes, using Tomey measurements, for a Emmetropizing Alcon IOL ACRYSOF WF IOL gave the following results; Holladay 19,5D -Haigis 20- D.Srkt 19 D-A 21,5 D lens was placed.

So, summarizing, a 20.5 D IOL would be a reasonable choice for emmetropia.

SURGERY

IOL implanted was; 21,5 D SN60WF. We aimed for safety; better some myopia than some hyperopia.

Postop: Dry eyes: UCVA 0,2-BSCVA 0,6 sf-0.25 cyl-3.5 Axis 55.The **result** was a sf.equivalent error of only -0.75 D.

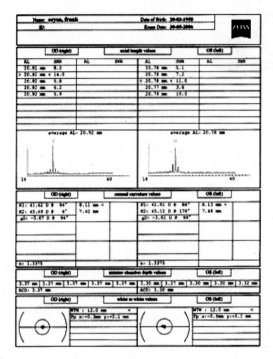

Fig. 1

4 weeks after surgery an "Enhancement LASIK. cyl. -3,5 D AXIS 55° "was performed and UCVA became 0,7-but still complaints about dry eyes.

CONCLUSION

1. After multiple surgeries the " dry eye" problem will becomes very important.

2. A refraction error, even with all best formulas possible, is to be foreseen in such a case-although the spherical equivalents was only 1 dptr off and we erred on the myopic side, which was good.

3. Use different formula's and look specifically at the Haigis formula which is performing well in these circumstances.

Chapter 29

Lens Surgery after Previous Refractive Surgery

Frank Goes (Belgium)

INTRODUCTION

We would like to share with you our clinical experience of more than 100 cataract and lens Implant surgeries in eyes that had previous refractive surgery such as -**Radial keratotomy - Excimer laser (LASIK-EpiLASIK-LASEK-PRK) - LTK – CK.**

DIAGNOSIS-DECISION MAKING –THE SURGERY – IOL CALCULATION –THE OUTCOME

* We started Radial keratotomy in 1981 and performed more than 1300 surgeries.
* We started Excimer laser surgery in 1991 and have performed more than 13.000 cases until now.
* We started LTK in 1998 and have performed 450 cases.
* We started CK in 2005 and have experience of 40 cases.

We have probably a better follow-up of cataract surgery after previous refractive surgery than any other clinic in the **world since we are in Excimer laser business since 1991 and have an excellent follow-up in our own private clinic.** (F.Goes Sr-F.Goes Jr.-C.Verschueren-N.Marien-A.Hoste-A.Lefebvre).

We will review three different groups:

* Lens surgery after previous **Myopic Excimer laser surgery**
* Lens surgery after previous **Hyperopic Excimer laser surgery**
* Lens surgery after previous **Radial keratotomy surgery**

DEMOGRAPHICS

In our database we included **108 eyes with sufficient follow-up**: 77 lens surgeries and IOL implantation after previous refractive surgery for **myopia** and 30 after previous refractive surgery for **hyperopia.**

The majority of lens surgeries were carried out in eyes with primary **PRK as a** Refractive procedure 58 eyes: 37 eyes had previous **LASIK** surgery-7 eyes had previous **RK** surgery – 4 **LTK** Surgery and 2 had **CK** surgery.

In the whole group there were **72 female** and **35 male** eyes; this corresponds with the distribution of patients coming in for refractive surgery purposes.

DECISION MAKING

Lens surgery was discussed whenever we felt that this procedure could solve the problem of a patient coming in with **visual complaints** after previous refractive surgery or **progressive refraction change** with a decrease of his UCVA and or BSCVA.

When all other reasons of visual deterioration were explored and regression after previous refractive procedure or the lens opacification were the only reasonable explanations for the complaints then the decision to replace the lens was made. When in doubt one has to follow the patients for 3-6 months repeat the topographies in order to arrive to a correct diagnosis document eventual progression and exclude all other possible reasons for a refractive change or a decrease of BCVA -after having performed Oct- Angiography –Topography-Careful fundoscopy- and visual field analysis

The main indication and reason for surgery in this group was **visual loss** or **subjective disturbances** caused by cataract formation-or **regression** in eyes after previous hyperopic surgery.

In case of regression after hyperopic refractive surgery we would decide faster for refractive lens exchange than in an eye with previous myopic surgery since we know that a retinal detachment after eventual Yag Laser Capsulotomy is infrequent or inexistent in short hyperopic eyes and is more frequent than normal in myopic eyes.

In case of regression after previous myopic surgery we proposed an enhancement when enough tissue was still available and when the natural lens was still healthy.

In the eyes that developed cataract after previous myopic laser surgery we nearly always found an ongoing myopization reaching sometimes values as high as -10 dptr. One can imagine that it becomes very difficult to use the history method in these cases as a basis for IOL power calculation, since the endpoint after the first laser surgery is difficult to determine. Often these patients had still reasonably good objective visual acuity but of course a lot of subjective complaints as glare and halos caused

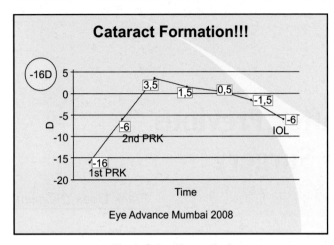

Fig. 1: Calcualtion method

by the change in lens index and the burden of a need to change spectacles frequently because of the ongoing myopization caused by the nuclear sclerosis.

IOL CHOICE

Since we performed our first cataract surgery after previous refractive surgery in1999! most of the eyes in the study were operated before the area of aspheric and multifocal IOLs.

The majority had silicone or acrylic **monofocal** IOL implanted and the early cases even had 6 mm IOLs. We would not implant a **multifocal IOL** in a post RK eye with more than four incisions since they have too many aberrations. I would not hesitate to implant a multifocal like the Tecnis MF in a post excimer laser surgery cataractous eye. However, I would warn the patient that they might need an enhancement because of imperfect IOL power calculation.

The preferred lens in case a monofocal IOL becomes the option would be an aspheric lens whenever possible. The choice of asphericity would be adapted according to the previous surgery and specifically in eyes with previous Hyperopic LASIK an aspheric neutral IOL would be the choice otherwise the AMO Tecnis monofocal or the Alcon Natural wave would be good choices.

SURGICAL CONSIDERATIONS OF CATARACT SURGERY AFTER PREVIOUS REFRACTIVE SURGERY. HOW TO PROCEED?

It is interesting to mention that the literature **not one article** was found describing the surgical approach and eventual tricks to apply when performing surgery in this group of patients. Only in the bible of Chang's book these items are discussed.

In our whole group not one complication or adverse effect occurred during or after surgery.

Radial Keratotomy

We performed phacosurgery in these eyes, using a clear corneal 3.0 to 3.2 mm incision exactly in between two radial incisions. In **8 incisions RK** eyes there is usually enough space to place a

clear corneal incision between the RK incisions. After having entered the eye, routine phacoemulsification was performed and the appropriate IOL was implanted. In two eyes one of the radial incisions opened and we had two place two corneal sutures; these sutures were removed after 6 weeks without causing any astigmatism.

In order to avoid an unstable wound or peroperative trauma we would advise a scleral tunnel approach in eyes treated with **16 or more radial incisions**. This scleral tunnel incision will not need suturing.

In the seven eyes operated after previous RK We have never seen a permanent instability of the cornea during the procedure or some ongoing refraction change in the postoperative period that could have been attributed to the earlier surgical trauma.

Excimer Laser

In the group of cataractous eyes after previous refractive excimer laser surgery also a clear corneal incision with a 3.0 mm.size was the preferred way. According to our subtraction he thinnest cornea of these eyes measured 400 micron centrally. We have never seen any abnormal reaction of the eye in these cases, except for the fact that long myopic eyes have a low scleral rigidity so that focusing during phacosurgery may become very difficult.

IOL POWER CALCULATION AFTER PREVIOUS CORNEAL REFRACTIVE SURGERY

Determining the IOL power in a cataract patient has **always been challenging**, but became a lot tougher lately. Thanks to refractive surgery, more and more individuals with cataracts have altered corneas that make it difficult to provide an acceptable outcome for cataract surgery. Many surgeons have tried to solve this problem, but so far the result has been a proliferation of formulas and methods with not one solution rising to the top.

As said in the introduction the topic of this chapter is not to discuss formula's. Nevertheless it is interesting to say that we, in our local meetings, **already from 1999** on highlighted the difficulty of IOL power calculations after previous refractive surgery.

Now in the literature, more than 100 papers have been published on this topic and the predictability of Iol power calculation improved enormously. We are, however, still convinced that the routine cataract surgeon did not always find the right approach for this complicated problem. That's why we have added in this book an important section on the new approaches of iol power calculation after previous refractive surgery.

Figure 1 shows a nice example of the problems that could be encountered in earlier days when we had to rely on the "Clinical History Method". Since most of the cataracts in these myopic eyes after previous Excimer laser surgery are nuclear cataracts, causing a myopisation of the eye, it was not always easy to determine the endpoint of stabilization after the first Excimer laser surgery (Fig 1).

160

Calculating IOL power after refractive surgery is **tough for several reasons** discussed in different sections of the book.

1. Most keratometers do not measure the central cornea where the effective corneal power is.
2. LASIK and PRK change the index of refraction between the front and back surfaces of the cornea;
3. Many modern formulas predict IOL position using the axial length and corneal curvature.

Kenneth J. Hoffer, MD (see section) has recently created a spreadsheet containing all of the formulas that would automatically do the calculations for every formula incorporating the data the surgeon can provide. According to Dr. Hoffer there are currently about 24 formulations in use. They can be divided into two major categories. "The **first group** tries to predict the true power of the patient's cornea base on multiple factors. These formulas give you a different K-reading to plug into your IOL power calculation. The **remaining methods** say, 'OK, your direct K-reading may not be accurate, but go ahead and calculate the IOL power; we'll give you a way to fudge or adjust that power to make up for the error.' Each of these groups can be subdivided into those that require some preoperative historical data and those that don't."

Even when all the pre-refractive surgery measurements are available, determining the correct IOL power with certainty can **still be difficult or impossible.** Since topographers and keratometers only measure the front surface of the cornea, "To calculate corneal power, you need to know the ratio of the front surface to the back surface. In a virgin eye, the front surface curvature is sufficient to give you a close approximation of corneal power because the ration of the back to front surface radii is about 82 percent (6.32/7.70) in the vast majority of normal eyes. **Refractive surgeries such as LASIK or PRK change only the front surface, altering the ratio**. Determining the correct ratio becomes a second source of error.

Since Wolfgang Haigis introduced a new Haigis L formula in connection with the IOL master measurement. (see his chapter) the task has become much easier.

A CASE REPORT

We will illustrate the currently existing problems with a case report.

A 43 years old lady (DS Nicole) had Excimer PRK in 1994 for -14 Dptr: t K values before surgery K1 43, 9 –K2 42 Dptr-Axl 30.86 mm.

Emmetropia was achieved in 1997. Due to a progressive nuclear sclerosis subjective complaints of glare and halos and visual deterioration became too important so that cataract surgery and IOL implantation was decided.

Using the routine IOL measurement data for calculation with a measured K1 32,6 D and K2 34 D with the autokeratometer- the emmetropizing IOL would have been **14 D according to SRK T,16 D according to Haigis,** and **20 D according to the Haigis L**. Using a corrected K value of 31,81 D according to the clinical history method –with the **SrKT formula 15,5 D** would have been the emmetropizing IOL. We implanted a 19 D IOL aiming for some myopia and came (with some luck)out at -0,5 D. So **differences up to 6 D** were found when using different formulas-. When relying on the newer formulas again **differences up to 4,5 D.** were still present.

In our whole series –going back 10 years with my first case done- the mean refractive error using a mix of approaches was a maximum error of 8 Dptr in the early days and 7/77 eyes in the myopia group needed a piggy back.

This has changed importantly recently since we can now use IOL master measurements with updated calculations formula's by Prof. Haigis or Pentacam measurements and calculate from these data without a need for clinical history.

In hyperopia the problems are less important since we change the cornea's less in the centre and we limit ourselves to maximum 5 dptr.

IN CONCLUSION

1. Look **at least at two formulas.**
2. Take the least corneal power the formulas produce and then use the Iol that has **the highest power.** It is much safer to err on the negative side- since these patients will still able to read without glasses- than the- opposite-erring on the plus side since this will give bad near and bad distance vision. When in doubt aim **for some (-1.0 Dptr.) myopia.**

We will review clinical outcomes in three different groups:

- Lens surgery after previous **Myopia Excimer laser surgery**
- Lens surgery after previous **Hyperopia Excimer laser surgery**
- Lens surgery after previous **Radial Keratotomy surgery.**

CLINICAL OUTCOMES - RESULTS—FOLLOW-UP

In this section we will analyze the outcomes of visual acuity and accurate IOL power calculation.

All our reviewed eyes were measured with the IOL master.

Table 1 shows the results of Bscva before the primary refractive surgery in the myopia and hyperopia group as well as the values for BSCVA before and after lens or cataract surgery.

Table 1: Comparing BSCVA Values			
BSCVA	Pre-refractive surgery	Pre-cataract surgery	Post-cataract surgery
Hyperopia SD	0,790,24	0,600,22	0,750,20
Myopia SD	0,650,23	0,450,18	0,750,,21

The BSCVA dropped of course before cataract surgery but this was less important in the hyperopia group since here the indication for surgery was often regression or progressive hyperopia. After cataract surgery the BSCVA improved in all eyes.

Remember that in an important number (30) of eyes in the myopia group and in the hyperopia group (5) the maximum BSCVA was only 0.5(20/40) before IOL surgery.

Comparing the BSCVA values before and after cataract surgery we found not a single patient with a loss of lines and in 33/77 eyes of the myopia group and in 5/30 eyes of the hyperopia group there was a gain of at least 3 lines.

- *Axial length:* in the myopia group the mean Axl was 27,9+/-1,87 mm with extremes between 25,7 and 36,8 mm. In the hyperopia group. The mean Axl was 22,71+/-1,4 mm with extremes between 20,8 and 24,86 mm.
- The **dioptric power** necessary for emmetropia in the myopia group was 18,85+/-1,4 Dptr. extremes....12-27..... (but that is the case where we had the hyperopic 8 dptr surpise:-24D at the start. So, in these highly myopic eyes (mean -10 D.) the dioptric power of the IOL implanted was only slightly inferior to the value for emmetropic normal eyes.

In the hyperopia group the values were: mean **23,8+/-3,2** Dptr -extremes 19-31 dptr.

Since nearly all cataracts after previous myopia surgery were nuclear cataract it is not surprising to see that the mean refractive anomaly before surgery was **-3,86 Dptr.** in the myopia group.

	Myopia	Hyperopia
Axl Mean and SD	27.9(1.87)	22.71(1.4)
Axl extremes	25.7-36.8	20.8-24.86
Emmetropizing IOL: Mean and SD	18.85(1.4)	23.8(3.2)
Emmetropizing IOL: Extremes	12-27	19-31

After cataract surgery and after eventual piggy back surgery the mean and extreme values for Sf.Eq. were -0,35 +/-1,34 D(extremes +2,75 to -3,75) in the myopia group and -0,48+/-0,87(extremes -2 to +3) in the hyperopia group. In the myopia group 44/77 eyes came out between +/-1,0 Dptr and in the hyperopia group this was 19/30. This outcomes are much lower than outcomes in virgin eyes. This learns us also that the calculation was much easier after hyperopic compared to myopic refractive surgery[29] since the outcome was better in hyperopia. However, the pre-existing refractive anomaly was much higher in myopia than in hyperopia.

	Myopia	Hyperopia
Mean sf. equivalent	−0,35	−0,48
Extremes	,-3,75 - +2,75	,-2 - +3
Outcome +/−1 dptr.	,44/77=57%	20/30=67%

In the myopia group -using a standard Haigis formula the mean IOL calculation error was -2,4+/-0,6-using a Srk Th it was -4,2+/-1,6 using the Holladay II formula with the clinical history method the error was only -0,75+/-1,5 Dptr. The Results of Haigis L are discussed in prof.Haigis chapter and were excellent and outperformed the above mentioned results.

	Myopia
MEAN Calculation Error	
Haigis Standard	,_2,4/+/_0,6
Srk Th.	,-4,2+/_1,6
Holladay Cl History	,-0,75+/-1,5

FOLLOW-UP AND SECONDARY PROCEDURES AFTER CATARACT SURGERY

We started Excimer laser surgery in 1991 and at that time very high myopic eyes were treated.

The mean **follow-up** after cataract surgery in the **myopia** group was 1201+/-980 days with the longest follow-up being 4951 days :18 eyes had a follow-up of at least 5 years.

The mean **follow-up** in the **hyperopia** group was 668+/-660 days and /11/30 hyperopic eyes had a fup of more than 3 years.

YAG CAPSULOTOMY

During the follow up in this whole group: **26/108 eyes needed a YAG laser capsulotomy**: 21/77 in the myopia group and 5/30 of in hyperopia group.

During this follow up 19 eyes needed a supplementary touch up with LASIK in order to correct residual refractive errors-spherical or astigmatic: 14/77 eyes of the myopia group and 5/30 eyes of the hyperopia group.

No complication at all was encountered in this follow-up period after Yag ND.

A PIGGYBACK IOL

Since we know that there is a learning curve in calculating the refractive errors after previous surgery it is not a shame to admit that we needed to add an extra IOL in the sulcus in 8 eyes of the myopia group-these were eyes operated in the early years 1998 -2002 and in one eye of the hyperopia group; the power of these IOLs was between -4 and +9 D. All piggy back IOLs in the myopia group except one were plus lenses. The mean value of the plus lenses was 5,6 +/- 1,6 D.The primary myopia of the eyes that needed a piggyback lens was always more than _10 D.mean -14,5 Dptr. So, be aware of an eventual problem in high myopes.

The secondary surgery itself was always without any problem; the extra IOL was placed in the sulcus. When looking back at these data please remember that some of the earlier implantations after previous refractive surgery were done in already 1999.

IN SUMMARY

1. Cataract surgery and IOL implantation after previous refractive surgery is extremely rewarding.
2. Technically, there are no hazards on condition to take the routine precautions for this particular type of surgery.
3. Cataract surgery after previous myopic refractive laser surgery was performed at a younger age compared to the hyperopia population.
4. Exact IOL power calculation may still pose a problem nowadays.

Chapter 30

Phaco in Hard Cataracts Grade-IV

Mahipal S Sachdev, Charu Khurana (India)

Phacoemulsification in a hard cataract with Grade-IV nucleus can be a challenging case even for the most experienced surgeons. Greater energy is required to break the nucleus with subsequent damage to the cornea and surrounding structures in the anterior chamber causing loss of endothelial cells and greater inflammatory response. Various maneuvers have been described by different surgeons to define the best technique for such a situation.

The following steps will help to overcome the problems faced during phacoemulsification in a hard cataract.

- Obtain a good mydriasis with 1% tropicamide and 10% phenylephrine eye drops
- Though topical anesthesia is adequate in most cases, we prefer to give a peri-bulbar injection of 2% lignocaine in very hard cataracts
- A 2.8 mm clear corneal incision is made and a side port opening made 30 degrees from the main incision
- Trypan blue dye maybe used to stain the anterior capsule to make visualization during the capsulorhexis
- A 5-5.5 mm capsulorhexis is created. Dispersive viscoelastic is used
- Hydrodissection is done and the nucleus is rotated in the capsular bag to ensure it is completely free
- The phaco parameters that we follow are: energy 40 %, vacuum 650 mm Hg and aspiration flow rate 60 ml/min (Figs 1 to 11)

- Phacoemulsification begins with the tip positioned with the bevel downward so that it is embedded deep into the substance of the hard nuclear fibers
- The chopper is introduced through the side port into the capsular bag till it lies opposite the phaco-tip
- If the hard posterior plate and dense epi-nucleus does not break completely, several pieces of the nucleus are chopped in the whole circumference by rotating the lens
- If the epinuclear plate is still intact, each chopped nuclear fragment is held against the phaco-tip with vacuum, pushing it slightly and pulled into the pupillary or iris plane. At the same tip, the chopper is held with its tip horizontal and parallel to the posterior capsule and placed below the nuclear/ epinuclear segment. The hook is moved centripetally and the epi-nucleus separated. It is then emulsified and aspirated using high vacuum and low power
- All other pieces are removed in the same manner repeating the steps as described above
- The entire procedure is completed using low power, high vacuum with minimal endothelial damage and reduced stress on the capsule and Zonular fibers
- Despite the advent of various high end phaco machines, the most important tool still remains the surgeon's skill when dealing with hard cataracts.

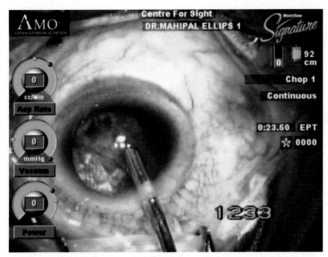

Fig. 1: Trenching in hard cataract

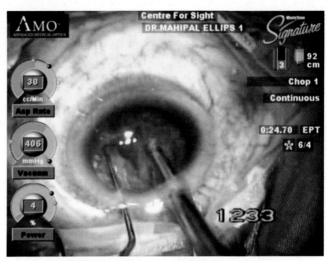

Fig. 4: Separation completed (high vacuum)

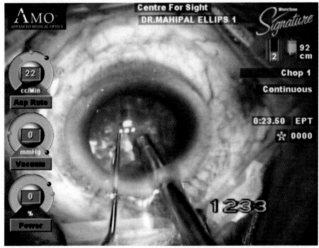

Fig 2: Cracking the nucleus

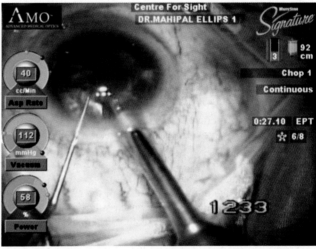

Fig. 5: Chopping the nuclear fragment

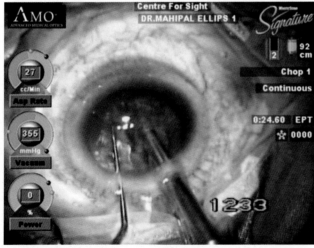

Fig. 3: Separating the 2 nuclear halves using high vacuum

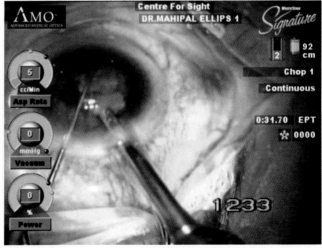

Fig. 6: Breaking up the nuclear fragment into smaller parts

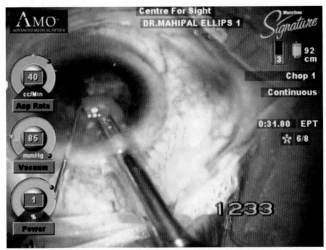

Fig. 7: Emulsifying the smaller fragment

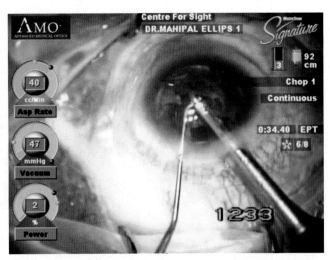

Fig. 9: Emulsification being completed

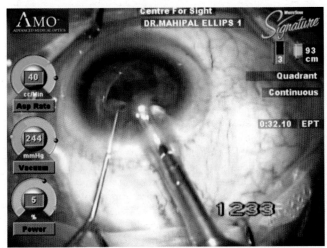

Fig. 8: Chopping the remaining nuclear pieces (high vacuum)

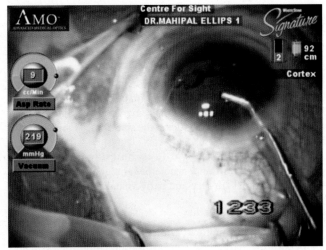

Fig. 10: Irrigation and aspiration

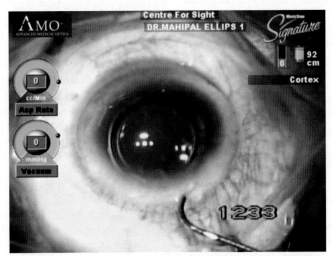

Fig. 11: IOL implanted. Note clear cornea at end of surgery

Chapter 31

How to Do the Microincision Cataract Surgery (MICS) with White Star Technology and Insertion of the New Accommodating IOL- Crystalens

Shui H Lee (Canada)

INTRODUCTION

New Surgical Technique

Since Dr Charles Kelman has invented phacoemulsification, it has undergone plenty of modifications for the last few years. The recent trend is toward less traumatic cataract surgery and early visual rehabilitation. This has emerged new phacoemulsification technologies for reducing the size of incision and using less phaco energy.

One of MICS surgical technique is **bimanual phacoemulsification** and it has met the goal of toward less traumatic cataract surgery and early visual rehabilitation.

Bimanual Phacoemulsification

It differs from conventional phacoemulsification by:
1. Separating irrigation from aspiration came forward and removing the cataract through two stab incisions. In conventional phacoemulsification, irrigation through the same tip helps to keep the temperature down of the phaco tip, thus preventing wound burn.
2. In Bimanual Phaco Machine, such as White Star-from AMO, White Star micropulse technology is a software modification that allows extremely short bursts of ultrasound energy. Thus decreases heat build-up with the retained efficiency of continuous ultrasound. The Signature Phaco Machine from AMO, so called the " Cool Phaco " machine is one of the favorable machines to do bimanual phaco.

THE ADVANTAGES OF WHITE STAR TECHNOLOGY

Chatter and Microchatter

Chatter is a phenomenon, in which ultrasound energy along with irrigation flow pushes a nuclear fragment away from the tip. The harder the nuclear fragment, the more evident the chatter. Pulsing technology in White Star helps to eliminate chatter. We know that "contact" is critical in the removal of nuclear fragments. During the down-time in White Star, the aspirational flow brings the particle back to the ultrasound tip here contact again occurs which is necessary for removal of nuclear fragment.

Jackhammer Effect and Cavitational Energy

Ultrasound creates a mechanical Jackhammer effect from the oscillation of the tip, and also creates cavitational energy. Cavitation is the formation of vacuoles in a liquid by a swiftly moving solid body such as the ultrasound tip. The collapse of the vacuoles releases energy that vaporizes and crushes lens material. Cavitational effect is more important of the two in emulsifying nucleus fragments.

With conventional ultrasound, cavitational energy is greatest when the ultrasound is first turned on and drops after a few milliseconds of utilization due to air dispersal and depletion from water (the sourse of cavitation). White Star ultrapulse technology, but turning off so fast, can minimize this decrease and more efficiently use cavitational energy than contineous ultrasound.

Fragment Followability

Increased followability wherein nuclear fragments stay with the emulsification tip and does not bounce off, has been reported. Followability is certainly related to a decrease of microchatter, with the off time allowing aspirational forces to more efficiently hold the particles in place for eventual emulsification, and this the one of the feature of White Star Technology.

Surgical Instruments

Those blades from MST make precise size corneal side incision, and are either made with stainless steel or diamond elements.

Other instruments on the tray will be cannula for hydrodissection and hydrodelineation. In general, less instruments are required for bimanual phaco than conventional phaco as the irrigation handpiece will have the chopper with it.

SURGICAL TECHNIQUE

A. *Topical Anesthesia:* All of my patients are operated under topical anesthesia.- Xylocaine 4% eye drop and, gel, and Lidocaine 1% intracamerally.

B. *Clear corneal incision:* Two side port incisions are created with the MTS blades about 75 degree aparts

After side ports corneal incisions are made, viscoelastic is injected into anterior chamber. The soft shell technique with two viscoelastic is favorable- Cohesive-Healon-GV, (AMO) and Dispersive- Viscoat (Alcon)

The sharp tip of the micro-rhexis forcep is used to make initial puncture into the anterior capsule and the forceps to grab the flap to make the tear circumferentially. The combined central and tangential vector forces to tear the capsule circumferentially.

Hydrodissection and hydrodelineation

Hydrodissection is to mobilize the nuclear-epinuclear complex within the capsule bag.

It is essential after hydrodissection and hydrodelineation, the epinuclear and nuclear complex are freely mobile within the capsular bag.

NUCLEAR DIVISION WITH WHITE STAR TECHNOLOGY

With White Star technology, phaco power is used to a much less energy, and irrigation chopper is used to maintain anterior chamber depth, and at the same time to do chopping of the nuclear fragments. The smaller the nuclear fragment, the easier it will be aspirated.

The setting of the parameters will be the surgeon's preference. Some will set the vacuum high and some will set it low, and the flow late show be high, and the phaco power is usually low except in hard nucleus.

Bimanual I/A will allow easy cortical clean up, and even at subincisional area. Complete cortical clean up leads much less postoperative inflammation.

NEW IOL TECHNOLOGY

Accommodative- IOL, from B&L, to reduce the dependency of reading glasses.

After a 3-mm corneal wound is made between the two side ports, or one of the side port is enlarged to 3 mm in size with slit knife, the Crystalens is inserted into the capsular bag, and it is rotated to 6 and 12 O'clock position.

The Crystalens is relatively easy to insert , just like the other foldable IOL. No learning curve is required.

Note that the optic of the IOL is vaulted backward after the insertion

PATIENT SELECTION

The Crystalens and other accommodating IOLs will have the ability to "fix" three things: a cataract; refractive error; and loss of accommodation. The ideal candidate, therefore, is someone who will get all three benefits—perhaps a 60-year-old, +5D hyperope with cataracts. Patients over 45 with significant refractive error but not much lens opacification are also good candidates. Younger plano presbyopes, on the other hand, are probably better served by corneal presbyopic procedures.

Patient counseling is extremely important in setting appropriate expectations prior to implantation of an accommodating IOL. I expect Crystalens patients to be a blend of cataract and refractive patients, but I have found that they are what I like to term "extreme refractive surgery" patients. The surgeon must carefully manage their expectations and do a lot of handholding both pre- and postoperatively to make sure they understand the lens, the procedure, and potential outcomes.

I tell my patients to expect that the procedure can fix their cataract and their hyperopia or myopia, but that there is no guarantee they will have the eyes of a 20-year-old. I explain that about 25 percent of my patients still need to wear glasses some of the time, so that patients are not disappointed if this happens. However, I am also very clear in explaining that there is no downside to an accommodating lens compared to a regular IOL.

POWER OF IOL CALCULATION

Power calculations should be done using the SRK-T formula for eyes with an axial length of ≥22 mm, and the Holladay II formula for eyes < 22 mm in length. One of the reasons to be so precise is that the Crystalens is available in more precise units of 0.25 D, compared to the 0.5 D steps available in other IOLs.

Postoperative Medications and Follow-up

About five minutes after implantation, I instill atropine 1%. In addition to the typical post-cataract eye shield, steroids, NSAIDs and antibiotics, patients should use cyclopentolate q.i.d. for one to two weeks. The resulting cycloplegia gives the lens a chance to fixate without vaulting in the early postoperative period.

Provided that the refractive result is close to emmetropia, patients should get the accommodative effect of the lens as soon as they are no longer cyclopleged, although the accommodative effect will improve over time. We have found there to be some improvement even after one year, perhaps due to better cortical adaptation or renewed utilization of the ciliary body.

BIBLIOGRAPHY

1. Agarwal A, Agarwal A, Agarwal S, et al. Phakonit: Phacoemulsification through a 0.9 mm corneal incision. J Cataract Refract Surg 2001;27:1548-52.
2. Chang D. 400 mmHg High-Vacuum Bimanual Phaco Attainable with the Staar Cruise Control device. J Cataract Refract Surg 2004;30:932-33.
3. Chang DF. Can cold phaco work for brunescent nuclei? Cataract and Refractive Surgery Today 2001;1:20-23.

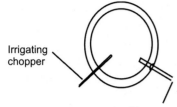

Irrigating
chopper

Phacoemulsification tip without
irrigation sleeve

Fig. 1

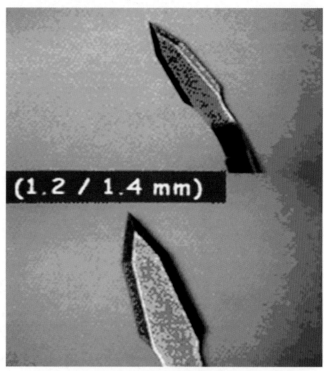

Fig. 3: 1.2 or 1.4 mm side port incision blades from MST
(microsurgical technology- duet system)

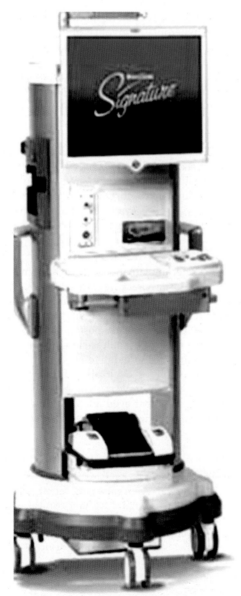

Fig. 2: The signature phaco machine from AMO

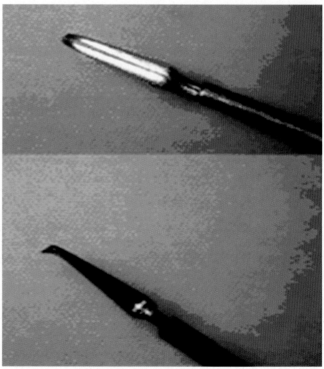

Fig. 4: Microrhexis forceps from MST

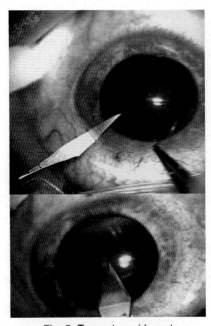

Fig. 5: To create a side port

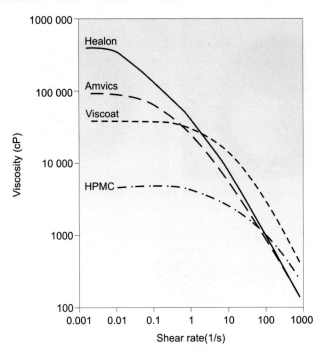

Fig. 7: Different viscoelastic' viscosity vs shear rate. Cohesive (Healon) has high viscosity and is good for maintaining surgical space, and easy to remove, Dispersive (Viscoat) has low viscosity, good to coat and protect the endothelium of the cornea but difficult to remove. The plant exract-Hydroxypropymethylcellulose (HPMC) such as Occoat, has the lowest viscosity, and hence is not as good as Cohesive agent to maintain the surgical space which is important for doing the rhexis

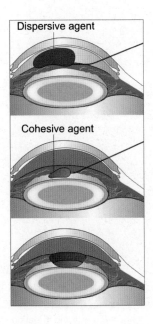

Fig. 6: Soft shell technique with injection of dispersive agent first and then cohesive agents into the anterior chamber

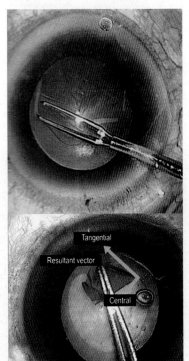

Fig. 8: Then with microrhexis forceps, a circular anterior capsulectomy is created

169

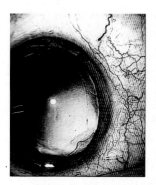
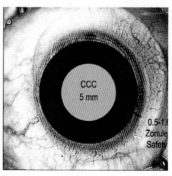

Fig. 9: An ideal 5-6 mm anterior capsulectomy is created

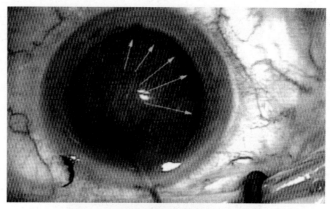

Fig. 12: Wave of fluid dissect the cortex from the epinucleus

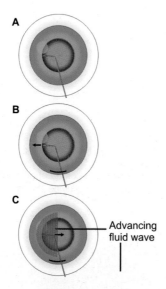

Hydrodissection

Figs 10A to C: The cannula is passing behind the edge of capsulorhexis to the peripherally to inject small amount of BSS solution to create wave form behind the back surface of the lens to dissect the cortex from the epi-nuclear complex

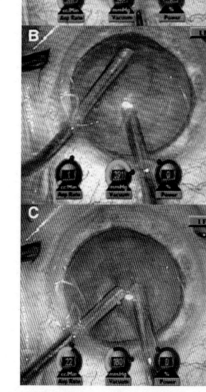

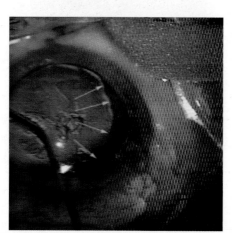

Fig. 11: Hydrodissection has created the cleaverage between cortex and epi-nuclear complex

Figs 13A to C: Horizontal chop with the irrigation chopper, and phaco hand piece to aspirate the nuclear fragments bimanual phaco with White Star technology

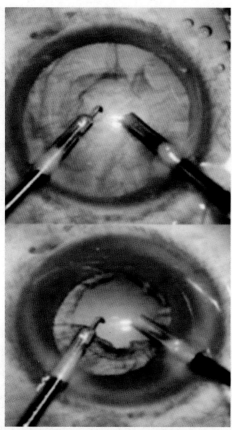

Figs 14: Once the nucleus is divided into large fragments, the fragments can be further divided into smaller fragments, as to facilitate aspiration by the phaco tube

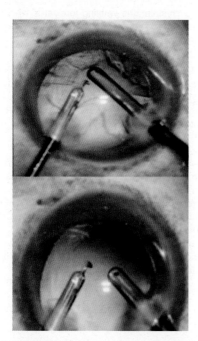

Figs 15: Final cortical clean up can be achieved with irrigation chopper and aspiration tube or the bimanual I/A set

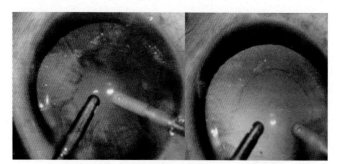

Fig. 16: Cortical cleaned up with bimanual I/A

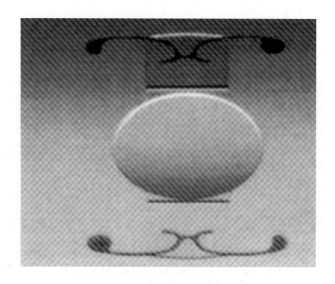

Fig. 17: New IOL technology

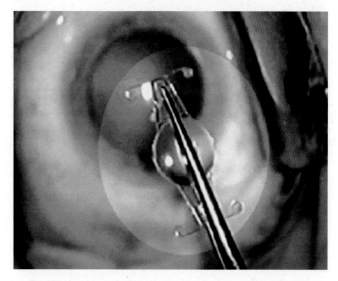

Fig. 18: Insertion of IOL- Crystalens is removed from its case

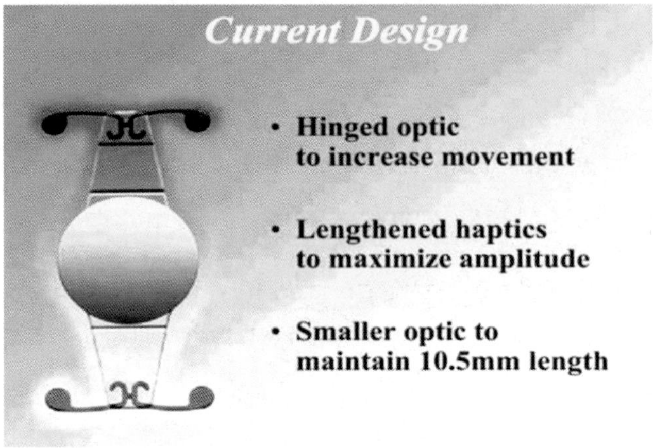

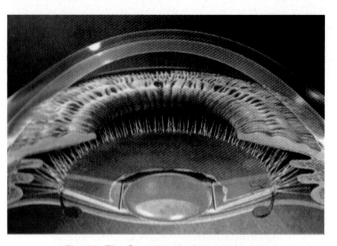

Fig. 19: Design of Crystalens and the lens in the capsular bag with optic vaults backwards

Fig. 22: The Crystalens is the capsular bag

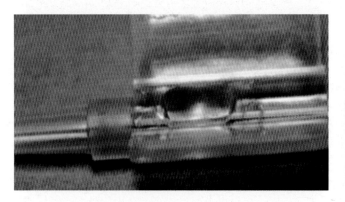

Fig. 20: The new cartage for insertion of Crystalens

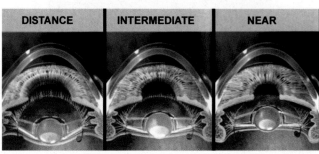

Fig. 23: The crystalens is vaulting forewards when the ciliary muscles contract when focusing at near

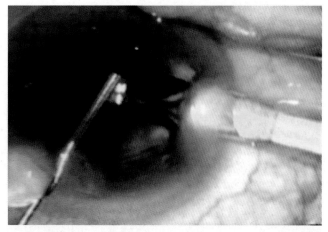

Fig. 21: Insertion of Crystalens

4. Chang DF. Chapter 18. Bimanual Phaco Chop – Fluidic Strategies. In: Phaco Chop: Mastering techniques, optimizing technology, and avoiding complications. Slack Inc, 2004.
5. Donnenfeld ED, Olson RJ, Solomon R, et al. Efficacy and wound-temperature gradient of White Star phacoemulsification through a 1.2 mm incision. J Cataract Refract Surg 2003;29:1097-1100.
6. Soscia W, Howard JG, Olson RJ. Bimanual phacoemulsification through 2 stab incisions. A wound-temperature study. J Cataract Refract Surg 2002;28:1039-43.
7. Soscia W, Howard JG, Olson RJ. Microphacoemulsification with WhiteStar. A wound-temperature study. J Cataract Refract Surg 2002;28:1044-46.
8. Tsuneoka H, Shiba T, Takahashi Y. Ultrasonic phaco-emulsification using a 1.4 mm incision: Clinical results. J Cataract Refract Surg 2002;28:81-86.

Chapter 32

Management of White Cataract

Sanjay Chaudhary (India)

There are six monsters to slay to successfully perform Phacoemulsification of white cataract. They are:
1. Absence of red glow
2. Pressurized capsular bag
3. Liquid cortex
4. Large brown nucleus
5. Weak zonules
6. Absence of epinucleus with thinned posterior capsule.

By addressing each of these phacoemulsification can be performed smoothly.

ABSENCE OF RED GLOW

Largest challenge is removal of mature cataract is absence of red fundus reflex when the cataract is viewed through the operating microscope. Surgeons have used several approaches to improve visualization of the anterior capsule in absence of red reflex.

- Employing oblique illumination
- Use of anterior capsular stains

Fluorescein sodium 2% weakly stains the anterior capsule on the exterior surface. Gentian violet and Methylene Blue are toxic to the endothelium.

ICG and Trypan Blue have been to be both safe and effective. Both techniques apply the dye under the cover of air bubble that fills anterior chamber in order not to dilute the dye. The use of ICG may be limited by its cost. But Trypan Blue have is not a viable option in children and pregnant females in which ICG may be useful.

PRESSURIZED CAPSULAR BAG

The pressure in the bag can lead to immediate extension of capsular incision across entire capsule resulting in gash of exposed lens across the center from one side of iris to other with a swath of stained capsule on either side of of gash. This striped appearance of capsule-lens-capsule resembles flag of Argentina.

LIQUID CORTEX

Liquid Cortex obscures the view of capsule through liquid cortex mixed with the viscoelastic in the anterior chamber. One solution is to use manual irrigation and aspiration cannula but there is always a danger of causing argentina flag. So it should be done in a controlled manner or liquid cortex can be removed by introducing viscoelastic in the anterior chamber with the posterior lip depressed at the same time.

LARGE BROWN NUCLEUS

In relatively young patient with an intumescent cataract, hydration that opacifies the cortex will also lead to softening of the nucleus. In elderly patients, the nucleus is often quite sclerotic and hard. To the surgeon's surprise hard brown cataract beneath white cataract is noticed on the operative table. Sculpting a central crater to allow the phaco tip to have better control during chopping is desirable. Also it decreases the volume of the nucleus to be emulsified. Stop and chop technique for Phacoemulsification in such situations comes in handy.

Weak Zonules

As soon as clinically significant zonular weakness is suspected, placement of morcher capsular tension ring is placed.

ABSENCE OF EPINUCLEUS POSTERIOR WITH THINNED CAPSULE

Absence of epinuclear cushion along with thinned and flaccid capsule makes it prone to come up to phaco tip and be ruptured. Useful step is to inject dispersive, non-cohesive viscoelastic behind the nucleus one or more times during phacoemulsification to provide artificial epinucleus cushion.

With the advent of staining of anterior capsule to assure visibility during surgery and with increasingly atraumatic phacoemulsification techniques along with use of viscoelastic, capsular tension ring ,the removal of mature cataract is a surgical challenge that frequently has a successful outcome.

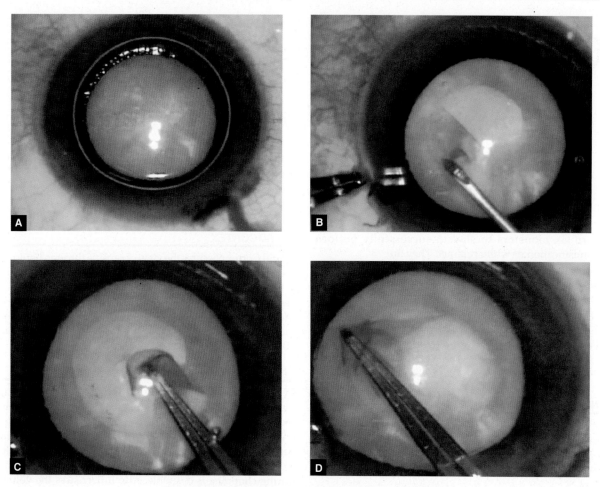

Figs 1A to D: Large capsulorhexis in white brown cataract

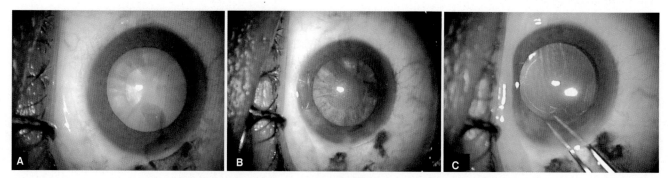

Figs 2A to C: Small capsulorhexis enlarged after IOL implantation in white cataract

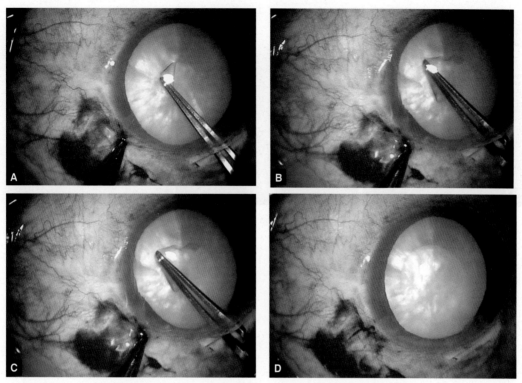

Figs 3A to D: Small capsulorhexis enlarged by spiralling out

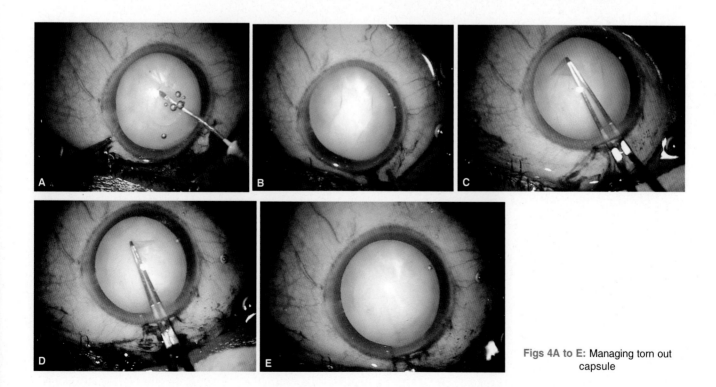

Figs 4A to E: Managing torn out capsule

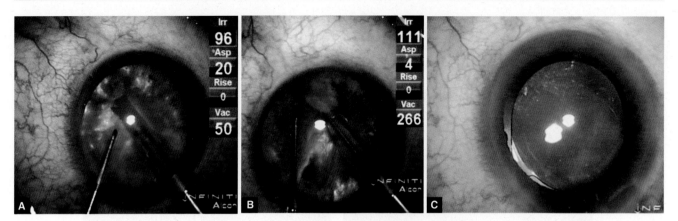

Figs 5A to C: Stop and chop in white with brown cataract

Chapter 33

Phaco Surgery in Highly Myopic Eyes

David F Chang (USA)

Whether performed for cataracts or refractive lens exchange, phacoemulsification in highly myopic eyes entails several challenges. Because these eyes are already at increased risk of pseudophakic retinal detachment, avoiding posterior capsular rupture is critical.[1] It is therefore important to understand the operative difficulties unique to these eyes and how to overcome them. Along with vitreous syneresis, myopic eyes tend to develop nuclear and oil drop cataracts at a younger age than the general population.[2-6] Some have hypothesized that vitreous syneresis allows more oxygen from the choroid to reach the hypoxic lens, and that this may be the primary cause of the myopic nuclear cataract.[7]

IOL Selection

The first challenge in myopic eyes is proper IOL power selection.[8] Although the advantages of non-contact biometry are widely acknowledged, myopic eyes (> 26 mm long) pose the unique problem of how to measure the appropriate axial length in eyes with a staphyloma.[9] Immersion ultrasound typically locates the posterior-most point of the globe, but will not measure the distance to the fovea if it is located on the slope of the staphyloma. Partial coherence interferometry, such as with the Zeiss IOL Master, is the only non-contact technology available that specifically measures the distance from the cornea to the fovea, and is the preferred biometric methodology in myopic eyes.

The IOL formulae are generally less accurate for eyes with extremely long or short axial lengths. Assuming that the axial length measurement is accurate, many lens formulae assume certain linear relationships between axial length and effective lens position (ELP). Holladay has shown that this assumption of a deeper ELP in increasingly longer eyes is not always correct, and his proprietary Holladay 2 formula uses other parameters besides axial length to predict ELP.[10] Hoffer has shown that of the modern regression formulae, the SRK/T formula is more accurate in long eyes, compared to the Hoffer Q or Holladay 1 formulae.[11]

Extremely myopic eyes may require very low or even negative power IOLs. Fortunately, several manufacturers now provide lens powers in the minus to low plus range. Even if the calculated power is very low or zero, it is still advisable to implant a posterior chamber IOL. Once it becomes shrink wrapped by the capsular bag, the IOL will reduce the chance of capsular fibrosis and opacification, and will serve as a barrier to vitreous prolapse should a YAG capsulotomy ever be necessary.[12] The SRK/T formula tends to lead to a hyperopic overcorrection when negative-powered IOLs are implanted, and one should aim for a 1.00–2.00 diopter more myopic target refraction.[13]

Anesthesia and Incisions

Because of the elongated globe and decreased scleral thickness, the increased risk of scleral perforation is an important concern with any regional injection anesthetic.[14] Using a peribulbar technique alone does not negate this risk. Topical anesthesia, with or without intracameral lidocaine supplementation, has the obvious benefit of avoiding a blind needle injection in these cases. Topical anesthesia, however, will not block the pain induced by lens iris diaphragm retro-displacement syndrome (LIDRS) which causes significant stretching of uveal tissues.[15] Avoiding and reversing LIDRS, as described below, is important if one is to employ topical anesthesia.

Proper incision architecture can be more difficult to attain in myopic eyes because of the thinner peripheral cornea and reduced scleral rigidity. A clear corneal tunnel must be appropriately long in order to be self-sealing. The surgeon must therefore avoid the tendency to penetrate Descemet's membrane too soon when the peripheral cornea is thinner than usual. Use of an interrupted suture should always be considered if the integrity of a clear corneal incision is in doubt at the conclusion of surgery.

Capsulorhexis

The difficulty of controlling the anterior capsule flap if the anterior chamber becomes shallow during the capsulorhexis step is well recognized. The same is true, however, if the anterior chamber becomes excessively deep, such as in a highly myopic or vitrectomized eye. The amount of ophthalmic viscosurgical device (OVD) needed to adequately pressurize the globe prior to creating the incision will often displace the lens very posteriorly. In this situation, the capsular flap often tends to veer peripherally as the capsulorhexis is performed, presumably

177

due to excessive zonular traction. These traction vectors are directed both anteriorly and peripherally when the lens is posteriorly displaced by OVD or irrigation infusion.

Aside from avoiding complications such as capsular rupture, a capsulorhexis that circumferentially overlaps the optic edge for all 360 degrees is the most important anatomic consideration for minimizing the risk of retinal detachment. Along with thorough cortical cleanup and a truncated IOL optic edge, an overlapping capsulorhexis significantly reduces the probability of capsular opacification requiring a YAG capsulotomy.[12, 16] The latter in turn elevates the risk of retinal detachment, particularly in young myopic men.[1]

Proper capsulorhexis sizing is difficult, however, because we rely solely upon visual clues to gauge the appropriate size. Because of the larger corneal diameter and anterior segment of a myopic eye, surgeons unintentionally tend to make a larger diameter capsulorhexis in these patients. If the capsulorhexis extends beyond the optic edge, the lens epithelial cell blocking capsular bend described by Nishi will not occur.[16] Parallax also makes it difficult to perfectly center the capsulorhexis.

Recognizing this, the solution is to err on making the primary capsulorhexis on the small side (Figs 1A and B). Following IOL implantation the diameter can always be enlarged but not reduced. A short oblique cut with capsule scissors creates a new flap that can be grasped with forceps (Figs 2A to D). The cut should be oblique, rather than radial, to better incline the resulting flap to tear in a circumferential direction. Curved Uthoff-Gills capsulotomy scissors with blunt tips (Katena K4-5126) have the perfect shape for creating an initial curved cut to either side of the phaco incision. If the anterior chamber is extremely deep, it helps to burp out some OVD so that the capsulorhexis becomes level with, and not posterior to the iris plane (Fig. 3).

Lens Iris Diaphragm Retro-displacement Syndrome

Initially described in 1994 by Wilbrandt, the lens iris diaphragm retro-displacement syndrome (LIDRS) is commonly encountered as soon as the irrigation infusion commences during phacoemulsification in high myopes and in vitrectomized eyes.[17] Cionni used intraoperative endoscopy to elegantly show that LIDRS is caused by reverse pupillary block as the iris becomes circumferentially pinned against the lens by the hydrostatic infusion pressure.[15] Lifting the iris off of the lens with an instrument tip breaks the pupillary block and allows equilibration of the hydrostatic forces anterior and posterior to the iris.

Although the pupil widens, the excessive anterior chamber deepening from LIDRS causes sudden discomfort for patients under topical anesthesia and exerts significant traction on the zonules. Nuclear emulsification is more difficult with an excessively deepened anterior chamber because the instruments and phaco tip must approach the lens from a much steeper angle. If the reverse pupillary block abruptly breaks during phacoemulsification, the iris will suddenly constrict creating a pupil diameter that is often much smaller than it was preoperatively. Cionni hypothesized that this might be due to

prostaglandin release caused by the excessive ciliary body stretching.

To prevent LIDRS, one can insert the phaco tip into the OVD-filled anterior chamber while in foot position zero. Next, the surgeon lifts the iris in the contra-incisional nasal quadrant using the phaco tip before initiating inflow with foot position one (Figs 4A and B). Alternatively, one can simply lift the pupil edge with a second instrument before initiating irrigation inflow. Either maneuver can also be utilized following the onset of LIDRS to gradually break the reverse pupillary block. These steps allow irrigation fluid to circulate into the posterior chamber, thereby equilibrating the hydrostatic forces both in front of and behind the iris. The hydrostatically widened pupil will then gradually constrict as the pupillary block is broken.

Phaco and IOL Insertion Technique

It is difficult to sculpt a nuclear trough with an excessively deep anterior chamber. Recognizing and managing LIDRS is therefore particularly important for the divide and conquer or stop and chop phaco techniques. The smaller nuclear and oil droplet cataracts typical of younger high myopes are well suited for both chopping and supracapsular flipping techniques.

To minimize the clear corneal incision size while injecting the IOL, it is important to have a relatively firm globe. Because of the increased volume of the anterior segment, there is frequently insufficient OVD remaining by this stage to tense the globe (Fig. 5A). An alternative to opening a new vial of OVD is to inject saline into the back of the capsular bag in the presence of a dispersive or retentive OVD (Fig. 5B). Because the latter will not burp out of the eye the globe will become firmer, which should facilitate insertion of the injector tip.

REFERENCES

1. Lois N, Wong D. Pseudophakic retinal detachment. Surv Ophthalmol 2003;48:467-87.
2. Kaufman BJ, Sugar J. Discrete nuclear sclerosis in young patients with myopia. Arch Ophthalmol 1996;114:1178-80.
3. Chen SN, Lin KK, Chao AN, et al. Nuclear sclerotic cataract in young patients in Taiwan. J Cataract Refract Surg 2003;29:983-88.
4. Tuft SJ, Bunce C. Axial length and age at cataract surgery. J Cataract Refract Surg 2004;30:1045-48.
5. Lin HY, Chang CW, Wang HZ, Tsai RK. Relation between the axial length and lenticular progressive myopia. Eye 2005; 19:899-905.
6. Kubo E, Kumamoto Y, Tsuzuki S, Akagi Y. Axial length, myopia, and the severity of lens opacity at the time of cataract surgery. Arch Ophthalmol 2006;124:1586-90.
7. Harocopos GJ, Shui YB, McKinnon M, et al. Importance of vitreous liquefaction in age-related cataract. Invest Ophthalmol Vis Sci 2004;45:77-85.
8. Pierro L, Modorati G, Brancato R. Clinical variability in keratometry, ultrasound biometry measurements, and emmetropic intraocular lens power calculation. J Cataract Refract Surg 1991;17:91-94.
9. Bose LT, Moshegov CN. Comparison of the Zeiss IOL Master and applanation A-scan ultrasound biometry for intraocular lens calculations. Clin Experiment Ophthalmol 2003;31:121-24.

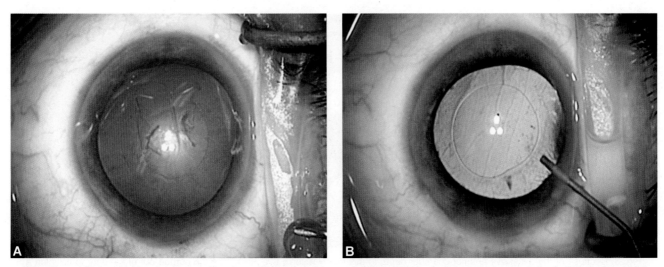

Figs 1A and B: In a highly myopic eye with a large diameter cornea, a conscious effort is made to make a capsulorhexis that appears to be smaller than usual. (A) View prior to hydrodissection. (B) View after cortical clean up

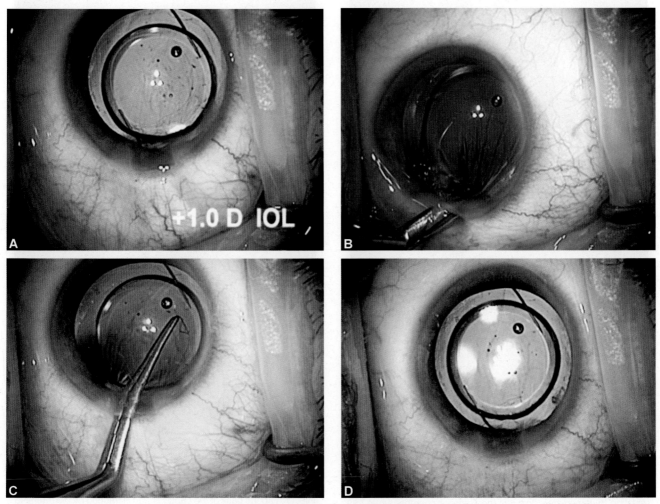

Figs 2A to D: Small diameter capsulorhexis is enlarged with forceps after creating a new flap with an oblique micro-scissors cut

179

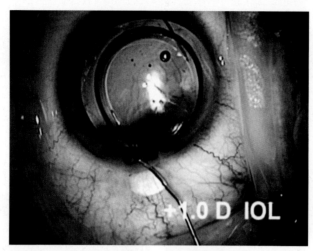

Fig. 3: Because of the excessive anterior chamber depth in this highly myopic eye, some OVD is burped out of AC prior to initiating a secondary capsulorhexis enlargement

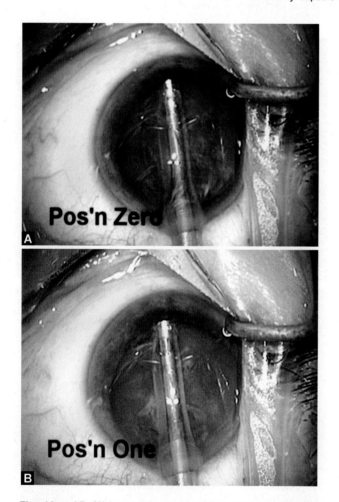

Figs 4A and B: (A) In order to prevent LIDRS, the phaco tip lifts the contra-incisional iris edge while in foot position zero. (B) This allows irrigation to immediately flow into the posterior chamber when foot position one is activated

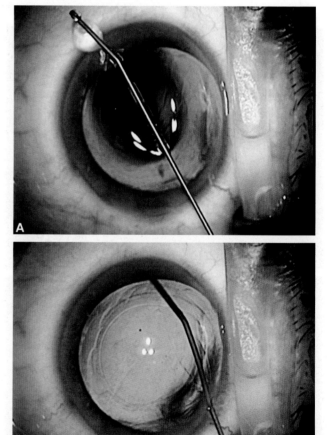

Fig. 5A and B: (A) Globe is still soft after the remaining OVD has been injected. (B) Globe becomes tense after balanced salt solution injected into the back of the capsular bag is trapped by the retentive OVD (Amvisc Plus, Bausch and Lomb)

10. Hoffer KJ. The Hoffer Q formula: a comparison of theoretic and regression formulas. J Cataract Refract Surg 1993;19:700-712. ERRATA 1994;20:677 and 2007;33:2-3.

11. Hoffer KJ. Clinical results using the Holladay 2 intraocular lens power formula. J Cataract Refract Surg 2000;26: 1233-37.

12. Ram J, Pandey SK, Apple DJ, et al. Effect of in-the-bag intraocular lens fixation on the prevention of posterior capsule opacification. J Cataract Refract Surg 2001;27:367-70.

13. MacLaren RE, Sagoo MS, Restori M, Allan BD. Biometry accuracy using zero- and negative-powered intraocular lenses. J Cataract Refract Surg 2005;31:280-90.

14. Gadkari SS. Evaluation of 19 cases of inadvertent globe perforation due to periocular injections. Indian J Ophthalmol 2007;55:103-07.

15. Cionni RJ, Barros MG, Osher RH. Management of lens-iris diaphragm retropulsion syndrome during phacoemulsification. J Cataract Refract Surg 2004;30:953-56.

16. Nishi O, Nishi K, Wickstrom K. Preventing lens epithelial cell migration using intraocular lenses with sharp rectangular edges. J Cataract Refract Surg 2000;26:1543-49.

17. Wilbrandt HR, Wilbrandt TH. Pathogenesis and management of the lens-iris diaphragm retropulsion syndrome during phacoemulsification. J Cataract Refract Surg 1994;20:48-53.

Chapter 34

Toric Bag-in-the-Lens (BIL) Implantation: Why and How to Implant?

Marie-José Tassignon, L Gobin, JJ Rozema (Belgium)

INTRODUCTION

Based on the current trends in intraocular lens (IOL) implantation, correction of the spherical equivalent (SE) of the patient's refractive error is no longer the only concern of the surgeon.

Correction of the corneal astigmatism at the level of the lenticular plane has gained more importance presently.

However, it is very ambitious and even risky to implant complicated IOL optics while the most important burden in current cataract surgery is not yet solved. We do all agree that the proliferation and differentiation of lens epithelial cells is the most common postoperative complication after uneventful cataract surgery and IOL implantation. As part of the healing process these cells can proliferate into clusters or a homogeneous layer scattering the incoming light, a condition called posterior capsule opacification (PCO). PCO can be treated by capsulotomy using a series of high intensity Nd:YAG laser pulses targeted at the posterior capsule.

The rate at which a Nd:YAG laser capsulotomy is required after the implantation of an IOL is called the Nd:YAG rate and it has been shown in the literature to depend on a number of lens specific factors, such as lens material,[1-4] size of the optical zone,[5] type of the IOL haptics,[6] edge of optical zone,[4,7,8] presence of capsular tension ring,[9] contact area of the capsular bag with the IOL and size of the anterior rhexis.[10,11] This leads to widely varying Nd:YAG rates between different IOL models.

The detrimental effects of PCO and subsequent capsular changes on the different aspects of visual quality include a reduced best-corrected visual acuity,[12] an increased retinal straylight,[12] and reduced contrast sensitivity.[13,14] After Nd:YAG laser capsulotomy, all these parameters are improved considerably.[12,13]

It has also been shown by Casprini et al.[15] who recently demonstrated that the wavefront quality after a 2.5 mm Nd:YAG laser capsulotomy is inferior to that of pseudophakic eyes that never developed PCO.

Bag-in-the-lens (BIL) implantation technique has been introduced in our department since 2000 and routinely used since 2004.

It has been published (I. Leysen)[16] in 2006 that early PCO rate when using this lens is zero. From our clinical experience with more than 2000 surgeries with adult eyes spread over a span of 9 years (2000-2009) the incidence of PCO was zero.

An additional advantage of the IOL is the ability to align according to the patient's visual axis. Alignment is a major issue, whilst implanting more complicated lens optics like toric and aspheric lenses.

Surgeon control, centration is not an option in the more traditional IOL implantation techniques but the BIL offers this distinct advantage!

The technique of implantation is illustrated herewith:

Our clinical experience is based on 13 cases with regular astigmatism ranging from 2.5 D to 6.5 D (mean 4.0 D).

The final orientation of the implanted BIL is then adjusted by aligning the Purkinje images along the cylindrical axis.

Using this technique, we found a mean residual astigmatism of which corresponds to the physiological amount of astigmatism making the patient spectacle-free.

Based on these very first encouraging data we can conclude that this lens is not just a solution to obviate PCO, but also allows perfect surgeon-controlled alignment of more complicated IOL optics.

REFERENCES

1. Kugelberg M, Wejde G, Jayaram H, Zetterström C. Posterior capsule opacification after implantation of a hydrophilic or a hydrophobic acrylic intraocular lens: one-year follow-up. J Cataract Refract Surg 2006;32(10):1627-31.
2. Findl O, Menapace R, Sacu S, Buehl W, Rainer G. Effect of optic material on posterior capsule opacification in intraocular lenses with sharp-edge optics: Randomized clinical trial. Ophthalmol 2005;112 (1):67-72.
3. Hayashi K, Hayashi H. Influence on posterior capsule opacification and visual function of intraocular lens optic material. Am J Ophthalmol 2007;144(2):195-202.
4. Heatley CJ, Spalton DJ, Kumar A, Jose R, Boyce J, Bender LE. Comparison of posterior capsule opacification rates between hydrophilic and hydrophobic single-piece acrylic intraocular lenses. J Cataract Refract Surg 2005;31(4):718-24.

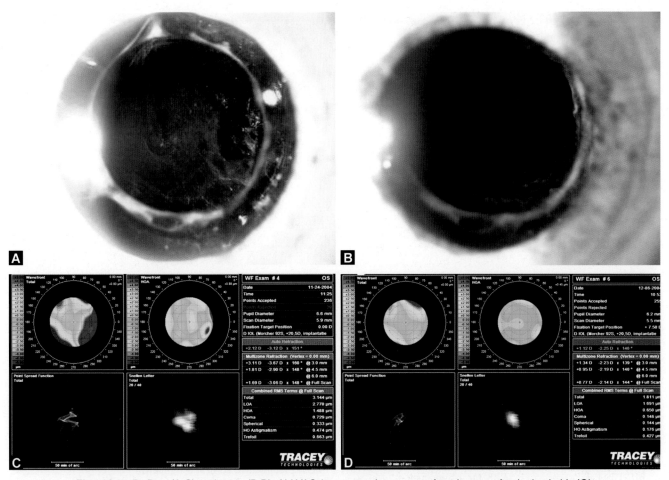

Figs 1A to D: Pre- (A-C) and post- (B-D) Nd:YAG laser capsulotomy wavefront images after hydrophobic IOL implantation (Alcon) showing an improvement of the quality of the image after Nd:YAG laser, but still not the perfect image

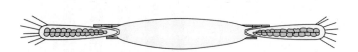

Fig. 2: Is a schematic side-view of the BIL with both capsules sandwiched in the groove defined by both haptic flanges

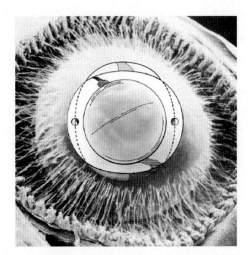

Fig. 3: Schematic illustration (anterior view) of the optimal position of the BIL as shown by scanning electron microscopy in a postmortem donor eye

183

Table 1: Refractive error of the 13 first eyes of patients who were implanted with a toric BIL				
Identification	Lens power	Astigmatism	@	Axis
BIL-T 001	16.5 D	5.0	@	136
BIL-T 002	-0.5 D	3.0	@	12
BIL-T 003	23.0 D	4.0	@	157
BIL-T 004	27.5 D	3.5	@	162
BIL-T 005	17.5 D	2.5	@	175
BIL-T 006	16.0 D	2.5	@	171
BIL-T 007	22.5 D	3.0	@	8
BIL-T 008	28.0 D	3.5	@	12
BIL-T 009	25.0 D	5.0	@	7
BIL-T 010	7.0 D	5.0	@	14
BIL-T 011	10.0 D	3.0	@	174
BIL-T 012	13.0 D	6.0	@	6
BIL-T 013	9.5 D	6.5	@	2
Mean	**16.5 D**	**4.0**	**@**	**80**

Table 2: Ocular history of all 13 eyes of 9 patients implanted between September 1st, 2007 and March 6th, 2008	
Identification	Ocular history
BIL-T 001	DTK
BIL-T 002	Aphakic eye since 2004
BIL-T 003	Amblyopic eye
BIL-T 004	IOL exchange
BIL-T 005	Nuclear cataract
BIL-T 006	Nuclear cataract
BIL-T 007	IOL exchange
BIL-T 008	Nuclear cataract
BIL-T 009	Amblyopic eye
BIL-T 010	PRK for astigmatism
BIL-T 011	PRK for astigmatism
BIL-T 012	Congenital cataract
BIL-T 013	Congenital cataract

Table 4: Pre- and postoperative visual acuity after toric BIL implantation	
Mean spherical refraction (D)	1.04
Standard deviation (D)	0.90
Mean astigmatism (D)	−0.92
Standard deviation (D)	0.88
Aimed refraction (D)	0.00
Mean preoperative visual acuity	0.53
Standard deviation preoperative visual acuity	0.16
Mean postoperative visual acuity	0.82
Standard deviation postoperative visual acuity	0.19
Mean preoperative corneal astigmatism	−3.92
Standard deviation preoperative corneal astigmatism	1.27
Average IOL astigmatism	4.03

Table 3: Ocular history of all 13 eyes of 9 patients implanted between September 1st, 2007 and March 6th, 2008	
Number of eyes with TORIC bag-in-the-lens	13
Mean follow-up (months)	4.07
Follow-up standard deviation (months)	2.89
Follow-up maximum (months)	11.49
Follow-up minimum (months)	0.92
Mean age at surgery (years)	59
Standard deviation (years)	21

Table 5: Age at surgery

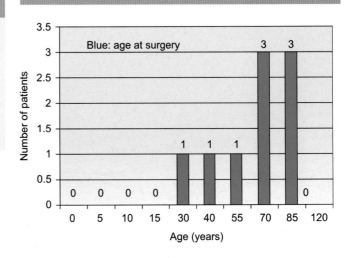

184

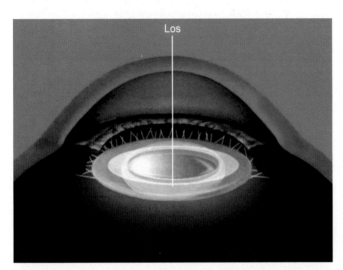

Fig. 4: Schematic drawing illustrating the positioning of the lens along the visual axis as determined by the surgeon using the principle of the Purkinje images of the light of the microscope. Quality of the image after Nd:YAG laser, but still not the perfect image

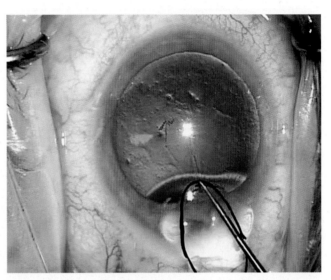

Fig. 5: Shows the insertion of the ring caliper to mark and center the plane of anterior capsulorhexis, based on the Purkinje images (only Purkinje image I is visible)

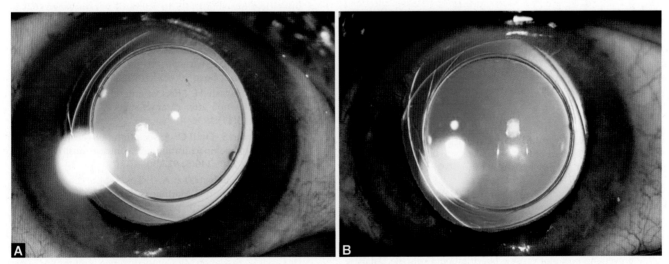

Figs 6A and B: Postoperative slit-lamp images depicting the centration of the implanted toric BIL

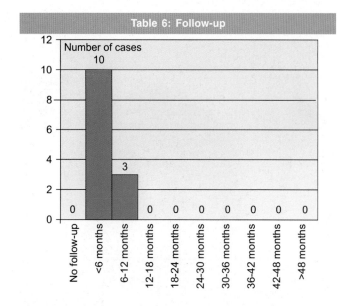

Table 6: Follow-up

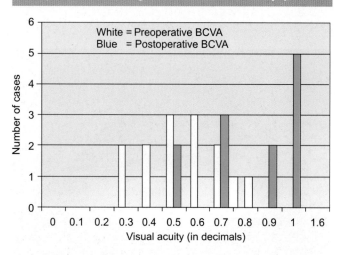

Table 8: Postoperative visual acuity. These cases included patients with congenital cataract and amblyopia

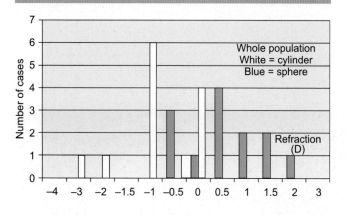

Table 7: Postoperative refraction (astigmatism and spherical correction)

5. Mamalis N, Crandall AS, Linebarger E, Sheffield WK, Leidenix MJ. Effect of intraocular lens size on posterior capsule opacification after phacoemulsification. J Cataract Refract Surg 1995;21(1):99-102.

6. Hwang IP, Clinch TE, Moshifar M, Malmquist L, Cason M, Crandall AS. Decentration of 3-piece versus plate-haptic silicone intraocular lenses. J Cataract Refract Surg 1998;24(11):1505-08.

7. Findl O, Buehl W, Bauer P, Sycha T. Interventions for preventing posterior capsule opacification. Cochrane Database Syst Rev 2007;18 (3):CD003738.

8. Kohnen T, Fabian E, Gerl R, Hunold W, Hütz W, Strobel J, Hoyer H, Mester U. Optic edge design as long-term factor for posterior capsular opacification rates. Ophthalmol 2008;115(8): 1308-14.

9. Kim JH, Kim H, Joo CK. The effect of capsular tension ring on posterior capsular opacity in cataract surgery. Korean J Ophthalmol 2005;19(1):23-28.

10. Ravalico G, Tognetto D, Palomba M, Busatto P, Baccara F. Capsulorhexis size on development of posterior capsule opacification. J Cataract Refract Surg 1996;22(1):98-103.

11. Aykan U, Bilge AH, Karadayi K, Akin T. The effect of capsulorhexis size on development of posterior capsule opacification: small (4.5 to 5.0 mm) versus large (6.0 to 7.0 mm). Eur J Ophthalmol 2003;13(6):514-45.

12. van Bree MC, Zijlmans BL, van den Berg TJ. Effect of neodymium: YAG laser capsulotomy on retinal straylight values in patients with posterior capsule opacification. J Cataract Refract Surg 2008;34(10):1681-86.

13. Hayashi K, Hayashi H. Effect of anterior capsule contraction on visual function after cataract surgery. J Cataract Refract Surg 2007;33(11):1936-40.

14. Buehl W, Sacu S, Findl O. Association between intensity of posterior capsule opacification and contrast sensitivity. Am J Ophthalmol 2005;140(5):927-30.

15. Casprini F, Balestrazzi A, Tosi GM, Lazzarotto M, Malandrini A, Lepri F, Martone G, Caporossi T, Caporossi A. Optical aberrations in pseudophakic eyes after 2.5-mm Nd:YAG laser capsulotomy for posterior capsule opacification. J Refract Surg 2008;24(7):702-06.

16. Leysen I, Coeckelbergh T, Gobin L, Smet H, Daniel Y, De Groot V, Tassignon MJ. Cumulative neodymium:YAG laser rates after bag-in-the-lens and lens-in-the-bag intraocular lens implantation: comparative study. J Cataract Refract Surg 2006;32(12):2085-90.

Chapter 35

Phacosection: A Manual Small Incision No Stitch Cataract Extraction Technique

Peter G Kansas (USA)

MODERN SUTURELESS MANUAL SMALL INCISION CATARACT SURGERY TODAY

Now several years into the 21st century, the vast majority of cataract surgery is performed by phacoemulsification. However, there are numerous times in advanced centers when, for any number of reasons, ultrasound can not be used (malfunction) and even more likely there are facilities where this technology is simply not available. For whatever reason, it is advantageous to have an alternative small incision technique at ones disposal. The ability to perform manual small incision sutureless cataract surgery is a great benefit. This alternative manual small incision pathway has been available for over two decades. Phacosection is a viscoelastic dependant technique that can be performed safely with the proper utilization of viscoelastics. Phacosection (manual fragmentation) has proven to be a safe, reliable small incision sutureless technique which allows excellent astigmatism control and rapid recovery similar to phacoemulsification. A well done, well healed phacosection procedure will be difficult to if not impossible to distinguish from a similarly well healed phacoemulsification procedure.

I started to develop a manual small incision technique in the early 80's as an alternative to phacoemulsification with which I was struggling to master. The first renditions were with 7.0 to 7.5 mm incisions (superior scleral tunnels after Kratz) combined with fragmenting the nucleus into two pieces (nucleus bisection). These incisions were usually closed with one or two sutures. Encouraged by the good results, I went on to develop the instruments to fragment the nucleus into three pieces thus allowing the incision to be predictably 6 mm. During this period, one piece and three piece 6 mm PMMA IOL's were available.

When McPherson described his 6 mm superior sutureless scleral tunnel technique in 1990, I quickly made the necessary dissection adjustment to combine this wound architectural advance with the Kansas manual small incision cataract extraction technique.

Incision

The Basics of Incision Construction

The incisional technique employed will have a profound affect on intraoperative wound behavior, self sealing predictability and postoperative astigmatism stability. A superior incision will tend to reduce the vertical meridian curvature and a temporal incision will reduce the horizontal meridian curvature. Radial sutures will have the opposite effect, i.e. steepening the meridians in which they are placed. (To minimize sutural effect, very shallow bites should be taken or horizontal sutures utilized)

The maximum flexibility in incision construction is achieved by working superiorly. A frown type incisional configuration is placed 1.5 to 2.0 mm behind the corneal-conjunctival border. The frown configuration brings each end of the incision further from the limbus thus enlarging the lamellar intrascleral interface area. The greater the interface area, the greater the postoperative would stability. Therefore, if a wider tunnel is needed, then a compensating adjustment can be performed for astigmatism control by bringing the groove further posterior. Koch's rule (Figs 1 and 2). The incision width can be decreased over time as the surgeon becomes comfortable with the procedure. Alternately, a superior straight line groove up to 4 to 6 mm can be utilized. A straight line groove beyond 4 mm will induce flattening in the corresponding meridian. Therefore, to avoid or minimize this response, the ends of the groove need to be sharply angulated so that each end of the incision is further from the limbus (Fig. 3).

Lamellar scleral—corneal dissection is performed with a crescent type scalpel and carried 1 mm into clear cornea (Figs 4A and B).

Anterior chamber entry. A clear cornea entry creates a prominent posterior lip which in turn is important to assure intraoperative anterior chamber stability as well as postoperative wound stability. A vitally important point (Figs 5A to C and 6). The internal entry into the anterior chamber is made slightly larger (wider) than the external groove. The resultant tunnel profile is trapezoidal. The internal widening is accomplished by cutting on the IN stroke. A sawing type motion is to be avoided. Another important caveat, if the nucleus is expected to be larger, as in an elderly patient with dark brunescent nucleus, the nucleus has not only a longer diameter but is also thicker. So the cross section volume of the tunnel most be larger. The 6 mm tunnel needs to be wider, sometimes vary much larger, up to 8 mm. In the presents of Fuchs corneal dystrophy, the tunnel always needs to be wider (6 to 7 mm is the safest). A wider tunnel tends to be more predictable since it will offer less resistance to fragment extraction, thus less trauma.

After the anterior chamber is entered, the anterior chamber is stabilized with 2% methylcellulose or a viscoelastic of the surgeons choice. A lateral and nasal paracentesis are created with a 15 degree blade (Fig. 7). These openings are 1.75 mm and are self sealing and astigmatism neutral. These paracentesis will allow 360 degree access to the anterior chamber thus providing better anterior chamber stability during I/A of the anterior and posterior epinucleus.

Anterior Capsulotomy

Following anterior chamber entry, the anterior chamber is stabilized with a viscoelastic. Although any viscoelastic will do, 2% methylcellulose is adequate for the capsulotomy since it will get washed out during the next step (hydrodissection). I prefer doing the capsulotomy with a bent 22 g needle and a straight shaft. I feel I have maximum control as compared to the popular capsulorhexis forceps (Figs 8, 9A and B). There are any number of patterns that are possible but the important point is the size of the opening. If it is too small, it will promote capsulophimosis. There is absolutely no advantage to a small capsulotomy. It is an unwanted side affect of capsulorhexis forceps usage. Since today's typical IOL diameter is 6 mm, a 5 mm rhexis opening is probably best. This size allows shrink wrapping of the IOL edge and helps retard posterior capsule opacification.

Another important consideration in regards to the capsulotomy size is that the delineated nucleus needs to be prolapsed through the capsulotomy and if it is too small it may tear the capsulotomy edge and disrupt the posterior capsule. Of course it is self evident that avoiding the anterior zonular insertions while performing capsulorhexis is also important.

Hydrodissection

Because of its simplicity, this is one of the more elegant steps in cataract surgery. A 27 G cannula on a 5 cc syringe is positioned well under anterior capsulotomy edge at 6 o'clock as BSS is injected (Fig. 10A). This dissects the posterior cortex and posterior epinucleus from the posterior capsule. This is followed by injecting into the more central anterior epinucleus for further delamination. Usually this can be repeated so that an onion skin affect is accomplished. The final hydrodissection step is nucleus delineation by simply injecting as centrally as possible to delineate the smallest diameter nucleus possible. Occasionally, a brightly illuminated ring or corona around the delineated nucleus is experienced (Fig. 10B).

Anterior Cortex/Epinucleus Removal

The rational for removal the anterior epinucleus at this point is to maximize visualization of the delineated nucleus. Visualization is greatly enhanced and greatly facilitates nucleus prolapse. Nucleus prolapse is an important precursor to nucleus fragmentation.

The anterior cortex and epinucleus is removed using a Kansas I/A hand piece which has a Simco type double barrel configuration with a 0.4 mm aspirating end opening on one cannula and an irrigating beveled opening on the other cannula (Figs 11 and 12). This hand piece fits snugly through the 1.75 mm paracentesis and provides a stable anterior chamber. I emphasize that the aspirating opening needs to be at least 0.4 mm and no smaller. This size allows good aspiration of both epinucleus and cortex.

Incidentally, this 0.4 mm end opening aspirating port works well with soft cataracts where ultrasound is not needed.

Nucleus Prolapse

Following the completion of epinucleus removal, the anterior chamber is stabilized with a visco dispersive viscoelastic such as Viscoate, Discovisc, Amvisc plus or a thick viscocohesive as Healon 5.

Using two blunt modified Kuglen hooks (Kansas), the nucleus is displaced inferiorly with one hook until cleavage along the edge of the superior pole is visualized (Figs 13A to C). The 2nd Kuglen hook is inserted into the cleavage, then gently sliding it posteriorly behind the nucleus. As the nucleus becomes lose from the posterior epinucleus, the two hooks are repositioned to alternately rotate the nucleus anteriorly. If the anterior chamber shallows before the nucleus is in the pupillary plane, the hooks are withdrawn and viscoelastic is injected behind the nucleus to complete the prolapse followed by injecting in front of the nucleus to deepen and stabilize the anterior chamber.

Phacosection

At this critical junction, it is important for the anterior chamber to be stabilized to its maximum depth with a viscodispersive viscoelastic. Now, through the scleral tunnel, the trisector is positioned first on the anterior surface of the nucleus (Fig.14). [Placing the trisector first, prevents the nucleus from being displaced toward the endothelium when positioning the vectis (cutting board) behind the nucleus. Now the vectis is insinuated behind the nucleus while keeping the trisector stable and not letting the nucleus drift upward toward the posterior corneal surface (Figs 15A and B). The trisector is pressed through the nucleus while the posteriorly positioned vectis supports the nucleus thus accomplishing the fragmentation of the nucleus into three pieces (Figs 16A and B). The middle fragment usually remains captured in the trisector and both are withdrawn together (Fig. 17). If it starts to float toward the endothelium, the vectis is removed and viscoelastic is injected anterior to the 1st fragment to avoid endothelial touch. After the fragment is stabilized, it can be removed with the with a Kansas fragment

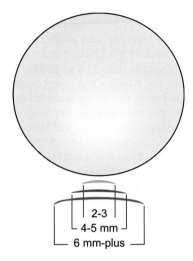

Fig. 1: Variable width

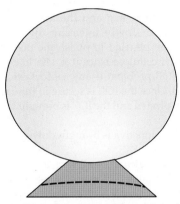

Koch's incisional triangle incisions placed within this triangle will have comparable stability

Fig. 2: Koch's triangle

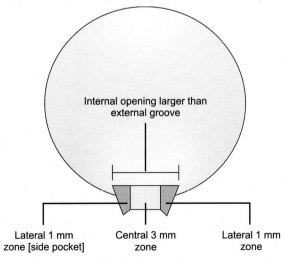

Lateral 1 mm zone [side pocket]   Central 3 mm zone   Lateral 1 mm zone

Fig. 3: Wound zones

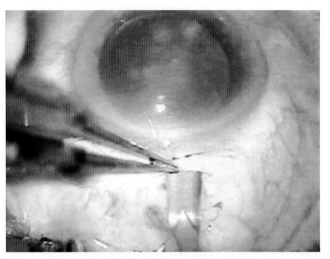

Fig. 4A: Scleral tunnel

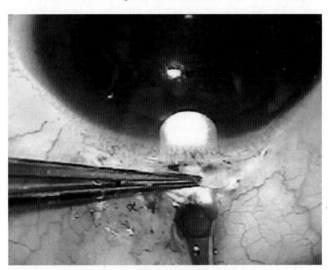

Fig. 4B: Into clear cornea

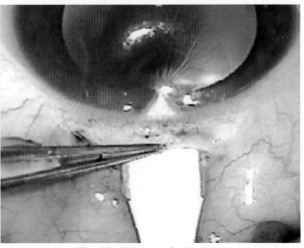

Fig. 5A: Keratome dimple down

forceps that has been especially design for this task (these forceps have 8 mm tynes lined with two rows of teeth on each tyne.

Now that fragment one has been taken care of, fragments two and three remain to be removed. The anterior chamber is deepened with more viscoelastic. Fragment 2 is grasped by the fragment forceps (Kansas) (Figs 18 and 19). A little lift of the superior tunnel roof with a fine toothed forceps is usually helpful while extricating fragments. As the fragments are extracted through the scleral tunnel, very light posterior pressure on the back wall of the tunnel will facilitate fragment removal. Finally fragment 3 is removed after the anterior chamber is redeepened with viscoelastic (Figs 20A and B). If the remaining fragments or fragment seem too large for the width of the existing tunnel, then the fragments can be further subdivided using the bisector (Kansas). In fact, the total fragmentation can be performed with the bisector but that necessitates more passes.

Sectioning with the bisector requires similar maneuvers as used with the trisector. In fact the surgeon may opt for any number of reasons to just bisect the nucleus from the beginning but this requires a 6 to 7 mm tunnel. The wider tunnel still allows stable self sealing but it most likely will induce some degree of against the rule astigmatic change. A 6 or 7 mm tunnel may trigger one to one and half diopters of astigmatic change. The wider tunnel can of course still enjoy the advantage of having sutureless architecture. If the surgeon desires to maintain the smallest possible wound then fragmenting with the bisector requires multiple steps, multiple fragmentations. Frequent replenishment of viscoelastic will be likely. Fragmenting can start from the center and work out or start on the end and fragment sequentially toward the center from left to right or right to left (similar to bread slicing).

Bisection combined with a 7 mm tunnel allows successful cataract removal in a Fuchs patient with a low cell count and still retain a clear cornea. Because phacosection is primarily is a viscodependent procedure, it requires dramatically less irrigation thus less trauma to the endothelium.

Posterior Epinucleus and Cortex

The remaining epinucleus and posterior cortex can be hydrodissected with a 19 g angulated cannula and prolapsed into the anterior chamber (Figs 21A and 21B). This is followed by removal with the Kansas I/A hand piece through the previously created nasal and lateral paracentesis' as described for removing the anterior cortex and epinucleus. Alternately, these remaining layers are further hydrodissected with BSS followed by injecting viscoelastic between the posterior cortex and posterior capsule, thus adding additional posterior capsule protection. Now the I/A of the epinucleus/cortex complex can proceed with decreased danger to the posterior capsule. Moderate to low vacuum is advised so as not to aspirate posterior capsule.

IOL Implantation

If the resultant tunnel is less than 6 mm the IOL can be folded and inserted with a forceps or it can be injected using a cartridge (Figs 22 and 23). The implantation by either method is preceded by filling the capsular bag and the anterior chamber with viscoelastic. While slowly injecting the viscoelastic, the viscoelastic tip can be used to polish the posterior capsule. I prefer 2% methyl cellulose since it is less likely to produce a postoperative IOP problem if any viscoelastic inadvertently remains behind. Once the IOL is secure in the capsular bag the viscoelastic is aspirated and the IOP is brought to normotensive levels with BSS.

Finally, the conjunctiva is brought down and coapted with wet field cautery.

Phacosection, manual small incision no stitch cataract removal has been utilized in many areas of the world where phacoemulsification has not been available or is cost prohibited. This technique is the modern way to do extracapsular cataract surgery. There is absolutely no need now in the 21st century do perform 180 degree incisions with 10 nylon suture closures. There is no need to subject any patient to the prolonged and somewhat risky postoperative course of large incision recovery.

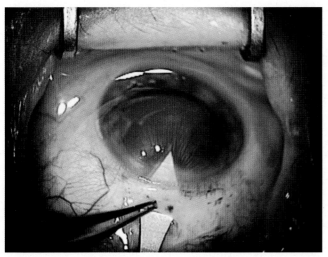

Fig. 5B: AC clear corneal entry

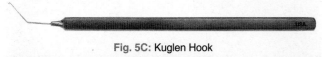

Fig. 5C: Kuglen Hook

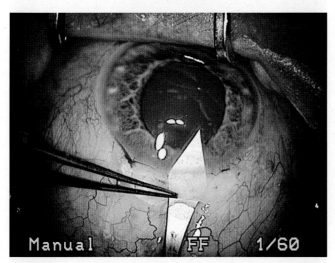

Fig. 6: Enlarging internal opening

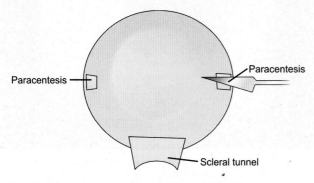

Fig. 7: Nasal and temporal paracentesis with a 15 degree blade

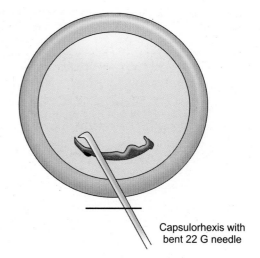

Capsulorhexis with
bent 22 G needle

Fig. 8: Rhexis

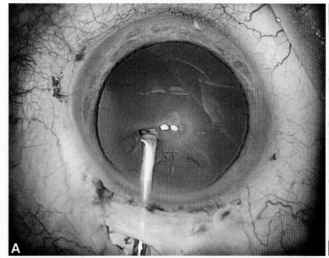

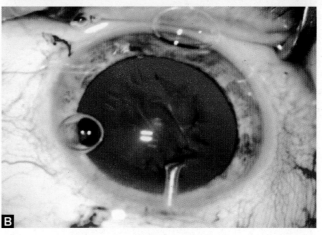

Figs 9A and B: (A) Start rhexis (B) End capsulorhexis

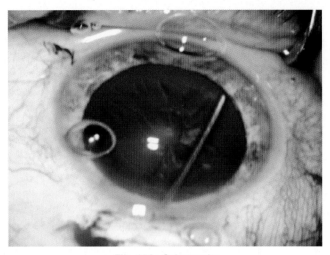

Fig. 10A: Subcapsular

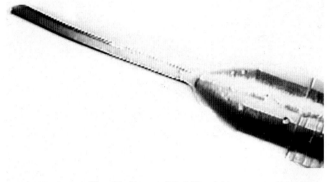

Fig. 12: Kansas-I & A Handpiece

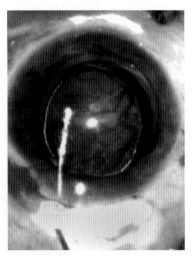

Fig. 10B: Corona

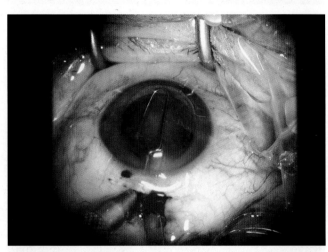

Fig. 13A: Lifting superior pole

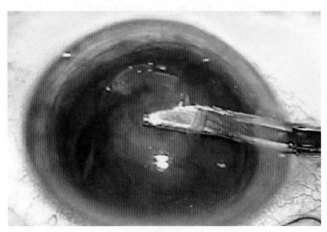

Fig. 11: Anterior epinucleus aspiration

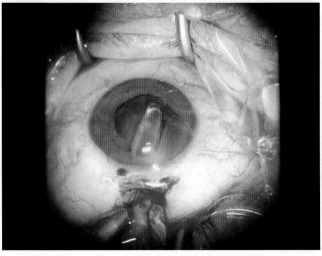

Fig.13B: Prolapsing into anterior chamber

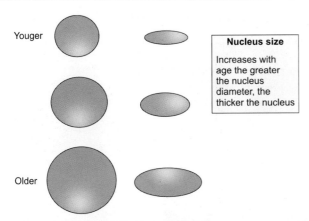

Youger

Older

Nucleus size

Increases with age the greater the nucleus diameter, the thicker the nucleus

Fig. 13C: Nucleus size to age

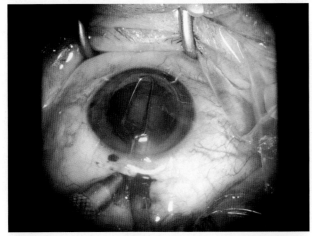

Fig. 14: Trisector positioned on anterior face of nucleus

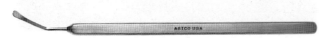

Fig. 15A: Kansas Vectis (cutting board)

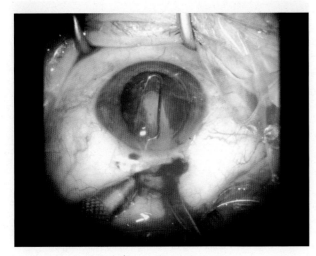

Fig. 15B: Vectis behind nucleus

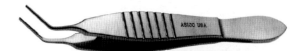

Fig. 16A: Kansas fragment forceps

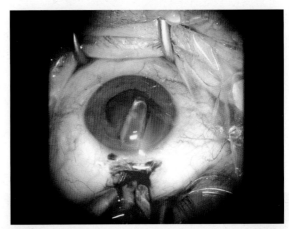

Fig. 16B: Trisection completed with middle fragment ensnared

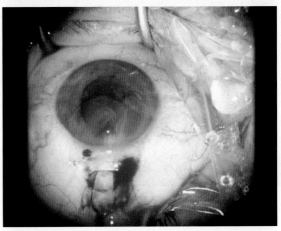

Fig.17: Removing trisector with fragment #1

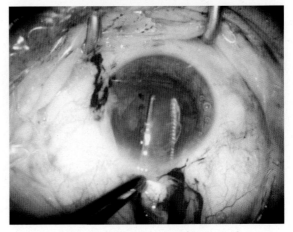

Fig. 18: Forceps removal fragment #2

193

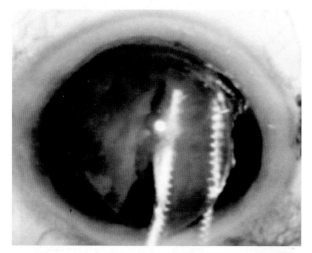

Fig. 19: Removal fragment #2

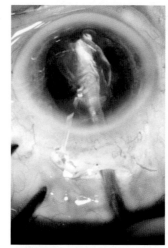

Fig. 21A: Hydroexpression of epinucleus

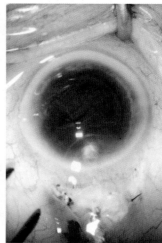

Fig. 21B: hydroexpressed nucleus in tunnel

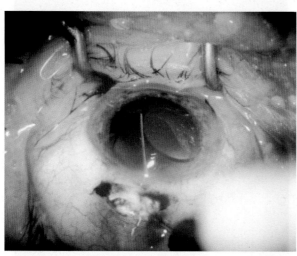

Fig.20A: Forceps removal fragment #3

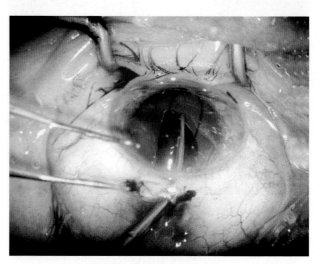

Fig. 22: Foldable lens implant

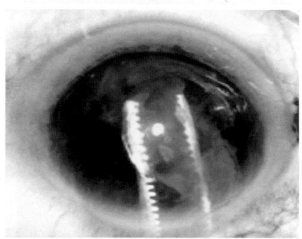

Fig. 20B: Fragment 3 removal

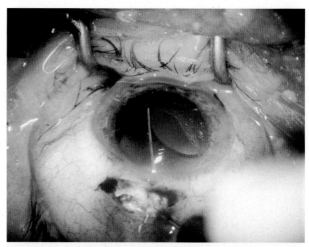

Fig. 23: Positioning of trailing haptic with Kuglen

Chapter 36

Sutureless Cataract Surgery with Nucleus Extraction "Fishhook Technique"

Albrecht Hennig (Nepal)

BACKGROUND

In 1997, I met Prof. Michael Blumenthal during a conference in Nepal and learnt about his mini-nuc technique, which I introduced in our Lahan Eye Hospital in southeast Nepal. Being a busy eye hospital with often 300-350 cataract surgeries per day, performed by four surgeons, there was need for a different, more simplified technique. Instead of anterior chamber maintainer and hydroexpression of the nucleus we use a small hook for nucleus extraction. From 1998 till August 2003, more than 160,000 sutureless cataract operations with nucleus extraction have been performed at Lahan. In the meantime, this technique has spread to many Asian and African countries and even some surgeons in Germany use it when phacoemulsification is not appropriate. It is named "Lahan Technique", "Hennig Technique" or more often "Fishhook Technique". In 2000, a video of this technique was honoured with a Special Award during the Annual Meeting of German Ophthalmic Surgeons (DOC).

THE HOOK

The hook is made of a 30G ½ inch needle, bending it with fine pliers or a needle holder. There are two bends:
1. The tip of the needle (Fig. 1), which will insert into the central nucleus.
2. A slight bend between the tip and the plastic mount (Fig. 2) to assure an easy insertion between the lower part of the nucleus and the posterior capsule.

The hook is mounted on a 1 ml tuberculine syringe and can be re-autoclaved and used for hundreds of nucleus extractions.

THE TECHNIQUE

Tunnel Construction

After fornix-based conjunctival preparation and scleral cauterization, the sclerocorneal tunnel can be done at 12 o'clock or temporal, ideally at the steepest corneal meridian to keep the postoperative astigmatism at a minimum. Scleral fixation with a good catching forceps, e.g. Pierse or Paufique, helps to perform a controlled corneoscleral tunnel with a minimum of 1 mm into the clear cornea. We start with a scleral Frown incision (Fig. 3) with a central distance of at least 2 mm behind the limbus (Fig. 4). The width of the tunnel depends on the age of the patient and the size of the nucleus. Very big brown nuclei may require an inner opening to the anterior chamber of at least 8 mm (Fig. 5).

For beginners we recommend conventional tunnel instruments. Experienced surgeons may use a diamond knife (double lancet with sharp sides), which enables them to perform the three tunnel steps as well as a linear capsulotomy with the same instrument.

Capsular Opening

A linear capsulotomy is either done with the keratome after preparing the inner corneal opening, or with a diamond knife. Preferred is a continuous curvilinear capsulorhexis (CCC) of 6-7 mm diameter (Fig. 6). However, CCC may be difficult in various advanced cataracts.

Hydrodissection and Nucleus Mobilization

After linear capsulotomy a forceful hydrodissection separates the capsule from the rest of the crystalline lens. Using the same irrigating cannula, the nucleus plus cortex is mobilized and slightly lifted up at the tunnel opening site.

In case of CCC, a careful hydrodissection is done on one side. If the CCC is large enough the cortex plus nucleus will tilt and partly prolapse mostly contra lateral to the hydrodissection side. Then the elevated cortex-nucleus part is rotated towards the tunnel opening position (Fig. 7).

Nucleus Hook Extraction

After placing some viscoelastics between nucleus and posterior capsule and into the anterior chamber, the bent 30G needle hook (Fig. 8) is inserted between nucleus and posterior capsule with the sharp needle tip pointing to the right side. Then the hook is turned and slightly pulled back, so that the needle tip is engaged into the central lower portion of the nucleus (Fig. 9).

195

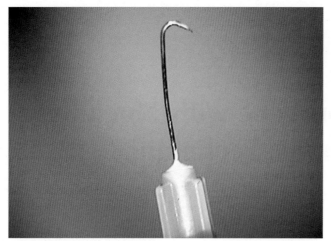

Fig. 1: "Fishhook", showing the bent tip of the 30G ½ inch needle

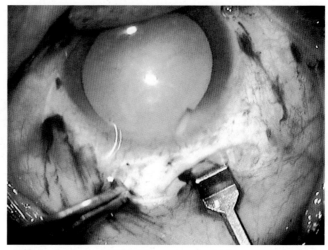

Fig. 4: Sclerocorneal tunnel

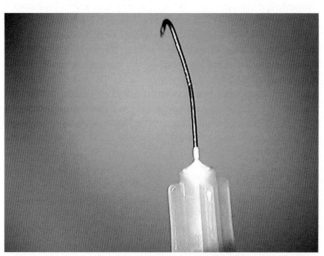

Fig. 2: "Fishhook", side view

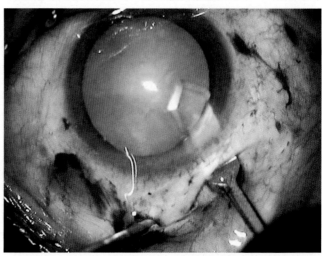

Fig. 5: Opening of the anterior chamber

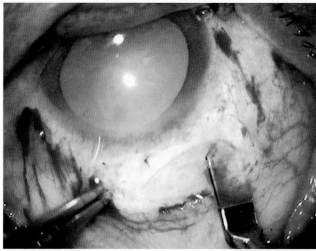

Fig. 3: Frown incision

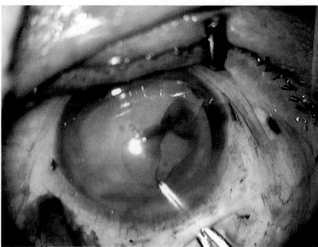

Fig. 6: Continuous curvilinear capsulorhexis

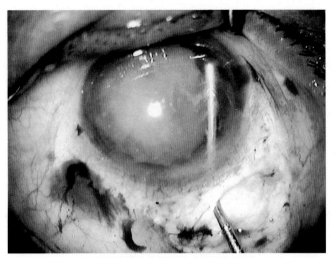

Fig. 7: Hydrodissection and nucleus mobilization

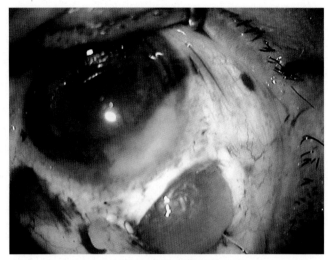

Fig. 10: Hook extraction of the nucleus out of the capsular bag

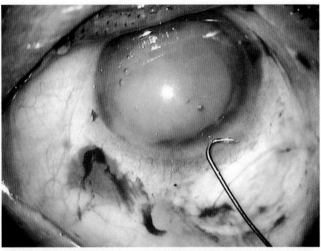

Fig. 8: The hook before insertion

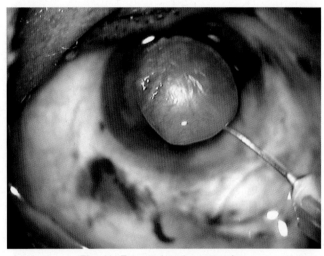

Fig. 11: Extracted nucleus, top view

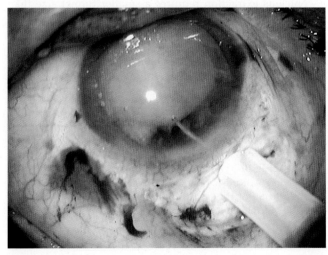

Fig. 9: Insertion of the hook between nucleus and posterior capsule

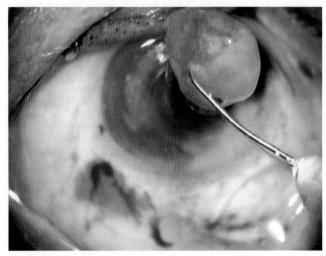

Fig. 12: Extracted nucleus, side view

197

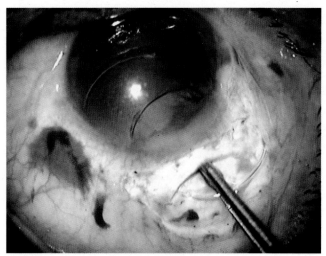

Fig. 13: Insertion of IOL

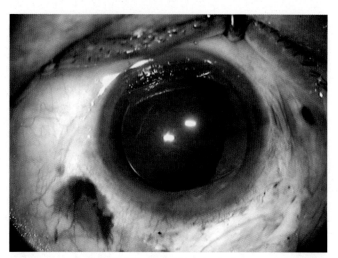

Fig. 14: IOL placed in capsular bag

Without lifting, the nucleus is pulled out of the capsular bag and through the tunnel (Fig. 10). Cortex remains in the anterior chamber, acts as a cushion and thus protects the endothelium from any contact with the nucleus.

Once the tip of the hook is correctly inserted into the nucleus, there is no risk to damage any part of the eye, nor does the nucleus rotate or tilt while being extracted (Figs 11 and 12).

Completing the Surgery

After hydroexpression of remaining cortex and removal with a Simcoe cannula, a 6 mm optic PMMA IOL is inserted into the capsular bag (Figs 13 and 14).

In case of linear capsulotomy, two small cuts are done with fine scissors on both sides of the anterior capsule, and the anterior capsule removed.

OUTCOME

In the hands of experienced surgeons sutureless cataract surgery with nucleus hook extraction has a very low surgical complication rate and provides excellent immediate uncorrected postoperative visual acuity.[1]

This is underlined by another outcome study on high volume surgery where six surgeons performed 2,111 sutureless cataract surgeries within six days.[2]

LEARNING CURVE

Sutureless tunnel surgery is more difficult to learn than ab-externo ECCE/PC IOL with sutures. Ophthalmologists without surgical experience may start with sutured ab-externo ECCE/PC IOL. Once they achieve consistent good results with a low surgical complication rate, a step-wise conversion to sutureless surgery is advised.

There is a much shorter learning curve for experienced phaco surgeons. They just need to learn the preparation of a larger tunnel and have to get familiar with the nucleus hook extraction. Once this technique is mastered, experienced eye surgeons at our hospital are able to perform 15-20 sutureless cataract operations per hour.

Do's and Don'ts

The sutureless cataract surgery with nucleus hook extraction is a safe, fast and inexpensive technique, which provides immediate good visual outcome.

The only additional instrument needed is a 30G needle, bent to a hook.

Among all other sutureless cataract surgical techniques, our technique is the only one where the nucleus is extracted straight from the capsular bag through the tunnel, avoiding corneal endothelium touch.

Nucleus extraction requires a smaller tunnel size than nucleus removal by hydroexpression.

With more than 160,000 sutureless cataract surgeries performed in Lahan and many more in other eye centers around the world, the nucleus hook extraction is one of the techniques most often used in sutureless non-phaco cataract surgery.

REFERENCES

1. Hennig A, Kumar J, Yorston D, Foster A. Sutureless cataract surgery with nucleus extraction: Outcome of a prospective study in Nepal. Br J Ophthalmol 2003;87(3):266-70.
2. Hennig A, Kumar J, Singh AK, Singh S, Gurung R, Foster A. World Sight Day and cataract blindness. BrJ Ophthalmol 2002;86:830-1.

Chapter 37

Chop-Multisection and Chopsticks Technique: Chopper, Spatula and Small Incision Cataract Surgery

Jorge Alvarez-Marin (Spain)

INTRODUCTION

I started to use the manual phacofragmentation techniques around 1993. Initially, I had begun with the Blumenthal Mininuc technique and later I also used also the Kansas technique, but I found that working in the anterior chamber with large instruments was awkward and clumsy. I wanted to reduce the large size of the incision and I began to use the Handle technique of Keener, modified by Quintana, using a nylon handle instead of a steel one. Finally, in 1995 I began to use the Nagahara chopper and a Barraquer vitreous spatula to divide the nuclei in the anterior chamber. Initially I divided it in two pieces, later in three and four pieces, and finally in multiple fragments.

I had developed a manual phacofragmentation technique carried out in the anterior chamber using a chopper and a spatula. I called this technique the "Chop-Section Technique", that is Chop-Bisection, Chop-Trisection or Chop-Multisection, as the nucleus is cut into two, three or more fragments. According to the number of fragments that we divide the nucleus into, and depending on their hardness and size, we are able to make an incision from 6 mm (Chop-Bisection in very hard and big nucleus) to 2.8 mm (by means of Chop-Multisection in a nucleus of any degree of hardness).

To take away the fragments I used hydro, viscoexpression, a vectis, and finally the same chopper and spatula that I used to divide the nuclei. I called this technique the "Chopsticks Technique".

INSTRUMENTATION

The instruments to carry out this technique are available in any set of instruments for phacoemulsification.
- **Chopper:** I use a "Nagahara", but any chopper can be used. It is advisable that the chopper has a cutting angle between 30 and 45° to facilitate the section and the fracture of the nucleus.
- **Spatula:** I use a Barraquer vitreus spatula, because it gives better control ot the nucleus during the section.

I have designed a chopper and a spatula to make the technique easier. Rumex international has made the second prototypes and I hope that soon the final product will be in the market (Fig. 1).

SURGICAL TECHNIQUE

Preoperative Management

We use sodium Cyclopentolate and Phenylephrine drops to dilate the pupil, and non-steroid anti-inflammatory drops. During the manipulation in the anterior chamber miosis may take place, however this doesn't affect phacofragmentation as we are working above the pupil. During irrigation-aspiration (IA) we can recover mydriasis, using an adrenaline infusion.

Anesthesia

This technique can be carried out under different types of anesthesia according to surgical experience and the degree of the patient collaboration. Once you are experienced in carrying out the technique, **Topical anesthesia (**1 drop three times every 5 min 15 min before the surgery) with **Intracameral** Lidocaine 0,75%, would be the best.

Incision

In three planes. We carry out a temporal (or on the sharpest curved meridian in case of astigmatism) blue-line preincision in the sclerocorneal limbus. We adapt the preincision size to the technique that we will use, 4.5-6 mm for the Chop-Bisection, 3.5-5 mm for the Chop-Trisection and 2.5 to 4.2 mm for the Chop-Multisection. If necessary, once the nucleus is broken into fragments, we can enlarge the incision to the desired size, maintaining its shape.

Capsulotomy

We carry out a capsulorhexis (CCC) with a cystotome or with Corydon forceps through the paracentesis or the incision. This capsulorhexis should be sufficiently wide (approximately 5.5 to 6.5 mm.) to allow the easy luxation of the nucleus to the AC. Even if you do not reach the CCC, you can still continue with the same technique.

Hydrodissection and Luxation of the Nucleus

Once the CCC is reached, we inject a balanced saline solution (BSS) between the anterior capsule and the córtex at 3h using a Charleux or Rycroft 27G cannula through the incision.

We inject the BSS gently in order to get the hydrodissection, we then hydrodelineate the hard nucleus and separate it from the epinucleus. We aspirate the cortex over the hard nucleus, we luxate it to the AC using cannula or viscoelastic, leaving the epinucleus in the capsular bag, in order to free up space in the AC.

Nuclear Fragmentation

Once the hard or primitive nucleus has been luxated to the AC, we inject high density viscoelastic around the nucleus filling in the AC. We introduce the Barraquer vitreous spatula between the nucleus and the posterior capsule and then the chopper between the cornea and the nucleus (Figs 2 to 5).

Then we continue with the Bisection/Trisection/Multisection, cutting with the chopper from 6h to 12h, creating counter pressure with another instrument, like the Barraquer spatula. In the Trisection we carry out a second incision parallel to the first one (Figs 6 and 7). In the Multisection we carry out as many incisions as necessary, until we obtain the desired size of nuclear fragments. An angle of about 40° should be maintained between both instruments in order to avoid vertical movement of the nucleus. In the final part of the trajectory section, we separate each of the instruments one to 3h and the other to 9h, to fracture the nucleus (Figs 8 and 9). Once divided, we adjust the final size of the incision (2.8 to 6 mm) in relation to the size and hardness of the fragments obtained.

Extraction of the Cortex and Nucleus Remained

The internal lip of the incision should be larger than the external one, creating an exit type cone that facilitates the exit of the nuclear fragments. Their extraction may be carried out by means of hydro or viscoexpression, with the help of a vectis (Fig. 10), with the sandwich technique, or using the Dr. Gutiérrez Carmona nucleotome and his spatula. These are very useful for very hard nuclei or in those with sharp edges.

In nuclei of medium to high hardness we pinch together the fragments laterally using the spatula and the chopper which hold the fragments (Fig. 11). I have called this technique "The Chinese Chopsticks Technique" (Fig. 12). It allows us to take advantage of the triangular free space that is on both sides of the nuclear fragment, between the limits of the fragment and the extreme edge of the incision. Using this method we achieve a better adjustment between the size of the incision and the size of the nuclear fragments, as we don't introduce the instruments from above or below the fragments as we do when using the vectis or the sandwich technique.

Once the nuclear fragments are extracted, we luxate the epinucleus into the AC and we hydroexpulsate it. Then we aspirate the cortex fixed to the capsule with a Simcoe cannula, and polish the capsular bag with a Kratz cannula irrigating profusely.

IOL Implant and Incision Closure

We expand the capsular bag by injecting viscoelastic and we implant a foldable lens (Fig. 13). We close the incision without stitching by hydrating the edges of the incision. We suture (Nylon 10/0) whenever the least minimum doubt of Seidel exists.

Postoperative Management

Eye-drops: Antibiotic-corticoid 2 drops every 4 hours for two weeks, NSAIDs 2 drops every 6h for four to six weeks.

Shortening the Learning Curve

The learning curve is similar to that of phacoemulsification. In order to shorten the learning curve, you should consider the next items:
1. Practising the phacosection with the chopper on the nucleus we have extracted using EEC. (Ab- externo).
2. Initially select patients without corneal problems and with soft nucleus.
3. Begin using wide incisions and progressively reduce their size as our expertise increases.
4. Make large capsulorhexis (6 to 7 mm).
5. Hydrodelineate and hydro or viscoexpulsate the hard nuclei to the AC.
6. Use dispersive or high density viscoelastics over and under the nuclei to enlarge the AC and to protect the endothelium, the iris and the incision.
7. Make sure that the incision is completely closed if we prefer not to stitch.

COMPLICATIONS

In a comparative study analyzing about the first 70 cases in each group (Chop-Bisection, Chop-Trisection, Chop-Multisection and phacoemulsification14 (that is including the learnig curve), I have not found significant differences in their frequency (Fig. 14).
- Capsular rupture (We found a smaller risk of fragments luxation to the vitreous as we do not work with positive pressures in the AC. Only one case in phacoemulsification group)
- Transient corneal edema and endothelial trauma
- Endothelial decompensation
- Iris trauma
- Iris prolapse and endothelial damage at the fragments extraction time when we make incisions disproportionate to the fragments size and hardness.
- Zonule dialysis
- Bleeding in the AC.
- Descemet's stripping.

ADVANTAGES AND DISADVANTAGES OF THE TECHNIQUE (Do's and Don'ts)

Advantages

- This is a simple technique for medium and small incision carried out by using simple instruments and no device is required.

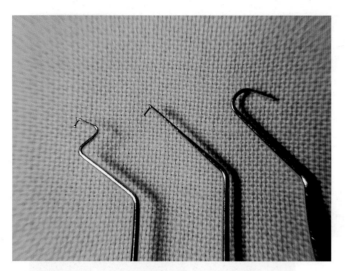

Fig. 1: Chop-Multisection surgical prototypes made by Rumex International: (from right to left) spatula for hard nuclei, spatula for medium and soft nuclei, and arcuate chopper

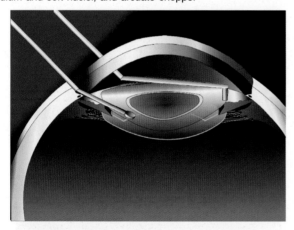

Fig. 2: Lateral view of the chopper and spatula

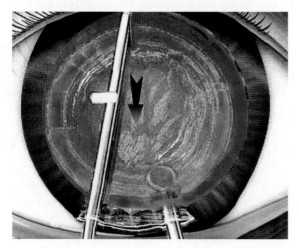

Fig. 3: Chopper slidding direction and angulation between both instruments

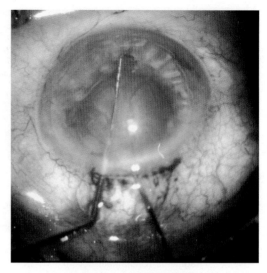

Fig. 4: Instruments position

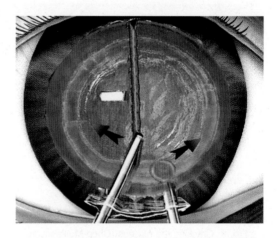

Fig. 5: Breaking force towards 3 and 9 h at the end of the cut

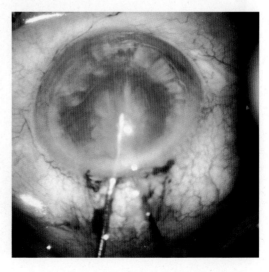

Fig. 6: Cracking the nucleus (Chop-Bisection)

201

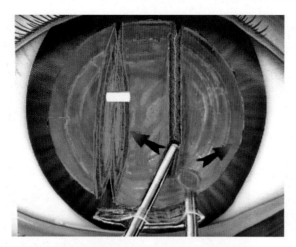

Fig. 7: Parallel cuts can be made to get 3 (Chop-Trisection) or more fragments (Chop-Multisection)

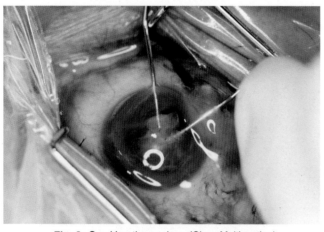

Fig. 8: Cracking the nucleus (Chop-Multisection)

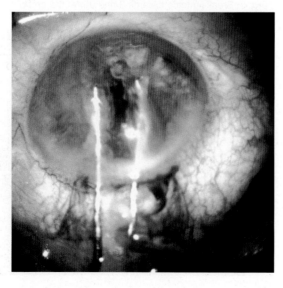

Fig. 9: Nucleofracture (Chop-Bisection)

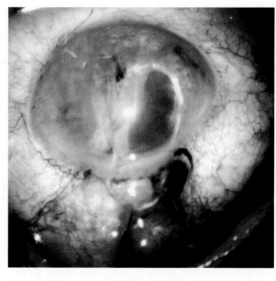

Fig. 10: Fragments extraction with the vectis (Chop-Bisection)

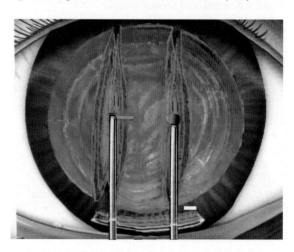

Fig. 11: Extraction of the fragments with the chopper and a spatula (Chopsticks technique)

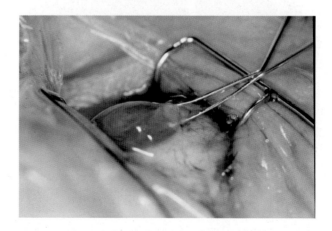

Fig. 12: Chopsticks technique

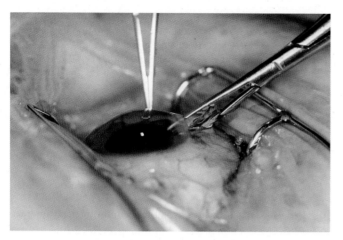

Fig. 13: Foldable IOL implantation

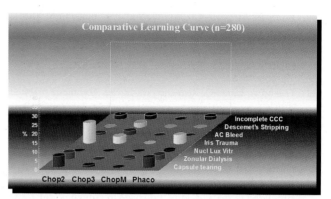

Fig. 14: Surgical complications in a comparative study between Chop-Bisection, Chop-Trisection, Chop-Multisection and Phacoemulsification 3

- We can work through incisions between 2.8 and 5 mm.
- We can fracture any hardness nucleus.
- Nucleus extraction using lateral free space between the fragments and the limits of the incision (chopsticks technique), instead of the superior and inferior used in the sandwich technique or with the vectis.
- This technique may be performed under intracamerular anesthesia, through a temporal incision (if desired, depending on the astigmatism) and with no stitches (similar to phaco).
- We have lower risk of capsule rupture compared to phacoemulsification as we work in the AC and we also have lower risk of nucleus luxation to the vitreous, as we work under low pressure in the AC.
- The practise of this technique facilitates learning the chopper use, the control of the hardness and dimensions of the nucleus and the AC (Helpful in phaco learning).
- This technique allows maintaining incision length in case of conversion from phaco to EEC.

Disadvantages

- Chop-Multisection requires a greater amount of viscoelastic than phacoemulsification, but if we use a chamber maintainer we need less viscoelastic.
- In very hard nuclei it can be difficult to maintain the necessary stability of the nucleus at the time of cutting it (Must maintain 40° between the instruments to avoid this complication).

CONCLUSION

With this manual phacofragmentation technique, we have:
- Simplicity and low cost.
- Fast visual recovery and low astigmatism.
- Excellent results on nucleus of any hardness.
- Convertion from phaco without enlarging incision.
- Similar results to phaco without the sophisticated and expensive technology.

For your information: Dr. Alvarez-Marin does not have any direct financial interest in the manual phacofragmentation system and is not linked financially or otherwise to any of the companies mentioned.

BIBLIOGRAPHY

1. Alvarez-Marín J, Abreu Reyes P. Facofragmentación Bimanual en cámara anterior con choper y espátula. Una alternativa de facofragmentación manual. Arch Soc Esp Oftalmol 2000;75:563-68.
2. Alvarez-Marín J, Hernández Brito A, Pérez Silguero MA, Delgado Miranda JL, Abreu Reyes P: Chop-bisección /Chop-trisección y técnica de los palillos chinos para extracción de los fragmentos nucleares. Arch Soc Canar Oftalmol, 1986-1998,9:123-29.
3. Alvarez-Marín J, Pérez Silguero MA, Abreu Reyes P: Estudio comparativo entre 5 técnicas de cirugía de pequeña y mediana incisión. Resultados Prefínales. Arch Soc Canar Oft, 1986-1998;9:93-100.
4. Alvarez Marín J, Abreu Reyes P. Chop-bisección: Una nueva técnica de facofragmentación manual. Libro de resúmenes del LXXII Congreso de la Sociedad Española de Oftalmología. Madrid; 1996:63.
5. Alvarez Marín J, Abreu Reyes P. Chop-bisección: Estudio comparativo con facofragmentación con asa de nailon. Primeros resultados. Libro de resúmenes del LXXII Congreso de la Sociedad Española de Oftalmología. Madrid; 1996:35.
6. Ardiaca R, Ferreruela R, Gómez X et al. Diferencias en el astigmatismo postoperatorio producido con la sutura de nailon 10-0 en puntos sueltos y en sutura continua. Microcirugía Ocular 1995;3:78-81.
7. Ashkenazi I, Avni I, Blumenthal M.: Maintaining nearly physiologic intraocular pressure levels prior to tying the sutures during cataract surgery reduces surgically induced astigmatism. Ophthalmic Surg 1991;22:284-86.
8. Beirouty ZA, Barker NH, Shanmugam NS. Sutureless one-handed small incision cataract surgery by manual nucleosuction - a new technique for cataract extraction. Eur J Implant Refract Surg 1995;7:295-98.

9. Boyd B. Atlas de Cirugía Ocular.Panamá: Highlights of Ophthalmology; 1995;V:60-64.

10. Bucher P. Manual phaco-fragmentation. A small incision cataract operation technique. Basel: University Eye Hospital; 1992.

11. Galand A, Garza O. Reduction du noyau. Technique manuelle d'ECCE avec incision moyenne. An Inst Barraquer (Barc) 1995;25:81-83.

12. Gómez A, Rentería C, Somavilla M y Saiz B. Asa de nailon y división nuclear. Microcirugía Ocular 1995;3(2):88-89.

13. Gutiérrez Carmona FJ. Nueva técnica e instrumental de facofragmentación manual para incisiones esclerales tunelizadas de 3, 5 mm. Libro de resúmenes del LXXII Congreso de la Sociedad Española de Oftalmología. Madrid; 1996:36.

14. Heaven CJ, Davison CRN, Boase DL. Learning phaco-emulsification: The incidence of complications and the outcome in theses cases. Eur J Implant Refract Surg 1994;6:324-27.

15. Howard V, Gimbel MD, Jonathan P, Ellant MD, Patrick K, Chin MD. Divide and conquer nucleofractis. Ophthalmol Clin of North Am 1995;8:457-69.

16. Naus NC, Luyten GP, Stijnen T, de Jong PT. Astigmatism and visual recovery after phacoemulsification and conventional extracapsular cataract extraction. Doc Ophthalmol 1995;1:53-59.

17. Olsen T, Bargum R. Outcome monitoring in cataract surgery. Acta Ophthalmol Scand 1995;73:433-37.

18. Quintana M. Pequeña incisión en EEC. Microcirugía Ocular 1993;1:24-32.

19. Rozakis GW. Alternative small incision techniques. Cataract surgery. NJ Slack; 1990.

Chapter 38

Manual Small Incision Cataract Surgery with Chevron Incision

CS Dhull, Sumit Sachdeva (India)

Manual small incision cataract surgery has been proving to be a boon for the surgeons world over. No doubt phacoemulsification is the procedure of choice for cataract surgery, but the steep learning curve, relatively lesser safety margin and expensive equipment have made it a procedure for the affluent especially in third world countries where most of the population who require cataract surgery come from the lower economic strata. It is here that manual small incision cataract surgery scores over phacoemulsification, in that it is easy to learn, can be performed in all types of cataracts, gives consistently good results and above all is very cost effective for the patients.

Technique

The technique involves creating a fornix based conjuctival flap, making a 6-7 mm long self-sealing partial thickness sclera tunnel with the help of a crescent knife and entering the anterior chamber with the help of 3.2 mm keratome.

Then the steps like capsulorhexis, hydrodissection are performed and nucleus is rotated out of the bag into the anterior chamber.

The nucleus can then be taken out of the AC by various techniques which can be modified according to the surgeons need. The cortical matter is then aspirated and the IOL is implanted in the bag. The conjunctiva is then reposited back.

Role of Incisions

The only concern associated with an otherwise excellent technique of manual SICS was the problem of astigmatism. Though significantly less than a conventional ECCE, it was still found to be more when compared with that in a phcoemulsification surgery. This was especially true for straight incisions given superiorly. Geometric shape of the external incision affects the astigmatism significantly which is explained by incisional tunnel. Any incision made within this tunnel will be astigmatically stable.

Over the time it was found that a frown incision gave better results than a straight incision which obviously goes out of the funnel.

But lately it has been found that a chevron incision is best amongst all the incisions for manual SICS. This involves giving an inverted V shaped incision with an angle of approximately 120° (range 100-120°) between the two arms, and the apex about 1.5 mm from the limbus. According to the amount of cataract and size of the nucleus of the lens different size of a 5.5 mm, 6 mm, 6.5 mm, 7.0 mm external incision are recommended for GR-I, GR-II, GR-III, GR-IV nuclear sclerosis respectively.

The main advantage of this incision was that it was very stable and gave excellent reduction in surgically induced astigmatism over the frown or a straight incision. Even in hard brown cataracts this incision gives significantly better results in terms of stability and astigmatism as compared to a straight or frown incision.

Conclusion

Thus whenever or wherever phacoemulsification is not feasible or available, manual small incision with chevron incision gave excellent results for all types of cataract, which meets every challenge for early postoperative rehabilitation and management of astigmatism.

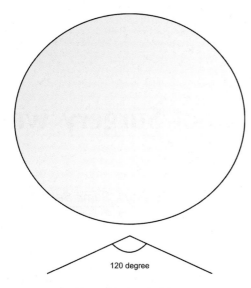

Fig 1: Chevron incision

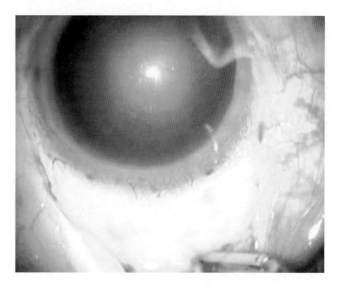

Fig 2: Conjunctival flap with wetfield cautery

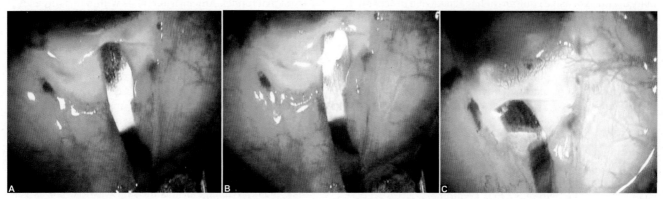

Figs 3A to C: Chevron incision. Scleral tunnel being made

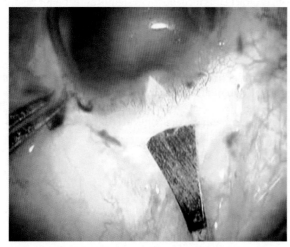

Fig. 4: AC entry with 3.2 keratome

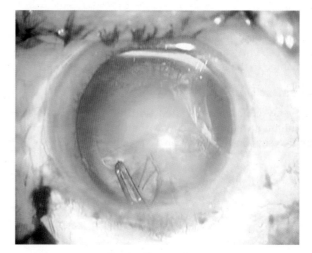

Fig. 5: Capsulorhexis

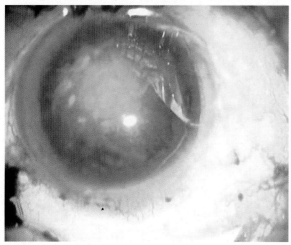

Fig. 6: Nucleus prolapsed in AC

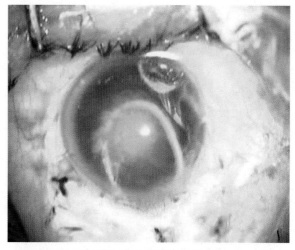

Fig. 7: Nucleus delivered out with irrigating wire vectis

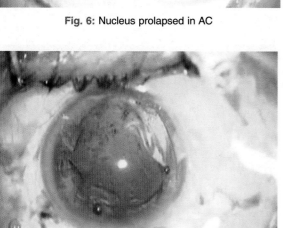

Fig. 8: Nucleus delivered out

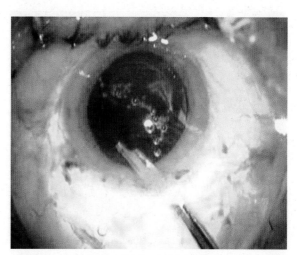

Fig. 9: Irrigation and aspiration

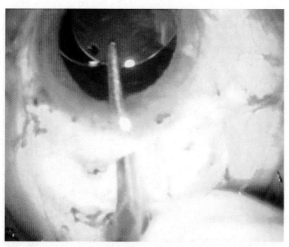

Fig. 10: IOL implantation

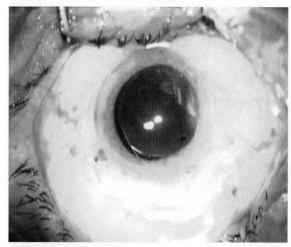

Fig. 11: IOL in the bag

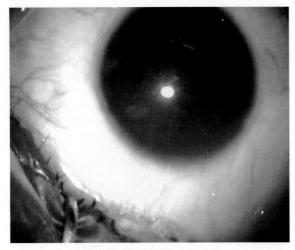

Fig. 12: Hard brown cataract

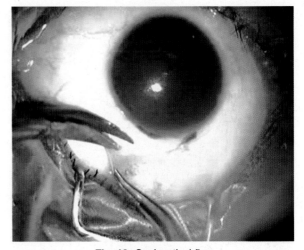

Fig. 13: Conjunctival flap

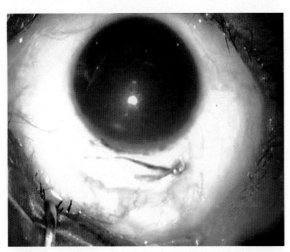

Fig. 14A: Chevron incision (note the angle is increased to accommodate large nucleus)

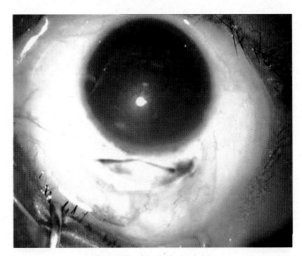

Fig. 14B: Chevron incision

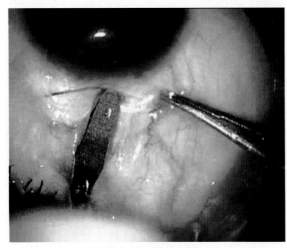

Fig. 15: Sclera tunnel

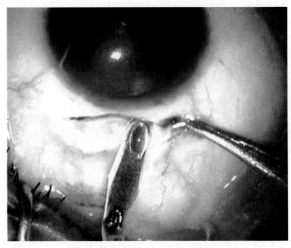

Fig. 16: Scleral tunnel making

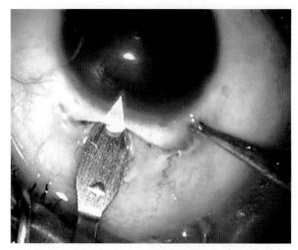

Fig. 17: AC entry

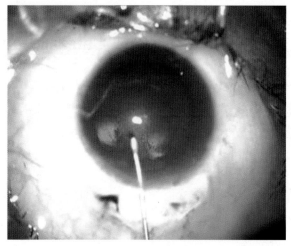

Fig. 18: Capsulotomy

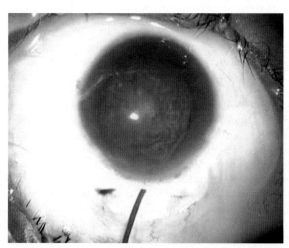

Fig. 19: Hydrodissection

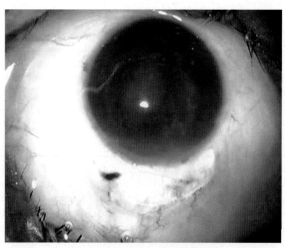

Fig. 20: Nucleus prolapsed in AC

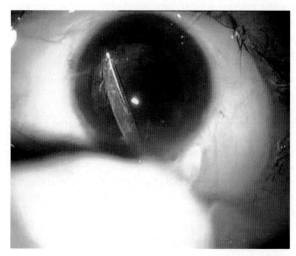

Fig. 21: I and A

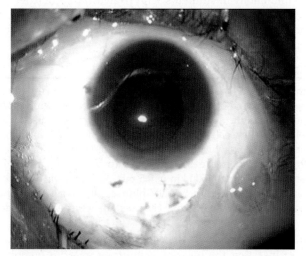

Fig. 22: IOL implanted in the bag

Chapter 39

Glued IOL

Amar Agarwal, Dhivya A, Soosan Jacob,
Athiya Agarwal, Chandresh Baid, Ashok Garg (India)

INTRODUCTION

We devised a new surgical technique for implantation of a posterior chamber intraocular lens (IOL) in eyes with deficient or absent posterior capsule with the use of biological glue. We used a quick acting surgical fibrin sealant derived from human blood plasma, with both hemostatic and adhesive properties.

SCLERAL FIXATED IOL

Intraocular lens implantation (IOL) in eyes that lack posterior capsular support has been accomplished in the past, by means of iris fixated IOL,[1,2] anterior chamber intraocular lens and transscleral IOL fixation[3-12] through the ciliary sulcus or pars plana. Surgical expertise, prolonged surgical time, suture induced inflammation, suture degradation, and delayed IOL subluxation or dislocation due to broken suture are some of the limitations in sutured scleral fixated intraocular lenses (SFIOL). It is also difficult and time consuming requiring minute and perfect adjustment of suture length and tension to ensure good centration of SFIOL.

FIBRIN GLUE

Fibrin glue[13-15] has been used previously in various medical specialities as a hemostatic agent to arrest bleeding, seal tissues and as an adjunct to wound healing. The fibrin kit we used was ReliSeal™ (Reliseal, Reliance Life Sciences, India). It is available in a sealed pack, which contains freeze dried human fibrinogen (20 mg/0.5 ml), freeze dried human thrombin (250 IU/0.5 ml), aprotinin solution (1500 kiu in 0.5 ml), one ampoule of sterile water, four 21G needles, two 20G blunt application needles and an applicator with two mixing chambers and one plunger guide.

SURGICAL TECHNIQUE

After inserting the infusion cannula or anterior chamber maintainer, localized peritomy is done. Two partial thickness limbal based scleral flaps about 4 mm × 4 mm are created exactly 180 degrees diagonally apart (Fig. 1) and about 1.5 mm from the limbus. This is followed by vitrectomy via pars plana or anterior route to remove all vitreous traction. Two straight sclerotomies with a 22G needle are made about 1.5 mm from the limbus under the existing scleral flaps. The sclerotomies are positioned such a way that the superior one lies close to the upper edge of the flap and the inferior one close to the lower edge of the flap. A scleral tunnel incision is then prepared about 2 mm from the limbus for introducing the IOL. While the IOL is being introduced with the left hand of the surgeon using a McPherson forceps, an end gripping 25G microrhexis forceps (Micro Surgical Technology, USA) is passed through the inferior sclerotomy. The tip of the leading haptic is then grasped with the microrhexis forceps, pulled through the inferior sclerotomy following the curve of the haptic (Fig. 2) and is externalized under the inferior scleral flap. Similarly, the trailing haptic is also externalized through the superior sclerotomy under the scleral flap (Fig. 3). Then, the reconstituted fibrin glue thus prepared is injected through the cannula of the double syringe delivery system under the superior (Fig. 4) and inferior scleral flaps. Local pressure is given over the flaps for about 10 to 20 seconds for the formation of fibrin polypeptides (Fig. 5). The anterior chamber maintainer or the infusion cannula is removed. Conjunctiva is also closed with the same fibrin glue.

In case of those patients who had a luxated IOL, similar lamellar scleral flaps as described earlier were made and the luxated IOL haptic was then grasped with the 25 gauge rhexis forceps and exteriorized and glued under the scleral flaps (Figs 6A to E). The haptic of the IOL if protruding beyond the scleral flap can be tucked in a tunnel created in the sclera (Fig. 7). Our follow-up anterior segment OCT (Figs 8A and B) showed postoperative perfect scleral flap adhesion as early as day 1 and continues to remain well maintained at one week and one month.

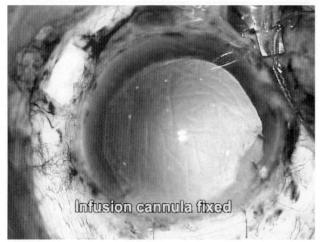

Fig. 1: Scleral flaps prepared 180 degrees diagonally apart. Note the infusion cannula fixed in and eye without any capsule

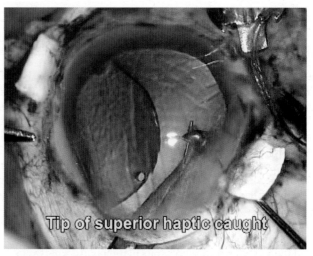

Fig. 3: Superior haptic grabbed by the 25 gauge microrhexis forceps (MST, USA) and then externalized under the scleral flap

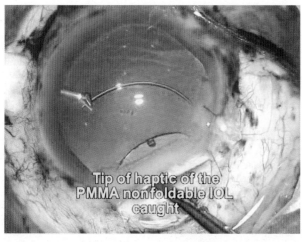

Fig. 2: Tip of the haptic grabbed by the 25 gauge microrhexis forceps (MST, USA) and then that haptic is externalized under the scleral flap

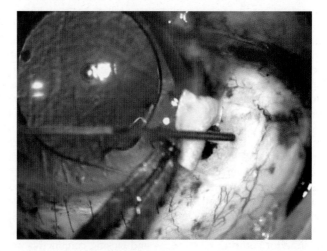

Fig. 4: Fibrin glue applied. Note the haptic which is externalized

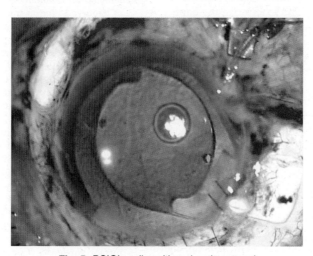

Fig. 5: PCIOL well positioned and centered

DISCUSSION

This fibrin glue assisted sutureless PCIOL implantation technique as described by us would be useful in a myriad of clinical situations where scleral fixated IOLs are indicated, such as, luxated IOL, dislocated IOL, zonulopathy or secondary IOL implantation. In dislocated posterior chamber PMMA IOL, the same IOL can be repositioned thereby reducing the need for further manipulation. Externalization of the greater part of the haptics along its curvature stabilizes the axial positioning of the IOL and thereby prevents any IOL tilt.[16] In the 12 eyes of our 12 patients, no complications like post- operative inflammation, hyphema, decentration, glaucoma or corneal edema were seen after a regular follow-up till now. We expect less incidence of UGH syndrome in fibrin glue assisted IOL implantation as compared to sutured scleral fixated IOL. This is because, in the former the IOL is well stabilized and stuck onto the scleral bed and thereby, has decreased intraocular mobility whereas in the latter, there is increased possibility of IOL movement or persistent rub over the ciliary body. Visually significant complications due to late subluxation[17] which has been known to occur in sutured scleral fixated IOL may also be prevented as sutures are totally avoided in this technique. Moreover the frequent complications[18] of secondary IOL implantation like secondary glaucoma, cystoid macular edema or bullous keratopathy were not seen in any of our patients. Another important advantage of this technique is the prevention of suture related complications[19-21] like suture erosion, suture knot exposure or dislocation of IOL after suture disintegration or broken suture. Chances of scleral melt[22-24] and haptic exposure are not increased by this technique except possibly, in high-risk patients like rheumatoid arthritis.

The other advantage of this technique is the rapidity and ease of surgery. Since all the steps of tying the difficult to handle 10-0 prolene suture to the IOL haptic eyelets, the time required to ensure good centration before tying down the knots as well as time for suturing scleral flaps and closing conjunctiva are done away with, the total surgical time is significantly reduced. It is also easier and does not require much surgical expertise to use the 25 gauge forceps to grasp and exteriorize the haptic. Fibrin glue takes only 20 seconds to act in the scleral bed and it helps in adhesion as well as hemostasis. Fibrin glue has been shown to provide airtight closure and by the time the fibrin starts degrading, surgical adhesions would have already occurred in the scleral bed.

The commercially available fibrin glue that we used is virus inactivated and is checked for viral antigen with polymerase chain reaction, hence the chances of transmission of infection is very low. But with tissue derivatives, there is always a theoretical possibility of transmission of viral infections,[25] therefore it is mandatory to get informed consent from the patient before the procedure. Though the use of fibrin glue in ophthalmology is considered off-label, it has been successfully used in the eye since long. Its various uses in the eye include repair of lacerated canaliculi[28] to seal full thickness macular holes,[26,27] to seal cataract incisions,[32-35] corneal perforations , and traumatic lens capsule

perforations.[29] It has also been used for temporary closure of scleral flaps[31] after trabeculectomy in eyes with hypotony, conjunctival fistula closure,[30] conjunctival autografts,[31] and amniotic membrane transplantation.[36,37]

Gabor et al[38] have shown sutureless scleral IOL fixation by placing the IOL haptic in a scleral tunnel. Our technique differed from other sutureless methods[38, 39] by use of the fibrin glue which enhances the rate of adhesion with hemostasis. We also used scleral flaps as in conventional sutured SFIOLs and this makes the learning curve very simple. There is also no danger of intraocular infection gaining entry through the tunnel as the fibrin glue hermetically seals the flaps leaving behind no possible entry route for microbes. There was no glue induced intraocular inflammation in any of our patients and all 12 eyes had clear media on the postoperative visits. Scleral indentation performed in the operated eyes showed no change in the axial positioning of the IOL. After one month of follow-up, we found no IOL decentration or any other complications in any of the operated 12 eyes.

SUMMARY

Fibrin glue assisted sutureless PCIOL implantation is appropriate for eyes with deficient or absent posterior capsule and this can be performed easily with the available IOL designs, instruments and with less surgical time. However, a longer duration follow-up might be necessary to judge the long-term functional and anatomical results of the procedure.

REFERENCES

1. Zeh WG, Price FW. Iris fixation of posterior chamber intraocular lenses. J Cataract Refract Surg 2000;26:1028-34.
2. Lorencova V, Rozsival P, Urminsky J. Clinical results of the aphakia correction by means of secondary implantation of the iris-fixated anterior chamber intraocular lens Cesk Slov mol 2007;63(4):285-91.
3. Bleckmann H, Kaczmarek U. Functional results of posterior chamber lens implantation with scleral fixation. J Cataract Refract Surg 1994;20:321-26.
4. Holland EJ, Djalilian AR, Pederson J. Gonioscopic evaluation of haptic position in transsclerally sutured posterior chamber lenses. Am J Ophthalmol 1997;123:411-13.
5. Factors contributing to retinal detachment after transscleral fixation of posterior chamber intraocular lenses. J Cataract Refract Surg 1998;24:697-702.
6. Solomon K, Gussler JP, Gussler C, Van Meter WS. Incidence and management of complications of transsclerally sutured posterior chamber lenses. J Cataract Refract Surg 1993;19:488-93.
7. Teichmann KD, Teichmann IAM. Haptic design for continuous-loop, scleral fixation of posterior chamber lens. J Cataract Refract Surg 1998;24:889-92.
8. Chang S, Coll GE. Surgical techniques for repositioning a dislocated intraocular lens, repair of iridodialysis, and secondary intraocular lens implantation using innovative 25-gauge forceps AJO 1995;120(1):126.
9. Mensiz E, Avtulner E, Ozerturk Y. Scleral fixation suture technique without lens removal for posteriorly dislocated intraocular lenses. Can J Ophthalmol 2002;37(5):290-94.

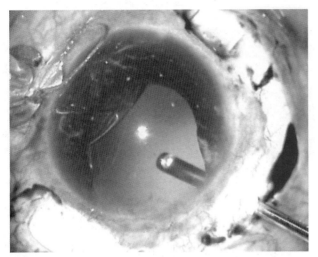

Fig. 6A: Subluxated IOL. Note the infusion cannula fixed and scleral flaps prepared. Vitrectomy being done

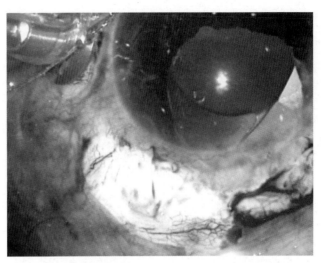

Fig. 6D: IOL haptic now glued by the fibrin glue

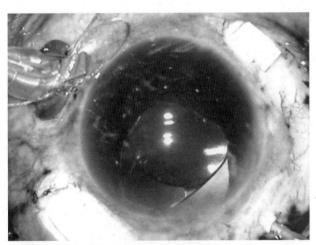

Fig. 6B: Haptics externalized under the scleral flaps and IOL well centered

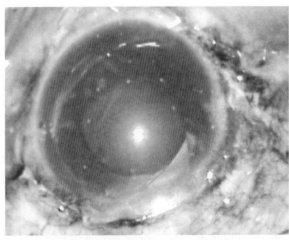

Fig. 6E: Fibrin glue seals the conjunctiva

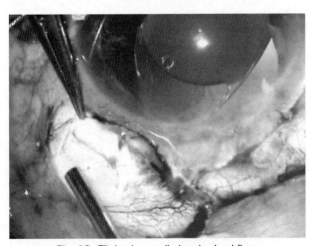

Fig. 6C: Fibrin glue applied and scleral flaps seal the haptic of the IOL

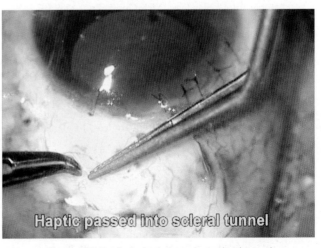

Fig. 7: IOL haptic tucked through a scleral tunnel

213

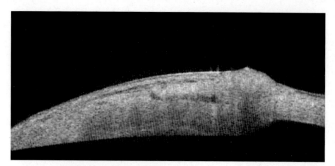

Fig. 8A: Anterior segment OCT of scleral flap

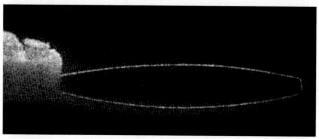

Fig. 8B: Anterior segment OCT of the IOL. Note IOL well centered

10. Mittelviefhaus H, Witschel H. Transscleral suture fixation of posterior-chamber lenses after cataract extraction associated with vitreous loss Ger Jr Ophthalmol 1995;4(2):80-85.

11. Scleral fixation technique using 2 corneal tunnels for a dislocated intraocular lens. J Cataract Refract Surg 2000;26(10):1439-41.

12. Oh H, Chu Y, Woong known O. Surgical technique for suture fixation of a single-piece hydrophilic acrylic intraocular lens in the absence of capsule support J Cataract Refract Surg 2007;33:962–65.

13. Fink D, Klein JJ, Kang H, et al. Application of biological glue in repair of intracardiac structural defects. The ann of thoracic surg 2004;77(2):506-11.

14. AF Matar, JG Hill, W Duncan, et al. Use of biological glue to control pulmonary air leaksThorax 45:670-74.

15. PD Mintz, L Mayers, N Avery, H, et al. Fibrin Sealant: Clinical Use and the Development of the University of Virginia Tissue Adhesive CenterAnn. Clin Lab Sci, January 1, 2001;31(1):108-18.

16. Teichmann KD, Teichmann IAM. The torque and tilt gamble. J Cataract Refract Surg 1997;23:413-18.

17. McCluskey P, Harrisberg B. Long-term results using scleral-fixated posterior chamber intraocular lenses. J Cataract Refract Surg 1994;20:34-39.

18. Biro Z. Results and complications of secondary intraocular lens implantation. J Cataract Refract Surg 1993;19: 64-67.

19. Heilskov T, Joondeph BC, Olsen KR, Blankenship GW. Late endophthalmitis after transscleral fixation of a posterior chamber intraocular lens. Arch Ophthalmol 1989;107:1427.

20. Mowbray SL, Chang S-H, Casella JF. Estimation of the useful lifetime of polypropylene fiber in the anterior chamber. Am Intra-Ocular Implant Soc J 1983;9:143-47.

21. Jongebloed WL, Worst JFG. Degradation of polypropylene in the human eye: A SEM-study. Doc Ophthalmol 1986;64:143-52.

22. Ahmed TY, Carrim ZI, Diaper CJM, Wykes WN. Spontaneous intraocular lens extrusion in a patient with scleromalacia secondary to herpes zoster ophthalmicus. J Cataract Refract Surg 2007;33:925-26.

23. Mamalis N, Johnson MD, Haines JM, et al. Corneal-scleral melt in association with cataract surgery and intraocular lenses: A report of four cases. J Cataract Refract Surg 1990;16:108-15.

24. Watson PG, Hayreh SS. Scleritis and episcleritis. Br J Ophthalmol 1976;60:163-91.

25. Schlegel A, Immelmann A, Kempf C. Virus inactivation of plasma-derived proteins by pasteurization in the presence of guanidine hydrochloride. Transfusion 2001;41:382-89.

26. Tilanus MAD, Deutman T, Deutman AF. Full-thickness macular holes treated with vitrectomy and tissue glue. Int Ophthalmol 1994/1995;18:355-58.

27. Olsen TW, Sternberg P Jr, Capone A Jr, et al. Macular hole surgery using thrombin-activated fibrinogen and selective removal of the internal limiting membrane. Retina1998;18:322-29.

28. Steinkogler FJ. Fibrin tissue adhesive for the repair of lacerated canaliculi lacrimales. In: Schlag G, Redl H (Eds). Fibrin Sealant in Operative Medicine, Ophthalmology-Neurosurgery. Berlin: Springer 1986;2:92-94.

29. Buschmann W. Progress in fibrin sealing of eye lens and conjunctiva. In: Schlag G, Ascher PW, Steinkogler F Stammberger H (Eds). Fibrin Sealing in Surgical and Nonsurgical Fields. Neurosurgery, Ophthalmic Surgery, ENT. Berlin, Springer-Verlag 1994;5:97-106.

30. Grewing R, Mester U. Fibrin sealant in the management of complicated hypotony after trabeculectomy. Ophthalmic Surg Lasers 1997;28:124-27.

31. Cohen RA, McDonald MB. Fixation of conjunctival autografts with an organic tissue adhesive [letter]. Arch Ophthalmol 1993;111:1167-68.

32. Grewing R, Mester U. Radial suture stabilized by fibrin glue to correct preoperative against-the-rule astigmatism during cataract surgery. Ophthalmic Surg 1994;25:446-48.

33. Mester U. Wound closure with fibrin adhesive in cataract surgery. In: Schlag G, Ascher PW, Steinkogler FJ, Stammberger H (Eds). Fibrin Sealing in Surgical and Nonsurgical Fields. Neurosurgery: Ophthalmic Surgery, ENT. Berlin, Springer-Verlag 1994;5:123-32.

34. Rauber M, Mester U, Zuche M. Fibrin adhesive for wound closure in small-incision cataract surgery. In: Schlag G, Ascher PW, Steinkogler FJ, Stammberger H (Eds). Fibrin Sealing in Surgical and Nonsurgical Fields. Neurosurgery: Ophthalmic Surgery, ENT. Berlin, Springer-Verlag, 1994;5:116-22.

35. Henrick A, Kalpakian B, Gaster RN, Vanley C. Organic tissue glue in the closure of cataract incisions in rabbit eyes. J Cataract Refract Surg 1991;17:551-55.

36. Lagoutte FM, Gauthier L, Comte PRM. A fibrin sealant for perforated and preperforated corneal ulcers. Br J Ophthalmol 1989;73:757-61.

37. Duchesne B, Tahi H, Galand A. Use of human fibrin glue and amniotic membrane transplant in corneal perforation. Cornea 2001;20:230-32.

38. Gabor SG, Pavilidis MM. Sutureless intrascleral posterior chamber intraocular lens fixation. J Cataract Refract Surg 2007;33(11):1851-54.

39. Maggi R, Maggi C. Sutureless scleral fixation of intraocular lenses. J Cataract Refract Surg 1997;23(9):1289-94.

Chapter 40

PCIOL Scleral Suturing Using Endoscopy

Boris Malyugin (Russia)

The endocapsular placement of an IOL is undoubtedly anatomically preferable. However, the presence of an unstable capsulo-zonular complex or its partial absence, as with pseudoexfoliative syndrome, ocular trauma or hereditary conditions, pre-empts endocapular fixation of the IOL (Figs 1A to C and 2). The necessity of alternative techniques of IOL fixation arises in aphakia, or when the IOL-capsule complex has subluxated postoperatively, which usually occurs secondary to pseudoexfoliation (Fig. 3).

One of the options is to suture posterior chamber IOL to the sclera. This type of fixation has an advantage, in that it may be performed in the presence of significant structural abnormalities of the anterior chamber.

In 1986, Malbran and coauthors were the first to describe trans-sulcus fixation of PCIOLs (Fig. 4). The placement of sutures involves either an abinterno or abexterno technique. The former is technically easier, whereas the latter facilitates the increased accuracy of suture placement.

Further variations in technique differ in the method of securing the haptic with fixation suture, the number of points of PCIOL fixation, and the method by which to avoid erosion of the suture/knot. The latter is one of the most significant complications in late postoperative period.

Currently, scleral fixation has been described using a rigid PMMA lens with eyelets and foldable three-piece acrylic lenses. Single-piece, all-PMMA lenses are ideal, as the greater plastic memory of PMMA loops better resists external forces and hence decentration (Figs. 5A to B).

Sulcus sutured IOL is placed more anteriorly and 1 to 1.5 diopters should be subtracted from the calculated IOL power to prevent a myopic shift.

Suturing of the lens to the ciliary suclus is a common but difficult procedure.

The surgeon who implants a sulcus-fixated IOL will need to know the exact location of the ciliary sulcus in relation to the corneoscleral limbus. It is not possible to observe the sulcus through an operating microscope, and most of the surgeons use indirect scleral landmarks for its location (Figs 6A to E).

R Duffey et al (1989) determined that the average scleral exit site of a suture passed from inside of the eye perpendicularly to the ciliary sulcus was 0.94 mm posterior to the surgical limbus in the vertical axis, 0.87 mm in the oblique meridians, and 0.50 mm in the horizontal axis (Fig. 7).

The ideal position for the haptics is when they are positioned in the ciliary sulcus (Fig. 8). In reality, sulcus position varies between patients and is not always easily located. In some instances, the IOL haptic may be decentered and located anteriorly or posteriorly to the sulcus (Fig. 9A). These IOLs may also be tilted because the suture did not pass through the sulcus, but rather through some other part of the ciliary body (e.g. pars plana or pars plicata) (Fig. 9B).

Posterior tilting of one haptic results in the anterior tilting of the other and could cause localized pushing of the iris, which would result in segmental angle closure and uveitis-glaucoma-hyphema syndrome (Fig. 10).

It is recommended to evaluate ciliary sulcus with an ultrasonic biomicroscopy (UBM) to locate abnormalities in cases of malpositioned IOLs. Figures 11A to C demonstrate the examples of abnormalities including posterior synechiae (A), irido-ciliary angle smoothening (B), residual cortical material (C) and capsular remnants (D). Abnormalities such as those mentioned above are clearly seen during ultrasonic biomicroscopy. When discovered, the surgeon may avoid these areas in the hopes that the lens will not dislocate postoperatively.

The attempts to visualize the ciliary body during the operation with the help of the mirrors were done by Kozawa (1994), Tsai (1996) and Kim (2006). Endoscope-assisted suture fixation of PCIOLs was first described by Eguchi and Araie (1990) (Fig. 12). According to them it could help ease the technical difficulty of implanting these lenses. The main advantage of endoscopy is that it allows direct visualization of the ciliary sulcus (Figs 13A and B).

Endoscope can enter the globe through either the corneal (Figs 14A to C) or the scleral incision (Figs 15A and B).

There are two methods to the endoscopic approach. In the first, bimanual method, the surgeon holds the instrument in one hand (Fig. 16) and penetrates the scleral wall with the other. At all times, one can see the ciliary sulcus on an endoscope screen much like that of a television screen.

There are two variatons of bimanual method. In "ab-externo" variation the surgeon can see how the bent 27 gauge needle is passed through the outer wall of the sclera directly in

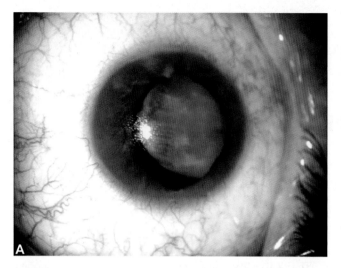

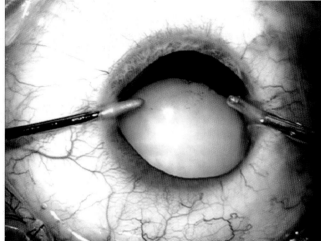

Fig. 2: Bimanual anterior vitrectomy is being performed in case of traumatic cataract with zonular rupture

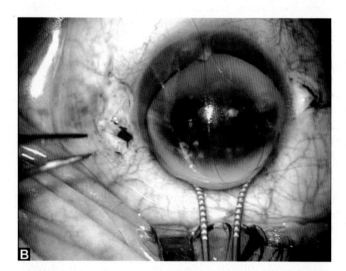

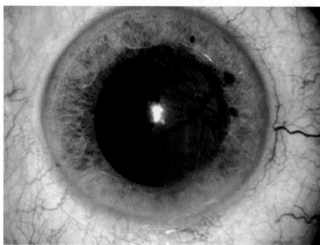

Fig. 3: Foldable PCIOL decentration

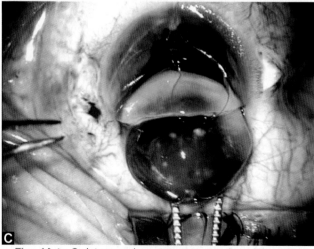

Figs 1A to C: Intracapsular catataract extraction with vectis in patient with lens subluxation

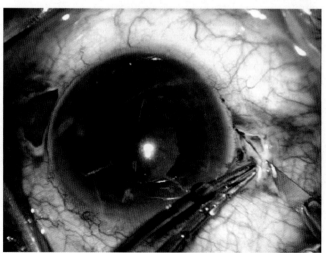

Fig. 4: Limbal-based triangular scleral flaps formation for scleral UIOL suturing

the sulcus (Figs 17A to D). In order to bring out the needle we "dock" the tip of the needle in a bent 27G needle and push them back until the tip of the needle is out.

The other case is an "ab-interno" variation. In this case the needle goes through the ciliary sulcus from inside of the eye outside (Figs 18A to C). The surgeon passes the needle posterior to the iris but anterior to the capsular bag and ciliary processes at the same time controlling the process with endoscopy (Figs 19A to C).

There is a downside to the bimanual method; it is very hard to coordinate the both hands movements and to view where your tips are exactly located during the surgery (Fig. 20).

Surgical Technique

In 2005, we developed an original technique of PCIOL scleral suturing with the help of microendoscopy. In this one-handed technique endoscope is used not only to visualize tissues but also as an active surgical tool. In the new technique, a needle is attached by a silicone sleeve to the endoscopic probe (Figs 21A to C). Therefore, the needle and point of penetration are viewable on the endoscope screen (Figs 22A to C).

The direct visualization provides the correct position of the suture and correct position of the IOL in the postoperative period, which is the most important thing (Figs 23A to E).

Ciliary sulcus is examined with the endoscope to locate possible abnormalities. In the Figure 24, you can notice the presence of residual lens capsule and cortical material.

The presence of any vitreous, lens and cortical remnants should be dealt with prior to IOL implantation by automated vitrectomy. On the screen of the endoscope the surgeon can clearly see vitrectomy probe tip inserted through pars plana approach (Fig. 25). With endoscopy the surgeon can directly visualize the posterior surface of the iris with pseudoexfoliative covering the ciliary processes (Fig. 26).

After tying the suture to the lens haptics, the surgeon grasps the needle fixated to the IOL haptic and attaches it to the endoscopy probe. The latter passed through the surgical incision, and via the pupil behind the iris. The tip of the needle goes out through the sclera posterior to the corneo-scleral limbus. Needleholder is used to catch the needle while it is being passed through the sclera (Figs 27A to C).

For cases of plate haptic IOL dislocation we developed the "Two string" suturing technique. With this technique the lens is "suspended" on the two parallel sutures passed through the ciliary sulcus in four points (Figs 28A to I).

The endoscopic probe is guided behind the lens optic. The thread passing through the eyelet in the haptics is visible with the endoscope (Fig. 29).

One of the most common intraoperative complications of trans-scleral lens suturing is bleeding (Figs 30A and B). This can occur in both the endoscopic approach as well as the traditional approach to scleral IOL fixation. For the most part, however, these complications are reduced with endoscopy because it does not induce extra manipulation in the eye.

One of the drawbacks of the endoscopic technique is the absence of a stereoscopic view (providing depth of focus), the surgeon is familiar with having when looking through an operating microscope. The image on the endoscope screen is flat.

The surgeon must get acquainted with landmarks that signify the distance from the tissue. The magnification on the screen of the endoscope indicates the distance from the tissue structures of the eye (Figs 31A to E). That is why there is a learning curve associated with the endoscopic approach.

CONCLUSION

In many scenarios, individual surgeons' comfort in performing various IOL fixation techniques may dictate the approach used. We are widely using endoscopy for transscleral suturing of PCIOLs and believe that its popularity will continue to grow, as the one-handed endoscopy technique significantly reduces the risk for complications and is superior to the traditional techniques.

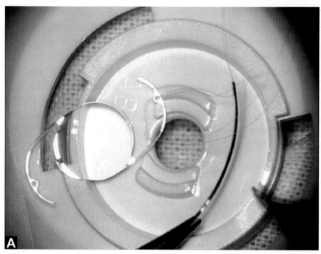
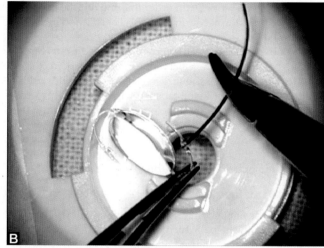

Figs 5A and B: Fixation of the suture to the eyelet in the haptics of PMMA IOL

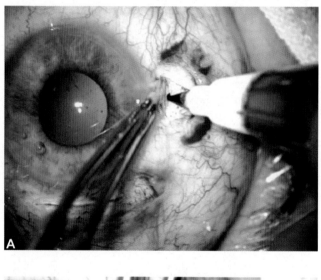
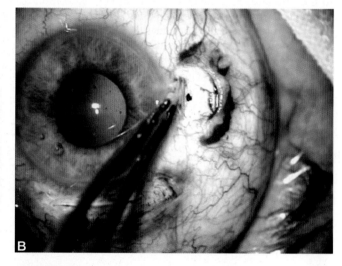
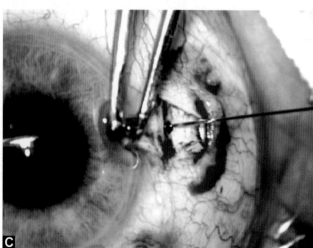
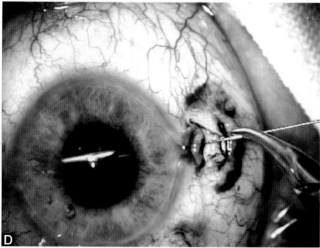

Figs 6A to D

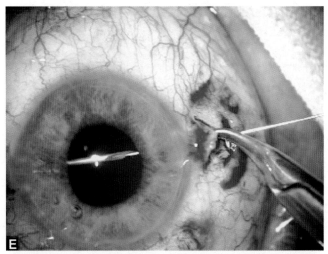

Figs 6A to E: Marking the site of the sutures pass through the sclera in ab-externo scleral suturing

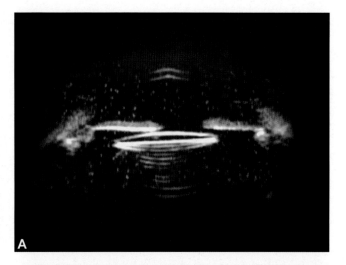

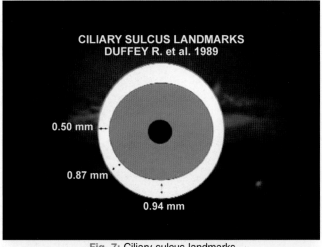

Fig. 7: Ciliary sulcus landmarks

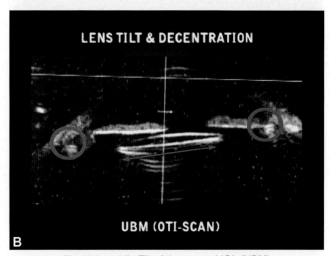

Figs 9A and B: Tilt of the sutured IOL (UBM)

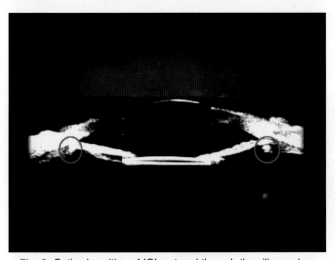

Fig. 8: Optimal position of IOL sutured through the ciliary sulcus (assessed with ultrasonic biomicroscopy - UBM)

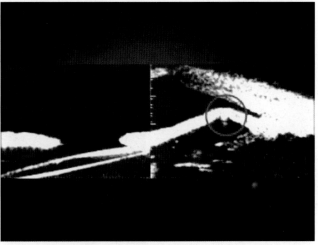

Fig. 10: Partial anterior chamber closing by the IOL haptic (UBM)

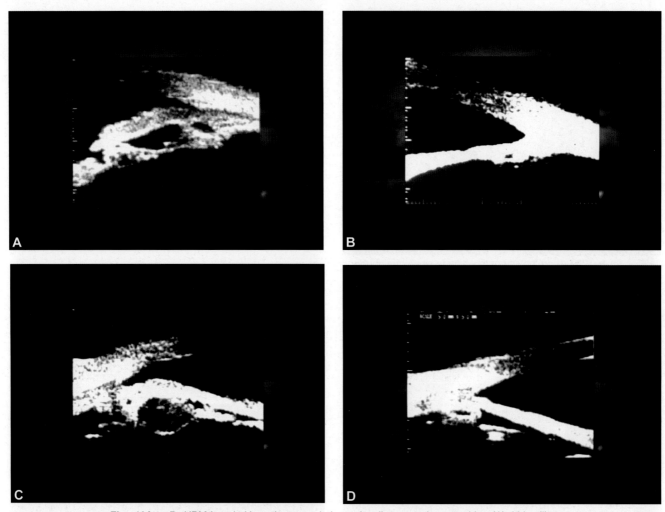

Figs 11A to D: UBM in aphakic patients can help to visualize posterior synechiae (A), irido-ciliary angle smoothening (B), residual cortical material (C) and capsular remnants (D)

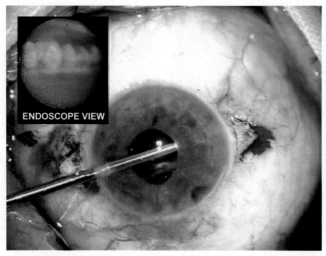

Fig. 12: Direct ciliary sulcus examination can be achieved with the endoscope

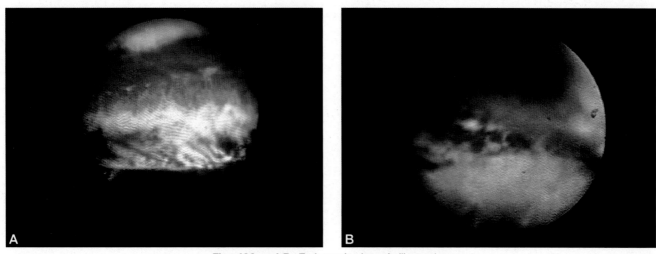

Figs 13A and B: Endoscopic view of ciliary sulcus

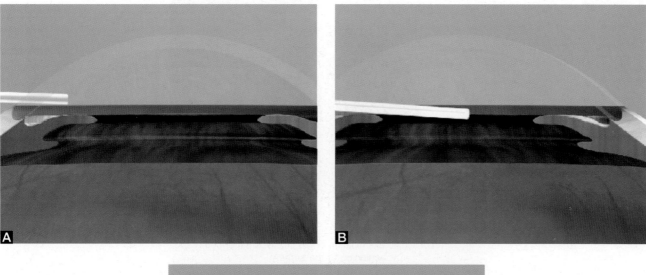

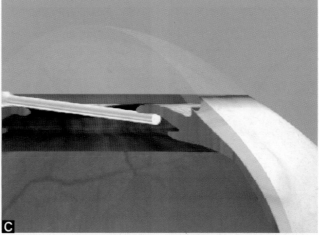

Figs 14A to C: Insertion of the endoscopic probe through the
corneal paracentesis

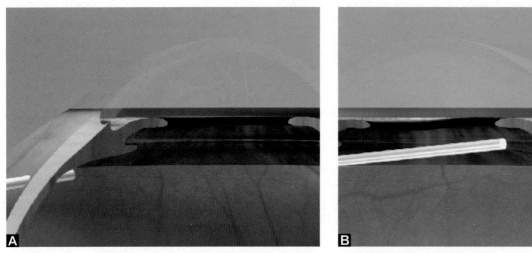

Figs 15A and B: Insertion of the endoscopic probe through the sclerotomy in the pars plana region

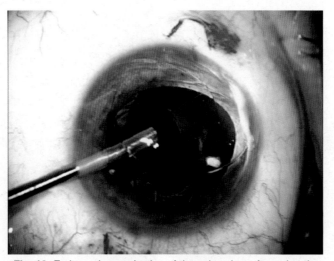

Fig. 16: Endoscopic examination of the sulcus is performed at the
beginning of the surgery

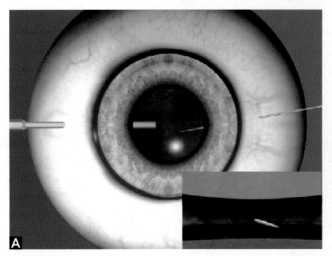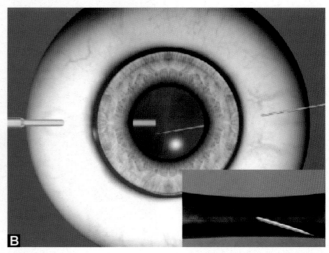

Figs 17A and B

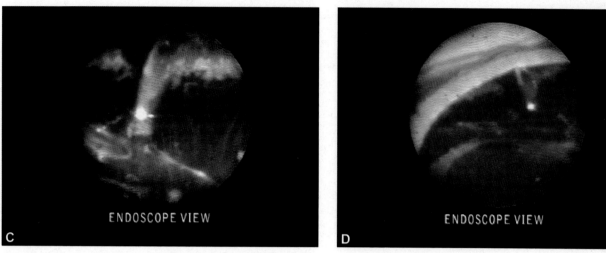

Figs 17A to D: "Ab-externo" variation of bimanual endoscopy technique

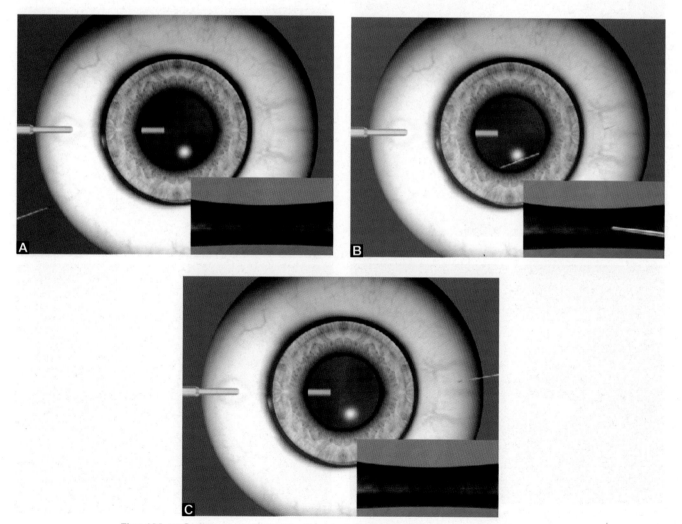

Figs 18A to C: Schematic view of the "ab-interno" variation of bimanual endoscopy technique

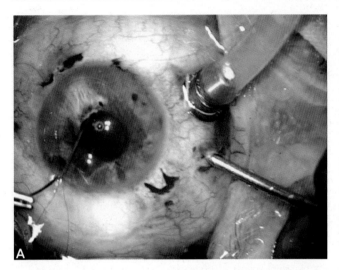

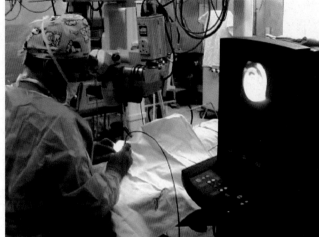

Fig. 20: Surgeon is observing the eye on the screen of the endoscope

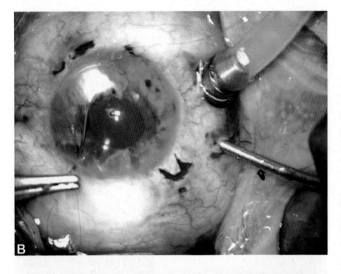

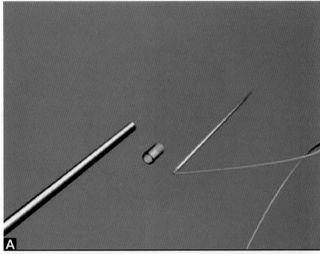

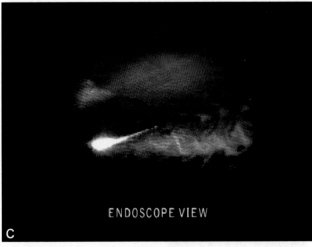

ENDOSCOPE VIEW

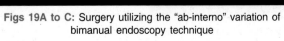

Figs 19A to C: Surgery utilizing the "ab-interno" variation of bimanual endoscopy technique

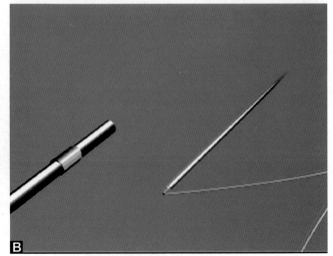

Figs 21A and B

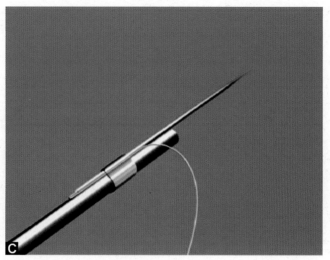

Figs 21A to C: Attaching the endoscopic probe and the needle in one-handed technique

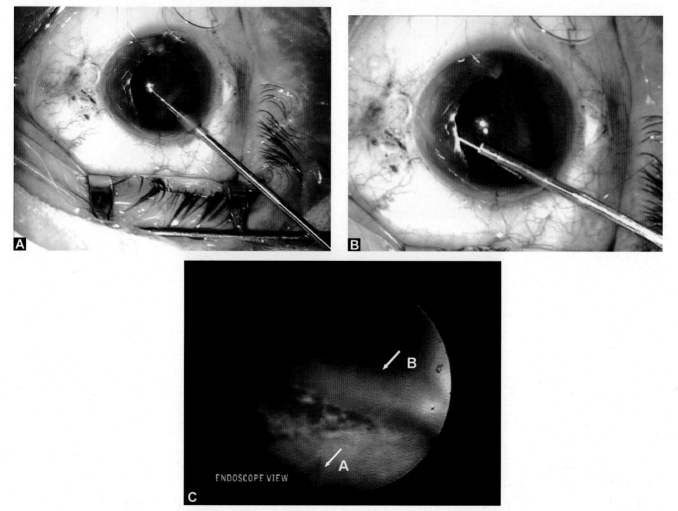

Figs 22A to C: Endoscopy in one-handed technique. The tip of the needle (A) and the point of penetration – ciliary suclus (B) are viewable on the endoscope screen (C)

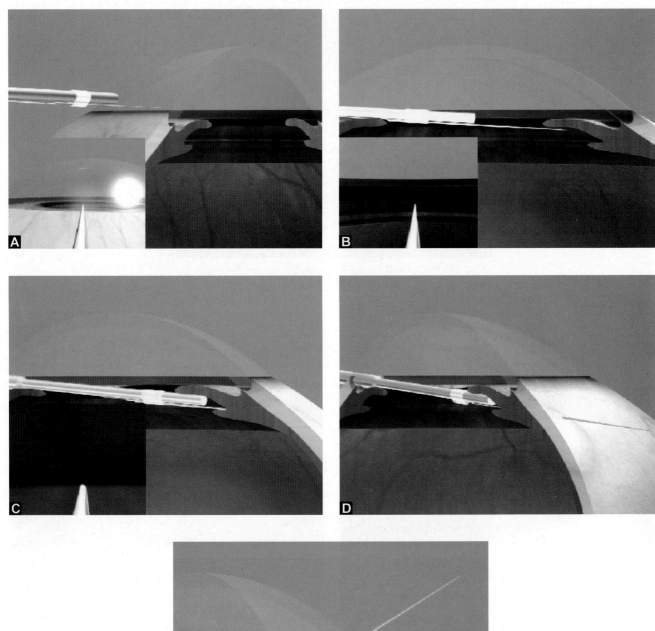

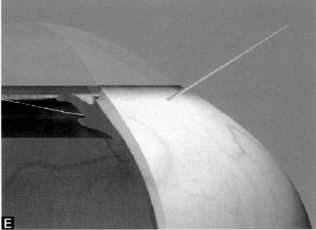

Figs 23A to E: Schematic representation of needle passing through the ciliary sulcus with the help of the one-handed endoscopy technique

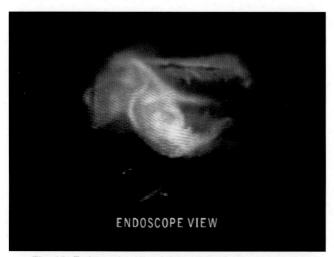

Fig. 24: Endoscopic view of the residual lens capsule and cortical material

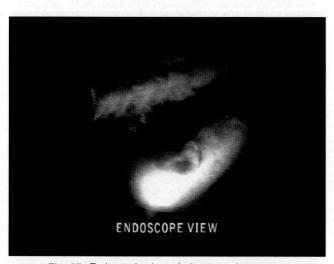

Fig. 25: Endoscopic view of vitrectomy in progress

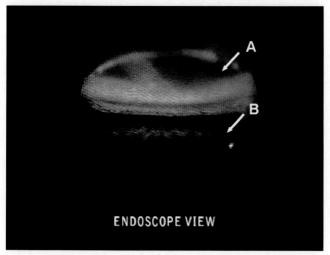

Fig. 26: Endoscopic view of the pupil (A) and ciliary processes (B)

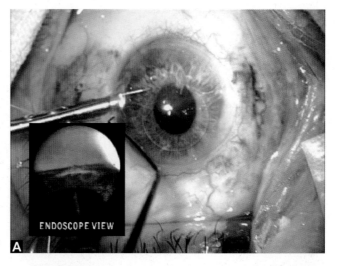

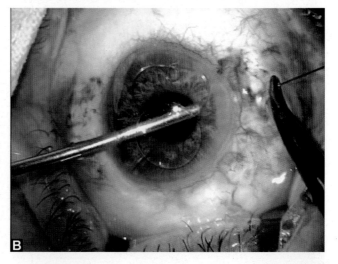

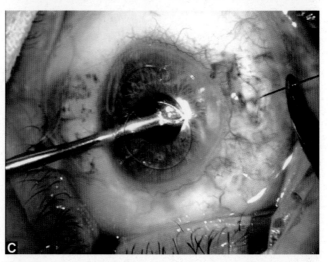

Figs 27A to C: Surgical steps of passing the needle through the sclera (A). Needleholder is used to catch the needle while it is being passed through the sclera (B, C)

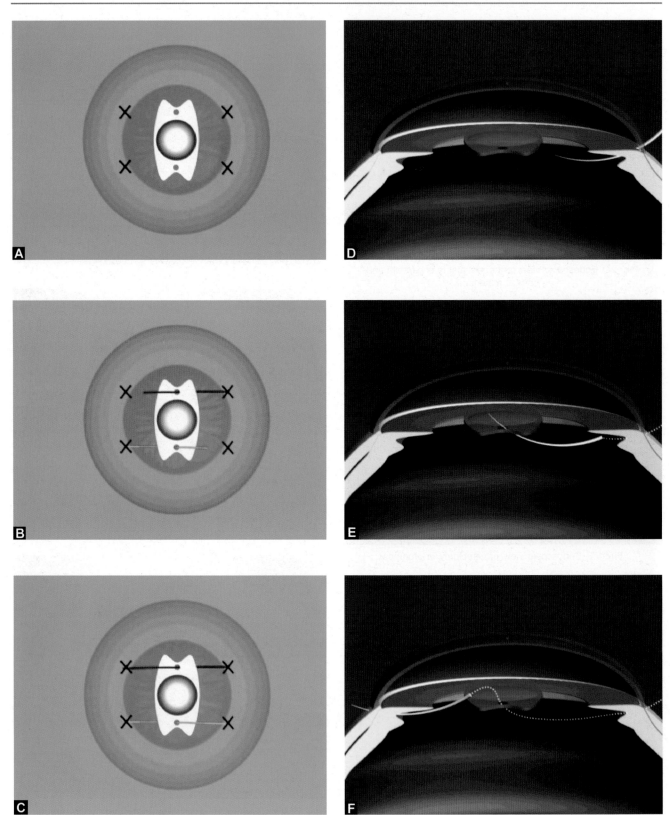

Figs 28A to F

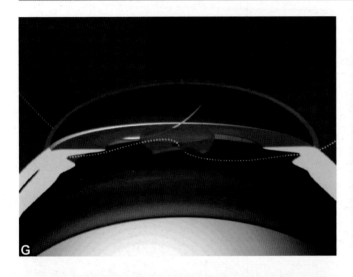

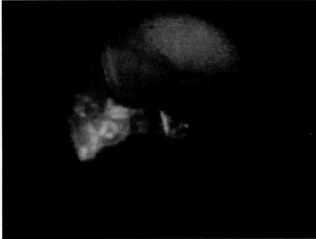

Fig. 29: Endoscopic view of the IOL haptic fixated to the sclera

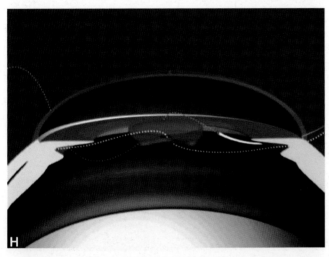

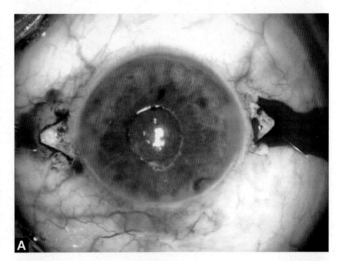

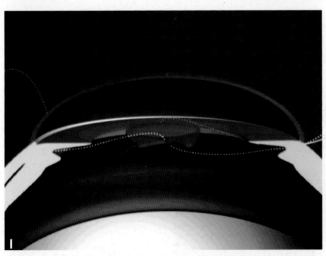

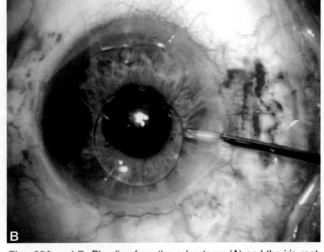

Figs 28A to I: Schematic representation of the "Two string" technique of the plate haptic IOL suturing. Side view (A to C) and lateral view (D to I).

Figs 30A and B: Bleeding from the sclerotomy (A) and the iris root (B) during lens suturing

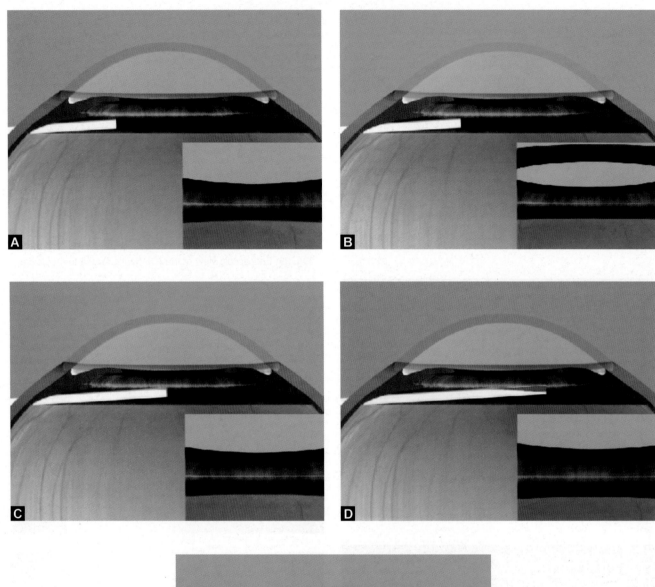

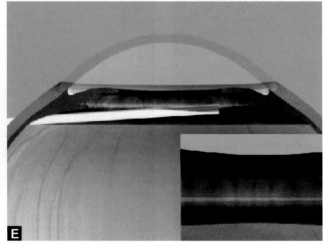

Figs 31A to E: The magnification on the endoscope screen can help to identify the distance from the tissue (ciliary body)

Chapter 41

Bimanual Microincision Phacoemulsification for Difficult and Challenging Cases

I Howard Fine, Richard S Hoffman, Mark Packer (USA)

The advantages of bimanual microincision phacoemulsification have been elaborated in a variety of papers within the literature.[1-6] We believe that the technique has distinct fluidic advantages because by separating inflow from aspiration and phaco, all of the fluid is coming in through one side of the eye and exiting through the opposite side of the eye, so there are never competing currents at the phaco tip. In addition, it is easier to achieve a nearly closed system because of the tightness of the incisions and we can address certain cases that would be less advantageous, or even impossible, with the use of a coaxial phaco tip.

High Myopia

In highly myopic eyes, we are able to achieve a situation in which we can maintain the anterior chamber in a completely stable configuration, never trampolining the vitreous face, by keeping the irrigating handpiece in the eye throughout the case. Chopping can take place in the usual manner, and with the completion of chopping, we can keep the irrigating chopper in the eye, remove the phaco needle, place viscoelastic, remove residual cortex, and then place viscoelastic for the implantation of the intraocular lens (IOL) without ever shallowing the anterior chamber. We believe that there may, eventually, be a documented decreased incidence of retinal detachment in high myopia as a result of non-trampolining of the vitreous face during phaco, and the implantation of IOLs that fill the capsule, such as dual-optic IOLs or IOLs that arch posteriorly, such as the crystalens.

Posterior Polar Cataract (Fig. 1)

In the situation of posterior polar cataracts, 35 percent have defective posterior capsules and almost all of them have weakened capsules, so it is very important to not over-pressurize the eye and perhaps force nuclear material through the defective posterior capsule. By the same token, it is important to not shallow the chamber and have the nucleus come forward, and possibly open the defect in the posterior capsule. These cases are advantageously done with bimanual microincision phacoemulsification.

We do hydrodelineation, without hydrodissection, and then carefully chop the endonucleus into pie-shaped segments and evacuate them from the eye. Once the endonucleus is removed, we viscodissect the epinucleus up from its position against the cortex without removing the irrigating chopper. In this way, we have a layer of cortex and viscoelastic under the epinucleus when we evacuate it, so should the capsule open, it is less likely that we will spill nuclear material into the vitreous. Once the epinucleus is gone, we leave the irrigation system in the eye, remove the phaco needle, and add viscoelastic. We viscodissect the cortex up into the plain of the capsulorhexis, in the same way and remove it while having a thick layer of viscoelastic on top of the fragile posterior capsule. We never polish the posterior segment of the capsule prior to the IOL implantation, but would rely on YAG laser if there were opacities within the visual axis, post-operatively.

Posterior Subluxed Cataracts (Fig. 2)

For posterior subluxed cataracts, which are hinged to a small zone of attached zonules, we will go through a pars plana incision and prolapse the lens, in its capsule, up into the anterior chamber and then add viscoelastic under the lens. We will then phaco the lens with bimanual microincision instrumentation utilizing an irrigating cannula in the left hand and a phaco needle in the right, keeping the irrigation on top of the viscoelastic, but below the nucleus. We don't try to disassemble these nuclei, but phaco them from the outside in. In general, with the irrigation under the nuclear material, we have a system in which there is fluid circulating in a circuitous pattern on top of the viscoelastic, and chips that are liberated from the mass of the nucleus tend to circulate entirely within the anterior segment and not get deposited into the vitreous. After removal of the cataract, we do a partial anterior vitrectomy and implant, through a 2.5 mm incision, a foldable intraocular lens, with the haptics under the iris and the optic on top. This allows the haptics to indent the undersurface of the iris and be easily identifiable. We then suture the haptics to the iris and nudge the optic beneath the pupillary margin. We have had great success with this technique.

Mature Cataract with Zonular Dialysis (Fig. 3)

In cases in which there was a dialysis of the zonular apparatus during phacoemulsification, as in a case of unrecognized pseudoexfoliation in the presence of a dense cataract, we can hold the nucleus with the phaco tip, remove the irrigating chopper, place viscoelastic under the lens, and then put the irrigating handpiece, without a chopper, under the lens and again phaco the lens entirely within the plain of the capsulorhexis. Nuclear material can be mobilized from the posterior chamber with an unsleeved phaco tip because there is no irrigation going along with the phaco tip, as in coaxial phaco, which would force the nuclear material into the vitreous cavity. This is not possible with a coaxial phaco tip. In these cases we also see chips that circulate in the fluid above the viscoelastic sitting on top of the vitreous, but we do not see chips that move posteriorly. Once this has been completed, we will do a bimanual microincision partial anterior vitrectomy, or a pars plana 25 gauge microincision vitrectomy, and implant an anterior chamber lens, or a posterior chamber lens, and suture it to the iris.

Punctured Posterior Capsule (Fig. 4)

In the case where the capsule is punctured during the course of phacoemulsification, we can keep the irrigation going high in the anterior chamber and go back into the endolenticular space with the unsleeved phaco tip, and complete the phacoemulsification without further enlarging the puncture in the posterior capsule. Without removing the irrigator, we then remove the cortex, and then instill more viscoelastic. We then implant the lens into the capsular bag or into the ciliary sulcus. Residual viscoelastic should be removed with a vitrector to avoid the possibility of bringing vitreous to the wound. This procedure would be impossible with a coaxial phaco tip because a continuously changing fluid wave from the phaco sleeve would enlarge, or extend, the capsular tear out to the periphery of the capsule, with loss of lens material into the vitreous.

Posterior Capsule Rupture (Figs 5 and 6)

In an extensive posterior capsule rupture, we can bring the entire endonucleus up into the anterior chamber by holding it with the phaco tip. Very little fluid leaks out of the incision when we remove the irrigator, place viscoelastic under the nucleus, and replace the irrigator under the lens. We then proceed with phacoemulsification in the plain of the capsulorhexis or in the anterior chamber, with the irrigator beneath the nucleus as we carousel, or phaco, it from the outside in. We can then proceed with cortical clean-up in a similar manner, or first perform a partial anterior vitrectomy, either through the pars plana, or through side-port incisions bimanually. Once all residual cortex has been removed, we implant a posterior chamber lens into the ciliary sulcus.

Pseudoexfoliation (Fig. 7)

In post-filtration surgery, in the presence of pseudoexfoliation, we like to use a endocapsular tension ring that we can introduce through a side-port with an injector. The injector does not enter the incision; it is just held against the incision, and the forces on the capsule as the endocapsular tension ring is being inserted are contained by the use of a Lester hook in the opposite hand. We then proceed with bimanual microincision horizontal chopping of the lens so as to not add any downward force on the lens which might stress the residual zonules. Cortical clean-up is facilitated in the presence of an endocapsular tension ring, by performing gentle cortical cleaving hydrodissection prior to the implantation of the ring. The lens is then implanted into the capsular bag through an incision between the two side-port incisions, which is our routine method for IOL implantation in the presence of two 1.1 mm phacoemulsification incisions.

Rock-Hard Nuclei (Fig. 8)

We can phacoemulsify rock-hard nuclei with the same facility and ease with which we do softer nuclei with bimanual microincision phacoemulsification, and we usually end up with average phaco powers under ten percent with effective phaco times under ten seconds, in spite of the density of these nuclei. This is an enormous advantage in terms of corneal, endothelial protection because of the great stability of the anterior chamber. We prefer a 30 degree phacoemulsification tip used with the bevel down. This allows the achievement of vacuum once the tip touches the endonucleus. A bevel-up tip must go deeply into the nucleus before occlusion and vacuum are achieved. With a bevel-down tip, we are also sending all of the energy toward the nucleus and none toward the endothelium or trabecular meshwork. Finally, one can mobilize pie-shaped segments from the level of the capsulorhexis up, rather than having to go deeply into the endolenticular space to achieve occlusion to mobilize these segments, as we would have to with a bevel-up configuration.

Switching Hands (Fig. 9)

In cases of zonular dialysis, another advantage of bimanual microincision phacoemulsification is that we can use the phaco tip with either hand. After inserting an endocapsular tension ring through one of the microincisions, we would hydroexpress the lens into the plain of the capsulorhexis and then utilize the phaco tip in either the right, or left, hand, depending on the zonular dialysis. For dialyses that are on the right side, we would use the phaco tip in the right hand, drawing material in the anterior chamber toward the area of weakened zonules, rather than away from it, which would stress the intact zonules. For dialyses that are on the left-hand side, we can use the phaco tip in our left hand and the irrigating chopper in the right to remove the nucleus, thereby closing the zonular dialysis with the activation of flow and vacuum toward the left side.

Microcornea or Microphthalmos (Fig. 10)

For very small eyes, such as microcornea or microphthalmos, the use of bimanual microincision phacoemulsification is enormously advantageous because the smaller size of the instruments allow us, through two clear corneal microincisions,

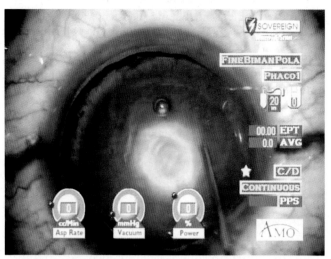

Fig. 1: Hydrodelineation of a posterior polar cataract

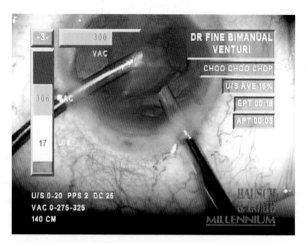

Fig. 4: Completing phacoemulsification in the presence of a punctured posterior capsule

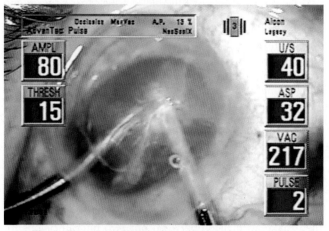

Fig. 2: Phacoemulsification of a subluxed cataract in the anterior chamber

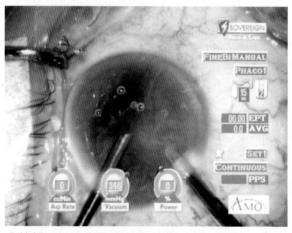

Fig. 5: Holding the nucleus with an unsleeved phaco tip prior to removing the chopper and adding viscoelastic under the nucleus in the presence of a large posterior capsule rupture

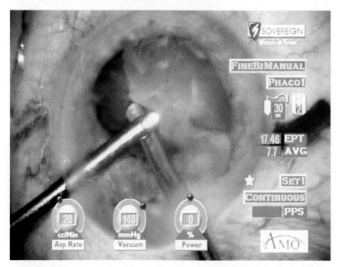

Fig. 3: Bringing nuclear material out of the posterior chamber with an unsleeved phaco tip in the presence of zonular dialysis

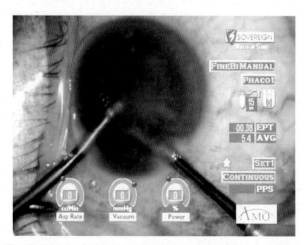

Fig. 6: Irrigating below the cataract in the presence of a capsule rupture

to maintain excellent visualization. A coaxial tip, which is much larger in size, would indent the cornea as it was manipulated and partially obscure the visualization of the intraocular structures. This has turned out to be especially advantageous in cases with a microcornea or a microphthalmic eye in the presence of an unusually large lens.

Post Malignant Melanoma (Fig. 11)

In one case in which 100 degrees of ciliary body and iris, with the exception of the sphincter, were excised for malignant melanoma, we were able to perform bimanual microincision phacoemulsification through two microincisions on each side of the 100 degree missing ciliary body and iris. The advantage here is that with the vitreous face open to the anterior chamber, we wanted to be drawing material toward the area of missing zonules, after having sequestered the vitreous in that area with Healon 5. Phacoemulsification performed in other locations would bring vitreous to the phaco tip and provide a much more challenging situation. The IOL was implanted nasally over the intact zonules to force the lens to push against the area of missing zonules, rather than to pull away from the area of missing zonules if it had been implanted in the temporal periphery.

Intraoperative Floppy Iris Syndrome (IFIS) (Figs 12 and 13)

We find bimanual microincision phacoemulsification enormously useful in cases of intraoperative floppy iris syndrome (IFIS). If we have adequate dilation in the presence of a floppy iris, we will perform gentle cortical cleaving hydrodelineation and hydrodissection, and then hydroexpress the lens into the plain of the iris. We will then carousel the endonucleus in the plain of the capsulorhexis with the irrigating cannula held high in the anterior chamber. Holding the irrigator high in the anterior chamber allows for a tamponading of the iris and disallows floppiness, or billowing, of the iris. After removing the endonucleus in the plain of the capsulorhexis, we see a fully intact epinuclear shell, which had been sitting on top of the iris, helping to hold it back. This is an extremely advantageous technique for nuclei of less hard densities that can be carouselled and phacoed in the anterior chamber without threatening the corneal endothelium.

For harder cataracts, and in the presence of pupils that will not dilate well, we will dilate the pupil with Healon 5, do a rather large capsulorhexis and then do one endolenticular chop. We then keep the irrigating chopper high in the anterior chamber and with the unsleeved phaco tip, bring nuclear material up to the chopper held high in the anterior chamber for further disassembly. This allows, once again, a tamponading of the iris and prevention of billowing or floppiness. We try to keep the phaco needle occluded and in foot position two or three, but with a clearance of occlusion, we go to foot position one in order to minimize evacuation of Healon 5, which is holding open the pupil.

After the endonucleus is removed in this way, we remove the epinucleus. Since it is harder to keep the tip occluded with

epinuclear trimming and flipping, there tends to be evacuation of Healon 5 and a reduction of the size of the pupil, although because of the irrigator held high in the anterior chamber, it does not billow. We then have to re-instill Healon 5 to redilate the pupil. Then, once again, holding the irrigator high in the anterior chamber, we keep the aspirating microincision handpiece occluded by going circumferentially around the capsulorhexis, removing the cortical material only from the fornix of the capsule, letting it sit as a cluster in the central portion of the capsule. After all of the cortex has been mobilized from the capsular fornix, we remove the residual cortex from the eye. In this way, we are able to keep Healon 5 in the eye and disallow miosis of the pupil until the case is complete.

Refractive Lens Exchange

We can do refractive lens exchange very easily, and safely, with bimanual microincision phacoemulsification. We do cortical cleaving hydrodissection and no hydrodelineation. We then hydroexpress the lens into the plain of the capsulorhexis, and carousel it, without any phacoemulsification energy for soft lenses, usually encountered in refractive lens exchange. We do an entirely fluidic-based extraction and then, because of cortical cleaving hydrodissection, we are able to evacuate the cortex by just tilting the phaco tip back into the posterior chamber where it jumps into the phaco tip as a single piece.

Refractive Lens Exchange in Post Radial Keratotomy (RK) (Fig. 14)

In cases where previous radial keratotomy (RK) has been performed, we can do bimanual microincision clear lens or cataract removal by going between two previously placed radials, making it much less likely that we will rupture the radial incisions during the course of the lens extraction. We then make an incision between our two microincisions for implantation of the IOL, but in the presence of previous RK, we make it through the posterior limbus for implantation of the IOL.

Intraocular Cautery (Fig. 15)

We have found that we can also, with bimanual microincision instruments, do intraocular cautery by using an irrigating cannula in one of the microincisions and a microincision bipolar cautery in the other. Pinching the irrigation tubing allows bleeding to take place, clearly identifying the point source because the eye softens and the bleeding points start to ooze. We cauterize them precisely with the bipolar cautery, and therefore minimize trauma to intraocular structures by avoiding more cautery than is necessary.

Bimanual Microincision Instruments (Figs 16 and 17)

There are a number of other instruments that have been developed for use through 1.1 mm microincisions. Iris reconstruction is very much easier utilizing intraocular forceps that stabilize the iris for suturing. New intraocular needle holders

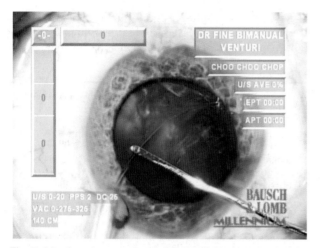

Fig. 7: Injection of a capsule tension ring through a microincision controlled by a Lester hook in the right hand

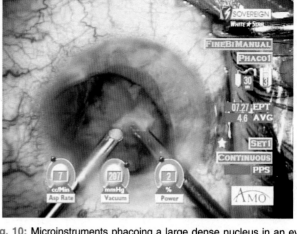

Fig. 10: Microinstruments phacoing a large dense nucleus in an eye with microcornea and iris coloboma

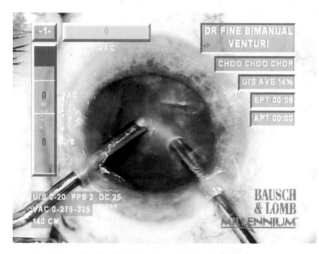

Fig. 8: Chopping a rock hard nucleus

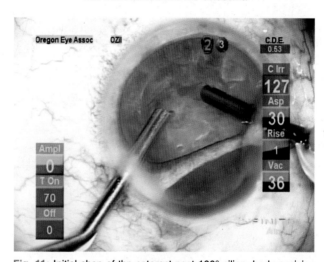

Fig. 11: Initial chop of the cataract post 100° ciliary body excision for malignant melanoma

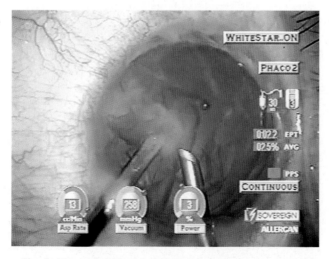

Fig. 9: Phacoemulsification in the left hand in the presence of zonular dialysis (surgeon's perspective)

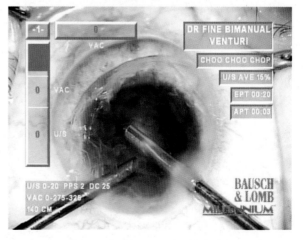

Fig. 12: Epinucleus holding the iris back after carouselling the endonucleus in the presence of intraoperative floppy iris syndrome (IFIS)

are also usable through a 1.0 mm incision. In this way, very fragile and atrophic irides can be sutured without putting excessive stress on the iris tissue. The knots are tied with a Seipser external tying mechanism, and the knots are cut with an intraocular microincision scissors, that is also admissible through a 1.0 mm incision.

For late reopening of capsular bags to recenter IOLs, we can enlarge a capsulorhexis in the late post-operative period by nicking the rhexis with intraocular scissors, and then tearing a larger opening with a microincision capsulorhexis forceps. Viscodissection of the lens, within the capsular bag, can be accomplished through microincisions which also allow for repositioning of IOLs without the need to make larger incisions to manipulate them intraocularly. There are currently additional microincision instruments under a state of development, including microincision Collibri forceps, microincision iris graspers, and microincision intraocular lens holders and cutters.

Conclusion

We believe bimanual microincision phacoemulsification is a technique that has a very short learning curve, is highly atraumatic, and is unquestionably the technique of the future.

For those who are willing to go through the short learning curve now, it represents the best and safest technique at present for the management of certain difficult and challenging cases.

REFERENCES

1. Tsuneoka H, Shiba T, Takahashi Y. Feasibility of ultrasound cataract surgery with a 1.4 mm incision. J Cataract Refract Surg 2001;27:934-40.
2. Agarwal A, Agarwal A, Agarwal S, Narang P, Narang S. Phakonit: phacoemulsification through a 0.9 mm corneal incision. J Cataract Refract Surg 2001;27(10): 1548-52.
3. Tsuneoka H, Shiba T, Takahashi Y. Ultrasonic phacoemulsification using a 1.4 mm incision: Clinical results. J Cataract Refract Surg 2002;28:81-86.
4. Tsuneoka H, Hayama A, Takahama M. Ultrasmall-incision bimanual phacoemulsification and AcrySof SA30AL implantation through a 2.2 mm incision. J Cataract Refract Surg. 2003 Jun; 29(6):1070-6.
5. Fine IH, Packer M, Hoffman RS. Power modulations in new technology: Improved outcomes. J Cataract Refract Surg 2004;30:1014-19.
6. Fine IH, Hoffman RS, Packer M. Optimizing refractive lens exchange with bimanual microincision phacoemulsification. J Cataract Refract Surg 2004;30:550-54.

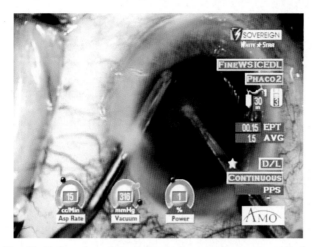

Fig. 13: Endonuclear disassembly in the anterior chamber with the irrigator tamponading the iris

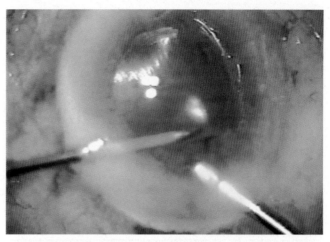

Fig. 15: Bipolar intraocular microcauterization with easy identification of the bleeding point by pinching the infusion tubing

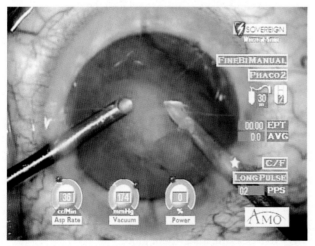

Fig. 14: Bimanual microincision phacoemulsification of a cataract between RK incisions

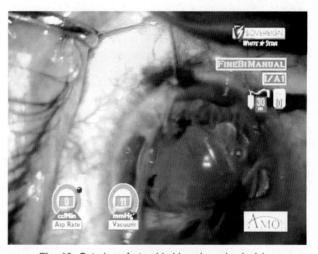

Fig. 16: Suturing of atrophic iris using microincision intraocular forceps

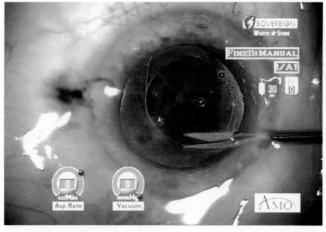

Fig. 17: Nicking the capsulorhexis with microincision scissors prior to enlarging the capsulorhexis

Chapter 42

Traumatic Cataracts

CS Dhull, Sumit Sachdeva (India)

TRAUMATIC CATARACTS

Cataract is the most common sequelae to a penetrating or mechanical ocular injury causing loss of vision. It can be an early or late manifestation after an episode of ocular trauma and needs to be assessed and managed properly for adequate visual rehabilitation of the patient. Besides cataract, ocular trauma can also induce lens subluxation and dislocation,and cause injuries to the cornea, iris, vitreous, and retina.

Pathophysiology

Traumatic cataracts occur secondary to blunt or penetrating ocular trauma. The blunt injury to the eye causes complications by coup and counter coup mechanism. Such injuries produce damage to the eye as a result of the sudden compression and indentation of the globe that occurs at the moment of impact. On the other hand penetrating injury causes cataract by disruption of lens capsule and opacification of cortex.

Management

There are two basic questions concerning the surgery of traumatic cataract: when and how a traumatic cataract has to be removed, if at all the intervention is decided. The greatest benefit of primary cataract removal is the surgeon's ability to inspect the posterior segment otherwise blocked by lens opacity. In general, primary cataract removal is recommended if the lens is fragmentized, swollen, or causing a pupillary block.

On the other hand secondary cataract removal gives us the benefit of better visibility, better chances of IOL power calculation and above all a patient in better frame of mind for surgery.

Key Points of Note

1. Wherever possible, proper evaluation on slitlamp is a must. A surgeon must try to look for following points:
   a. Is the lens extruded?
   b. Is the lens dislocated/luxated into the AC?
   c. What is the condition of cornea?
   d. Are there lens particles in the AC?
   e. Is the lens swollen?
   f. Has vitreous prolapsed into the AC? If yes, is it also incarcerated into the wound?
   g. Has the anterior capsule been breached?
   h. Is there an intraocular foreign body inside the lens?
   i. Is the lens cataractous? If yes, is it partial or complete?
   j. Has the posterior capsule been breached? If yes, has the vitreous prolapsed into the lens?
   k. Is the lens subluxated/luxated into the vitreous cavity? If luxated, is the lens fragmented?
   l. What posterior segment pathologies are present?
   m. What additional anterior segment pathologies are present? What is the IOP?
2. Try to assess the integrity of globe.
3. Never ignore the other eye.
4. Proper investigations like ultrasound and CT scan has to be carried out to know the extent of injury.
5. And above all before any intervention proper written and informed consent has to be taken from the patient or relatives about the procedure and its potential consequences.

Conclusion

Proper evaluation and management of traumatic cataracts can go a long way in restoring functional vision to the patient and proper counseling can further help in his rehabilitation.

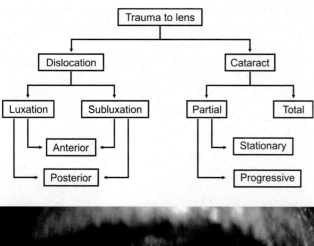

Fig. 1: Traumatic cataract with sealed corneal perforation

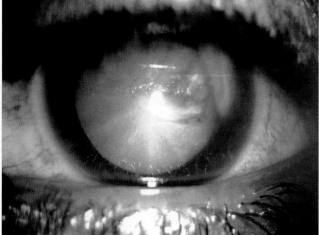

Fig. 2: Traumatic cataract with sealed corneal perforation (Disruption of lens capsule)

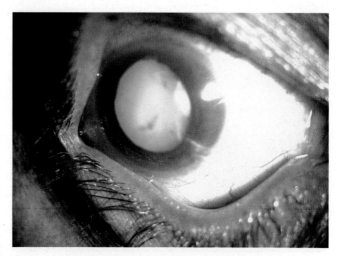

Fig. 3: Traumatic cataract due to blunt injury

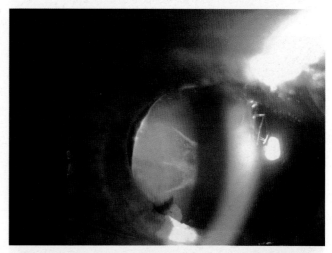

Fig. 4: Rosette cataract with subluxation of lens with organized blood clot in AC

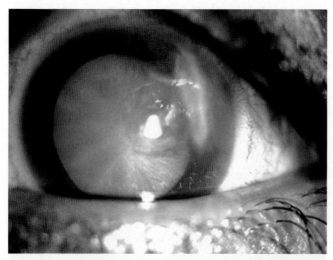

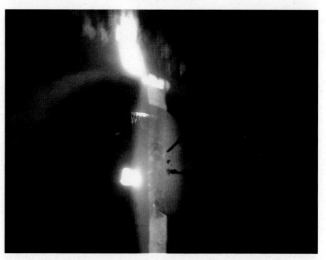

Fig 5A: Traumatic cataract (due to blunt trauma) with posterior synechiae

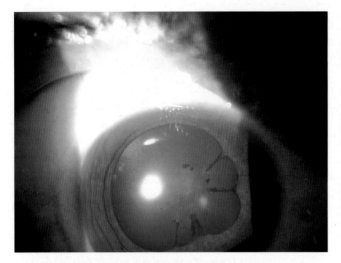

Fig. 5B: Traumatic cataract with post synechiae with partial vossius ring

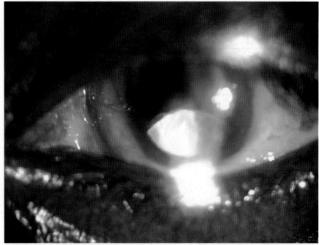

Fig. 7A: Inferior subluxation of traumatic cataract

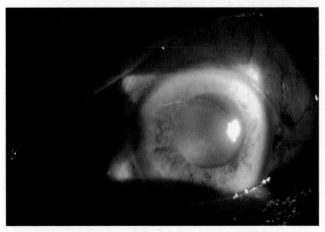

Fig. 6A: Traumatic cataract with subluxation of lens

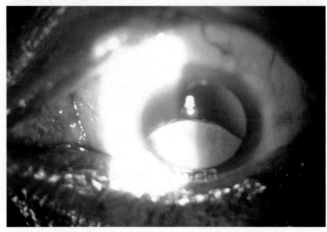

Fig. 7B: Inferior subluxation of traumatic cataract

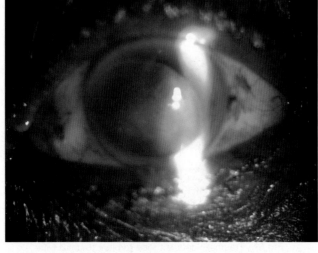

Fig. 6B: Traumatic cataract with anterior subluxation of lens (Note the anterior tilt)

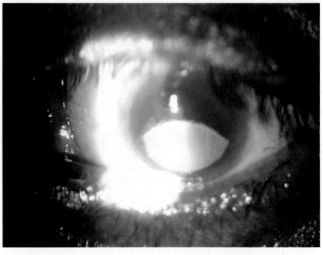

Fig. 7C: Inferior subluxation of traumatic cataract

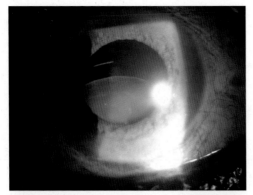

Fig. 8: Traumatic subluxation of crystalline lens

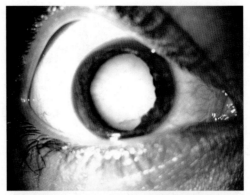

Fig 11: Traumatic milky white cataract

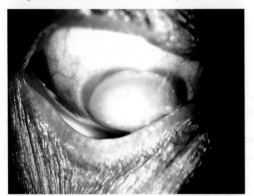

Fig. 9: Traumatic cataract with anterior dislocation

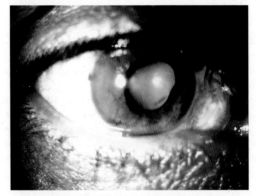

Fig. 12: Traumatic subluxation of lens

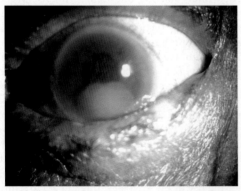

Fig. 10: Partially absorbed traumatic cataract with anterior dislocation

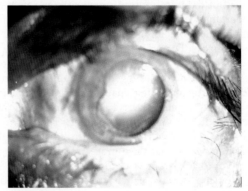

Fig. 13: Traumatic cataract with post synechiae

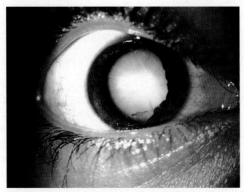

Fig. 14: Traumatic cataract with pigment dispersion on lens

Chapter 43

Complicated Cataract Surgical Procedure

Bojan Pajic, Brigitte Pajic-Eggspuehler (Switzerland)

MANAGEMENT OF THE SMALL PUPIL IN PHACOEMULSIFICATION

Good mydriasis is one of the necessary conditions to perform safe cataract surgery. However, there are situations when pupils do not dilate or dilate poorly.

Recently advancements have happened, and a number of techniques were developed to provide good mydriasis for surgery. Besides surgery facilitation, the main objective of these techniques is to allow the normal functioning of the pupil without causing functional or esthetic changes that can compromise the final results.

Preoperative Considerations

Assessment of the pupil during preoperative examination is very important. We are referring to an examination after the use of mydriatic drops for a diagnostic purpose, after 20 to 30 minutes the size of the pupil is evaluated. After assessment, the conclusions could be a pupil with optimal, good, regular, or poor reaction to the mydriatics agents or a pupil with no reaction to a mydriatic drug remaining small, unaltered. A small pupil is the one with a diameter under 4 mm that can be a cause of complication during phacoemulsification. The hyporeactive pupil dilates under pharmacological mydriasis but in an unsatisfactory way. They are more frequent among high hyperopic eyes, constantly medicated patients or elderly patients with those individual characteristics. The fixed pupil does not react during dynamic examination, and no reaction to mydriatic drugs has many causes, the most common being senile, inflammatory (after uveitis), traumatic, miosis following neurological diseases, and iatrogenic miosis (chronic usage of miotic drug for the treatment of glaucoma). Regardless of the cause, it is usual to attribute the presence of a structural change in these cases of small and fixed pupil of long duration. Among these structural changes are arteriosclerosis, hyalinization of the iris stroma, and dilator muscle atrophy.

Surgical Techniques

Hyporeactive Pupil

The "lazy pupil" is usually found in high hyperopic eyes (with axial length of less than 22.0 mm) or in patients with senile miotic pupil. In these cases, pharmacologic dilation yields a pupil of approximately 4 mm or less increasing the risk of complications during phacoemulsification (Fig. 1). The capsulorhexis will be very small, nucleus manipulation risky, and the intraocular lens (IOL) implantation will be more difficult than in a usual case. The following technique can be used for this challenging case.

Pharmacologic Treatment

If it is known after the preoperative examination that the pupil will be poorly dilated, it is proposed to use a combination mydriatics, that is the administration of Phenylephrine 10%, Tropicamide 1% and Ketorolac Tromethamine 0.5% three times (nine drops total) starting one hour prior to surgery, and maintenance of the patient in a dimly lit room. The use of cyclopentolate is not recommended because of its possible psychogenic side effects. Once at surgery if obtained mydriasis is less than 4 mm, 0.5 ml of unpreserved adrenaline 1:1000 diluted in 10 ml of BSS is introduced through the paracentesis incision. A 4 mm pupil does not constitute a contraindication for the experienced surgeon to perform endocapsular phacoemulsification. Capsulorhexis has to be at a diameter of minimum 5 mm to prevent its retraction (phimosis) postoperatively after IOL implantation. In these cases it is very important the use of the bimanual technique with the iris manipulator to see capsulorhexis flap at its total diameter.[1]

If after the use of the viscoelastic agent, a 5 to 6 mm stable pupil is obtained, the bimanual and endocapsular phacoemulsificadon technique will be quite safe. Failure of the above mentioned methods led us to the use of mechanical forms of treatment, as iris hooks.

Phaco Chop Technique at Small Pupil

Mechanical Treatment with Iris Hooks

Iris hooks, in soft and flexible nylon, are introduced after four symmetrical incisions placed at 10, 2, 5, and 7 o'clock positions (Fig. 2). After the scleral or corneal tunnels are developed and the viscoelastic material injected, these secondary incisions should be performed with the symmetrical introduction of the hooks. Pupillary margins are hooked, and then its retraction is carefully forced towards the iris periphery, where it will be

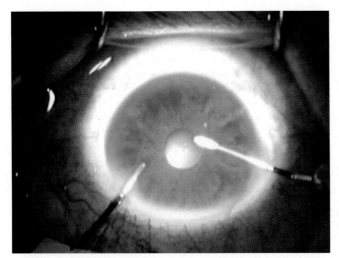

Fig. 1: Miotic pupil of less than 4 mm

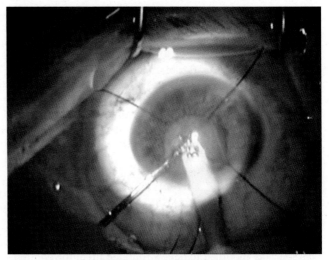

Fig. 4: Phacoemulsification with the stop and chop technique is the safest method at a small pupil

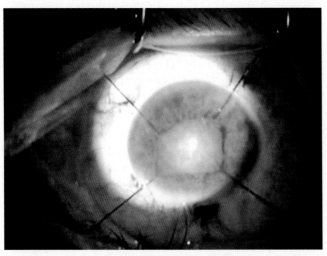

Fig. 2: Iris hooks placed through four symmetrical incisions

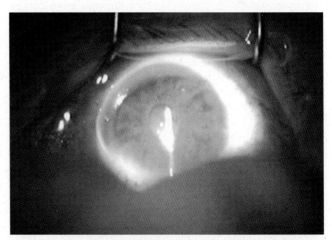

Fig. 5: Hydrodissection through main corneal access

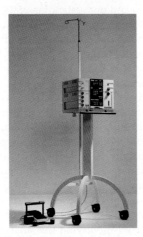

Fig. 3: OS 3 (Ophthalmic Small-incision Surgery System) machine from Oertli Instruments AG Switzerland

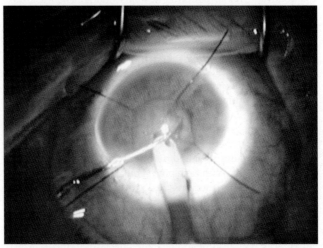

Fig. 6: The nucleus has to be rotated about 45 degrees clock-wise

fixated with the help of the hook s adjusting silicone sleeve. After good positioning of the hooks and assessment of the mydriasis are obtained, the surgery is performed in its usual sequence. Immediately after IOL implantation, the hooks are carefully removed (very flexible, nontraumatic) and self sealing closure of the incisions is evaluated.[2-5] During the capsulorhexis the stability of lens has to be evaluated. If there is any zonulolyses then the iris hooks can be used for maintaining the lens stability with fixation at the capsulorhexis edge. All phacoemulsification procedures are done with a OS 3 (Ophthalmic Small-incision Surgery System) machine from Oertli Instruments AG Switzerland (Fig. 3).

Phaco Chop Technique
The next step is to perform the phacoemulsification with the stop and chop technique. It is the safest technique to perform the phacoemulsification at a small pupil (Fig. 4). A lens hook was specially modified to have a rounded tip at the end to be sure, that the capsule is safe during the manipulation. Before beginning phacoemulsification it is very important to carry out the hydrodissection comprehensive through main corneal access (Fig. 5). So there is no danger of hydrogenate the vitreous. Then phaco tip is placed in the eye and put in the superior nucleus. While the phaco tip is just held there, the phaco chopper is placed through the sideport incision and stuck into the nucleus down at six o clock. The phaco tip just sits there like a chopping block and the phaco chopper is pulled up toward the phaco tip, effectively chopping the nucleus in two. As it approaches the phaco tip, the two instruments are separated, one to the left and the other to the right. The nucleus is split in two pieces. The nucleus is rotated and the phaco-chop is repeated, breaking each nuclear half into quarters that can be easily emulsified. But it takes much time to perform the phacoemulsification with this technique and with the small pupil there could be too much tension on the capsular bag. Thus more room in the bag is necessary. Begin the procedure as though it were a four quadrant cracking procedure. Enter the eye with the phaco tip and begin to sculpt down a deep trench toward six o clock. A little space for quadrant manipulation is now just made. Then a groove can be made that will let you crack the nucleus into halves. The chopper will be placed into the eye, put the tip right down into the depths of the groove, and pull the left half toward the sideport incision. The phaco tip supports the right half and can even push a little bit to the right. The nucleus cracks into two halves very easily. Important is to be enough deep during the cracking procedure. From stage you can go on with chop. The nucleus has to be rotated about 45 degrees clockwise (Fig. 6). Slightly put the phaco tip one-third of the way across the nucleus half and hold it there. Put the chopper in the periphery of the nucleus at the same spot and pull it towards the phaco tip. The nucleus will split. With each piece you get off of the bag you get more room with consecutive less capsular tension. When the chopper reaches the phaco tip, pull the chopper to the left and push the tip to the right. A small piece of nucleus will be chopped off and will be stuck on the phaco tip. Emulsify gently and the small piece will disappear. Place the phaco tip in the middle of the remaining 2/2 of a half of nucleus and hold it there. Put the

phaco chopper in the periphery and pull towards the tip, chopping off another small piece, which will be stuck to the phaco tip. Then go on to the next piece. Each nuclear half can be chopped up into three or four small bite-sized pieces easily with this technique. Each of the pieces is stuck on the phaco tip and can be removed just by stepping on the footswitch. Manipulation of the piece within the eye is not usually necessary. You don t have to push, pull, or otherwise manipulate the nucleus piece before removing it. After each chop the piece to be removed is already stuck on the phaco tip, bagging to be emulsified. This is a bit tougher in the extreme cataracts. After one or two chops in a soft nucleus the whole thing wants to collapse into the middle of the bag and be removed. In a real hard nucleus you may have to chop the thing into eight or ten small pieces. It s reasonably easy to chop off small pieces and emulsify them with short bursts of energy. At the end there is a perfect result with IOL implantation in the bag. (Fig. 7).

Postoperative Considerations

The manipulation of a small pupil during cataract surgery can present some problems. Among the most common are an increase in inflammation of the anterior segment observed during the immediate postoperative period, light bleeding without clinical translation, light ocular hypertension secondary to the inflammatory reaction, temporary or permanent mydriasis, aesthetical changes, and a decrease in visual acuity because of glare.[6]

Finally, the use of the better viscoelastic agents, good instruments, diversity of techniques and experience, and popularization of phacoemulsification techniques among ophthalmologists have made possible that the results obtained in small pupil cataract surgery are similar to those obtained in normal sized pupils.

PHACOEMULSIFICATION IN SUBLUXATED CATARACTS

Surgical management of the cataract associated with zonular dialysis is a real challenge for the ophthalmic surgeon. Due to recent advances in equipment and instrumentation, better surgical techniques and understanding of fluidics, the surgeon will be able to perform relative safe cataract surgery in presence of compromised zonules. In presence of mild up to sever loss of zonular fibers, cataract surgery can be managed by conventional or advanced phacoemulsification and implantation techniques.[7] When more than 4 or 5 clock hours of capsular zonular support are missing, many surgeons prefer performing an intracapsular cataract extraction with implantation of an anterior chamber or sutured posterior chamber intraocular lens (IOL). Traditionally, congenital or acquired zonulocapsular pathology has not allowed implantation of a posterior chamber IOL in the capsular bag nor in the ciliary sulcus. For this reason, new techniques have been designed to correct the deficiencies of the natural support for the IOL, as with the use of endocapsular rings to expand the equatorial portion of the capsule, or artificially modifying this anatomical support by suturing the anterior capsule to the sclera. IOL in-the-bag suture is a new approach to zonular dehiscence.

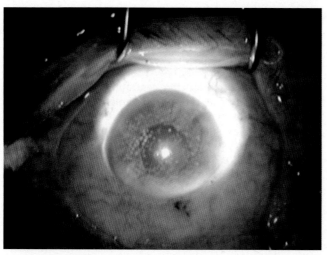

Fig. 7: Perfect result with IOL implantation in the bag

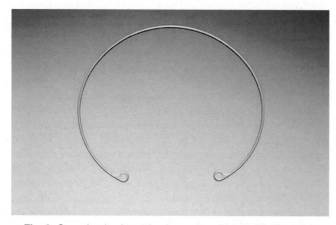

Fig. 8: Capsular ring is made of one-piece PMMA CQ UV C-F-M

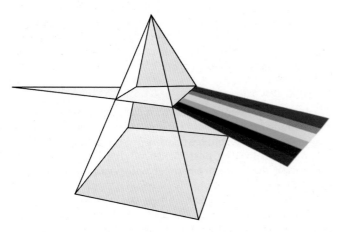

Fig. 9: Induction of aberration

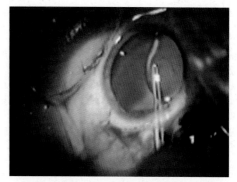

Fig. 10: Capsulorhexis

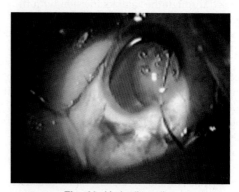

Fig. 11: Hydrodissection

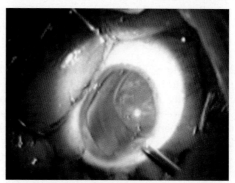

Fig. 12: Capsular ring

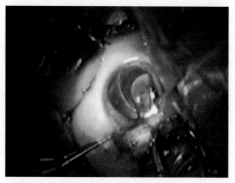

Fig. 13: IOL implantation

Capsular Ring

Description

The capsular ring is made of one-piece PMMA CQ UV C-F-M (Fig. 8) and is available in different sizes depending of their use in patients with emmetropia, low, or high myopia. Capsular ring has an haptic thickness of 0.15/0.20 mm, depended on the design and is used for the circular expansion of the capsular bag. Long-term studies have shown a properly expanded bag in myopic eyes.

Implantation Technique

After filling the capsular bag with viscoelastic material, the ring is introduced through the cataract incision with the convexity to the left or to the side in which the paracentesis was made to allow easier manipulation. Once the ring is being introduced in the bag, a buttonhole spatula is placed through the paracentesis guiding the ring and preventing the continuous circular capsulotomy from getting deformed. To complete implantation of the ring, it may be helpful to use a similar spatula, introduced through the phacoemulsification incision. This step is certainly more complicated and depends on the size and rigidity of the ring to be implanted.

Surgery Technique at Subluxated Cataracts

An early sign of zonular weakness is the presence of radial folds in the anterior capsule at the time the continuous circular capsulotomy is started. In this situation, a safe continuous circular capsulotomy will be difficult. Before beginning with phacoemulsification the calsular ring has to be implant. The surgeon should be able to finish the planned procedure without major complications.

To obtain pseudophakia in subluxated lenses the degree of subluxation have to be evaluated in a supine position. The presence and density of a cataract, iridodonesis, phacodonesis, and the opposite eye must be determined. A subluxated lens can induce optical aberrations difficult to correct with the use of contact lenses or glasses. The astigmatism is induced by the equator of the lens, the motion of this subluxated lens, or the lens shape irregularity as a result of the partial loss of the zonular fibers. The high myopia that is usually associated, can be caused by the high refractive power of the peripheral zone of the lens or by the increase of its curvature due to the absence of zonular fibers. This optical alteration can cause monocular or binocular diplopia, anisometropia, or amblyopia in children (Fig. 9). The use of the endocapsular ring would maintain the capsular bag and an IOL may then be inserted. The surgical technique is difficult, but if the intraocular compartments and pseudophakia are maintained, the risk of cystoid macular edema and retinal detachment frequently will be decreased.

The aim of the novel surgical technique is to preserve the capsule with implanting the IOL in the bag. The surgical technique is started with a small continuous circular capsulotomy with a needle or/and forceps (Fig. 10) where the anterior capsular folds can be observed. After the hydrodissection (Fig. 11) a capsular ring has to be implanted in the capsular bag

(Fig. 12). The surgeon should be careful during nucleus rotation preventing zonular tension. With low energy of phacoemulsification, stop and chop technique as described above can be used. One of the most important steps is to create more room in the capsular bag. The IOL implantation in the bag (Fig. 13) leads to a better centration, but it is often not sufficient (Fig. 14). The suture is fixed anterior and posterior the IOL haptic, capsular ring and lens capsule (Fig. 15) in the direction of the calculated optimal, main mathematical vector (Fig. 16). The next step is to prepare a sclerapocket 1 mm from the limbus (Fig. 17). With a insulin needle the suture is placed in the area of the scleralpocket (Fig. 18). A consecutive suture fixation can be done using a (Fig. 19). A perfect centration can be stated after surgery (Fig. 20), even after 1 year later (Fig. 21). The advantage of the novel surgery method is a long-term fixation und centering of chamber posterior IOL at the physiological space. The capsule is adherent with the ciliary body after months. The known disadvantages of the aphakia and chamber anterior IOL could be avoid. The surgical treatment of a congenital lens subluxation is sophisticated surgery method which shows excellent results.

PHACOEMULSIFICATION IN PSEUDOEXFOLIATION

Phacoemulsification in the presence of pseudoexfoliation of the lens presents surgeons with particular challenges. Intraoperative and postoperative complications such as zonular dialysis, capsule tears, vitreous loss, and IOL decentration may be avoided with careful attention to detail and elegant surgical technique.

Improvements in phacoemulsification technology, intraocular lenses, and new capsular supporting rings offer surgeons the capability of performing safer surgery in these patients. Cataract surgery in the presence of pseudoexfoliation of the lens presents surgeons with unusual challenges. In addition to a higher incidence of glaucoma, these patients have loss of zonular integrity occasionally associated with lens subluxation and pupils that dilated poorly. Although the use of phacoemulsification in experienced hands has resulted in a low incidence of intraoperative and postoperative complications such as zonular dialysis, capsule tears, vitreous loss, and IOL decentration,[8] special care should still be exercised when performing cataract surgery in these patients. Improvements in phacoemulsification technology, technique, and new capsular supporting rings will ultimately enable these patients to undergo cataract surgery with even fewer complications.

Capsulorhexis

Weak zonules present particularly challenging situations during phacoemulsification. Of utmost importance is not to challenge the integrity of the zonules by over-pressurizing the eye. This can occur following peri- or retrobulbar injection, over-expanding the anterior chamber with viscoelastic prior to capsulotomy, or utilizing an excessively high bottle height during phacoemulsification. During the capsulotomy, special care and attention are required, because traction on the capsule can unzip weakened zonules. If there are areas of missing zonules, centripetal traction on the capsular flap may result in

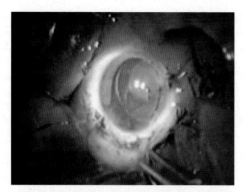

Fig. 14: Insufficient centration

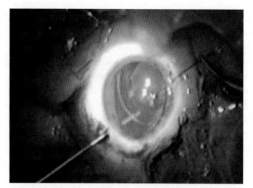

Fig. 18: Suture placing

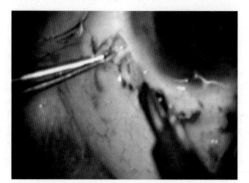

Fig. 15: Sclerapocket preparation

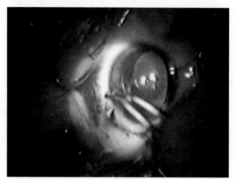

Fig. 19: Suture fixation

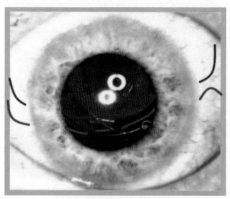

Fig. 16: Target suture area

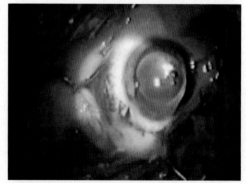

Fig. 20: Perfect centration

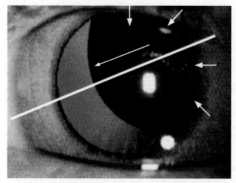

Fig. 17: Target zone vector calculation

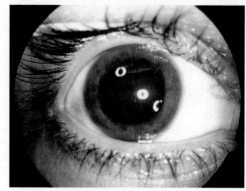

Fig. 21: Result after one year

247

further damage to the adjacent weakened zonules. Capsulorhexis size is extremely important in patients with pseudoexfoliation. Ideal capsulorhexis size is felt to be 5.5 to 6.0 mm or larger in routine patients.[9] We believe it should be at least 6.0 mm in pseudoexfoliaton cases, since a larger capsulorhexis leaves a smaller burden of lens epithelial cells postoperatively than smaller capsulorhexis. Residual lens epithelial cells participate in metaplasia and extracellular matrix deposition, ultimately resulting in capsular fibrosis.[10] Patients with pseudoexfoliation are particularly susceptible to marked shrinkage of the rhexis, because the strong forces of fibrosis and contraction are unopposed by strong zonular traction.[11] Thus, a larger capsulorhexis should decrease the incidence of symptomatic capsule contraction by decreasing the number of epithelial cells able to participate in the fibrosis process and allowing for a larger final rhexis diameter once capsule contraction has ultimately ceased to progress.

Hydrodissection and Hydrodelineation

Cortical cleaving hydrodissection[12] requires extremely careful maneuvers especially when one decompresses the bag after having performed the posterior fluid wave. It is important to do this very gently and to utilize multiple locations for partial cortical cleaving hydrodissection injections with gentle central lens decompression. This should alleviate the chances of depressing the lens with excessive forces which would tear zonules. Hydrodelineation is a useful technique in pseudoexfoliation, since it produces an epinuclear shell as an important added safeguard. During both hydrodissection and hydrodelineation, it is wise to keep the cannula in a position slightly depressing the posterior tip of the large 3.0 mm incision. This will ensure easy egress out of the eye for either viscoelastic or fluid should one overinflate the spaces with balanced salt solution.

Phacoemulsification

One must use extreme caution during manipulation of the lens as not to tear zonules. Two-handed rotations of the lens nucleus are wise, since the forces can be truly tangential and can be divided by utilizing opposite sides of the same meridian. Grooving also requires special care, since it is a tendency to put posterior pressure on the nucleus. High cavitation tips are great advantage, since they can obliterate nuclear material in advance of the tip without exerting forces on the lens or the lens zonules. For diminuation the tension bag it is necessary to create space. Already during the capsulorhexis there is possible to detect a lentodonesis (Fig. 22). If the zonulolysis is less than 90° there is possible to go on with a good hydrodissection (Fig. 23) and implantation of a casular ring (Fig. 8). Gently beginning with the phacoemulsification with the stop and chop technique (Fig. 24). If the zonulolysis is along of 270° (Fig. 25) then the phacoemulsification has to be stopped. Iris hooks have to be then fixed at the capsulorhexis ede (Fig. 26). Thus the capsule and lens are stable. There is possible to go on with the phacoemulsification (Fig. 27). I/A has to be performed very gently while the capsule is fixated with iris hooks (Fig. 28). There have to be concepted where the suture will be (Fig. 29). Scleral pocket has to be performed in 3 and 9h (Fig. 30). From the one side a needle goes through the scleral pocket (Fig. 31), behind the iris and through the capsule and from the other side a needle with a filum will be put through the scleral pocket, capsule and then diagonally through the camber anterior (Fig. 32). The filum has to be got out from the clear cornea opening. While the IOL is folded the filum will be sutured at the haptics (Figs 33A and B). Afterwards, the IOL will be implanted in the capsular bag (Fig. 34). The suture has to be fixated now at the scleral pocket till the IOL is centered (Fig. 35). The iris hooks can take away (Fig. 36). I/A will be performed (Fig. 37) with consecutive application of carbachol (Figs 38A and B). The same procedure is possible also with a PMMA IOL. The difference is that the chamber anterior opening has to be a frown incision if the trend is to a no stitch technique (Fig. 39).

Conclusions

Phacoemulsification in the presence of pseudoexfoliation presents aurgeons with the possibility of many complications which are less likely to occur in absence of pseudoexfoliation. Specialized techniques are available which should allow the surgeon to both avoid and cope with the various intraoperative difficulties which may become manifest during cataract surgery in these patients. One of the newest devices available to assist in managing these cases is the endocapsular ring. It offers the potential benefits of fewer intra and postoperative complications by means of capsular stabilization.

REFERENCES

1. Miller KM, Keener GT. Stretch pupilloplasty for small pupil phacoemulsification (letter). Am J Ophthalmol 1994;3:107-8.
2. De Juan E, Hickingbotham D. Flexible iris retractor (letter). Am J Ophtalmol 1991;11:776-77.
3. Fine IH. Phacoemulsification in the presence of a small pupil. In: Steinert RF (Ed). Cataract Surgery: Technique, Complications and Management. Philadelphia: W.B. Saunders; 1995;199-208.
4. Mackool RJ. Small pupil enlargement during cataract extraction: A new method. J Cataract Refract Surg 1992;18:523-26.
5. Nichamin LD. Enlarging the pupil for cataract extraction using flexible nylon iris retractors. J Cataract Refract Surg 1993;19:793-96.
6. Masket S. Relationship between postoperative pupil size and disability glare. J Cataract Refract Surg 1992;18:506-7.
7. Cionni R, Osher R. Endocapsular ring approach to the subluxated cataractous lens. J Cataract Retract Surg 1995;21:245-49.
8. Osher RH, Cioni RJ, Gimbel HV, Crandall AS. Cataract surgery in patients with pseudoexfoliation syndrome. EurJ Implant Ref Surg 1993,5:46-50.
9. Joo CK, ShinJA, Kim JH. Capsular opening contraction after continuous curvilinear capsulorhexis and intraocular lens implantation. J Cataract Refract Surg 1996;22:585-90.
10. Ishibashi T, Araki H, Sugai S, et al. Anterior capsular opacification in monkey eyes with posterior chamber intraocular lenses. Arch Ophthalmol 1993;111:1685-90.
11. Davison JA. Capsule contraction syndrome. J Cataract Refract Surg 1993;19:582-89.
12. Fine IH. Cortical cleaving hydrodissection. J Cataract Refract Surg 1992;18:508-12.

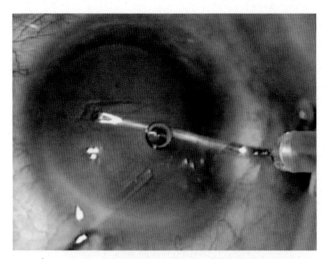

Fig. 22: Lentodonesis during capsulorhexis

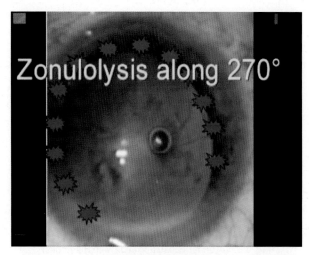

Fig. 25: Zonulolysis along 270°

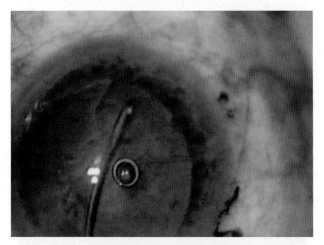

Fig. 23: Hydrodissection after detecting lentodonesis with zonulolysis of less than 90°

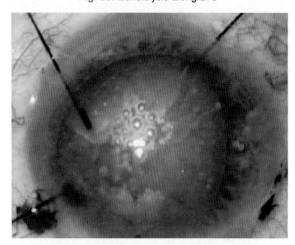

Fig. 26: Iris hooks at the ege of capsulorhexis

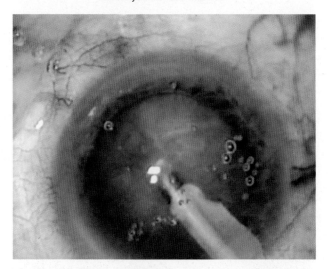

Fig. 24: Gently phacoemulsification if the zonulolysis is less than 90°

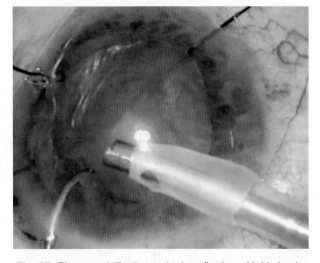

Fig. 27: Phacoemulsification under lens fixation with iris hooks

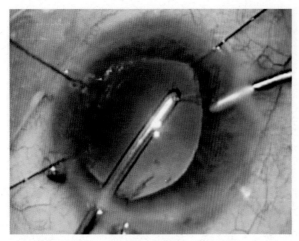

Fig. 28: I/A under capsule fixation with iris hooks

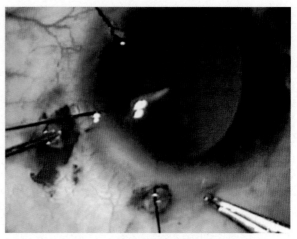

Fig. 31: Leading needle without filum

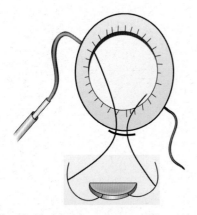

Fig. 29: Model of the suture and IOL position

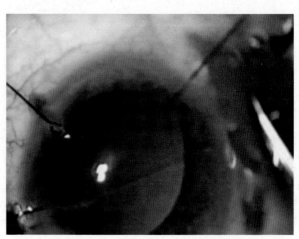

Fig. 32: Needle with filum will put through chamber anterior

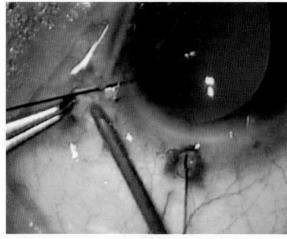

Fig. 30: Scleral pocket in 3 and 9h

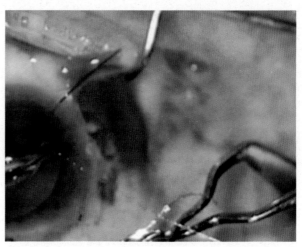

Fig. 33A

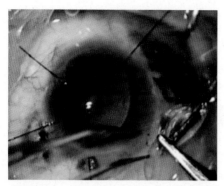

Figs 33A and B: Suture at the haptics of folded IOL

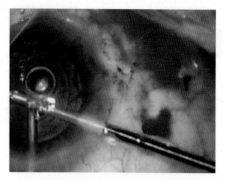

Fig. 37: I/A of the chamber anterior

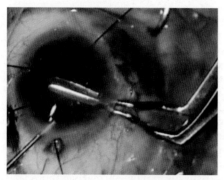

Fig. 34: IOL implantation in the capsular bag

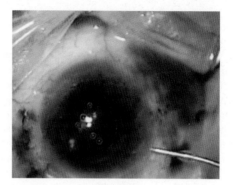

Fig. 38A

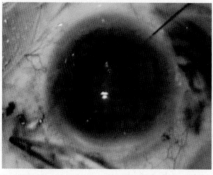

Fig. 35: Suture fixation till the IOL is centered

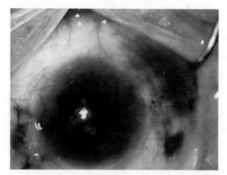

Figs 38A and B: Application of carbachol

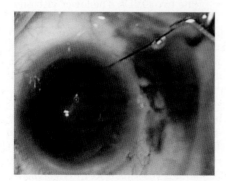

Fig. 36: Iris hooks take away

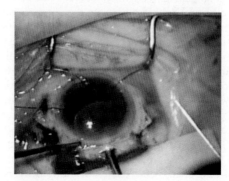

Fig. 39: PMMA IOL implantation through a frown incision

251

Chapter 44

Pearls for Small Pupil Phaco Surgery

Boris Malyugin (Russia)

Significant number of patients who present for phaco-emulsification cataract surgery have pupils that do not respond adequately despite several pharmacological attempts with different mydriatic agents.

Poor pupil dilation we can be observed in cases complicated by pseudoexfoliation syndrome, uveitis, posterior synechiae, trauma, previous intraocular surgery (Figs 1A and B).

Chang and Campbell (20055) recently described the intraoperative floppy-iris syndrome (IFIS) associated with systemic administration of the Ü-1A antagonist tamsulosin (Flomax). The intraoperative diagnostic triad of this symptom is fluttering and billowing of the iris stroma, a tendency to iris prolapse through the main and/or side-port incisions, and progressive constriction of the pupil during surgery.

The most significant problems for the surgeon to be mentioned are decreased visualization, iris trauma due to incarceration into the wound, iris chafing, pupillary margin damage by the phaco needle and some others (Figs 2A and B). All of these factors compromise the surgery and increase the risk for complications (Fig. 3).

Unfortunately present pharmacological approaches of managing a small pupil during cataract surgery have limitations. Intracameral mydriatics are an effective and safe addition to topical mydriatics in phacoemulsification (Figs 4A and B). In some cases their use can simplify preoperative patient's preparation and in certain high-risk groups, may reduce the risk for cardiovascular side effects.

There is no general recommendation or universal solution to the small pupil problem because the strategies for pupil enlargement greatly depend on surgeon skill and preferences, as well as on intraoperative situation.

Fortunately not every patient with the small pupil requires special dilation protocols. If the iris tissue is rigid and the diameter of the pupil is 4.0 to 4.5 mm an experienced surgeon can effectively remove cataract and to avoid significant trauma of the anterior segment tissues. To the contrary, even if the pupil is reasonably wide but the iris tissue is flaccid and atonic, like in IFIS, there is a significant risk of complications.

Allan (1995) described one of the critical factors of iris prolapse during phaco which relates to fluid velocity. His model considers the Bernoulli principle as the most important because

when the velocity of fluid passing through the anterior chamber increases, the force exerted on the iris increases by the square of the velocity.

The pupil often dilates poorly in atrophic irises, with significantly decreased iris tone unable to withstand the fluidic currents in the anterior chamber and maintain the correct position of the iris. In small pupil iris tissue is located closer to the zone of the high fluidic currents that is why it is more likely to be aspirated into the US or I/A handpieces. Decreasing of flow parameters is an important factor of preventing iris damage during phacoemulsification.

Not only reducing the flow can make an appreciable difference in these cases, but also central positioning and minimal movements of the handpiece are also important to prevent iris damage (Figs 5A to C). Endocapsular lens nucleus fragmentation is much safer because the areas of the highest fluidics currents are located inside the capsular bag away from the corneal endothelium and iris. With vertical phaco-chop technique of nucleus disassembly the manipulations are usually performed in the central part of the anterior chamber and the necessity of wider exposition of the anterior lens surface is diminished (Fig. 6).

VISCOELASTICS

Viscomydriasis with high viscosity viscoadaptive OVDs such as Healon5 (AMO) or Microvisc Phaco (Bohus Biotech) are very useful in small pupil phaco cases. S Arshinoff (2006) described a technique using ophthalmic viscosurgical devices to perform cataract surgery in patients with IFIS. This method uses a combination of the two OVDs. The lower-viscosity dispersive OVD which is highly retentive despite the presence of moderate fluid turbulence is injected in the periphery of the anterior chamber and covers the endothelial layer and the iris. The viscoadaptive central layer of Healon 5, according to S Arshinoff adds a relatively rigid OVD roof above the surgical space and adds rigidity to the OVD structure to keep the iris from moving and the Viscoat in place. The BSS layer just over the pupillary space and below viscoadaptive central layer provides working space for the phaco tip. The surgeon is working in the endocapsular space and Healon 5 is not attracted into the phaco tip and the OVD shell structure remains intact throughout the case. This technique gives satisfactory iris stability and permits uneventful surgery.

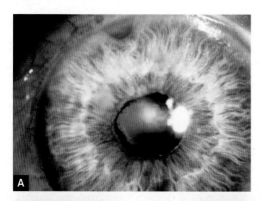

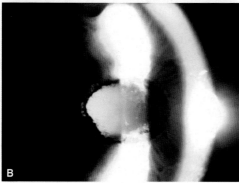

Figs 1A and B: Eye of the patient after glaucoma surgery. Small undilated pupil is associated with extensive posterior synechiae

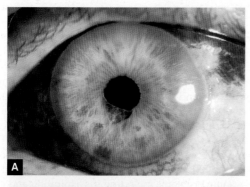

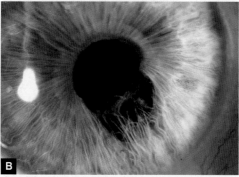

Figs 2A and B: Eyes of the patients with the minor (A) and significant (B) pupillary margin trauma after phacoemulsification due to small pupil

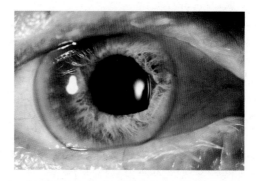

Fig. 3: Atonic dilated pupil after the phaco surgery due to excessive iris manipulations

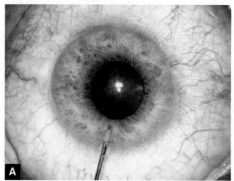

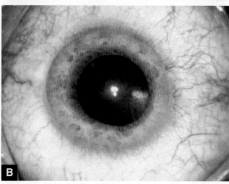

Figs 4A and B: Intracameral injection of phenylephrine (A) can help in achieving intraoperative pupil dilation (B) and iris tissue stabilization

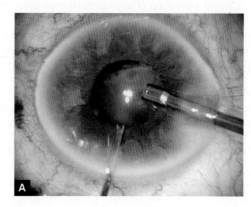

Fig. 5A

253

SYNECHIOLYSIS AND PUPILLARY STRETCHING

Most surgeons decide to dilate the pupil mechanically at the time of the surgery if pharmacological agents fail. There are four main dilation methods: synechiolysis, mechanical stretching, iris cutting and iris retraction.

During synechiolysis the surgeon separates adhesions between the iris and the lens capsule. Usually it is done with blunt instrument – spatula, nucleus manipulator, etc. (Figs 7A to D).

Mechanical stretching of the pupil was introduced by Miller and Keener (in 1994). It is usually effective for small pupils with the rigid iris tissue which is usually caused by prior miotic use, pseudoexfoliation, or posterior synechiae. Stretching can be achieved with the spatula, Sinskey or Kuglen hooks or a special instrument—Beehler pupil dilator. Usually a pair of hooks is introduced through 2 stab incisions in the cornea engage the iris sphincter. After that the hooks are pulled in opposite directions. This maneuver creates microscopic sphincter tears which enlarge the pupil aperture. The main advantage of this procedure is that it is relatively simple and requires no special instruments. Mechanical stretching of the pupil usually provides sufficient access to the lens and maintains the pupil diameter intraoperatively.

Sometimes iris stretching technique leads to instability of its pupillary margin, which can compromise cataract surgery. The drawback of this technique is that it is creating permanent damage of the iris sphincter and sometimes – bleeding (Figs 8A to F). The micro tears of the sphincter muscle are usually clinically asymptomatic but sometimes result in postoperative hyphema and pigment dispersion.

In some eyes and stretching technique fails to adequately expand the pupil. Stretching of the pupil is ineffective in IFIS because the iris pupil margin remains elastic and the pupil immediately snaps back to its original size following attempts at stretching it.

In the limited number of patients during synechiolysis and/ or iris stretching peripupillary membrane attached to the posterior iris surface can be identified. Its removal with forceps first presented by R.Osher in some cases effectively increases pupil diameter. On the Fig. 9 we present step-by-step approach to mechanical pupil enlargement including synechiolysis (Figs 9 A to C), pupil stretching (Figs 9 D to G) and peripupillary membranectomy (Figs 9 H to K).

Partial-thickness iris sphincter cuts made with micro scissors is not very common pupil enlargement technique nowadays. The cutting method requires multiple maneuvers of the scissors inside the anterior chamber which can result in corneal endothelial damage. The main disadvantages are the same as those with the stretching method, but more pronounced bleeding from the pupillary margin can be expected. I personally limit cutting techniques to the cases where it is necessary to release the anterior synechiae in strong irido-corneal adhesions.

IRIS HOOKS

Suboptimal pupil dilation in response to the preoperative mydriatic protocols and minimal efficacy of pupil stretching techniques is a usual indication to the intraoperative use of iris hooks or other mechanical pupil dilation devices.

Retracting the iris tissue rather than cutting it as in a classic sector iridectomy is much simpler and results in a much better postoperative pupil appearance. Mackool (1991) was the first one who described a 4-point iris retractor configuration for phacoemulsification. He developed metal iris retractors connected to small blocks of titanium. The latter allows for stabilization of the hooks during the retraction of the iris. This method was enhanced with the introduction of the flexible iris retractor by de Juan and Hickingbotham (1992).

Traditionally, 4 evenly spaced retractors are placed through limbal paracenteses 90 degrees apart from one another (Figs 10 and 11). The main cataract l incision is centered on 1 of the 4 sides of the square. Some surgeons use iris retractors in a triangular pattern decreasing the number of additional corneal incisions (Figs 12A to C).

Modification of the original square retractor configuration is described by Oetting T. and Omphroy L. (2002). The rotation of the square improves lens access in clear corneal phacoemulsification by orienting the phacoemulsification needle along the diagonal. This was called "diamond configuration" of retractors. Advantages of this technique include ease of conversion from phacoemulsification, optimal orientation of the maximum pupil diameter nucleus expression or intracapsular lens removal, and conservation of iris tissue.

Iris hooks are good for the patients with shallow chamber where implantation of the pupillary rings and other devices can lead to the endothelial trauma. They are also indicated for the complicated cases where conversion to the manual ECCE or even ICCE is likely.

During engagement of the pupillary edge with the iris hook, it may catch and damage the capsule, leading to an anterior capsule tear that may extend to the periphery. To avoid this problem, a drop of viscoelastic material should be injected between the iris and the capsule before the hook is inserted. The other useful technique is to keep the hook parallel to the iris plane during the insertion and to tilt it slightly posterior right near the pupillary edge to engage the iris only. The iris hooks may become loosened during surgery. Their tips may become dislocated, no longer holding the pupillary edge. This can cause some problems including iris aspiration and chafing from contact with the phacoemulsification needle.

Iris hooks should be avoided in patients with narrow lid fissures because of their tendency to get in the way of the lids.

Most of the surgical maneuvers for enlarging the pupil and preventing its intraoperative constriction are not safe enough. They can lead to an increased risk of iris sphincter tear, bleeding, iris damage, posterior capsule tears, and loss of the vitreous body. The postoperative complications can include an atonic pupil of irregular shape with poor cosmetic result, and photophobia.

PUPIL EXPANSION DEVICES

For the iris retraction several devices have been introduced into clinical practice. Graether (1996) developed a pupil expander

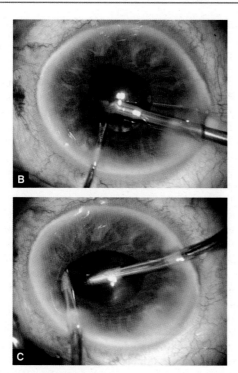

Figs 5A to C: C-MICS with Stellaris (Bausch and Lomb) through 1.8 mm incision in patient with the small pupil (A,B). The surgeon is retracting the iris with the bimanual irrigation handpiece (Duet, MST) to achieve better exposition of the equatorial portion of the capsular bag and access to the cortical material (C)

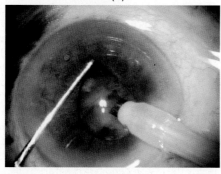

Fig. 6: Vertical phaco chop in patient with the small pupil. The chopper is used simultaneously to retract the iris and to cut the lens nucleus into pieces

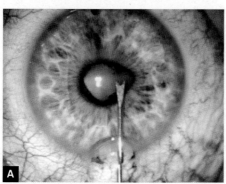

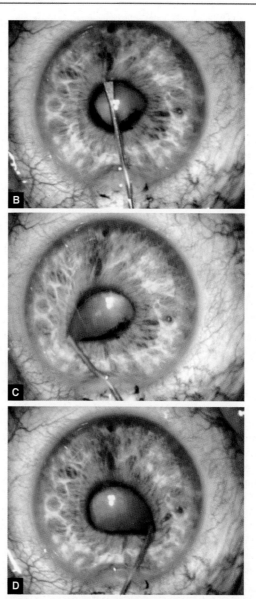

Figs 7A to D: Patient with cataract and posterior iris synechiae. The latter are being broken with help of Bechler nucleus manipulator

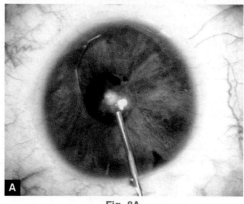

Fig. 8A

that according to his data is superior to other methods of pupil enlargement, causing less sphincter trauma and fewer cases of permanent pupil size alteration (Fig. 13).

Pupil dilation technique with the hydrogel ring reported by Siepser has a potential benefits but very limited clinical use.

The Perfect Pupil device (Milvella) is a disposable polyurethane ring with the 0.24 mm flanged groove throughout the length of the ring and an integrated arm that allows insertion and removal from the anterior chamber at the end of surgery (Fig. 14).

The main disadvantages of these devices include the bulkiness and rigidity. They are difficult to insert, remove, and manipulate through a small incision. Intaoperative iris manipulations may lead to severe postoperative fibrinoid reaction especially in eyes with pseudoexfoliation syndrome, chronic uveitis, glaucoma or diabetes. That is why cataract surgery in the presence of a small pupil remains one of the most difficult and challenging cases.

MALYUGIN RING

The Malyugin Ring is a relatively new pupil expansion device. It has one-piece design and square shape with four equidistantly located circular loops (Fig. 15). The loop at each angle has a gap to accommodate the iris tissue (Fig. 16). The basic concept of this device is the scroll principle of catching and holding the pupillary margin (Figs 17A to D).

The Malyugin Ring System produced by MST (Microsurgical Technology Inc., USA) consists of a pre-sterilized single-use holder containing the ring and inserter (Figs 18A and B). The dark blue Ring is located inside the holder and can be visualized through its upper portion (Fig. 19).

The introduction of the injection device was a great improvement with the significant impact on the easiness of the ring handling during the surgery. The hook of the injector catches one or the loops of the Malyugin Ring and is used to retract it inside the tube (Figs 20A to E).

The Malyugin Ring produced by MST comes with two sizes: 6.25 mm and 7.0 mm. The implantation and removal of the both versions is performed with the same insertion device. The advantage of the smaller ring is that it is easier to insert and to retract. The advantage of the 7.0 mm ring is that one can use it if the pupil starts of bigger, and also in IFIS cases. The 7.0 mm ring provides larger exposition of the lens nucleus and is preferable for the surgeons using phaco flip nucleus removal technique, and also for the 6.5 mm optics IOLs users. Evacuation of the cortical material with 7.0 mm Malyugin Ring is also easier and safer.

The Malyugin Ring System can be used effectively both with the conventional SICS (Small Incision Cataract Surgery) and MICS (Microincision Cataract Surgery).

SURGICAL TECHNIQUE WITH MALYUGIN RING IN SICS

After topical anesthesia is applied, clear corneal incision is performed and ophthalmic viscosurgical device (OVD) is injected in the anterior chamber to stabilize it and protect the corneal endothelium.

Surgical steps in SICS are demonstrated in the patient with the cataract complicated by pseudoexfoliation syndrome and small pupil. The ring is loaded in the inserter. Then it is inserted through an unenlarged 2.2 mm clear corneal incision. The tip of the inserter is positioned at the center of the anterior chamber. While pushing on the thumb button, the ring is released from the tip until the distal scroll is engaged with the distal iris (Fig. 21A). Both lateral scrolls will then start to emerge from the tube of the inserter and one (or both) of them simultaneously catch the iris margins (Fig. 21B).

The proximal scroll is expelled from the cannula/inserter, and the injector is moved until the inserter hook is no longer holding the ring. In this position, the proximal scroll is lying on top of the iris. The inserter is withdrawn from the eye, and the hook is used to engage iris margin with ring scrolls (Figs 21C and D).

In some cases it is useful to disengage the trailing scroll from the inserter with the help of the hook introduced through paracentesis. The surgeon may push the ring slightly to the side to allow the inserter to exit out of the eye.

Capsulorhexis is performed using microforceps (Fig. 21E). Hydrodissection and hydrodelineation are performed with BSS until the nucleus could be rotated freely inside the capsular bag. Phacoemulsification is done with the Millennium (Bausch and Lomb) utilizing a "quick chop" technique (Fig. 21F).

Bimanual irrigation/aspiration is used to clean residual cortical fibers from the capsular bag (Fig. 21G). The capsular bag is then filled with the cohesive OVD. Then foldable intraocular lens (IOL) is inserted using injector (Fig. 21H). The Malyugin Ring is then removed from the eye in the reverse order (Figs 21I and J). It is necessary to use plenty of viscoelastic at this stage in order to keep the anterior chamber deep.

In order to retract the Ring completely inside the inserter barrel, it is necessary to press with the side port instrument on the lateral scrolls when they merge together (Fig. 21K). With this maneuver the surgeon can avoid catching the rim of the inserter with the lateral scroll, which is located above, and subsequent twisting of the ring. Alternatively the surgeon can decide not to retract the ring completely in the inserter and withdraw it from the eye at the moment when half of the Ring is located inside the inserter and both lateral scrolls are merged. After Ring removal the pupil constricts spontaneously (Fig. 21L).

The number of scrolls (1, 2 or 3) that can simultaneously engage the iris margin during the initial steps of the Malyugin Ring insertion depends on the depth of the anterior chamber and configuration of the anterior lens capsule. If the lens capsule is flat it is possible to engage the iris margin first with the distal scroll and then at the same time with both lateral scrolls (Fig. 22A). If the shape of the anterior lens capsule is prolate, only the distal scroll is engaged with the contraincisional pupillary margin (Fig. 22B). Then the ring is fully released from the inserter and the remaining scrolls are positioned in place with the hook (Sinskey, Lester or Kuglen).

The other clinical case of using the Malyugin Ring in patient with the cataract, previously operated glaucoma, and

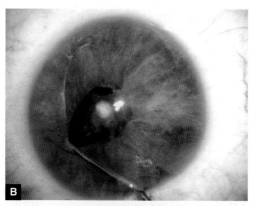

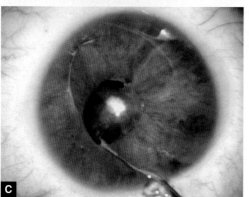

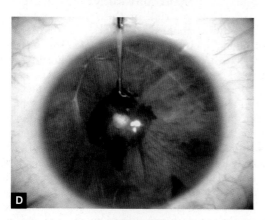

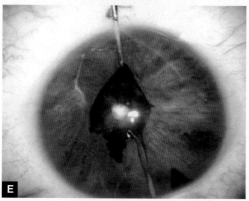

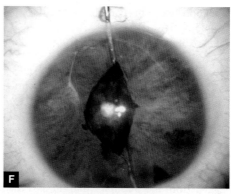

Figs 8A to F: Patient with chronic uveitis, anterior and posterior synechiae, intensive iris neovascularization and brown cataract with fibrosed anterior lens capsule. Synechiolysis (A to C) is combined with the iris stretching (D to E) which produced bleeding from the iris vessels

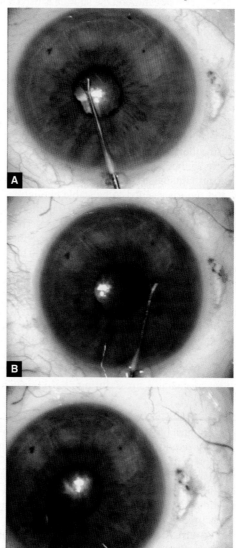

Figs 9A to C

257

pseudoexfoliation syndrome complicated by the small pupil is presented on Figs 23A to O.

Surgical technique with Malyugin Ring in 1.8 mm coaxial MICS.

In MICS with incisions less than 2.0 mm, the injector cannot enter the anterior chamber. Wound-assisted technique of the Malyugin Ring insertion is used in such cases (Figs 24A and B). The position of all four Ring scrolls is performed with the help of the hook (Figs 24C and D). Phacochop is being performed through the 1.8 mm incision with the Stellaris (Bausch and Lomb) (Fig. 24E).

After lens removal and IOL implantation, the ring scrolls are disengaged from the pupillary margin and the device is positioned on top of the iris (Figs 24 F and G). The hook inserted through the main incision, catches the proximal ring scroll and retracts the device from the eye (Fig. 24H). When both lateral scrolls comes close to the incision the spatula is used to depress the internal lip of the corneal tunnel in order to avoid catching it with the right lateral scroll (Fig. 24I). Then the ring is fully retracted from the eye with the forceps (Figs 24J and K).

SPECIAL CASES

The Malyugin Ring is more convenient than hooks in cases with narrow lid fissures because it does not involve additional external manipulations. It works very well in patients that are on alpha blockers (Flomax) and can be inserted in any stage of phacoemulsification.

On Figure 25 there is the fragment of the cataract surgery in a patient on tamsulosin. Initially pupillary diameter was sufficient and the iris seemed to be stable enough to proceed with phaco. But as soon as the Healon 5 left the anterior chamber iris started to billow and prolapse (Fig. 25A). The ring was inserted and a good exposition of the nucleus together with iris stabilization was achieved (Figs 25B and C). The case was completed successfully (Fig. 25D).

In eyes with zonular weakness some surgeons use iris hooks to fixate capsulorhexis edge to the papillary margin (Fig. 26). Stabilization of the iris-capsule complex can be achieved with the Malyugin Ring. The surgeon can temporarily clamp the edge of the anterior capsulorhexis to the pupillary margin, simultaneously providing a large pupillary aperture and zonular support (Figs 27A and B). The fixation is strong enough to withstand the mechanical stress during phaco (Fig. 27C).

CONCLUSION

Different techniques of nucleus disassembly in small-incision cataract surgery require a wide and unobstructed view of the anterior portion of the lens as well as the instruments inserted into the anterior chamber. The other important factor is sufficient manipulability of the instruments, which is critical for the successful completion of surgery. A pupil that fails to dilate makes cataract removal more difficult.

The Malyugin Ring is an important tool in phacoemulsification surgery. It adequately dilates the pupil and prevents iris sphincter damage. The easy to insert and remove

device expands the pupil, protects the iris sphincter during surgery, and allows the pupil to return to its normal shape, size, and function after the operation.

Clinical study of David Chang describing the use of the 6.25 mm Malyugin Ring produced by MST was published in Journal of Cataract and Refractive Surgery in 2008. He concluded: «The disposable Malyugin pupil expansion device was highly effective at maintaining an adequate pupil opening in eyes with IFIS. It is easier and faster to use than iris retractors and other pupil expansion rings and represents an excellent small-pupil strategy. We believe that iris retraction technique with the Malyugin Ring System (MST) has several advantages:

- The ring is as effective as other conventional iris hooks; however, compared with other commonly used iris retractors, it is friendlier to the eye due to its well-distributed stretching, gentle holding of delicate iris tissue, and the easier and less traumatic implantation. It has no sharp or pointed endings that can damage the eye;
- An equidistant positioning of the loops holds the iris tissue, ensuring correct position of the iris and preventing the effects of an overstretched pupil that are often observed in the incorrect positioning of iris hooks;
- The device applies pressure to the sphincter muscle over an area, which is wider than in cases of iris hooks. It is particularly useful in patients for which cutting or tearing of the iris tissue should be avoided, especially in the presence of rubeosis chronic anterior uveitis or systemic coagulopathy. The iris rim is safely fixed in the ring's loops, and there is no risk of the iris aspiration during phacoemulsification;
- Additional incisions are not required. This instrument is inserted through the one main incision, thus reducing surgical trauma and minimizing the risk of contamination and postoperative inflammatory reaction. In the technique, when the square pupil is formed by the conventional iris retractors, the iris can prolapse through the wound. This is particularly true in patients with relatively wide paracenteses and atonic and atrophic irises that seem particularly floppy;
- Sufficient room is available for nucleus fragmentation and removal. The device configuration allows a surgeon to work in the deep lens layers below the iris plane, and the square-shaped pupil formed by the ring. This provides enough space for grooving and cutting the nucleus and increases peripheral visualization during the chopping phase; and
- The ring is inserted and removed from the eye with a help of an inserter, thus reducing the risks of contamination and disturbance of the incision's architecture and wound integrity.

Careful intraoperative manipulation and insertion of the ring with liberal use of an ophthalmic viscoelastic device can help prevent complications. After surgery, most of our patients had pupils almost indistinguishable from their appearance before surgery, and functional activity was preserved. This device is likely to reduce postoperative abnormalities in pupil size and function.

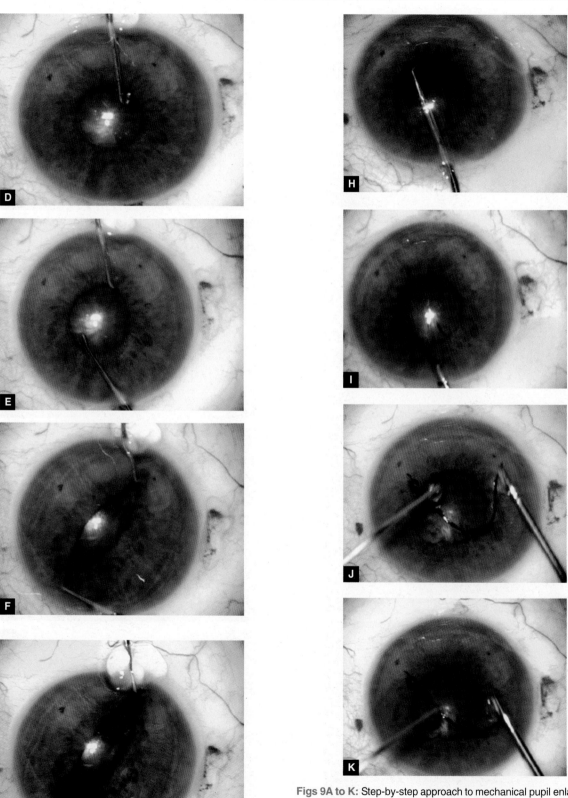

Figs 9A to K: Step-by-step approach to mechanical pupil enlargement: synechiolysis (A to C), pupil stretching (D to G) and peripupillary membranectomy (H to I). Membrane removed from the eye and positioned on top of the cornea (J and K)

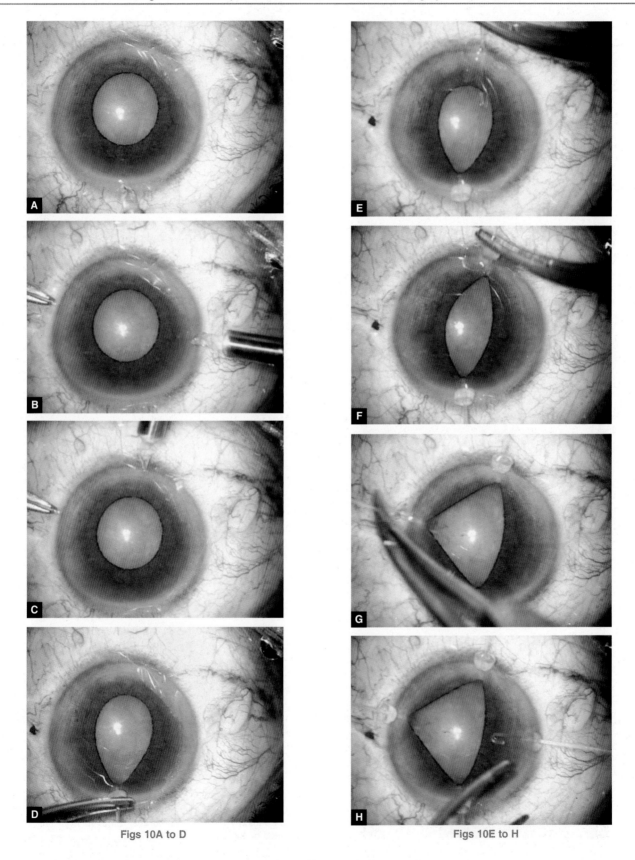

Figs 10A to D

Figs 10E to H

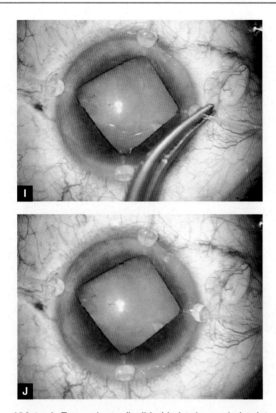

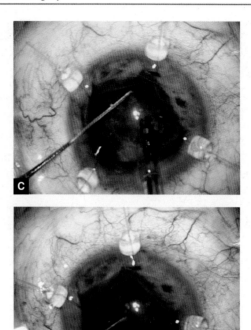

Figs 11A to D: Four flexible iris hooks are positioned in place. The pupil is not square but has trapezoidal configuration due to uneven spacing of the corneal paracenteses (A, B). This does not complicate nucleus removal (C, D), but may lead to overstretching of the iris and atonic pupil postoperatively

Figs 10A to J: Four polymer flexible iris hooks are being introduced through corneal paracenteses performed with the diamond knife

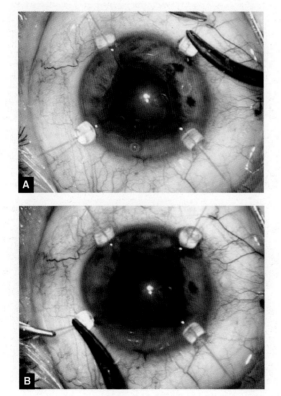

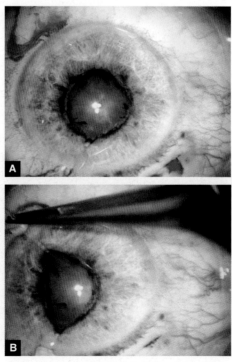

Figs 12A and B

261

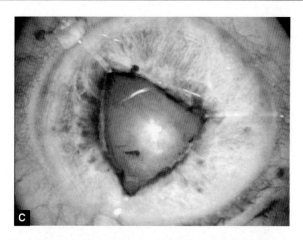

Figs 12A to C: Three polymer iris hooks inserted in triangular manner. Small bleeding from the pupillary margin vessels

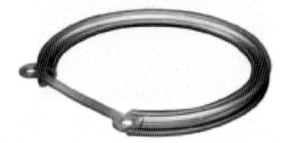

Fig. 13: The Graether pupil expander

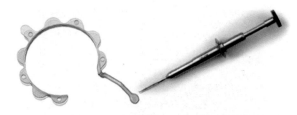

Fig. 14: The Perfect Pupil device (Milvella)

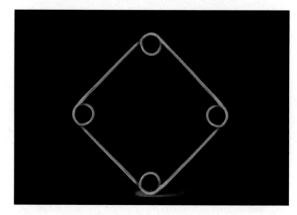

Fig. 15: The view of the Malyugin Ring

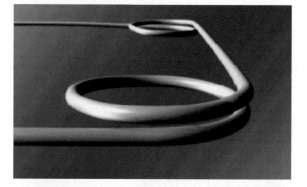

Fig. 16: The gaps of the ring loops are used to catch the pupillary margin

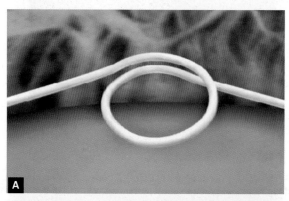

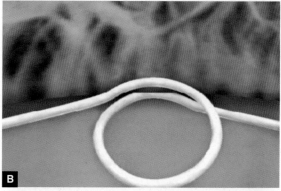

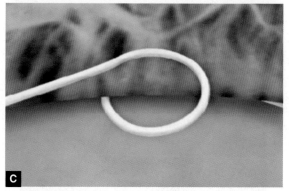

Figs 17A to C

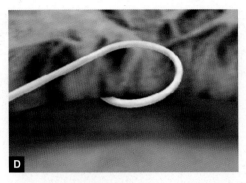

Figs 17A to D: The principle of pupillary margin fixation by the Malyugin Ring

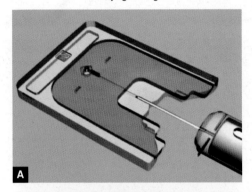

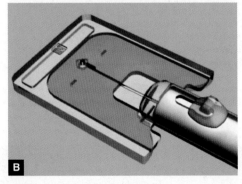

Figs 18A and B: Schematic view of the Malyugin Ring System produced by MST (assembly of the holder and inserter)

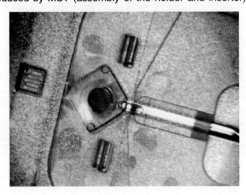

Fig. 19: The ring can be viewed through the semi-transparent upper part of the holder

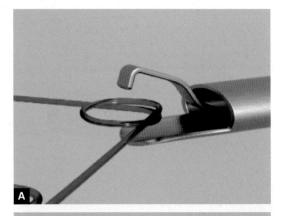

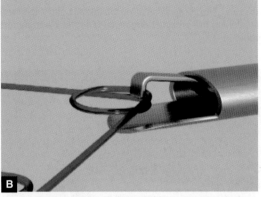

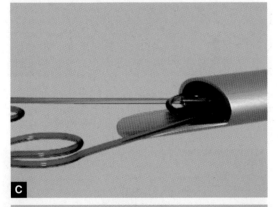

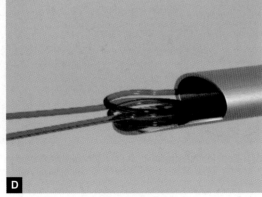

Figs 20A to D

263

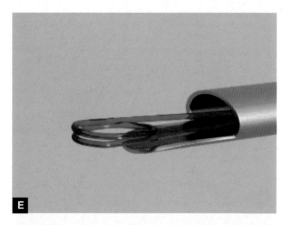

Figs 20A to E: The surgeon is pulling the thumb button and the inserter hook is catching the proximal ring scroll. The device is loaded inside the inserter

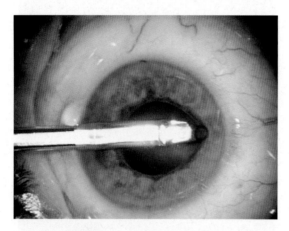

Fig. 21A: Malyugin Ring is inserted in the AC through the main clear corneal incision with a help of injector. The Ring is released from the tip until the distal scroll is engaged with the distal iris

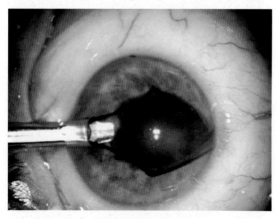

Fig. 21B: Both lateral scrolls starts simultaneously to emerge from the inserter tube. At the same time they catches iris margins

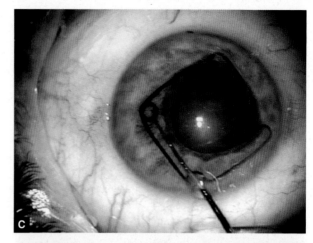

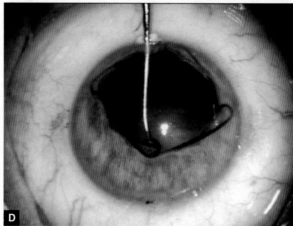

Figs 21C and D: The inserter is withdrawn from the eye and the iris hook is used to push the scrolls and engage the iris margin

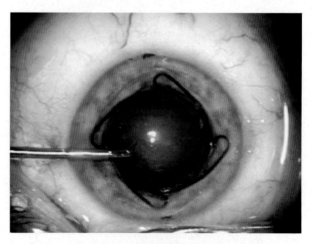

Fig. 21E: 7.0 mm Malyugin Ring is in place. Continuous curvilinear capsulorhexis is performed with the microforceps

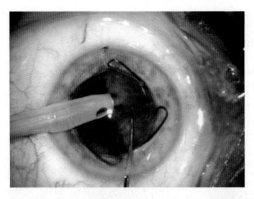

Fig. 21F: Removal of the lens nucleus with the US handpiece. Phaco chop is in progress

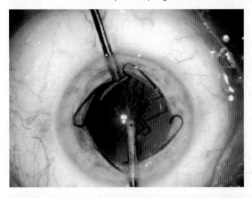

Fig. 21G: Irrigation-aspiration with bimanual system (Duet, MST)

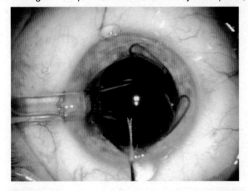

Fig. 21H: Hydrophylic acrylic IOL is implanted with injector

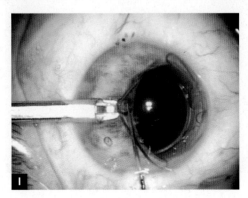

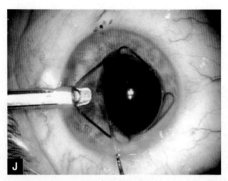

Figs 21I and J: Malyugin Ring is removed from the eye with the help of the inserter. Surgeon is to lifting the proximal ring loop with the second instrument helping the inserter hook to engage the proximal scroll of the device

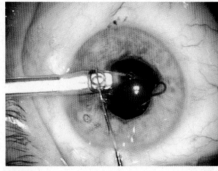

Fig. 21K: The surgeon is pressing on both lateral scrolls with the sideport instrument while retracting the device into of the inserter barrel

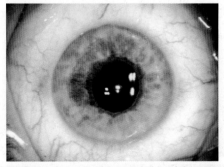

Fig. 21L: Patient's eye at the completion of the surgery

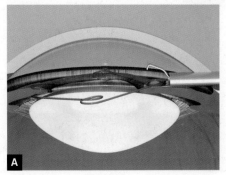

Fig. 22A

265

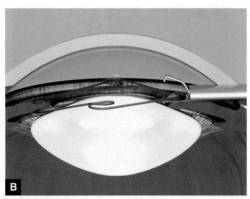

Figs 22A and B: The schematic side view of the anterior chamber in patient with the flat (A) and prolate (B) anterior lens capsule

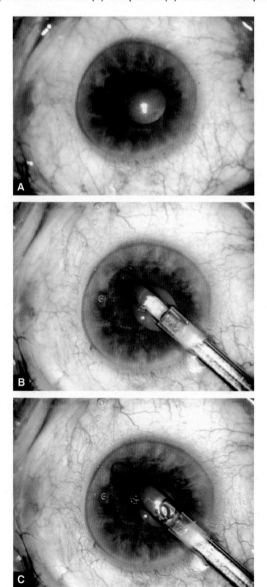

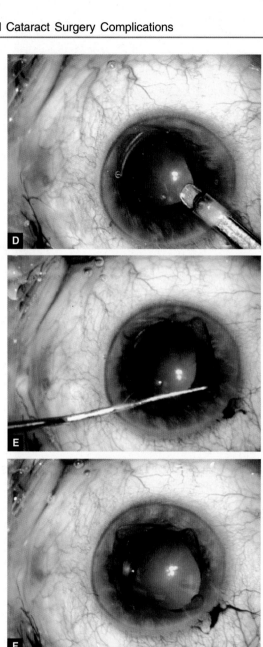

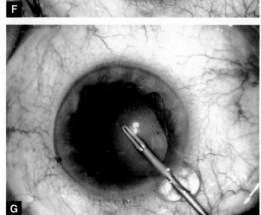

Figs 23A to C   Figs 23D to G

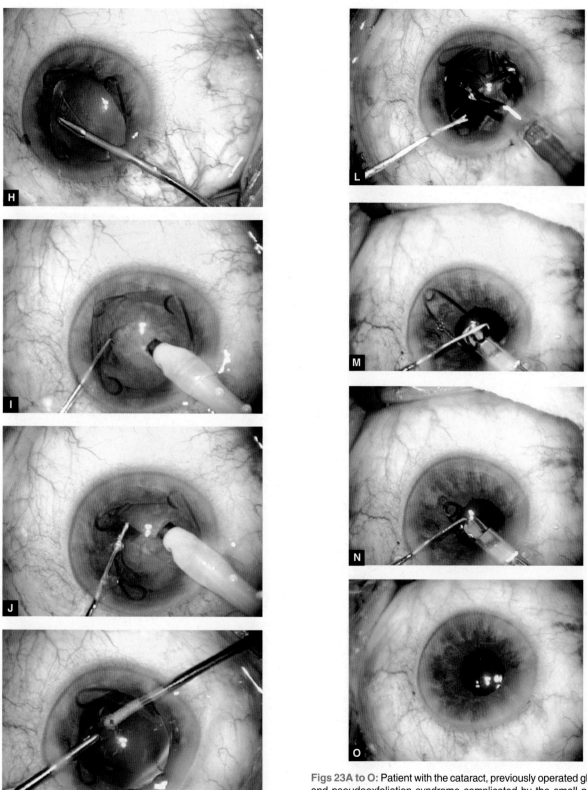

Figs 23A to O: Patient with the cataract, previously operated glaucoma, and pseudoexfoliation syndrome complicated by the small pupil. The surgery is performed with the help of the 6.25 mm Malyugin Ring System

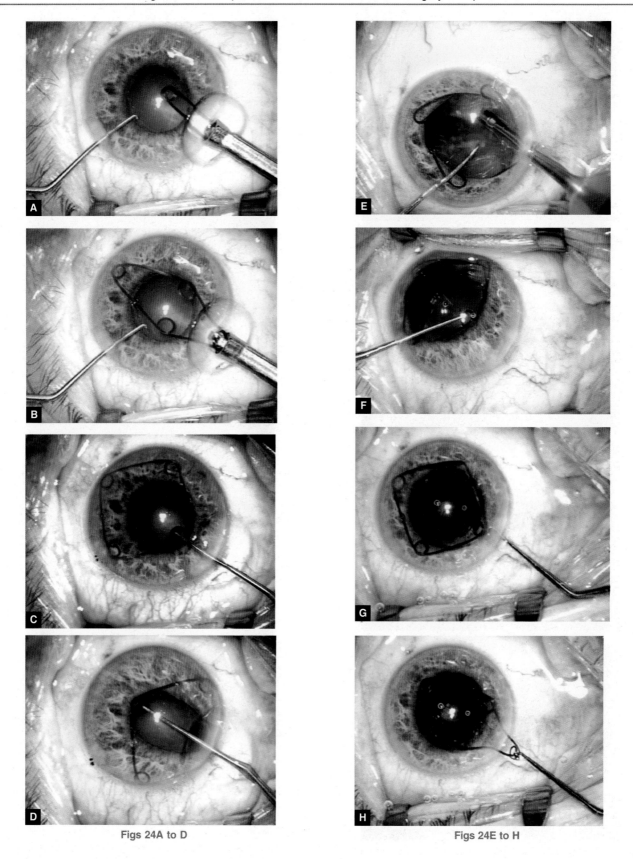

Figs 24A to D

Figs 24E to H

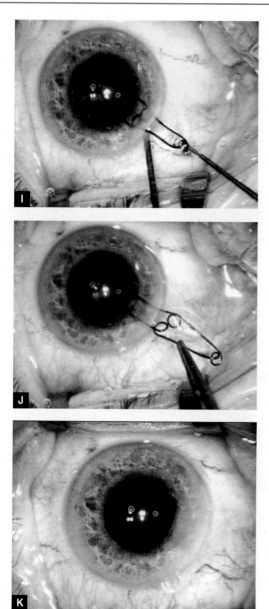

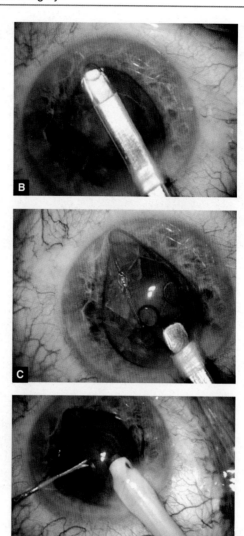

Figs 25A to D: Cataract surgery in patient with IFIS

Figs 24A to K: 1.8 mm C-MICS with 7.0 mm Malyugin Ring. Wound-assisted implantation and removal techniques

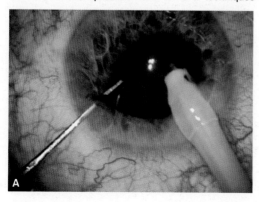

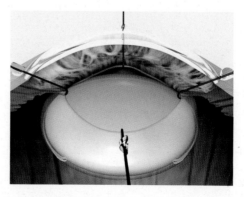

Fig. 26: Schematic view of the lens supported with iris hooks catching the capsulorhexis margin. Capsular tension ring is located in the equatorial zone of the capsular bag

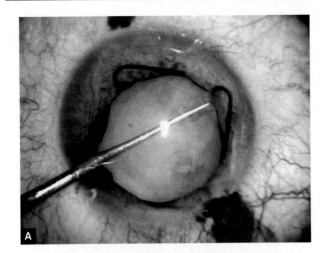 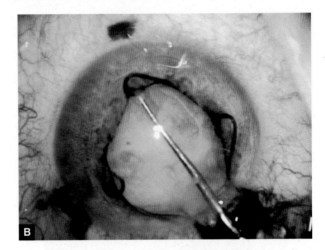

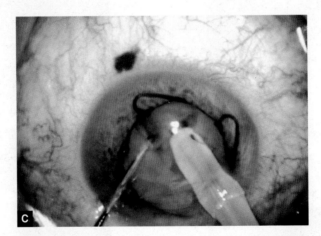

Figs 27A to C: Stabilization of the iris-capsule complex with the Malyugin Ring (A, B). The fixation is strong enough to withstand the mechanical stress during phaco (C)

Chapter 45

Management of IFIS with Biaxial Technique and Malyugin Ring

Robert J Weinstock, Neel Desai (USA)

INTRODUCTION

Intraoperative Floppy Iris Syndrome (IFIS), first described by Chang and Campbell in 2004, can rapidly turn a seemingly straightforward cataract surgery into a surgeon's nightmare with iris billowing, progressive pupillary constriction, and iris prolapse through the wounds. Though first described in the context of prior use of Tamsolusin (Flomax), IFIS has been more recently associated with other broad classes of drugs and even nutriceuticals. These include non-selective alpha-1 antagonists (e.g. Terazosin), angiotensin antagonists (lisinopril, losartan), certain muscle relaxants, and saw palmetto. This chapter will illustrate how the biaxial microincisional techniques, combined with pupil expanders like a Malyugin ring, can turn such cases into fairly routine cases with a little preoperative planning and preparation.

Several techniques to mitigate the symptoms of IFIS have been previously described. These include the use of mechanical pupil stabilizers like Grieshaber iris hooks and the Malyugin ring. In addition, many pharmacological agents have been suggested such as topical non-steroidal anti-inflammatories (NSAIDs) which are thought to potentiate pupil dilation, intracameral epinephrine and lidocaine (epi-Shugarcaine) which stiffen and dilate the iris, and specialized viscoelastics like Healon 5. Epi-Shugarcaine can be injected at or just below the iris plane prior to the injection of viscoelastics. Very often the periodic re-application of Healon 5 or similar viscoelastics is sufficient to stabilize the pupil.

However, over and above all of these techniques, we find that biaxial microincisional surgery carries the greatest advantage step-for-step during cataract surgery. Once viscoelastics have been injected and the pupil stabilized, the use of microincisional capsulorhexis forceps provide excellent control of the capsular tear since viscoelastics do not as easily egress from the wound. In IFIS cases, we feel it is especially important to provide a large capsulorhexis, even if construction requires tearing beyond the constricted pupil margin. This will aide in easy fragment and cortical removal without excessive blind hunting with an aspirator which is risky when faced with a constricted and floppy pupil. A larger capsulorhexis also facilitates a tilting of the nucleus out of the capsular bag during hydrodissection, where it can act as its own pupil dilator.

Cataract and cortex removal was performed with low flow, low ultrasound power, and low vacuum settings in order to minimize chatter and intraocular turbulence. Special attention was paid to keeping the phaco needle away from the floppy iris, central in the eye, and just below the iris plane. Using a bimanual technique in such cases offers the significant advantage of being able to maintain a consistent fluid dynamics above the iris plane with the irrigating chopper, regardless of how the phaco needle is maneuvered. The chamber does not collapse when the phaco needle is withdrawn slightly to access a sub-incisionally located fragment, and the iris does not billow when the phaco needle or aspiration port is torsionally rotated or moved to a different plane. The irrigating chopper can be used to gently push the iris peripherally to inspect the equator of the bag to ensure complete removal of all cortical material.

After IOL implantation, the Malyugin ring's distal loop should be disengaged from the pupil with a Kuglen hook, followed by the proximal subincisional loop to facilitate easier and less-traumatic removal. In cases of extreme IFIS, we will often pre-place, but not yet tie, a 10-0 suture in the wound just prior to viscoelastic removal since it is much easier to place the suture with viscoelastic still in the eye. Once viscoelastic removal is complete it is easy enough the tie the suture without risking chamber collapse and further iris prolapse. During viscoelastic removal with coaxial irrigation and aspiration, the bottle height is kept low to maintain a low intraocular pressure with low turbulence to minimize iris prolapse through the enlarged wound.

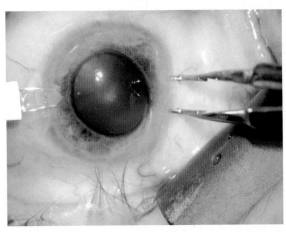

Fig. 1: Initial biaxial incisions are made with a trapezoidal shaped 1.4/1.6 mm diamond keratome matched for 19 gauge irrigating, phaco, and aspirating instruments

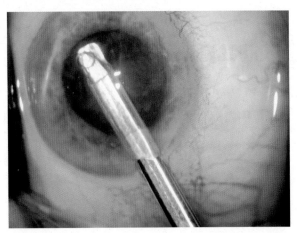

Fig. 4: Injector is placed well into the eye, need the distal iris

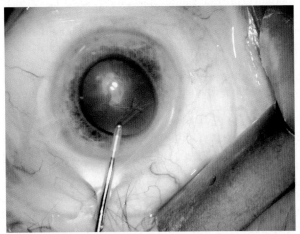

Fig. 2: After a cohesive viscoelastic is injected into chamber, a MST microcapsulorhexis forceps is used to create a rhexis. A well-controlled reasonably large rhexis, achieveable with microincisional techniques, will aide cortical removal in difficult cases

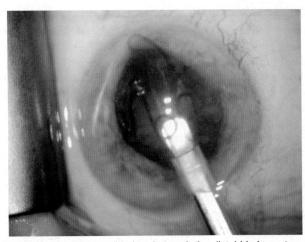

Fig. 5: As the injector slide is advanced, the distal iris is captured with the first loop

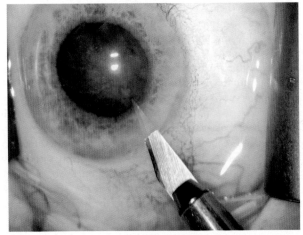

Fig. 3: One of the wounds is slightly enlarged to accommodate the injection system for the Malyugin ring

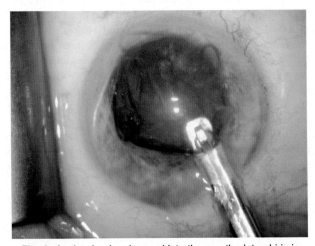

Fig. 6: As the ring is advanced into the eye the lateral iris is captured in the second and third loops

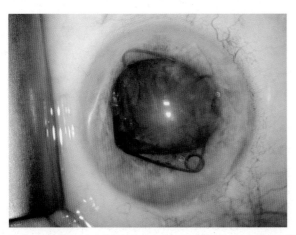

Fig. 7: The final loop is left in the chamber just above the proximal iris. It is often difficult to engage the final loop with the injector, necessitating the use of a hook

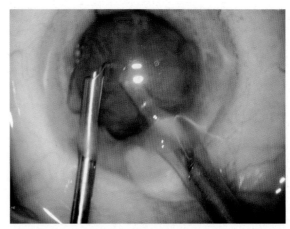

Fig. 10: 19 gauge biaxial phacoemulsification is used to remove the nucleus. Notice a silicone sleeve has been placed over the phaco needle to fully fill the wound and prevent iris prolapse. Recall the 1.6 mm wound was enlarged to 2.5 mm for the Malyugin ring injector

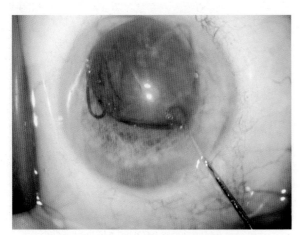

Fig. 8: A Kuglen hook is used to engage the final loop in the proximal iris

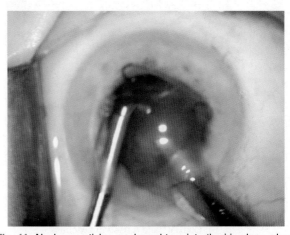

Fig. 11: Nuclear particles are brought up into the iris plane where there is good visibility and are phacoemulsified

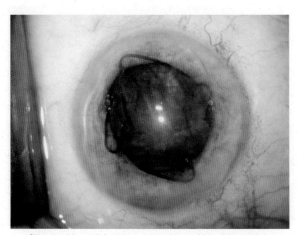

Fig. 9: After all four loops are in position the pupil is stabilized and in a good central position

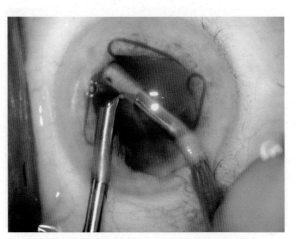

Fig. 12: Biaxial I and A is used to remove the cortex

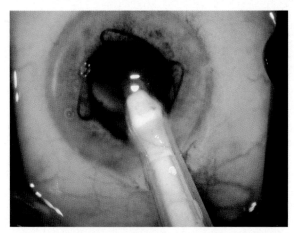

Fig. 13: After the capsule is filled with viscoelastic, A Bausch and Lomb LI61U 3-piece PCIOL is injected into the capsule

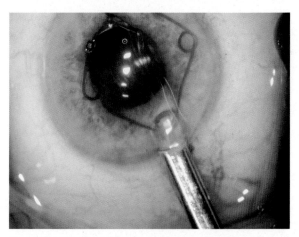

Fig. 16: The injector is placed in the eye and is used to grasp the proximal loop

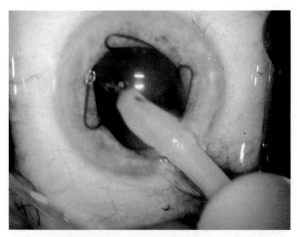

Fig. 14: Coaxial I and A used to evacuate the residual viscoelastic

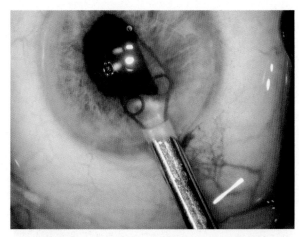

Fig. 17: As the ring is retracted into the injector, the other 3 loops are disengaged from the iris

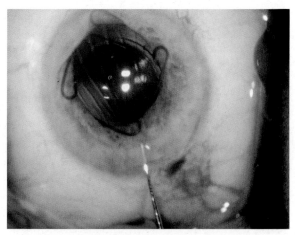

Fig. 15: A Kuglen hook is used to disengage the proximal loop from the iris

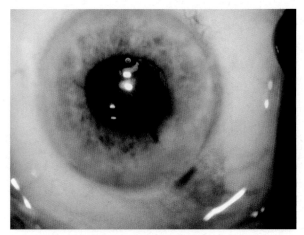

Fig. 18: At the completion of the case the iris is left round and undamaged

Chapter 46

Managing Intraoperative Floppy Iris Syndrome

David F Chang (USA)

In 2005, John Campbell and I first described a new small pupil syndrome associated with systemic tamsulosin that we named intraoperative floppy iris syndrome (IFIS).[1] In addition to a tendency for poor pupil dilation, we identified a triad of intraoperative signs that characterize IFIS — iris billowing and floppiness, iris prolapse to the main and side incisions, and progressive intraoperative miosis[1] (Fig. 1). Particularly when such iris behavior is unexpected, the rate of complications such as posterior capsule rupture, vitreous loss, and iris trauma is increased with IFIS.[1, 2]

Tamsulosin (Flomax), a systemic alpha-1 antagonist, is the most widely prescribed treatment worldwide for benign prostatic hyperplasia (BPH), which is characterized by increased urinary frequency. Systemic alpha-1 antagonists improve the lower urinary tract symptoms of BPH by relaxing the smooth muscle in the prostate and lower bladder wall. By allowing more complete emptying of the bladder, these medications decrease night-time urinary frequency. Alpha-1 receptors also mediate contraction of the iris dilator muscle, and we proposed that loss of dilator muscle tone and rigidity was the cause of the floppy iris. Furthermore, we postulated a semi-permanent effect because of several cases of IFIS in patients who had discontinued tamsulosin several years before surgery. Indeed, in a prospective trial, stopping tamsulosin preoperatively did not prevent or decrease the severity of IFIS.[2]

Since our initial report, it has become clear that other systemic alpha-1 blockers such as doxazosin (Cardura), terazosin (Hytrin), and alfuzosin (Uroxatral) can also cause IFIS. However, the frequency and severity of IFIS is much less with these nonspecific alpha-1 antagonists, as compared with tamsulosin.[3] This difference may relate to the much greater affinity and specificity of tamsulosin for the alpha-1A receptor sub-type that predominates in both the prostate and the iris dilator muscle.[2, 4]

IFIS can be classified as being mild (good dilation; some iris billowing without prolapse or constriction), moderate (iris billowing with some constriction of a moderately dilated pupil), or severe (classic triad and poor preoperative dilation). In a prospective study of 167 eyes in patients taking tamsulosin, the distribution of IFIS severity using this scale was as follows: 10%

no IFIS, 17% mild, 30% moderate, and 43% severe.[2] There can be significant variability in the severity of IFIS between different patients, and even between two eyes of the same patient. This makes it difficult to determine whether one pupil management strategy is superior to another. In fact, the various IFIS techniques discussed in this chapter can be combined and it is therefore helpful to master several complimentary approaches.

As general surgical principles for IFIS patients, one should make a well constructed shelved incision, perform hydrodissection more gently than usual, and reduce the irrigation and aspiration flow parameters if possible. Bimanual microincisional cataract surgery may be helpful, particularly for mild to moderate IFIS.[1] This technique utilizes water tight incisions and allows the surgeon to dissociate the irrigation and aspiration currents. Keeping the irrigation inflow anterior to the iris can lessen the iris billowing and prolapse.

In our original report, we noted that mechanical pupil stretching, performed with or without partial sphincterotomies, did not prevent iris prolapse or pupil constriction with IFIS.[1] Excessive iris manipulation may in fact worsen the iris prolapse in IFIS. Instead, we found that mechanical pupil expansion, such as with iris retractors, was far more effective. Subsequently, several other strategies for the surgical management of IFIS have been suggested, and are outlined below.

Because IFIS results from alpha-1 receptor blockade of the iris dilator muscle, a variety of pharmacologic strategies for managing IFIS have been proposed.[2, 4-10] As first suggested by Sam Masket, preoperative atropine drops (e.g. 1% tid for 1-2 days preoperatively) can provide sufficient cycloplegia to prevent intraoperative miosis.[2, 5, 6] However, as a single strategy atropine alone is often ineffective for more severe cases of IFIS.[2] Stopping tamsulosin preoperatively is of unpredictable and questionable value, and has the potential to cause acute urinary retention in patients with severe BPH. This is particularly true if preoperative atropine is used.

Direct intracameral injection of alpha agonist drugs is an excellent pharmacologic strategy for preventing or mitigating IFIS. Richard Packard first reported using intracameral phenylephrine,[7, 8] and Joel Shugar subsequently suggested using epinephrine for this purpose.[9] By presumably saturating the alpha-1A receptors, these agents can further expand the pupil (Figs 2A and B). Alpha agonists may also prevent billowing and prolapse by increasing iris dilator smooth muscle tone and maximizing iris rigidity. Preserved solutions should be avoided and one should use a diluted mixture (e.g. 1:1000 bisulfite-free epinephrine (American Regent) mixed 1:3 with BSS or BSS+) in order to buffer the acidic pH of the commercial preparation. Finally, Sam Masket reported excellent results with the synergistic combination of preoperative topical atropine with intracameral epinephrine in a small series patients taking tamsulosin.[6]

As first described by Bob Osher and Doug Koch, Healon 5 (Advanced Medical Optics) is a maximally cohesive ophthalmic visco-surgical device that is particularly well suited for viscomydriasis and for blocking iris prolapse in IFIS[2, 10] (Fig. 3). However, to avoid immediately aspirating Healon 5 the surgeon must employ low flow and vacuum parameters (e.g. < 175-200 mm Hg; < 26 ml/min). This strategy is therefore less suitable if a surgeon wishes to use high vacuum settings for denser nuclei. Wendell Scott has proposed injecting Healon 5 peripherally over the iris, and then filling the central chamber with a dispersive agent such as Viscoat (Alcon) to create a Healon 5 "donut". The Viscoat will better resist aspiration and delay the evacuation of Healon 5. For surgeons favoring high vacuum and flow settings, DisCoVisc (Alcon) has been advocated by Satish Modi.

A final set of strategies utilizes devices to mechanically expand and maintain the pupil diameter during surgery. Both the Morcher 5S Pupil Ring and the Milvella *Perfect Pupil* are disposable PMMA pupil expansion rings whose grooved contours are threaded alongside the pupillary margin using metal injectors (Figs 4A to C). In contrast, a disposable plastic injector is used to insert Eagle Vision's Graether disposable silicone pupil expansion ring. All of these rings are more difficult to position if the pupil is less than 4 mm wide or if the anterior chamber is shallow.

Iris retractors are a more popular mechanical strategy for pupil expansion in IFIS. Placement of the hooks in a diamond configuration has several significant advantages[11] (Figs 5A and B). The subincisional hook retracts the iris downward, and out of the path of the phaco tip. This maximizes exposure in front of the phaco tip while the nasal hook facilitates chopper placement. One millimeter limbal paracenteses are made in each quadrant, including a separate stab incision made just posterior to the temporal clear corneal incision. In this way, the subincisional hook and the phaco tip access separate entry tracks. If the pupil is fibrotic, overstretching it with iris retractors can cause bleeding, sphincter tears, and permanent mydriasis. This typically does not occur with the IFIS pupil, which is so elastic that it readily springs back to physiologic size despite being maximally stretched. Options include 6-0 nylon disposable retractors (Alcon) or reusable 4-0 polypropylene retractors (Katena, FCI). Being of the same size and rigidity as an IOL haptic, the latter are easier to manipulate and can be repeatedly autoclaved making them more cost effective to use.

It is much easier and safer to insert iris retractors and pupil expansion rings prior to creation of the capsulorhexis. If the pupil dilates very poorly or billows during injection of intracameral lidocaine, one should suspect severe IFIS and consider using these mechanical devices. Often, the pupil dilates reasonably well preoperatively, and it is not until after hydrodissection or during phaco that the prolapse and miosis occur. Healon 5 and intracameral epinephrine are excellent "rescue" techniques in this situation where it is difficult to visualize the capsulorhexis edge. If one chooses to insert iris retractors at this point, one should retract the pupil margin with a second instrument to avoid hooking the capsulorhexis margin with the retractors.

Eliciting a history of current or prior alpha-blocker use should alert surgeons to anticipate IFIS and to employ these alternative strategies either alone or in combination. A prospective, multi-center prospective trial using these techniques in 167 consecutive eyes from patients on tamsulosin demonstrated excellent outcomes and only a 0.6% posterior capsular rupture rate.[2] Because of the variability in IFIS severity associated with tamsulosin and other alpha-1 blockers, surgeons may consider using a staged approach in dealing with this condition.[8] Pharmacologic measures alone are often adequate for managing the pupil in mild to moderate IFIS cases. Even if they fail to expand the pupil, intracameral alpha agonists can reduce or prevent iris billowing and prolapse by increasing iris dilator muscle tone. If the pupil diameter is still inadequate, viscomydriasis with Healon 5 can further expand it for performing the capsulorhexis. Finally, mechanical expansion devices insure the most reliable and optimal surgical exposure for severe IFIS, and should be considered when other complicating risk factors (e.g. dense nuclei, narrow angles, posterior synechiae, weak zonules, pseudoexfoliation, etc.) are present.

REFERENCES

1. Chang DF, Campbell JR. Intraoperative floppy iris syndrome associated with tamsulosin (Flomax). J Cataract Refract Surg 2005;31:664-73.
2. Chang DF, Osher RH, Wang L, Koch DD. A prospective multicenter evaluation of cataract surgery in patients taking tamsulosin (Flomax). Ophthalmology 2007;114:957-64.
3. Blouin M, Blouin J, Perreault S, et al. Intraoperative floppy iris syndrome associated with Alpha-1 adrenoreceptors. Comparison of tamsulosin and alfuzosin. J Cataract Refract Surg 2007;33:1227-34.
4. Chang DF. Chapter 10: Intraoperative floppy iris syndrome. In Agarwal A, ed. Phaco Nightmares. Conquering Cataract Catastrophies. Slack Publishing Inc 2006.
5. Bendel RE, Phillips MB. Preoperative use of atropine to prevent intraoperative floppy-iris syndrome in patients taking tamsulosin. J Cataract Refract Surg 2006;32:1603-05.
6. Masket S, Belani S. Combined preoperative topical atropine sulfate 1% and intracameral nonpreserved epinephrine

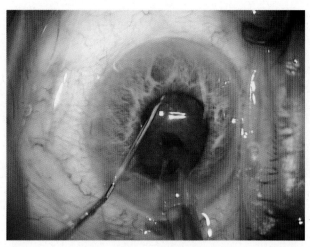

Fig. 1: Intraoperative floppy iris syndrome in a patient taking tamsulosin. In addition to iris prolapse to the phaco and side port incision, the pupil has constricted limiting visibility

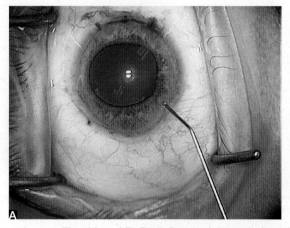
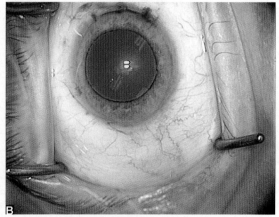

Figs 2A and B: Pupil diameter in tamsulosin patient before (A) and after (B) injection of 0.2 ml of intracameral epinephrine solution (bisulfite-free 1:1000 mixed 1:3 with BSS)

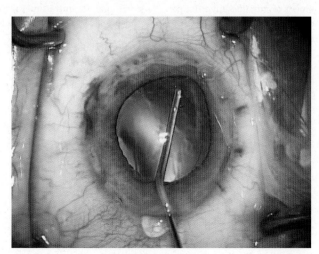

Fig. 3: Healon 5 viscomydriasis in a patient with IFIS following removal of the cortex

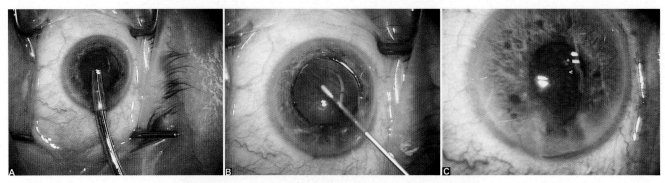

Figs 4A to C: Management of IFIS using a Morcher PMMA pupil expansion ring. (A) Ring is inserted with an injector. (B) Ring is threaded along pupil margin to maintain a constant diameter. (C) Following removal of the ring, iris prolapse and pupil constriction occur during removal of the viscoelastic

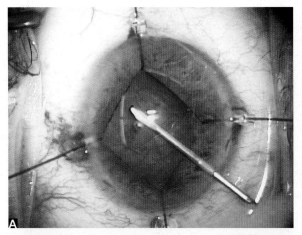
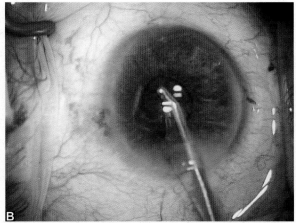

Figs 5A and B: Management of IFIS using 4-0 prolene iris retractors in a patient taking tamsulosin. (A) Retractors placed in a "diamond" configuration, with the sub-incisional retractor placed directly behind the clear corneal phaco incision. (B) Pupil constriction and iris prolapse occurring after removal of the iris retractors

hydrochloride 1:2500 for management of intraoperative floppy iris syndrome. J Cataract Refract Surg 2007;33:580-82.

7. Gurbaxani A, Packard R. Intracameral phenylephrine to prevent floppy iris syndrome during cataract surgery in patients on tamsulosin. Eye 2005;[Epub ahead of print].

8. Manvikar S, Allen D. Cataract surgery management in patients taking tamsulosin. J Cataract Refract Surg 2006;32:1611-14.

9. Shugar JK. Intracameral Epinephrine for Prophylaxis of IFIS [letter]. J Cataract Refract Surg 2006;32:1074-75.

10. Arshinoff SA. Modified SST-USST for tamsulosin-associated intraocular floppy iris syndrome. J Cataract Refract Surg 2006;32:559-61.

11. Oetting TA, Omphroy LC. Modified technique using flexible iris retractors in clear corneal surgery. J Cataract Refract Surg 2002;28:596-98.

Chapter 47

Modern Phaco in Complicated Cases

Jes Mortensen (Sweden)

As a micro surgeon you are often reminded of the old Greek Philosophy telling you not to commit hybris or you will be punished by Nemesis. You may feel happy doing a lot of cataract surgery for a long-time without any unexpected incidents, feeling that your surgery is perfection, then suddenly the patient with the unexpected complication turns up and destroys your day if you are not prepared to cope with that challenge.

I shall try to show the precautions I take when operating a complicated cataract. Obstacles to deal with are the physiognomy of the patient, such as a small orbit and deeply positioned eyes, different ethnic distinctions such as epicantus and the anatomy of the eye; mature, hard lens, shallow anterior chamber, small pupil, floppy iris and not least abnormalities of the lens.

At the end of the chapter I shall describe how I perform scleralfixation of the lens using an injector to minimize the incision to the normal size of 2.5 to 2.75 mm.

The Physiognomy of the Patient

Many cataract surgeons use the temporal approach, which often helps, if that is not sufficient the eye can be lifted with a subtenonal injection of an anesthetic like Xylocain®. If the pressure in the orbita is high after the subtenonal injection do not forget canthatomy. Good anesthesia of the eye is mandatory in surgery for complicated cataracts, the more fixated the eye is the better control of the surgery.

The Anatomy of the Eye

The Anterior Chamber

A shallow anterior chamber is a challenge for phacoemulsification. The ultrasound probe can severely damage the endothelium if it is not taken into account. The depth of the AC is a function of the eye's anatomy and the size of the lens. Pressure from the vitreous is another parameter seen in phacomorphic glaucoma. During phacoemulsification the vitreous can be hydrated shallowing the AC, and increasing the intraocular pressure.

If the AC is shallow due to anatomy of the eye or a big lens you have to first think of the endothelium and protect it with Viscoat®. You can even increase the infusion pressure to mechanically increase the depth of the AC. Another way is to start a deep sculpturing of the lens in the center to create room for the manipulation, again refilling the AC liberally with Viscoat® during the phacoemulsification.

If the cause of the shallow AC is from the posterior segment the problem is bigger. Thanks to the small incision in modern phacoemulsification the problem can be solved without too high a risk.

Phacomorphic glaucoma is due to that the swelling of the lens reduces the iridocorneal angle, it can also be secondary to pupillary block. It is common in developing countries, seldom seen in a modern western country.

The AC is extremely shallow and the IOP is high. A technique that can be used is to deepen the AC by a pars plana vitectomy, followed by phacoemulsification.

Phacolytic glaucoma can present in the same way with high IOP, but the diagnosis can be made by the inflammation in the AC and that the lens is often ballooned, if the capsule has not spontaneous ruptured. If it has the AC is filled with a milky substance. Pars plana vitrectomy is not needed here, an easier technique is to reduce the IOP with oral glycerol or intravenous Mannitol to reduce the vitreous volume. When the IOP is reduced you can often do the phacoemulsification, as soon you have punctured the lens capsule the AC will deepen and you will often see a reduced nucleus.

If the AC shallows during operation and the IOP increases you have two options; choroid swelling (bleeding or hydration) or hydration of the vitreous. It is most important to differ. If ophthalmoscopy is possible you can use the 60 diopters lens under the operating microscope, if not you have to use the B-scan. If choroidal bleeding is evident or suspected, close the incision and end the operation. If hydration of the vitreous is the problem you can stop the operation and dehydrate the vitreous by orally glycerol or intravenous Mannitol and wait until the pressure is reduced and the AC is reformed, then the operation can safely be continued.

The Lens with Normal Zonular Support

If the lens has its normal zonular support even very hard, mature lenses are often not a problem with the new phaco machines. If the phaco time is expected to be long, you should start with

Viscoat® and refill the anterior chamber during phacoemulsification; by doing this the risk of permanent damage to the endothelium will be reduced.

If you feel uncomfortable with the phaco time used, you might reconsider and carefully express the reduced nucleus before damage is overt, the price to pay is a larger incision. The gray, brittle nucleus is no problem often easy to "divide and conquer"; the brown to black nucleus is often difficult to separate as the lens fibers are cross-linked. ECCE might be the better alternative. If you have planned for ECCE stick to the plan and do not start with phaco as converting is often an inferior alternative to a well conducted ECCE.

The Lens with Reduced Zonular Support

The zonulae of the lens can be totally absent or reduced due to trauma, exfoliation syndrome or congenital abnormalities such as seen with ectopia lentis. In Sweden exfoliation syndrome is seen in almost every second patient, the zonulae have not only few but also fragile and the lens capsule is thin especially in the posterior part. I shall show some cases operated by myself and my colleagues to illustrate the various approaches used to get the best result. First a discussion of the instruments we use. The pupil is normally very small and rigid in the exfoliation syndrome, if the pupil is easily dilated it is a positive sign that the zonulae of the crystalline lens are normal. If zonular defects and a loose lens is suspected it is always prudent to be prepared.

The iris hooks were first used in doing vitrectomy in the beginning of the 1990s and were later adopted by the cataract surgeons. The first hooks were of metal and non disposable. Later the disposable nylon hooks were developed. In the beginning these were used only to enlarge the pupil. Later after the capsular rhexis was introduced they were even utilized to stabilize the capsular bag. The next big step was the introduction of the capsular tension ring. Different types of the tension ring have developed making it possible to directly sclerally fixate the tension ring or like the Ahmed Capsular Tension Segment to stabilize the capsular bag with more profound zonular dialysis.

The surgical cases demonstrate the technique used to successfully cope with a loose lens, congenital ectopia lentis and ectopia after trauma.

The best way to learn is to see how difficult cases have been managed:

The first case is an illustration of a traumatic cataract with dehiscence of the zonulae. It was operated several years ago, before capsular tension rings were available. The use of a PMMA lens is still a less expensive choice in many countries.

Case Number One (Traumatic Zonular Dehiscence)

The patient was a 50 years old man who, 12 months before the cataract operation, was struck in his right eye by a piece of wood immediately causing hyphema and localized zonular dehiscence. Later traumatic cataract followed. Iris hooks were used to stabilize the capsular bag. The nucleus was quite soft and could more or less be irrigated out of the Anterior Chamber

with the phaco probe. A Heparin Coated PMMA IOL (Pharmacia) was implanted to stabilize the bag. Today you would have used a modified Morcher ring designed by Dr. Cionni with an eyelet allowing it to be sutured to the sclera as the zonular dehiscence was almost 180 degrees. But this eye had healthy residual zonulae so the IOL is still in place after 15 years. If the zonulae had been weak you probably have seen a dislocation of the IOL, which is more and more common even if a capsular tension ring is used in cases with severe zonular weakness, e. g. severe exfoliation syndrome (Figs 1 and 2).

The next two cases will illustrate bilateral congenital subluxation of the lens due to dehiscence of the zonulae.

Case Number Two (Ectopia Lentis in One Eye)

A young boy 10 years old with one eye with congenital subluxation of a small lens in one eye. A synechia was seen more or less centring the lens in mydriasis. The lens was without zonulae temporally and only half the normal size. The operation was performed due to development of cataract. Two scleral pockets were made in preparation for scleralfixation.

First the iris was retracted so the lens synechia could be cut with microscissors (Figs 3 to 5).

Capsular rhexis was performed with Corydon forceps. The flexible iris hooks were inserted around the margin of the capsular rhexis to make it steady.

The soft lens material could easily be removed with the I/A system. Healon 5® was injected into the bag and a capsular tension ring was placed. You can see that even the smallest ring is too big.

A single-piece SA60AT AcrySof® IOL (Alcon®) was injected and rotated into the capsular bag.

Miochol was injected followed by miosis and centration of the pupil.

The scleral pockets were not needed. Today you would have used a modified Morcher ring designed by Dr Cionni with an eyelet allowing it to be sutured to the sclera as the zonular dehiscence was more than 180 degrees and the healthy zonulas pulled the lens bag nasally leading to a dislocation of the IOL. Two years after the first operation a new operation was performed by which an anchoring suture was placed temporally through sclera and around the capsular tension ring relocating the IOL.

Case Number Three (Ectopia Lentis Bilateral)

A young woman in her thirties with congenital subluxated lens in both eyes with visual acuity 20/60 and 20/50; she has a sister with the same problem who has already had a successful surgery. The operation was performed by my young colleague, Dr. Öhman.

Cataract was the cause for operation in both sisters. The lens was of normal size and the zonulae dehiscence was from 3 to 6 o'clock making the lens subluxate temporally, no vitreous was seen in the anterior chamber. Operation was performed in general anesthesia. The mydriasis was good and allowed a safe capsule-rhexis with forceps to be performed. Two flexible iris

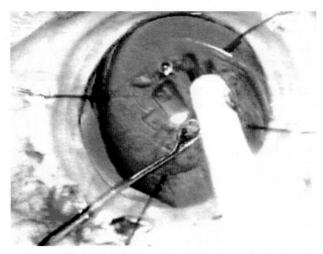

Fig. 1: Iris hooks were used to stabilize the capsular bag

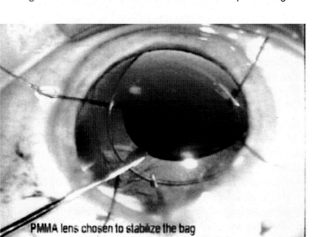

Fig. 2: A heparin coated PMMA IOL (Pharmacia®) was implanted to stabilize the bag

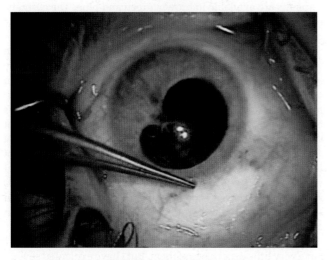

Fig. 3: A synechia was seen more or less centring the lens in mydriasis

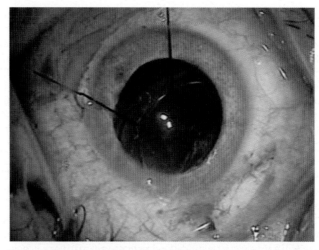

Fig. 4: A capsular tension ring was placed. You can see that even the smallest ring is too big

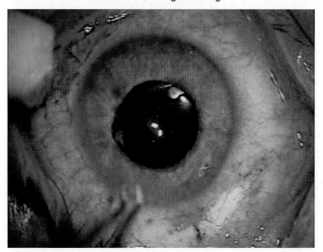

Fig. 5: The healthy zonulae pulled the lens bag nasally leading to a dislocation of the IOL

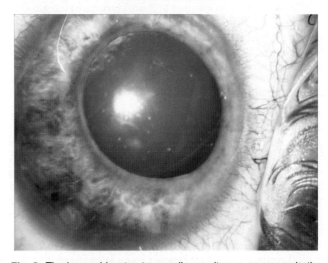

Fig. 6: The lens subluxates temporally, no vitreous was seen in the anterior chamber

hook retractors were inserted to support the capsular bag at the dehiscence. A scleral pocket was created at 6 o´clock in the dehiscence zone. A temporal clear corneal incision was made with the 2.75 mm keratome. Phacoemulsification (Alcon, Legacy®) was done with aspiration no ultrasound was needed. A modified Morcher ring designed by Dr Cionni with an eyelet was sutured to the sclera at the dehiscence area at 6 o'clock with double-armed 10-0 polypropylene suture (Ethicon STC-6, Johnson and Johnson Intl., Belgium). A single-piece SA60AT AcrySof® IOL (Alcon®) was implanted in the capsular bag.

When using the modified Morcher ring be sure that the sutures are placed over the capsular rim so the hook will be placed over the capsular rim. Perforating the bag with the needle might tear the capsular bag (Figs 6 to 8).

I have no follow-up on this patient so far, but if she does as well as her sister, who had inferior visual acuity preoperatively, she will gain a visual acuity allowing her to get a driver's license.

Case Number Four (Traumatic Cataract with Capsular Rupture)

A boy aged nine was hit by a rubber band with steel hooks in is right eye during play. Visual acuity was perception of light. A dehiscence of the iris was seen from 1 to 3 o'clock, and rupture of the lens capsule was suspected. Blood in the anterior chamber did not allow ophthalmoscopy. Surgical exploration was performed as rupture of the bulb was suspected, but no rupture was found. After 4 weeks a traumatic cataract had developed. The blood had cleared from the anterior chamber and synechia had developed in the dehiscenced area (Figs 9 and 10).

Vision Blue® was used and capsulorhexis could be performed utilizing the flexible iris hooks during the procedure. The capsule was ruptured from 1 o'clock till 4 o'clock; small scissors were used to cut the capsular rim free. The lens material could be washed out with the I/A. The cortical material sealing the rupture was left until a one piece Acrysof IOL had been placed in the capsular bag. As the pupil centred well and the iris dehiscence was small no repair was needed.

Visual acuity was low due to choroid rupture engaging the macula. The patient was however pleased as his expectations were very low. He had only had perception of light in the eye for 4 weeks and could now enjoy the full   periphery of the visual field.

Case Number Five (Riegers Syndrome)

The patient is a 60 years old man with Riegers syndrome diagnosed when he was in his thirties. He has three brothers and one sister. The sister has no abnormality in her eyes. One brother is severely afflicted and the two other brothers only modestly. The patient's left eye was already severely damaged by glaucoma when the diagnosis was made almost 25 years ago. In spite of glaucoma medication and trabeculectomy the right eye's visual acuity worsened so the patient had to retire before 50 years of age. When I saw the patient the left eye was amaurotic since decennia, the right eye had perception but not in all directions. A mature cataract and a synechia of the pupil were seen. The patient was informed that no guarantee could

be offered that the procedure could be done by a single surgery. The operation was performed to prevent the development of a hypermature cataract and in the hope that some improvement of vision might come (Figs 11 and 12).

The operation was performed under subtenonal anesthesia. Healon5® was used. First flexible iris hooks were placed and a test to rupture the fibrotic ring of the pupil was done, but the fibrotic ring could not be removed without endangering the iris, why small cuts were made 360 degrees round to let the pupil slowly dilate by the flexible iris hooks so as not to give big ruptures of the pupil rim. The Healon5® was washed out and Vision Blue® was injected into the AC. CCC was performed with Corydon Forceps. The flexible iris hooks were placed round the rim of the capsular bag. The lens was extremely hard why I choose to divide the nucleus into four quadrants. Healon5® was injected several times during the phacoemulsification to minimize the potential damage to the endothelium due to the long phaco-time. As the lens bag was found stable no tension ring was inserted. A single-piece SA60AT AcrySof® IOL (Alcon®) was implanted in the capsular bag.

The patient experienced that he was better able to localize the direction of the light and even to percept shadows of people in the room.

Case Number Six (Traumatic Cataract with Pupilloatinia)

A man in his forties suffered a trauma aged seven to his left eye in his childhood leaving him with cataract and traumatic maximal mydriasis. He was operated by one of my young colleagues, Dr Lassarén. This case will demonstrate the new possibilities of iris defect repair.

The lens was phacoemulsified in the usual way the rim of the capsular bag supported with the flexible iris hooks. The aniridia ring Type 50 C from Morcher was first placed in the capsular bag and then the single-piece SA60AT AcrySof® IOL (Alcon®). Lastly the Iris Prosthetic System (IPS®, designed by H. Hermeking, MD, Germany) was used. The elements are available for 3 mm and 4 mm pupils and Iris Reconstruction Implants are available in brown, green and blue. The cosmetic result is excellent and so was the rating by the patient of the procedure (Figs 13 and 14).

I shall end the chapter by a description of how scleralfixation with an injector is performed. I have chosen not to give any advice how to cope with the ruptured capsule. The broken capsule is the most difficult situation to cope with, first you must be honest with the patient and tell them when it has happened and even prepare the patient for the possibility that you might need to send him/her to a more experienced colleague to get the best result. I am not fond of the different techniques that involve the more or less blind injection of viscomaterial via a sclerotomy into the posterior chamber to support the ruptured capsule, at least not in an inexperienced surgeon's hand. The best result is if a posterior segment surgeon can clean up and a secondary implantation is possible.

I have not used an anterior chamber IOL, since 1989 so I have very little experience of them. But I have explanted several anterior chamber lenses due to decompensation of the cornea.

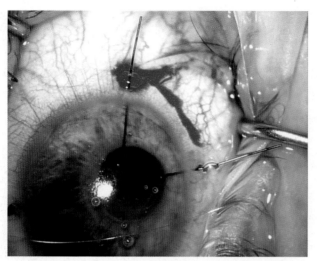

Fig. 7: A scleral pocket was created at 6 o'clock in the dehiscence zone

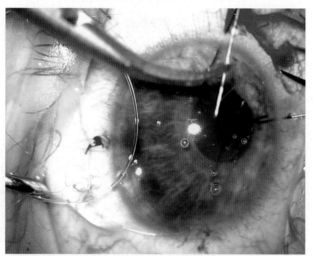

Fig. 8: A modified Morcher ring with an eyelet was sutured to the sclera at the dehiscence area at 4 o'clock with double-armed 10-0 polypropylene suture

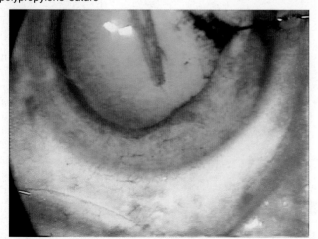

Fig. 9: Vision Blue® was used and capsular rhexis could be performed using the flexible iris hooks during the procedure

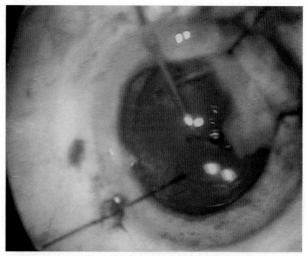

Fig. 10: The cortical material sealing the rupture was left till a one piece Acrysof® IOL had been placed in the capsular bag

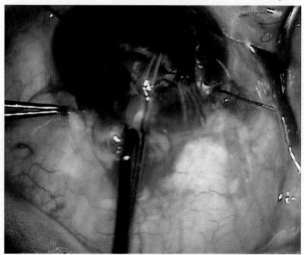

Fig. 11: Small cuts were made 360 degrees round to let the pupil slowly dilate by the flexible iris hooks

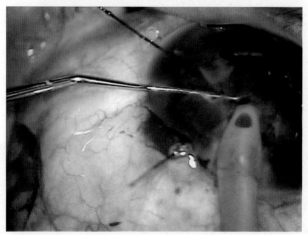

Fig. 12: The lens was extremely hard why the nucleus was divided into four quadrants

283

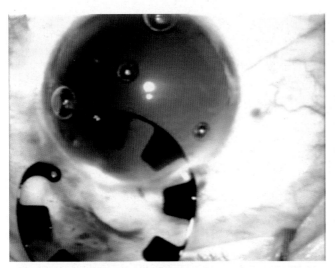

Fig. 13: The aniridia ring Type 50 C from Morcher was first placed in the capsular bag

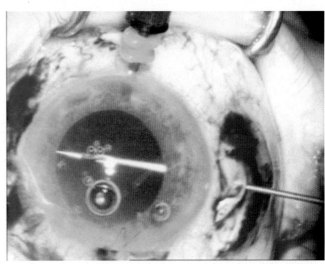

Fig. 16: A 25-gauge injection needle is inserted under the opposite scleral flap meeting the straight needle

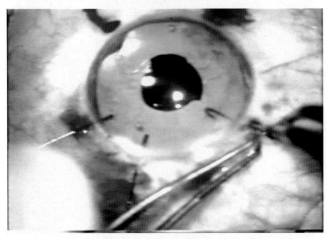

Fig. 14: At last the Iris Prosthetic System was used

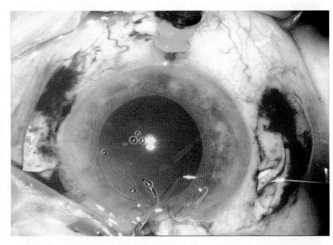

Fig. 17: The second prolene suture is guided out at the phaco incision at 12 o'clock using the 25-gauge injection needle

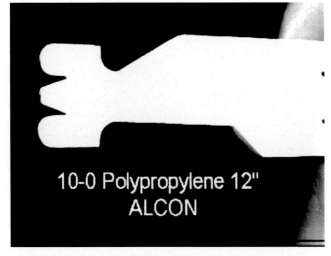

Fig. 15: A 10-0 polypropylene suture (Prolene)

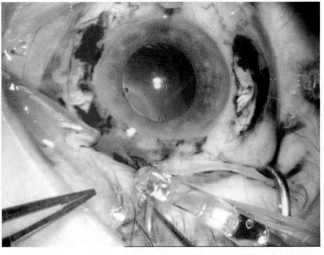

Fig. 18: The left prolene suture is then fixated to the leading haptic

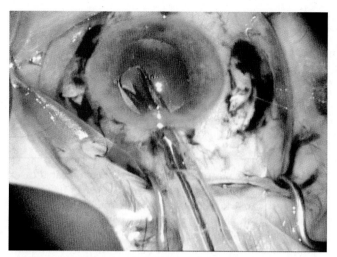

Fig. 19: The IOL is now injected into the AC and the left haptic is guided by pulling the prolene suture

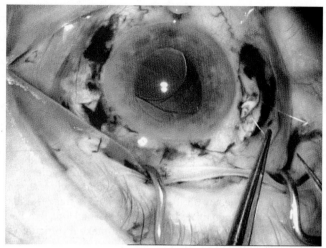

Fig. 21: The IOL is rotated in place by pulling the two sutures

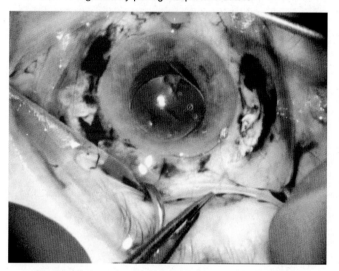

Fig. 20: Prolene sutures are knotted to the second haptic

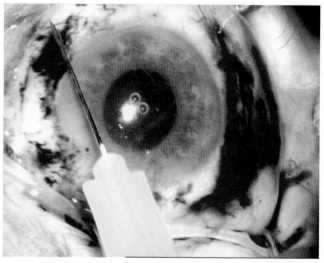

Fig. 22: At last the biological glue, Tisseel®, is used to glue the scleral flap and the conjunctiva

Quite often the cornea cleared up after the explantation and a scleralfixation of a posterior lens solved the problem. In many cases a penetrating keratoplasty was required. I have no experience of the new technique of suturing the posterior IOL to the iris, but I should hesitate to do that in a younger patient, remembering the problems with the iris sutured lenses, e.g. the Shamrock IOL; including UGH (uveitis, glaucoma and hemorrhage) syndrome.

Scleralfixation with an Injector

The scleralfixation of a posterior chamber lens is not a new procedure, but it initially had a bad reputation due to choroidal bleeding and retinal detachment. The most important thing to remember is never to penetrate the sclera in a soft eye. Today

I always use an infusion needle transcorneally at 6 o'clock and use the Acurus vitrector (Alcon®) to provide the intraocular pressure that can be raised to 60 mm Hg before penetrating the sclera with the suture needle. It is even most important that no vitreous is engaged when the IOL is injected into the eye. Thorough anterior vitrectomy is mandatory as a brisk insertion of the IOL may catch the vitreous still attached to the retina causing a dialysis of pars plana (Figs 15 to 22).

How to Do

Two scleral pockets are made at 9 and 3 o'clock. Bend the straight needle in the 25-gauge injector needle making it easier to guide the straight needle. Then the straight needle of the 10:0 polypropylene (Alcon®), Prolene suture penetrates the sclera under the preformed scleral flap 1.5 mm from limbus. A 25-gauge injection needle is inserted under the opposite sclera flap 1.5 mm from the limbus meeting the straight needle and the prolene suture is pulled through.

A site port incision is made at 2 o'clock to fill the AC with Healon5® to protect the endothelium. An incision is made by the 2.75 mm phaco knife at 12 o'clock. The Prolene suture is grasped and cut. If no capsule is left supporting the IOL a second Prolene suture is placed 2 to 3 mm from the first Prolene suture under the scleral flap. In a right eye temporally and in a left eye nasally. The second Prolene suture is guided out at the phaco incision at 12 o'clock using the 25-gauge injection needle.

A Hoya IOL is placed in the injector and slowly pressed forward in the injector till the leading haptic is free. The left Prolene suture is then fixated to that haptic. The Hoya lens has haptics with small knobs at the ends that make it difficult for the Prolene suture to slip off.

The IOL is now injected into the AC and the left haptic is guided by pulling the Prolene suture. The other haptic is outside the eye and the two right Prolene sutures are knotted to the second haptic. To make it easier I place the second suture over the first suture. The first prolene suture is first knotted to haptic, then the second suture making sure that no crossing of the two sutures occurs as that will prevent the stabilization of the IOL.

The haptic is then pushed into the AC using a Sinsky hook and the IOL is rotated in place by pulling the two sutures.

The two sutures can now be sutured together in one knot. The small curved needle on the Prolene suture is used to suture under the scleral flap.

The Healon® is removed with I/A and an antibiotic is injected into the AC. Finally the biological glue, Tisseel®, is used to glue the scleral flap and the conjunctiva.

CONCLUSION

In this chapter the management of different complicated cases in cataract surgery has been discussed. The use of flexible iris hooks and capsular tension rings is one of the biggest improvements in handling those cases with dehiscence of the zonulae and in managing cases with small pupils. The old extra-capsular technique should not be forgotten as very hard cataracts still are a problem; a successful operation followed by an decompensated cornea due to too much ultrasound may cause more problems for the patient than the cataract did.

The scleralfixation with an injector minimizes the incision to 2.5 to 2.75 mm reclining the risk of high astigmatism. I find scleralfixation a better choice in eyes with endothelial dystrophy and glaucoma than the anterior chamber IOL.

Chapter 48

Chandelier Illumination and Bimanual Vitrectomy Used to Remove a Dislocated IOL

Amar Agarwal, Soosan Jacob, Athiya Agarwal, Sunita Agarwal, Ashok Garg (India)

INTRODUCTION

Numerous advances in microsurgical techniques have led to highly safe and effective cataract surgery. Two of the current trends in the evolution of modern cataract techniques include increasingly smaller surgical incisions associated with phacoemulsification (e.g. sub 1.4 mm incisions as in phakonit with rollable IOL implantation)[1], as well as the movement from retrobulbar and peribulbar anesthesia to topical anesthesia, and even "no anesthesia" techniques.[2] Despite such advances, the malpositioning or dislocation of an intraocular lens (IOL)[3-5] due to capsular rupture or zonular dehiscence remains an infrequent but important sight-threatening complication for contemporary cataract surgery. The key to the prevention of poor visual outcome for this complication is its proper management.

MANAGEMENT OF A MALPOSITIONED IOL

Disturbing visual symptoms such as diplopia, metamorphopsia, and hazy images are associated with a dislocated intraocular lens (IOL) (Fig. 1). If not properly managed, a malpositioned IOL may also induce sight-threatening ocular complications, including persistent cystoid macular edema, intraocular hemorrhage, retinal breaks, and retinal detachment. Contemporaneous with advances in phakonit microsurgical techniques for treating cataracts, a number of highly effective surgical methods have been developed for managing a dislocated IOL.

CHANDELIER ILLUMINATION

Visualization is done using a Chandelier illumination in which xenon light is attached to the infusion cannula. This gives excellent illumination and one can perform a proper bimanual vitrectomy as an endoilluminator is not necessary for the surgeon to hold in the hand. (Fig. 2). A Reinverter system has to be used if one is using a wide field lens (Volk or Oculus). The supermacula lens (Fig. 3) helps give better steropsis so that one will not have any difficulty in holding the IOL with a diamond tipped forceps (Fig. 4). When one is using the Chandelier illumination system one hand can hold the IOL with the forceps and the other hand can hold a vitrectomy probe to cut the

adhesions of the vitreous thus doing a bimanual vitrectomy (Fig. 5). One can also use two forceps to hold the lens thus performing a hand shake technique (Fig. 6). The lens is then brought out anteriorly and removed through the limbal route (Fig. 7).

REINVERTER SYSTEM

When we use the wide field indirect contact vitrectomy lenses we have to use a reinverter as the image is seen inverted. The reinverter again makes the image erect so that the surgeon does not have difficulty in operating. The one we use is the one from Zeiss microscopes which has a foot switch connection. In other words on pressing the footswitch button the reinverter works.

The Volk Reinverting operating lens system is also present. It has a unique single-element prism design. This installs in the Zeiss and other microscopes. It offers surgical visualization ranging from high magnification of the macula to panoramic viewing upto and including the ora serrata.

WIDE FIELD INDIRECT CONTACT VITRECTOMY LENSES

These are essential for performing proper bimanual vitrectomy. When one is doing vitrectomy for dropped IOL we use the Mini Quad Volk lens or the Oculus lens. These lenses give the view of the retian upto the ora serrata. When one wants to pick up the IOL with the diamond tipped forceps then we use the Supermacula Volk lens. This lens gives very high magnification. Another advantage of this lens is the better steropsis so that you know exactly where the IOL haptic is in relation to the retina. These lenses come with a handle so that the assistant can hold the lens comfortably.

BIMANUAL VITRECTOMY

The advantage of the bimanual vitrectomy set up is that the hand which normally holds the endoilluminator is free and so one can use two instruments to manipulate the dropped IOL. The Chandelier illumination system we used was from Synergetics (USA) and the machine was the Photon.

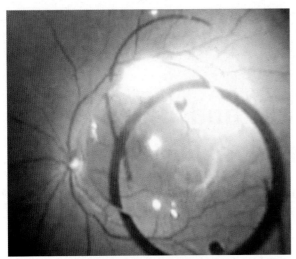

Fig. 1: Dislocated IOL on the retina

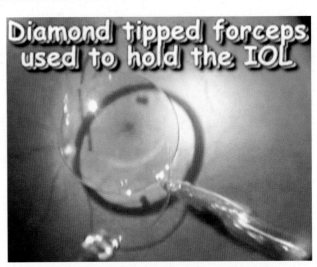

Fig. 4: Diamond tipped forceps lifting a looped IOL lying on the retina after a vitrectomy

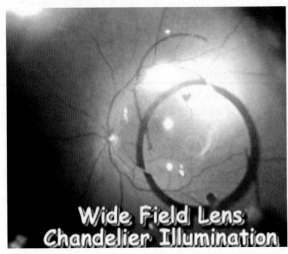

Fig. 2: IOL lying over the macula. Notice the wide field view of the retina. This is because of the wide field contact lens being used and the Chandelier illumination which is seen in the upper left hand corner

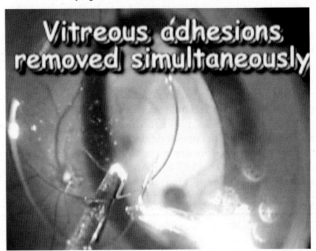

Fig. 5: Forceps holding the IOL and the vitrectomy probe cutting the vitreous adhesions. This is bimanual vitrectomy which is possible due to the Chandelier illumination

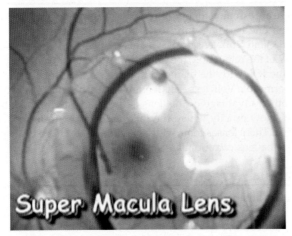

Fig. 3: View using the super macula lens. This gives better steropsis

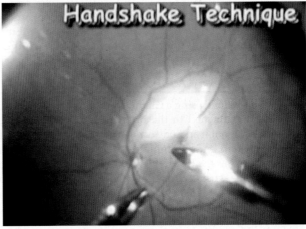

Fig. 6: Handshake technique. Using two forceps one can hold the IOL comfortably and bring it anteriorly

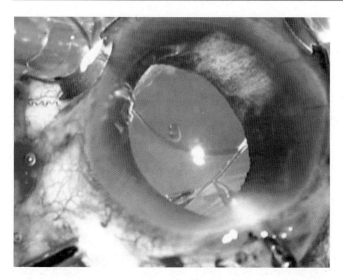

Fig. 7: IOL brought out anteriorly through the limbal route. Notice in the upper right and left corners infusion cannulas fixed. One is for infusion and the other for the Chandelier illumination. One can also have the same infusion cannula with the Chandelier illumination

Sophisticated filtering techniques within the Photon and its associated fiberoptics are used to provide higher illumination levels.

REFERENCES

1. Agarwal A, Agarwal S, Agarwal A. Phakonit: Lens removal through a 0.9 mm incision. In: Agarwal A Phacoemulsification, Laser Cataract Surgery and Foldable IOL's First edition. Jaypee Brothers 1998.
2. Agarwal A, Agarwal A, Agarwal S. No anesthesia cataract surgery. In: Agarwal a phacoemulsification, laser cataract surgery and foldable IOL's second edition. Jaypee Brothers 2000.
3. Chang S. Perfluorocarbon liquids in Vitreo-retinal surgery. International Ophthalmology Clinics-New approaches to vitreo-retinal surgery Vol 32, No.2, Spring 92:153-63.
4. Chan CK. An improved technique for management of dislocated posterior chamber implants. Ophthalmol 1992; 99:51-57.
5. Chan CK, Agarwal A, Agarwal S, Agarwal A. Management of dislocated intraocular implants. In: Ophthalmology clinics of North America, posterior segment complications of cataract surgery, December 2001; editors: PN Nagpal, IH Fine; WB Saunders, Philadelphia; p 681-693.

Chapter 49

Prevention of PCO

Frederic Hehn (France)

INTRODUCTION

PCO (Posterior capsular opacification) is caused by lens epithelial cells (LEC) retained in the capsular bag following surgery which then proliferate, migrate and transform to myofibroblasts. Interest in the prevention of PCO has centred around surgical technique, pharmacological methods to remove or destroy lens epithelial cells and changes in intraocular lens material and design.

Subject

Changes in surgical technique have little effect in prevention of PCO although a capsulorhexis size which lies on the optic diameter appears to be beneficial. Many different cytotoxic drugs and pharmacological agents have been used experimentally to prevent PCO but the problem has limited damage only to lens epithelial cells. So far, no method has been shown to be safe for clinical use. Current interest is centred once again on the intraocular lens itself, particularly the material that it is made from and changes in its edge profile.

A simple procedure called a YAG posterior capsulotomy is performed to restore vision lost from the clouded capsule. The well-known preventing factors of a PCO are: no IOL decentration, a 360° IOL overlapping of capsulorhexis, an ablation of visco-elastic behind the optic, a reduction of the retro-optical space, no folds on posterior capsule, the speed of the capsular bend formation, the adhesion between the optic and posterior capsule by fibronectin, IOL materials, and of course Square Edge IOL design. But only a total cleaning of anterior and equatorial LEC could be efficient to avoid the PCO.

The problem of PCO is not only the cost and the morbidity of Nd: Yag capsulotomy, but the real challenge is to keep a soft capsular bag . With a soft capsular bag, LEC free, it will be possible to restore accommodation in pseudophakic eyes with the "phacoersatz" and avoid practice anterior vitrectomy and PCCC* in children's cataract surgery.

There are only two ways to avoid PCO, Block LEC migration, or kill the LEC. Until we will be not able to take off or kill entirely the equatorial LEC, PCO occurs irreversibly from month to month after cataract surgery. Different systems can help to reduce PCO. Block LEC migration, in using a Square edge profile of the haptics and optic, in using a capsular ring.

The second way is to try to kill the LEC in using: Perfect Capsule™ system, which is able to kill the LEC by hypo-osmolarity, but there is some risk for endothelium if the suction leaks. Actually perfect casule device is not available for MICS** because it needs a 5.0 mm width cornea incision. Aqualase®: An hot hydrojet, able to lyse the nucleus of the crystalline, is there any possibilities to lyse the LEC in equatorial region? Actually aqualase is compatible with bimanual technique , but not with MICS because the needle of aqualase handpiece needs of 3.2 incision, the next generation of aqualase certainly will be compatible with MICS. Phaco-laser (the Dodick photolysis) is compatible with MICS, recently at ARVO 2004 meeting, it has been shown the possibility of direct LEC destruction by Nd yag laser on anterior capsule. CBJ: Cleanbagjet® Is a new phaco handpiece, which produce a micro hydrojet able to clean the LEC even in equatorial region, developed by Ioltech laboratories, first clinical results are attempted in ASCRS 2005.

CONCLUSION

PCO remains the really final frontier in cataract surgery, especially in pediatric cataract surgery.

Before three years old implantation is not recommended, and the classical technique with anterior and posterior CCC and anterior vitrectomy is still the consensus for congenital cataract management. But in this case, to let a good anterior capsule ring seems to be useful for a later IOL in the sulcus implantation. Some new device like CTR, aqualase, phacolaser, perfect capsule and clean bag jet seem to be useful to decrease or delay PCO. We hope that as soon as possible without PCO, we can recreate a natural accommodation in pseudophakic eye and perform cataract surgery as easily in children than in adult without anterior vitrectomy nor PCCC.

---

*   Post continuous circular capsulorhexis

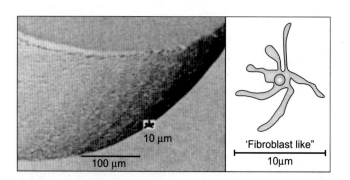

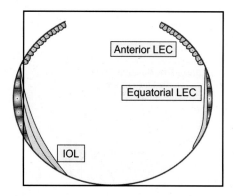

Figs 1 and 2: Prevention of PCO in one of the final frontier that eye surgery is not resolved. PCO is not very popular among ophthalmologists because the Nd: YAG capsulotomy is very efficient and lucrative so....for the both surgeons and laboratories. Nd: YAG capsulotomy procure an immediate visual improvement and only few complications, even they should be worst like a IOL displacement, retinal detachment, glaucoma, uveitis or an endophthalmitis. PCO in due to a metaplasia of residual equatorial LEC (lens epithelial cells) into fibroblastic cells induce fibrosis and pearls

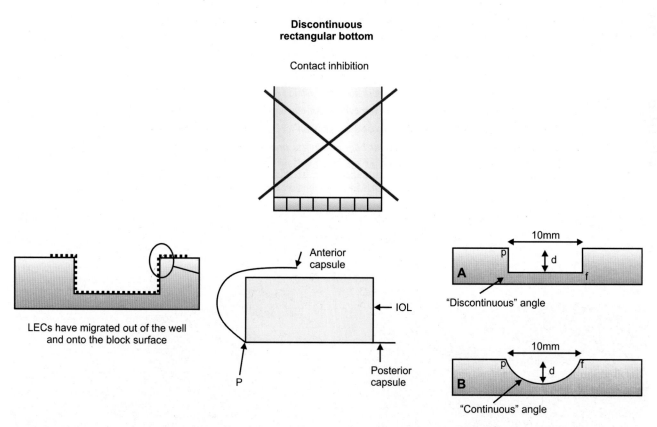

Figs 3 and 4: One of the most used technique is to build a square edge on the posterior edge of the IOL's optic to bloc LEC migration. This device is as efficient as possible if the IOL is harder than softer, then PMMA or hydrophobic acrylic are more efficient than hydrophilic acrylic in this way. In fact it's not the square edge shape itself which blocks LEC migration, but the square edge increase the pressure on the contact point between capsule and square edge. This pressure avoids the LEC progression behind the IOL's optic

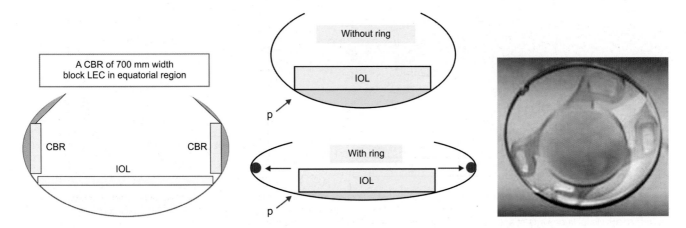

Figs 5 and 6: Another way, in the same idea, is to use a tension ring during the cataract surgery to make the square edge immediately efficient. But this technique is not popular due to the cost of the procedure

01: the CTR increases the pressure at the 'p' point and then the SEIOL design tension effect

02: the CTR reduces the retro-optical space too according to the no space no cell theory

03: the CTR increases the speed of the capsular bend formation

04: the CRT facilitates the adhesion between the capsule and the IOL according to the 'sandwich' theory

05: the CTR probably makes some equatorial LEC destruction by direct cell compression

06: the CTR prevents IOL decentration deformation and tilting with soft IOL

07: the CTR facilitates the equatorial LEC removal by an IOL rotation inside the capsular bag

08: the CTR facilitates the retro-optical viscoelastic ablation too, according to the 'no space no cell' theory

09: the CTR facilitates the anterior capsular bag cleaning to prevent capsular shrinkage

10: the CTR decreases the capsular folds of posterior capsule

Fig. 7: In this picture we relate all the properties of the tension ring which can help to avoid LEC migration

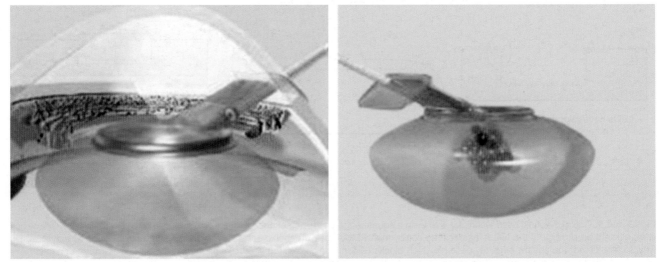

Fig. 8: An other way is the perfect capsule device: A difficult technique with a micro anterior capsulorhexis then collapse with a soft cup in using a air depression. Then inside the capsular bag an irrigation of different cytotoxic drugs can be used to kill the LEC. There are some risks of zonular breaking or damage of the both endothelium or retina (depends of the drugs used : 5FU, hypotonic water...)

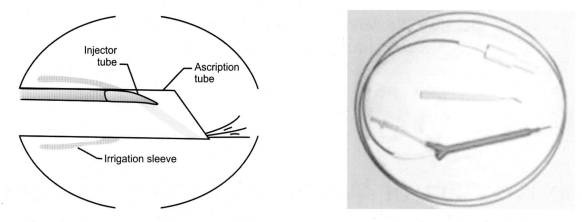

Figs 9 and 10: Aqualase ALCON system or phacolaser, are not able to kill all the LEC, and can't stop PCO

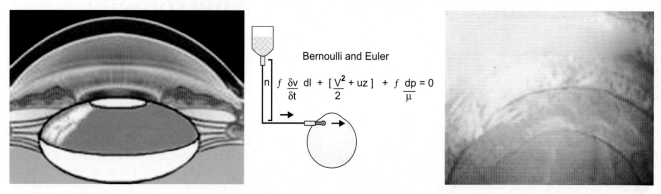

Bernoulli and Euler

$$n\left| f\ \frac{\delta v}{\delta t}\ dl\ +\ \left[\frac{V^2}{2}\ +\ uz\right]\ +\ f\ \frac{dp}{\mu}\ =\ 0\right.$$

Fig. 11: Another device called CLEANBAGJEJ CBJ®, can clean with safety the equatorial region of the capsular bag of the LEC, in using a micro waterjet. But this system of mine is unfortunately not now available. The big challenge is not to make or not an Nd: YAG capsulotomy, but avoid completely the PCO, to keep a lifetime soft capsular bag. Because a permanent soft capsular bag is the way to avoid PCCC (post continuous circular capsulorhexis) in childhood catatract surgery. The second challenge is to build further really accommodative IOLs, which absolutely need no at all PCO

Chapter 50

The New Era of Wavefront-Guided Cataract Surgery and Astigmatism Correction with the O Range Intraoperative Aberrometer

Neel Desai, Robert J Weinstock (USA)

As new technology in the cataract surgery arena emerges, particularly with regard to newer intraocular lenses for the correction of presbyopia and astigmatism, patient expectations continue to rise. As surgeons, we continuously strive to meet or exceed these expectations whenever possible by harnessing the power of the most cutting edge techniques and tools available in the modern era. The onus is on the surgeon, more than ever before, to hit specific refractive targets postoperatively with the increasing utilization of so-called premium lenses that demand premium outcomes. The unique optical properties of many presbyopia-correcting lenses are particularly sensitive to even small amounts of uncorrected or under-corrected astigmatism. In addition, the detrimental effects of off-axis placement of a toric lens has been well-documented—even 5 degrees of off-axis placement results in a 15% reduction in the corrective power of the lens. Furthermore, post-refractive surgery intraocular lens power calculations present an increasingly frequent challenge to cataract surgeons with a plethora of formulae and calculation methods to chose from, each with their own weaknesses and ambiguities. In each of these areas, from incisional astigmatism correction and toric lens placement to post-refractive IOL targeting, wavefront technology, like the Wavetec O Range intraoperative aberrometer, offers surgeons a tool to predictably improve visual outcomes for their patients.

Wavefront technology has measurably improved visual outcomes and the level of patient satisfaction by customizing our treatments for myopic and hyperopic astigmatism with excimer laser vision correction. The transference of wavefront technology from applications in astronomic telescopes to ophthalmology that produced wavefront-guided LASIK,

represented a transformational moment in the history and success of laser vision correction. We are now witnessing a similar ground-breaking transformation in cataract surgery with the advent of wavefront-guided cataract surgery.

The earliest manifestation of this trend toward wavefront-guided cataract surgery was in the development of aspheric intraocular lenses. With increasing understanding of the visual influence of higher-order aberrations, measurable by wavefront aberrometers, lens manufacturers aimed to reproduce the natural state of the youthful eye prior to the development of cataracts. The natural crystalline lens in a youthful eye imparts negative spherical aberration that offsets the positive spherical aberration of a prolate cornea. Placement of a prolate lens with positive spherical aberration produces an additive effect that has been thought to increase glare and halo in scotopic conditions. Implantation of lenses with zero or negative asphericity resets this balance.

With regards to astigmatism correction, the current practice of using preoperative keratometric data and visually placed axis marks on the corneal limbus falls short of our aim to deliver precise outcomes for many reasons. First, visually placed marks are inherently inaccurate because they often cover several degrees of arc, frequently fade before use, and are prone to parallax. When these marks at 12, 3, 6, and/or 9 o'clock are used to place other marks for LRI placement or toric lens alignment, this further compounds the error. These inherently inaccurate marks, then, only partially compensate for the significant error introduced by cyclotorsion of the eye when the patient is placed in a supine position. In addition, measurements of keratometric cylinder are centered on the corneal apex, not the visual axis where it counts most. When

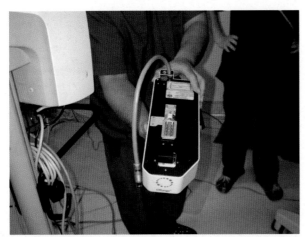

Fig. 1: The O Range intraoperative aberrometer is small in size and attaches to the bottom side of the head of the surgical microscope with a specialized mount

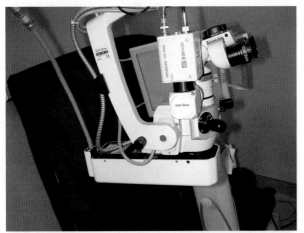

Fig. 2: Once attached to the microscope it is calibrated and the ready for use. It can be left in place indefinitely or removed if desired

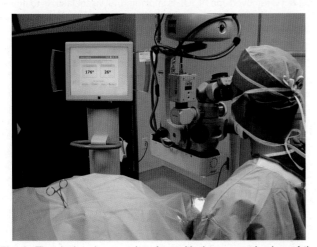

Fig. 3: The device does not interfere with the surgeon's view of the operative field and its small footprint does not hinder the surgeon in performing surgery

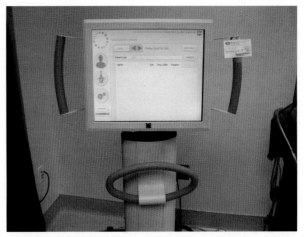

Fig. 4: The data captured by the device is sent via a cable to the O Range computer and touch screen display. The computer is also connected to the internet to transfer data to Wavetec for data collection, analysis and the utilization of nomogram databases

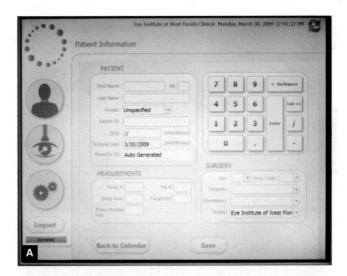

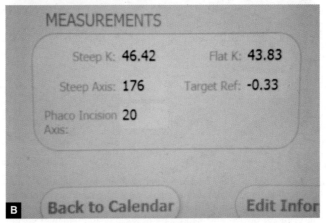

Figs 5A and B

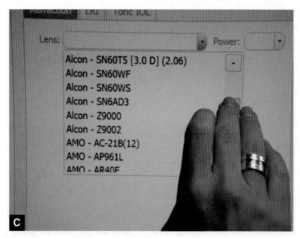

Figs 5A to C: The intuitive touch screen takes the user through a set of data entry pages that is entered prior to surgery. Patient demographics as well as refractive data such as, keratometric values, lens power, lens type, refractive target and incision axis are entered

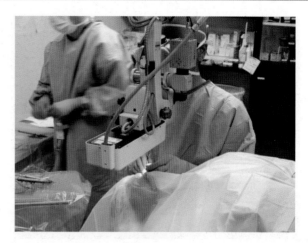

Fig. 7: The microscope with O Range attached is placed over the eye with the long axis of the device aligned along the 180 degree meridian of the eye. It is also positioned planar to the corneal apex and coaxial to the visual axis

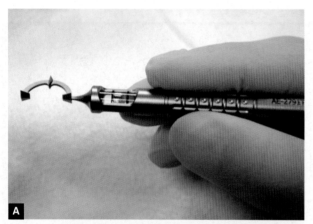

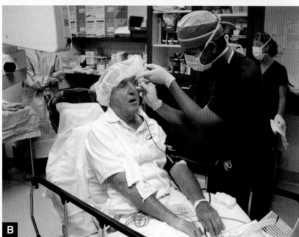

Figs 6A and B: Using a bubble marker with gentian violet dye, 90 and 180 degrees are marked at the limbus with the patient sitting upright and looking at a distance target. This helps in proper alignment with the O range device and avoidance of cyclotorsion variables in the supine position

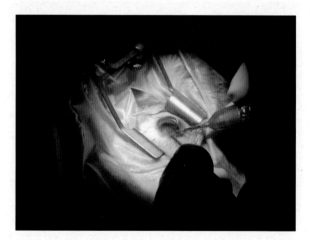

Fig. 8: Prior to capturing wavefront data for surgical guidance, the cataract is removed, the PCIOL is implanted, all viscoelastic is removed including any behind the implant and the eye sealed to give a normotensive intraocular pressure

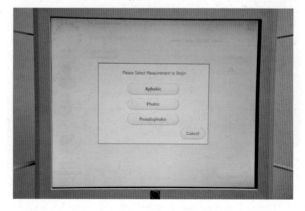

Fig. 9: The screen is a touch display and the initial menu prompts the user to select a category for the image to be taken

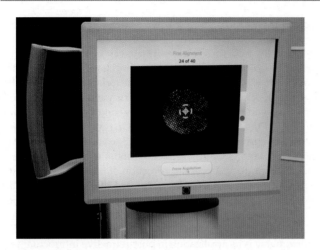

Fig. 10: Wavefront imaging is then obtained with O Range to determine the refraction of the eye and if the toric IOL is at the proper axis

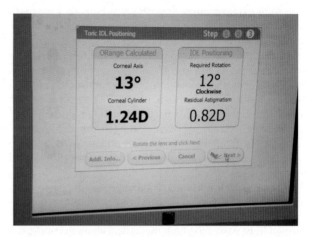

Fig. 11: The O Range software based on the wavefront autorefraction determines there is residual cylinder and toric IOL needs to be rotated 12 degrees clockwise to align with the steep axis of the cornea and further reduce the astigmatism present

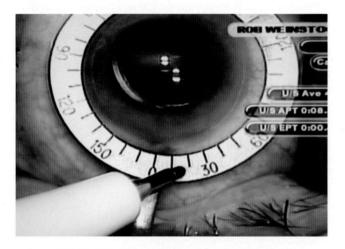

Fig 12: A Mendez gauge is used to help measure the 12 degree rotation

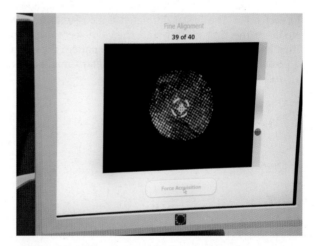

Fig. 13: After the toric implant is rotated 12 degrees, the eye is sealed and another wavefront autorefraction is captured with O Range

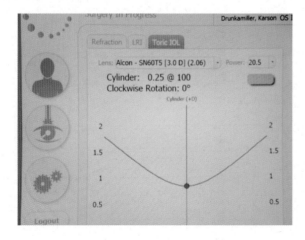

Fig. 14: The O Range data screen reveals that the lens is in the best possible position with neutralization of the cylinder to 25 diopters and no further lens rotation is needed. The patient and the surgeon can leave the operating room knowing the lens is placed at the proper axis and astigmatism has been eliminated

combining cataract surgery with simultaneous astigmatism correction with LRIs, AKs, and/or toric lenses, the wound-induced astigmatism is not only variable from surgeon to surgeon, but from wound to wound and eye to eye – not every eye will respond to a clear corneal wound in the same manner. Hence, pre-operative calculators that factor in a rather arbitrary value for induced-astigmatism, often 0.5 D, are prone to error as well. Intraoperative wavefront technology is currently being used by a limited number of elite cataract surgeons worldwide to completely avoid these weaknesses and make advantageous use of wavefront technology in order to provide superior outcomes.

When a wavefront image is taken, a narrow beam of light is directed into the patient's central visual axis and reflected off the retina, as they fixate on a provided laser target. As the reflected light passes through the optical elements of the eye is produces an aberrated wavefront which is collected by the WaveTec ORange intraoperative wavefront aberrometer, a Talbot-Moire based interferometer. The reflected wavefront is relayed through an internal optical system and directed through a pair of gratings set at a specific distance from, and angle off-set to, each other. The light is diffracted as it passes through the elements of the first grating and then the second grating, creating a fringe pattern. This Moire-effect pattern is captured by a camera and processed using proprietary mathematical algorithms to calculate refractive values. Increasing myopia, for instance, rotates the fringe pattern counter-clockwise where as increasing hyperopia rotates fringes clockwise. Unique fringe patterns also elucidate astigmatic errors based on the aberrated wavefront. Thus, each fringe is unique for a given eye, and the algorithmic processing of that pattern yields a truly custom refractive value. This enables the surgeon to make wavefront-guided surgical decisions regarding IOL power calculation and astigmatic correction intraoperatively. Specifically, it helps titrate the size, placement, and number of limbal relaxing incisions to ensure accurate and precise correction of corneal astigmatism. When toric intraocular lenses are placed, the ORange software provides wavefront-guided recommendations on lens rotation to maximize astigmatism correction.

A significant benefit of intraoperative wavefront aberrometry is its application in post-refractive intraocular lens calculations. As is becoming more frequent, all cataract surgeons have been challenged by lens calculations for patients who have had prior LASIK, PRK, or RK as they alter and mask the cornea's true keratometric power. The Wavetec intraoperative aberrometer is able to capture wavefront images of the aphakic post-refractive surgery patient. This information can be used to confirm or alter preoperative lens power decisions in these difficult circumstances, giving the surgeon increased confidence and the patient a better, more predictable, outcome.

Chapter 51

No Ultrasounds Phaco in CLE with Soft Nucleus

Roberto Pinelli (Italy)

TECHNIQUE DESCRIPTION

Phacoemulsification without ultrasounds is perhaps the best procedure in CLE (Clear Lens Extraction), where the nucleus is safe (refractive lensectomy).

Examining the whole procedure, in the first phase, after incision (Fig. 1), the capsulorhexis (Fig. 2) is not different compared to a classical cataract; it is necessary to put attention to the elasticity of the capsule of the young patient's eye because, due to the elasticity itself, the flap during rhexis is difficult to control.

During hydrodissection (Fig. 3) the best strategy is to perform also hydrodelamination in order to obtain a peripheral cortex able to protect the posterior capsule during suction.[1]

In our experience at ILMO (Istituto Laser Microchirurgia Oculare) in Brescia - Italy, we use an ACCURUS machine (Alcon Laboratories, Inc.-Fort Worth, Tx–USA).

During aspiration, phacoaspiration and not phacoemulsification in this case, we plan the vacuum at 500/550 mm Hg (under control) in linear way and we create a sulcus (Fig. 4), better if central; then with a spatula we penetrate it and we create another deeper sulcus in order to facilitate aspiration;[2] then we go to the periphery and, slowly and gradually, we aspirate (Fig. 5), before peripherally and after centrally, where the nucleus is a little bit more adherent (Fig. 6); hydrodelamination, previously performed, will help us to preserve the posterior capsule.

Finally we aspirate through I/A (irrigation-aspiration) maneuver (Fig. 7) the residual cortex.

In CLE hydrodissection and hydrodelamination are crucial because, if not properly performed, they leave tissue very adherent to the capsule and, consequently, the rotation of the nucleus can be very difficult.

In this technique (soft nucleus) the chopper is not useful and, consequently, we do not use it.

The ideal technique is, in this case, the "Phacofracture":[3] taking the spatula from behind the cortical mass to the center, the phaco can aspirate and "eat" the tissue; also during I/A maneuver we have to control the intimate adherence between capsule and cortex tissue.[4]

When we start the phaco usually we use ultrasounds during the creation of the sulcus; in CLE we do not use ultrasounds but we create a small sulcus in the center and then we aspirate (beginning at 40/50 mm Hg vacuum) because the nucleus is generally soft.

When the sulcus is performed, with a spatula we go into and take the lenticular mass close to the phaco.

Here the vacuum can go to 200/250 mm Hg and, in this delicate moment, it is necessary to control it very carefully because the tissue, here, has not a big resistance.

As far as hydrodissection, again, we have to be very effective because the lenticular tissue is very adherent to the capsule in young patients (in our experience candidate to CLE generally are around 40/45 years old).

We can perform phacoaspiration also with the I/A instruments (infusion/aspiration cannulas) but this maneuver is more complicated and it can take time and it is actually more risky because the control of the depth of the chamber is more hard to perform.

Once removed the central lenticular tissue, we will perform I/A on the more peripheral ones: here also concentration is crucial in order to take tissue to the center and, consequently, to aspirate it.

Also the CAP VAC maneuver is important and we cannot leave equatorial cells: we have to remove them in order to prevent the secondary cataract and, in this phase, an appropriate "screeping" is fundamental.

It is useful to perform CAP VAC not only to the posterior capsule but also to the posterior face of the anterior capsule, close to the rhexis.

Then, with a vacuum of 10/15 mm Hg, using a "sandlike" cannula, not completely smoothed, we perform a "cleaning" of the cells of the posterior part of the anterior capsule.

A different technique, actually very useful during hydrodissection, is to use also a viscoelastic agent after BSS (balanced salt solution), in order to luxate the nucleus and induce it to go closer to the anterior chamber: in this way the spatula can be more easily inserted between nucleus and cortex; if this manoeuvre is successful, we can avoid to perform the central sulcus again.

Using this alternative technique we can start with a vacuum around 200/250 mm Hg, different from machine to machine

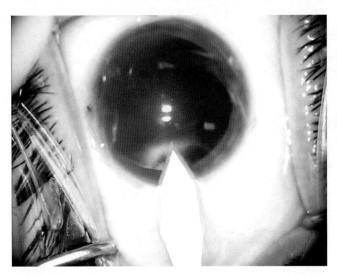

Fig. 1: Main incision is performed

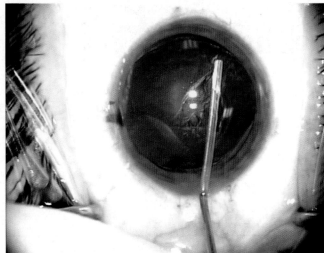

Fig. 3: Hydrodissection

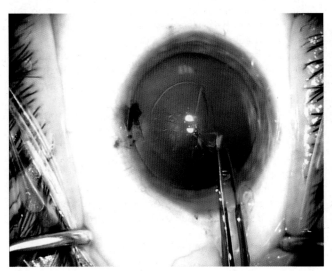

Fig. 2: Anticlockwise capsulorhexis is started

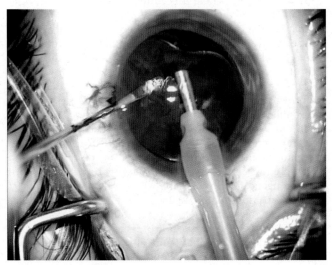

Fig. 4: Central sulcus is performed

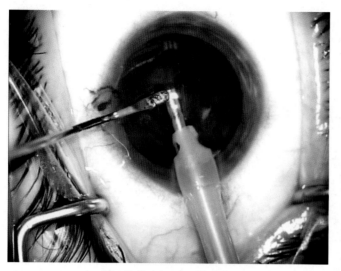

Fig. 5: Peripheral aspiration

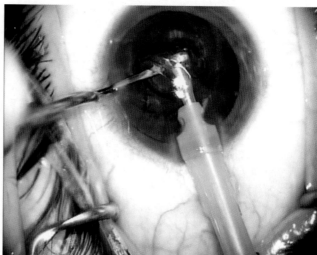

Fig. 6: Central aspiration

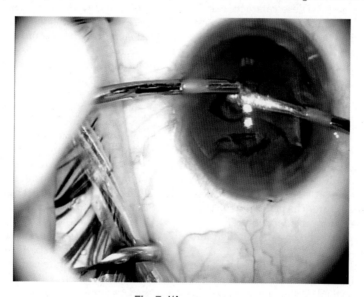

Fig. 7: I/A maneuver

(using ACCURUS we start with a 250 mm Hg vacuum and we have to remember that this phacomachine has a "Venturi" pump, not a peristaltic one).

CONCLUSION

In conclusion, not using ultrasounds helps also to preserve endothelial cells and, not less important, the risk of posterior capsule rupture is largely reduced.

The procedure of this technique is also described in the following sequence of images (Figs 1 to 7).

REFERENCES

1. Güell JL, Vàzquez M, Lucena J, Velasco F, Manero F.Phaco rolling technique. J Cataract Refract Surg 2004;30:2043-45.
2. Smith SG. Nucleus-splitting phacoemulsification technique. J Cataract Refract Surg 1991;17:632-36.
3. Vajpayee RB, Sabarwal S, Sharma N, Angra SK. Phacofracture versus phacoemulsification in eyes with age-related cataract. J Cataract Refract Surg 1998;24:1252-55.
4. Nishi O. Nucleus removal following circular capsulorhexis: surface cortex aspiration. J Cataract Refract Surg 1990;16: 372-76.

Chapter 52

Posterior Polar Cataract
Phacoemulsification: A Myth Exploded

Rohit Om Parkash (India)

Posterior polar cataracts are uncommon cataracts. These cataracts are autosomal dominant.[3] These cataracts can be congenital or acquired. These cataracts are usually bilateral. These patients are usually in the younger age group.

The Posterior Polar Cataracts can be diagnosed by onion whorl type lenticular opacification in the central part of the posterior capsule. In a good majority of patients there is no associated nuclear sclerosis.

The patients usually have good visual acuity on Snellens chart. However, the patients have problems while going out in the sun, driving at night and reading fine print. The patients become symptomatic when they enter the adulthood when the symptoms start interfering with the lifestyle.[6]

These cataracts are occasionally associated with defect in the posterior capsule. The Posterior Polar cataracts have a high incidence of posterior capsule rupture. The patients have to be explained the possibility of posterior capsular rupture.

The posterior polar cataracts can be broadly divided into two groups.

The first group is patients having a pre-existing defect or a hole in the posterior capsule, which can be conclusively diagnosed by the presence of particulate matter just behind the posterior capsule. These cataracts usually are progressing at a rapid rate.

In the second group are those cataracts, which have thinned posterior capsule without any rupture. This chapter is based in evolving a technique to manage the second group of Posterior Polar Cataracts. The incidence of rupture is still high in this group without posterior capsular defects.

The increased incidence of posterior capsule rupture can be attributed to one of the two logistic reasons.

Firstly, this group has an inherent vulnerability of the posterior capsule rupture. Therefore, in such a condition the incidence of posterior capsule rupture should be constant.

Secondly, there is a fallacy in the current techniques. Hence, an improvement in techniques should cause decrease in the incidence of posterior capsule rupture.

The incidence of posterior capsule rupture is different in different studies ranging from as low as 7%[5] to 36%.[1] This exaggerated difference in posterior Capsule rupture can be attributed to the fallacy in the current techniques. Now, let's critically try to pinpoint the weak link in the current techniques.

There are two questions that need to be answered. Firstly, at what step does the rupture occur? Secondly, Can we avoid this rupture?

Let's analyze the present techniques. In the present techniques a lot of preventive measures are being taken to prevent posterior capsular rupture.

1. A stable chamber setting with low height of the bottle is used to avoid any fluctuations in the chamber depth.
2. Slow motion Phacoemulsification is done.
3. Hydrodissection[5] and rotation of the nucleus is avoided.
4. Hydrodelineation is done to form a protective cushion of Epinucleus to avoid insult to posterior capsule.
5. Wide separation of nuclear pieces is avoided.
6. Sideport inflating of the chamber before removing the Ultrasonic handpiece.
7. Dry aspiration is done and Automated IA is avoided.

Let's analyze the steps in the present techniques when posterior capsule rupture can occur.

1. Hydrodelineation
2. Nucleus emulsification
3. Separation of the epinucleus from the posterior capsule
4. IA

Hydrodelineation is safe because we keep away from the posterior capsule. Hydrodelineation, on the contrary, forms a protective cushion for the weak thinned out posterior capsule.

The nucleus Emulsification is the safest possible with stable chamber settings and slow motion procedure. In other words, the nucleus management techniques can't be pinpointed as the weak link.

Dry IA is the safest procedure for cortical removal.
The only step where the thinned or weakened posterior capsule is insulted with a force is when Epinucleus is separated from the posterior capsule.

The following questions now need to be answered.

Firstly, is this separating force really a large force? The answer is yes.

Now how is it possible to reduce this force? Let's try to understand this analogy.

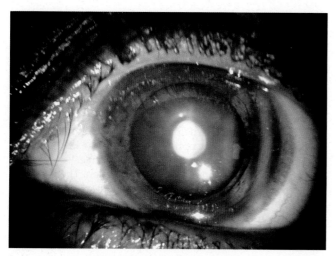

Fig. 1: Posterior polar cataract

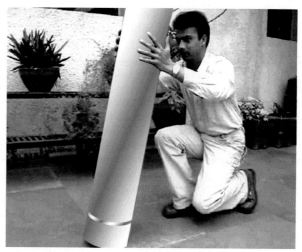

Fig. 4: It's easier to move the object by rotation than by linear pushing or pulling

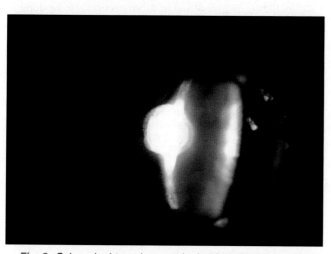

Fig. 2: Onion whorl type (concentric rings) usually there is no associated nuclear sclerosis

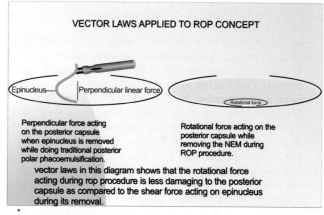

Fig. 5: Vector laws applied to posterior polar cataracts

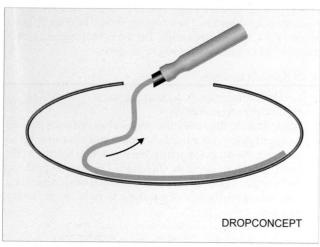

Fig. 3: Epinucleus being removed with high linear force

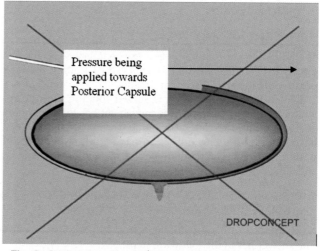

Fig. 6: Cortical decompression during hydrodissection causes a rent at the site of thinned central posterior polar cataract

Let's try to move a heavy object from its place. It is difficult to push it or pull it. It is easier to move by rotating it.

WHAT DOES IT PROVE?

Rotational force is more efficient than linear force as vindicated by vector laws.

Let's apply it on separating epinucleus from posterior capsule. While separating the Epinucleus there is a high linear force at the time of separation. This force can be reduced by using a rotational force that is lesser than the linear force. In other words, the trauma to the thinned out weakened posterior capsule would be dramatically reduced if the Epinucleus separates from the posterior capsule with a rotatory force.

Now, this is another problematic situation. Rotation is not possible without hydrodissection. Hydrodissection, as we know, has to be avoided because it itself causes posterior capsule rupture.

The solution to this predicament lies in doing modified hydrodissection.

MODIFIED HYDRODISSECTION

Hydrodissection has primarily two steps:
1. Squirting fluid with the hydrodissection cannulae
2. Cortical decompression

In the Dr Rohit Om Parkash concept for Posterior Polar cataracts, Modified Hydrodissection has to be done
1. The slow hydrodissection is to be done using the 25 Gauge cannula. One has not to rush in the wave formation. It has to be a slow process. In those situations, where there is a resistance to wave formation one may stop with hydrodissection. Over zealous attitude can give rise to sudden flow of fluid which can endanger the integrity of posterior capsule. This step gives partial separation of nucleus epinucleus mass from the posterior capsule.
2. Cortical decompression has not to be done because this is the part of the hydrodissection when there is stress directly on the posterior capsule. This is vindicated by the decreased incidence of posterior capsule rupture in the series of Dr. Fine where he viscodissects the Epinucleus from the posterior capsule.

MODIFIED ROTATION OF THE NUCLEUS

The advantage of rotation is that the complete separation of the nucleus epinucleus mass is achieved by putting the least possible stress on the posterior capsule.

The dilemma of rotation is solved rotating the nucleus without posterior pushing. The movement has to be in a non-aggressive manner in lateral direction. The initiation of rotation has to be done using non-aggressive trials. No posterior pushing is done. The rotation may be tried in both clockwise and anticlockwise directions. **Patience** is the key.

WHY SHOULD MODIFIED ROTATION BE DONE? IS'NT VISCODISSECTION, AS DESCRIBED BY DR. FINE, SUFFICIENT TO SEPARATE THE EPINUCLEUS?

The answer lies in the following steps:
- There is no doubt that viscodissection is much safer than the other methods of separation adopted by other authors.

However, the impact force by a viscoelastic is still large. The next hurdle is about finding a way that causes lesser stress (impact force) to posterior capsule while separating Epinucleus from posterior capsule.

Let's understand another basic aspect. "The separating force exerted by BSS is much lesser than a viscoelastic." This is because a substance with higher viscosity (more mass) exerts more impact force on contact.

This basic aspect helps conclude "separation force by BSS appears to be the option which puts the least stress on the weakened thinned out posterior capsule."
- BSS is used as in modified hydrodissection. There are two aspects to this modified hydrodissection:
  a. The separating force combination (fluid squirting and modified rotation) is comparable to the separating force of viscodissection.
  b. This combination force is applied in two steps that get divided. Subsequently the force is applied in parts that make insult to the posterior capsule still lesser.

Concluding, the modified hydrodissection is to be done. It is because the separating force combination of modified hydrodissection and modified rotation delivered in parts makes it the least insulting force applied to the already thinned out posterior capsule.

PHACOEMULSIFICATION OF THE NUCLEUS

The key features are the same as the current techniques for posterior polar cataracts. The bottle height is lowered. The flow rate/vacuum are decreased. The nuclear pieces have to be chopped into smaller pieces. The nuclear pieces are moved into the center of the pupil and emulsified. There has not to be wide separating force while dividing. After emulsification, the AC is kept inflated with viscoelastic so that there is no sudden collapse of AC. Dry aspiration with Gill's cannula is done. It is because sudden hydrodynamics can make posterior capsule give way.

However, a few points have to be borne in mind for the success of this technique.

GRADE ZERO NUCLEUS

This type of Posterior polar cataract forms the majority of Posterior polar cataracts. The sculpting should be done by going beyond the Capsulorhexis edge. Do the debulking and slowly emulsify. Modified rotation has to be done.

NUCLEAR SCLEROSIS

1. No Hydrodissection is done at the start.
2. Hydrodelineation is done.
3. While making the valley the nucleus has not to be pushed. A central valley is made. The chopper and ultrasonic tip are placed in the deepest part; partial separation is achieved by moving both in opposite direction. There is no posterior pushing. No aggressive movement is used while separating. The movement while separating is only in the lateral direction.
4. While chopping, the ultrasonic tip holds the nucleus piece and it is slightly lifted. The chopping is done. No movement or pressure is directed posteriorly.

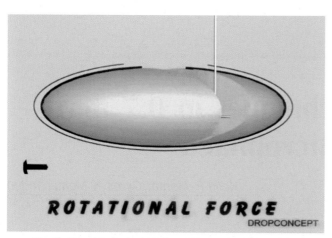

Fig. 7: Non aggressive rotation without posterior pushing

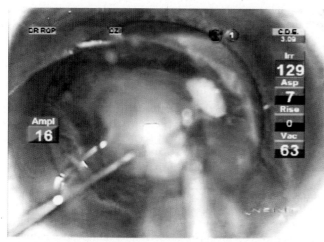

Fig. 8: Successful removal of nucleus Epinucleus mass with the posterior polar opacity

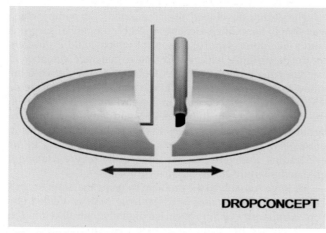

Fig. 9: Division of the nucleus with lateral movement without any posterior pushing. Wide separation is avoided

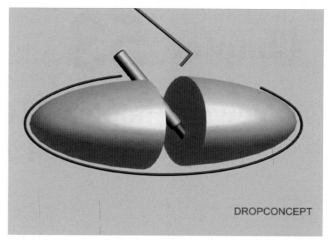

Fig. 10: Nucleus Epinucleus mass being lifted while chopping

5. The Modified Hydrodissection is done. Modified rotation of the Epinucleus is tried. If rotation is not possible, viscodissection is done.

AUTHENTICATION OF DR. ROHIT OM PARKASH CONCEPT

- The posterior capsule rupture rate is outstandingly low. However, in cataracts with nuclear sclerosis the change in the timing of modified Hydrodissection and rotation has helped in reducing the incidence of posterior capsule rupture.
- There is an instance of posterior capsule rupture while pushing Acrysof IOL posteriorly in an effort to adhere it to the Posterior capsule.
- There is an instance of posterior capsule rupture when automated IA is used because of sudden pressure.

Concluding, Modified hydrodissection, Modified rotation and division, planned nucleus emulsification and meticulous IA understanding explode the myth about posterior polar cataracts. On the contrary, the understanding of the vector laws help evade the fallacy which most of us share that the Epinucleus falsely protects the Posterior capsule.

REFERENCES

1. Vasavada A, Singh R. Phacoemulsification in eyes with posterior polar cataract. J Cataract Refract Surg 1999; 25:238-45.
2. Haripriya A, Aravind S, Vadi K, Natchiar G. Bimanual microphaco for posterior polar cataracts J Cataract Refract Surg June 2006; Vol 32 Issue 6:914-17.
3. Yamada K, Tomita Ha, Kanazawa S, Mera A, Amemiya T, Niikawa N Genetically distinct autosomal dominant posterior polar cataract in a four –generation Japanese family American Journal of Ophthalmology February 2000 (Vol. 129, Issue 2, Pages 159-65.
4. Vasavada A, S. Raj Inside- out delineation. J Cataract Refract Surg June2004 Vol 30 pg 1167-69.
5. Ken Hayashi, Hideyuki Hayashi, Fuminori Nakao, Fumihiko Hayashi Outcome of Surgery for Posterior polar cataract J Cataract Refract Surg Vol 29,Issue 1,P45-49, January 2003.
6. I Howard Fine, Mark Packer, Richard S Hoffman Management of Posterior Polar Cataract. J Cataract Refract Surg Vol 29 Issue 1 Page 16 to 19 Jan 2003.

Chapter 53

Newer Chopping Techniques in 0.7 mm Bimanual Microphaco

Keiki R Mehta, Cyres K Mehta (India)

A new generation of surgical instruments coupled with newer and better equipment with more sophisticated software has led to the gradual emergence of microphaco from an occasional procedure to soon join the mainstream of phaco. These newer techniques have led to excellent anterior chamber stability better protection to the ocular structures especially the endothelium.

Perhaps the first question which is asked when one talks of micro phaco, bimanual or co-axial is "does it make any difference in terms of refractive or astigmatic outcome and is the improve net really significant for one to change his surgical technique". The answer is that it not only decreases astigmatism (literally now zero astigmatic induction), but it significantly reduced optical aberrations.

One of the main bugbears, and dangers of microphaco or for that matter, any phaco is Surge. Surge tends to occurs when an occluded fragment is held by high vacuum and is then abruptly aspirated with a burst of ultrasound. Resultant fluid from the anterior chamber rushes out exiting via the phaco tip leading to a collapse of the anterior chamber.

If the inflow and outflow were a constant we would only have to balance the outflow from a 19 gauge needle (approx 40 cc/min) with 19 gauge inflow. However there is always a leakage from all the ports for the simple reason that we are putting in a round instrument, be it an inflow or outflow instrument, in a linear incision. In regular phako, to some extent the sleeve acts as a block to egress of fluids from the incision by molding itself to the edges, however, in bimanual microphaco there is no sleeve so leakage is an inevitable certainty.

Problem is the variable suction on the tip of the phacoemulsifier in contrast to with an constant inflow: (Note at 20 mm Hg in the A/C via a 19 G needle, we need 55+ cc/min to balance the outflow. Regular sleeved phaco pumps in 55-65 cc/min. While the high flow Alcon Infiniti sleeves average still more, almost still more > 75 cc/min.

Let us then rationalize the fluidics of microphaco. To balance the outflow through a 19 G needle we need to achieve a 55 cc/min inflow via a 19 G needle. In addition, the flow must be unrestricted (i.e. an open ended needle). If one needs to use a closed tip needle then the oval openings at the side will need a 18 G cannula to compensate for the end restriction.

The height of the fluid must be 2.8-3 meters above the surgical table which is well nigh impossible in most theatres with the low false ceilings now in most buildings in Mumbai.

It was this mismatch between irrigation and outflow which led to the concept of development of the "forced flow "concept. Since there is a limit to how high bottles could be raised. The obvious answer was a "force feed" fluid in the eye.

One of the ways in which the problem has been solved is by Dr Amar Agarwal who conceived of a fundamental solution by using a aquarium fish pump to pressurizes the fluid going in the eye. This to a tremendous extent seems to solve the problem. Surge was significantly reduced and the flat chamber became a thing of the past. However, the fish pump solved some problems but led to a host of other difficult situations. In a hypermature cataract putting on the air pump with even a moderate pressure has led to a posterior capsular blow out. In older persons with weaker zonules, high-pressure uncontrolled ingress of fluid led to dehiscence's occurring in the periphery of the capsule due to the sudden high pressure. It became almost impossible to operate a high myope as the nucleus seems to sink into the eye. The answer was to gradate the pressure to the eye. The quantum required often would vary from patient to patient.

The author developed the "regulated" air pump, which was simply a modified airpump used by the retinal surgeons with a microprocessor based control which could exquisitely control the pressure. It had the advantage that there was inherent safety for the posterior capsule. One could now decrease the inflow in deep chambered eyes like in high myopes and increase it is small chambered eyes and in those where the IOP is a bit on the high side. Again there was no sudden surge pressure tightness. The eye is very sensitive to sudden fluctuations in pressure which lead to an uncontrollably tight feeling in the eye leading to severe pain, at times quite severe. Having a gradated pressure solves all these problems.

Dr Jorge Alio solved the problem by using the *Alcon Accurus VGFI system which is used in the posterior chamber* Vented Gas Forced Infusion (VGFI®) system is a digitally controlled infusion system created by Alcon for instant access to the surgeon to elevate pressures in the posterior chamber and control retinal bleeds via the foot switch. In his hands it worked equally well.

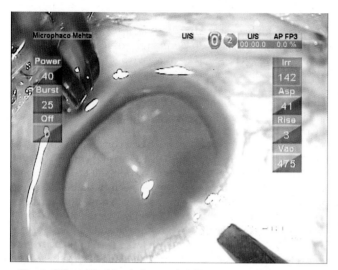

Fig. 1: Sideport incision being made with a 0.8 mm diamond knife

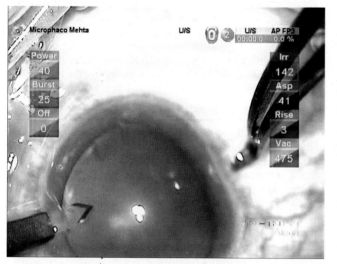

Fig. 2: Second sideport incision made

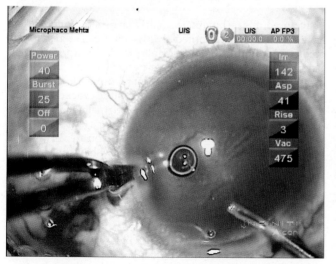

Fig. 3: Rhexis commenced with the Indo German microforceps

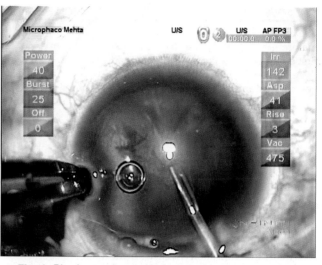

Fig. 4: Rhexis completed with the Indo German microforceps

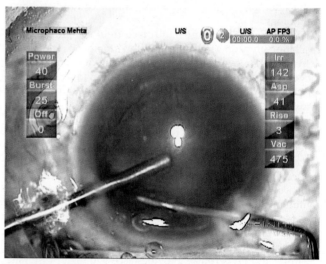

Fig. 5: Hydrodissection first horizontally

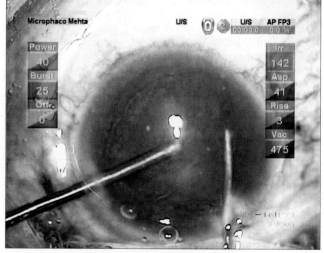

Fig. 6: Hydrodissection now vertically

THE ADVENT OF 0.7 mm PHACOEMULSIFICATION

The only problem with bimanual was always the difficulty in maintaining an adequate deep chamber. Dr Amar Agarwal first commenced using a 0.7 mm tip made by MST and having done successful phako spoke on the effectivity of this tip. He however continued to use the 'fish-pump' with the procedure.

The author who owes a great deal to Dr Agarwal for this concept started using the same technology. It became fairly obvious fairly fast the with the reduced output through a the 0.7 mm tip once could use higher vacuum pressure and thus hold the nucleus better and do faster phaco that with a 0.9 mm tip Dr Boveit using simple calculations of area ($A = \pi r^2$). The 0.9 mm tip has an area of 0.64 while a 0.7 mm tip has an area of only 0.38, virtually half the area. The application of a 700 u tip has solved the problem as utilizing the standard chopper made by MST gives a very stable chamber and combined with the Alcon infinity platform.

Another modification which has made microphaco still more effective is the advent of the torsional phaco or the OZil. Application of the OZil® Torsional handpiece to Microphaco technology.

The OZil® Torsional handpiece delivers side-to-side oscillating ultrasonic movement. With virtually no repulsion, it delivers a high level of followability. The unique movement of torsional phaco shears the lens material, providing decreased repulsion while improving the thermal safety profile over traditional ultrasound. Thus it is the decreased repulsion: Increased followability, reduced potential for turbulence, and increased cutting efficiency which would seem to make all the difference. Interestingly the Ozil uses a lower frequency of 32 kHz which thus induces less frictional movements and thus reduce the risk for thermal injury significantly especially in a tight wound. Thus it permits the use of sealed incisions and continuous torsional modes increasing surgical efficiency and thus facilitates the emerging trend of micro-coaxial phaco.

Naturally using the custom power modulations provide for a choices of energy options.

Pulse and Hyperpulse. Provides access to high pulse rates with customizable on times and variable, easy-to-understand duty cycles. The customized energy modulations allow for reduced repulsion and an improved thermal safety profile when compared to continuous ultrasound.

Smart pulse allows low energy delivery to complement and aid in traditional micropulse phaco settings below 20 ms.Linear

Burst adds control of energy power to the traditional burst mode—allowing increased precision, more instantaneous control and decreased repulsion based on lens densities. The customized burst off limit improves the thermal safety profile by providing modulation of ultrasound energy delivery.

SURGICAL TECHNIQUE

Two side ports incisions are made using standard 0.9 mm diamond knife at 10.00 o'clock and at 2.00 o'clock. Viscoelastic is perfused in. My personal preference is for Viscoat (Alcon) simply because it preserves the chamber well and at the same time protects well the endothelial cells . I have found using the 'soft shell' technique of Arshinov also useful especially in highly myopic eyes or eyes with deep chambers.

Rhexis is done with a MST (MicroSurgical Technology) rhexis forceps which easily slips in via a 0.9 mm opening or alternatively with the Indo German rhexis forceps designed in India. The rhexis needs to be at least 6.5 mm in size. The next step of hydrodissection is done at two planes, first horizontally and then vertically, repeated if necessary till the edge of the nucleus tips forward at the 5.00 o'clock position. This in my opinion is an essential step because it immediate simplifies all the procedure which will follow.

Though the flow is not so much of a constraint with the 0.7 mm tip, it is evaluated (bottle at least 3 feet higher than the eye).

First the MST chopper is introduced from the 2.00 o'clock port. And the nucleus is supported. It often needs a slightly screwing motion to get the chopper tip in smoothly in these tight incisions. A simple tip is to place a drop of Viscoelastic on the incisions prior introducing the chopper tip as it lubricates it and permits an easier entry. With the 0.7 tip in place, I prefer to use either the regular phaco handpiece or more recently the OZil handpiece with a vacuum of 450, a with a burst mode with 40% power for a Grade 3 cataract. The OZil® Torsional handpiece delivers side-to-side oscillating ultrasonic movement. With virtually no repulsion, it delivers a high level of followability. The unique movement of torsional phaco shears the lens material, providing decreased repulsion while improving the thermal safety. Usually after the first two chops I change to hyperpulse dropping the power. The phaco can proceeds as normal with no difficulty.

BIMANUAL MST HANDPIECES USED TO COMPLETE THE I/A

We still do not have access to IOL's which can take the advantage of the small incision. The insision now needs to be expanded to 1.6 mm using a 1.4-1.8 diamond knife. An acrysmart IOL (Acrytec) is my usual choice or the Care Groups. Micriol. Both give good results. To go through this tight incision, one has to implant the IOL using a smooth hook to take support from the side incision and simultaneously keeping the tip of the injector pressed tightly against the incision (assisted technique). Provided the procedure is followed carefully and the tip of the injector is invaginated into the superior lip of the incision the lens goes in easily.

Results

I have used this technique in a fairly large series of cases and have now virtually adopted this technique. The results are predictable. The opening is for all practical purposes a zero astigmatic incision, the eyes are very quiet the next day and the technology is similar to the standard phaco technique so adopting it is your practice needs only little practice with the assisted implantation but otherwise it is virtually the same. Just simply be careful in implanting higher powers (+25 and above) as the bulk of the lens increases and unless you are very careful the IOL will simply open outside the eye. I have never had a phaco burn and the average surgery time for the phaco component taking into account Grade 3 cataracts is 44.8 seconds over the last 140 serial cases done with the OZil. The average phaco power was 14% with true phaco time a virtually unbelievable 3.8 seconds.

Thus usage of the reduced 0.7 mm tip does not in any way compromise the length of the phako procedure or the endothelial cells.

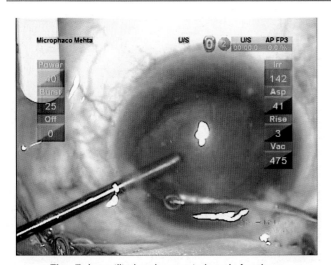

Fig. 7: Lens tilted and supported ready for phaco

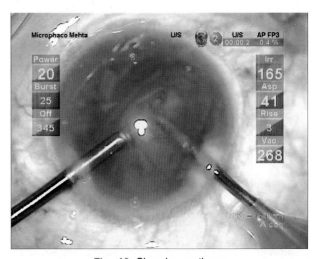

Fig. 10: Chopping continues

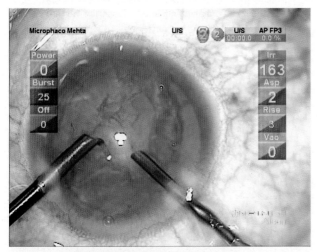

Fig. 8: MST Duet 20 G chopper and 0.7 mm
phaco tip onto an Infiniti phaco handpiece

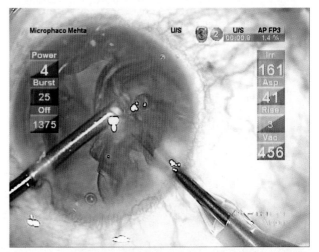

Fig. 11: Just simple stabilization with the chopper can permit the
fragments or be easily chewed off

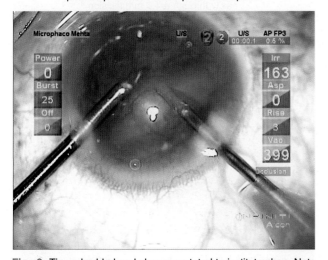

Fig. 9: Tip embedded and chopper rotated to institute chop. Note
that high vacuum can be used safely with the 0.7 phaco tip by MST

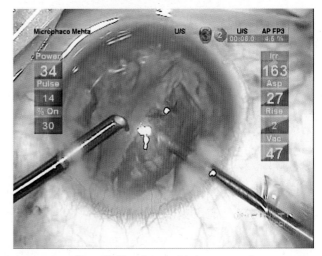

Fig. 12: Final fragment being removed

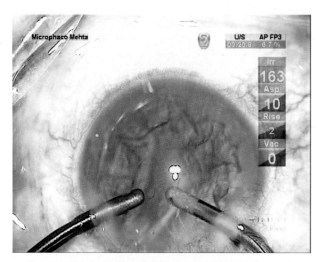

Fig. 13: Irrigation and aspiration using the MST instruments

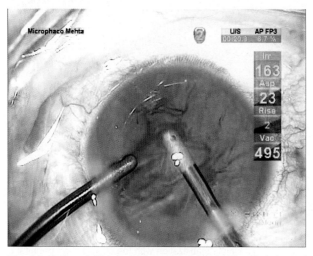

Fig. 14: Notice stable chamber as the inflow/outflow is balanced

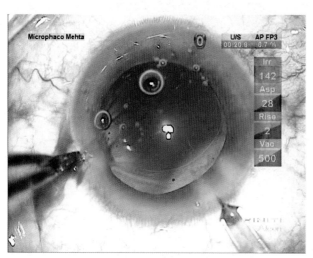

Fig. 15: Using the 1.4-1.8 mm diamond blade the incision is gradually opened

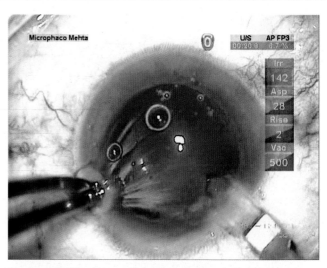

Fig. 16: Note that the combination blade is extended almost but not totally to the tip thus making it just a bit less than 1.8 mm incision

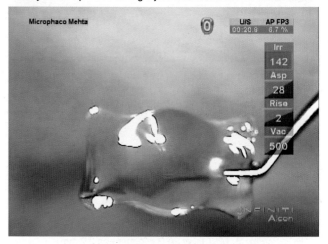

Fig. 17: The foldable Acrismart IOL which can pass easily through a 1.7 mm incision

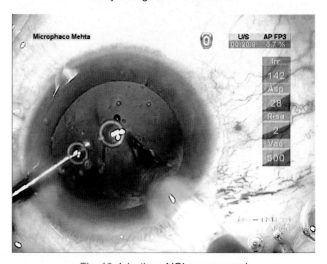

Fig. 18: Injection of IOL commenced

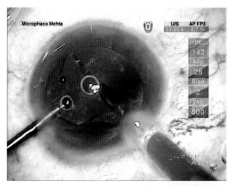

Fig. 19: Injection of IOL with the advancing tip under the rhexis

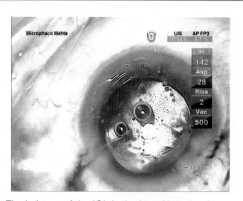

Fig. 23: Final picture of the IOL in the bag. Note the rings on the IOL

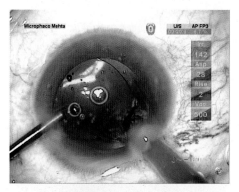

Fig. 20: Injection of IOL completed

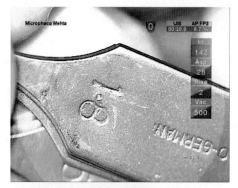

Fig. 24: An 1.8 mm gauge pictured

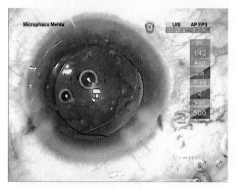

Fig. 21: Note though the inferior part of the IOL lies in the capsular bag. The proximal part lies anterior to the capsule

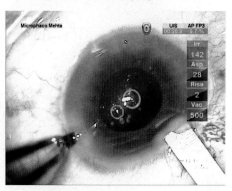

Fig. 25: Shows that the gauge does not enter indicating that the incision is a 1.7 mm or a tight 1.8 mm

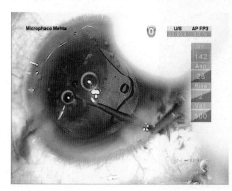

Fig. 22: The lens simply flexed into the capsular bag

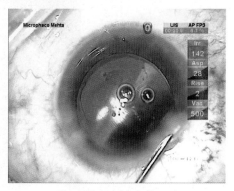

Fig. 26: Incision hydrated

311

Advanced Phaco Techniques: Soft Lens Removal and Implantation of ReSTOR Multifocal Lens

Ahmad K Khalil (Egypt)

Implantation of multifocal lenses is gaining popularity, and is pushing the lens removal age and degree further to the more active and visually demanding population with softer lenses. Soft cataracts/lenses pose difficulty in their removal by phacoemulsification. Commonly performed techniques involving division and chopping are not easy to perform in soft lenses, and the phaco probe can reach the capsule easier through the soft lens matter. Meanwhile, implantation of various forms of multifocal lenses pre-requires a more critical approach to various details of the phacoemulsification procedure to give optimum parameters for positioning and subsequent function of the lens.

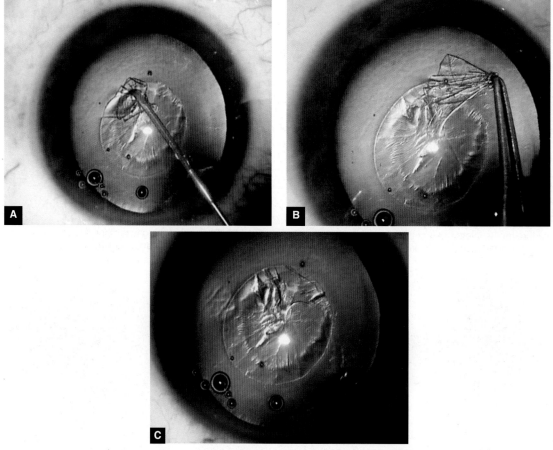

Figs 1A to C: A medium size rhexis to cover the lens edges and keep the diffractive rings of the lens uncovered

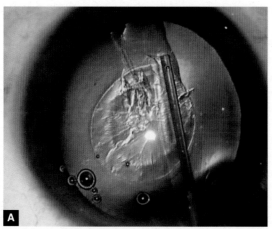
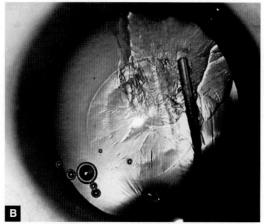

Figs 2A and B: Hydrodissection, by gently introducing the tip of cannula just beneath the edge of the capsulotomy, fluid is injected. Fluid wave should pass all the way around lens matter. This is a particularly important step in soft lenses, where lens cortical fibers are sticking to the inside of the capsule

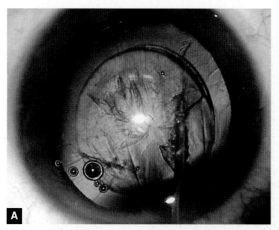
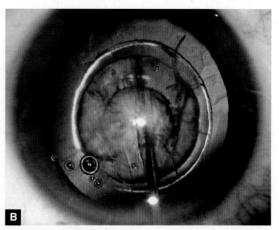

Figs 3A and B: Hydrodelineation to separate the lens cortex from the nucleus. Successful hydrodelineation is evidenced by the classical golden ring sign. Further hydrodelineation planes (as evidenced by the multiple rings here) are made at different depths of the soft nucleus to separate the inner nucleus from outer nuclear layers

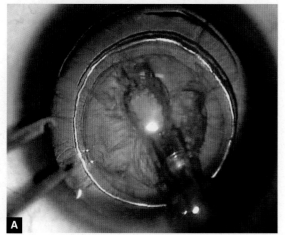
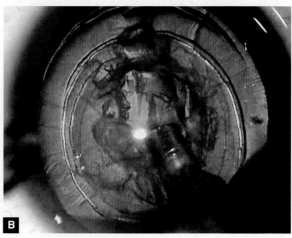

Figs 4A and B: Using low vacuum, low phaco power and low flow rate,
a central broad area of the lens nucleus is sculpted

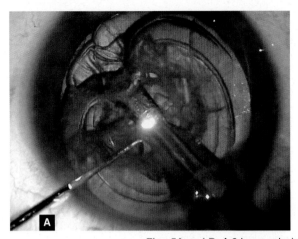 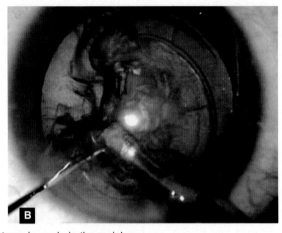

Figs 5A and B: A 2 hours relaxing nucleotomy is made in the periphery of the nucleus which eases the tension around the nucleus

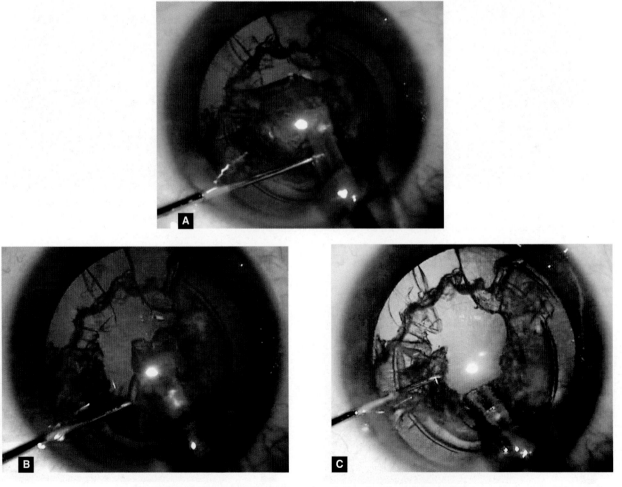

Figs 6A to C: The remaining inner nucleus is freed and emulsified easily out of the eye because of preliminary multilayered hydrodelineation

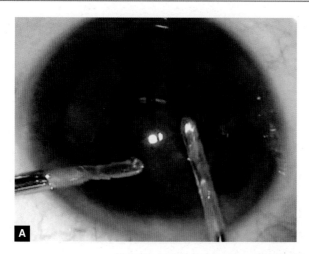

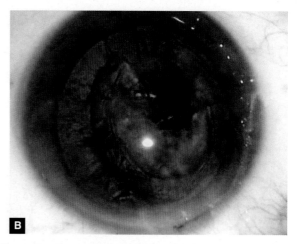

Figs 7A and B: Using bimanual irrigation aspiration probes, the remaining epinucleus is aspirated and pushed to be freed out of the bag at least one pole (one handle)

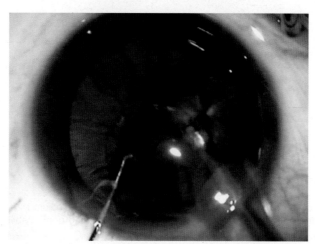

Fig. 8: Remaining epinucleus is safely emulsified and aspirated out of the eye

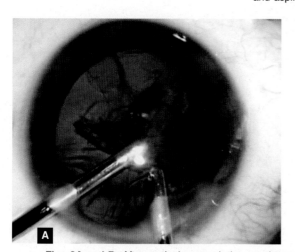

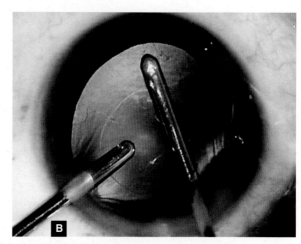

Figs 9A and B: After cortical removal, the anterior capsule is polished by gentle vacuuming to remove lens epithelial cells that can potentially cause anterior capsular opacification and phimosis

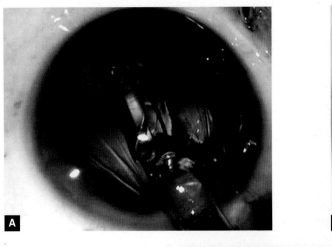

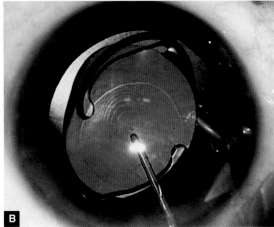

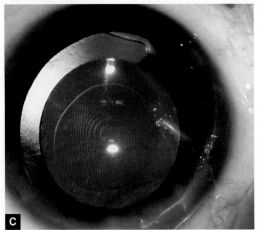

Figs 10A to C: Intraocular lens is injected in the bag. With the central medium size capsulorhexis and the smooth phaco procedure, the pseudophakos is well centered ensuring good stability and function of the multifocal technology

Chapter 55

Cataract Surgery in Complex Situations

Armando Capote, Marcelino Rio, Belkis Rodríguez (Cuba)

IRIS DISORDERS

Iris anatomy and function can be altered by congenital or degenerative conditions, as well as following trauma or certain infections, inflammation or toxicity. Tumors can be found affecting its tissue and the related structures. Iris integrity is quite important considering its purpose as diaphragm and particularly in cataract surgery and other Anterior Segment surgeries it is highly important to be able to manage its reconstruction and conservation.

Congenital Iris Anomalies

The Embryonic fissure closure defect can cause typical iris colobomas which are placed inferiorly. They can be partial like the small notch seen in Fig. 1, or complete, extending from the iris to the optic disc. The small coloboma in this figure does not need any kind of treatment.

Atypical colobomas are placed outside from the inferonasal quadrant, are not associated usually with posterior uveal colobomas and are caused by remnants of hyaloid system and pupillary membrane. This eye (Fig. 2) would need surgical iris reconstruction in case of cataract surgery.

CAPSULO-ZONULAR AFFECTIONS

The presence of anomalies in the position or form of the crystalline lens as well as in the integrity of the zonular complex still constitutes a challenge for the Anterior Segment surgeon that changes the surgical routine. The stability of the crystalline lens is affected during its extraction, Phacoemulsification or aspiration. The barrier provided by the lens capsule between

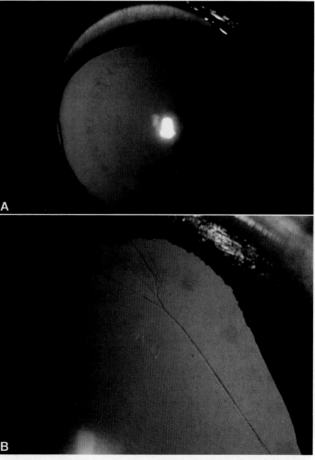

Figs 2A and B: Atypical iris coloboma. Vascular remnants are seen with blood cells circulating through them in 2B

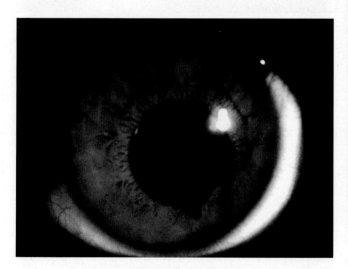

Fig. 1: Partial small iris coloboma

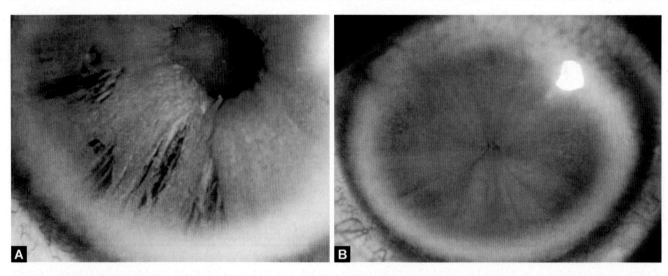

Figs 3A and B: Axenfeld-Rieger syndrome. Right (A) and left eye (B) from the same patient. Iris hypoplasia and mild dyscoria Right eye and Left eye has iris hypoplasia, microcoric closed pupil. Embriotoxon is present both eyes. Both eyes need particular care during cataract surgery due to the fragility of the iris and possible glaucoma; and left eye requires pupilloplasty

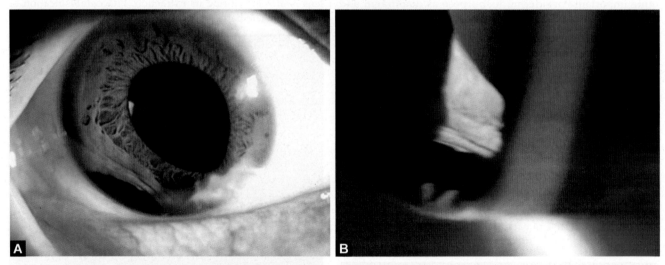

Figs 4A and B: Traumatic iris dialysis. The Ciliary processes can be observed under higher magnification

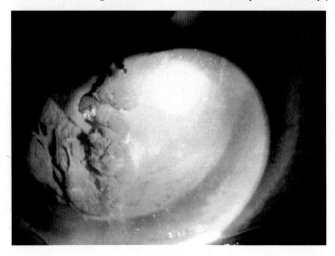

Fig. 5: Extensive traumatic iris dialysis, cataract and lens subluxation caused by severe blunt trauma of the eye globe. Large anterior segment reconstructive surgery is required

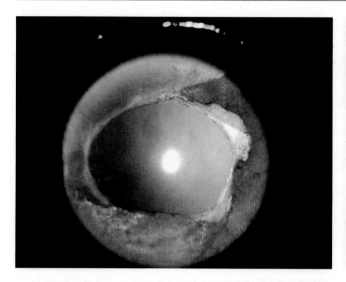

Fig. 6: Extensive traumatic iris defect and aphakia

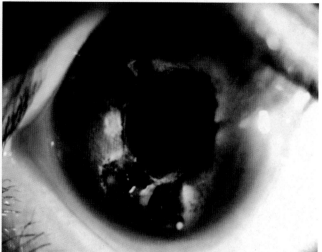

Fig. 7: Traumatic aniridia. Aphakia and abundant capsular remnants with central round hole. Cortical material among anterior and posterior capsules has developed a doughnut shape. The author's choice of election would be to clean the cortical material and implanting an aniridia intraocular lens

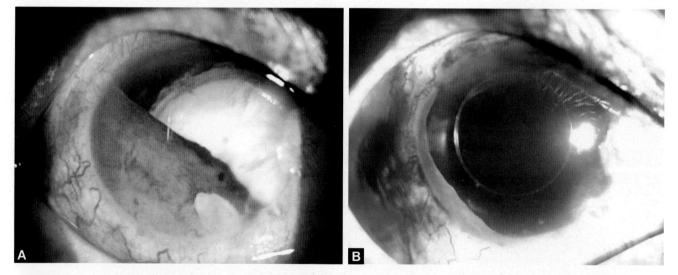

Figs 8A and B: Severe contusive ocular trauma caused extensive iris dialysis and lens opacification and subluxation. (A) Cataract extraction and implantation of a Morcher aniridia intraocular lens was performed as seen in the postoperative photograph on the right. (B)

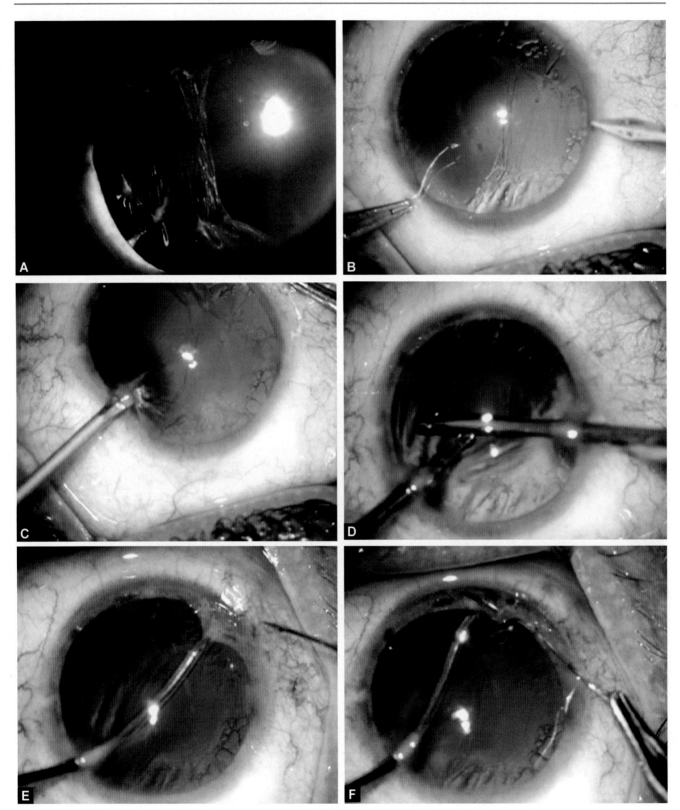

Figs 9A to F

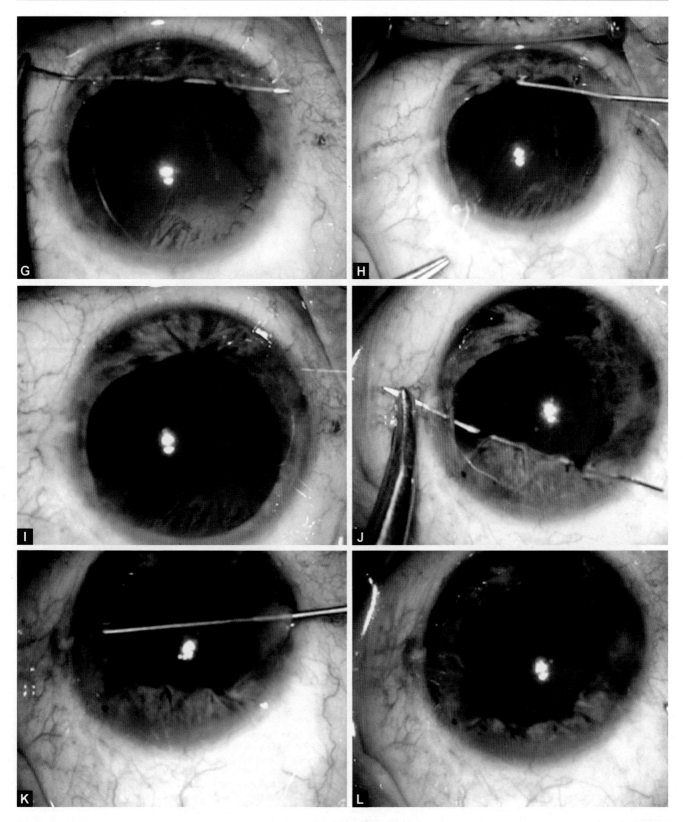

Figs 9G to L

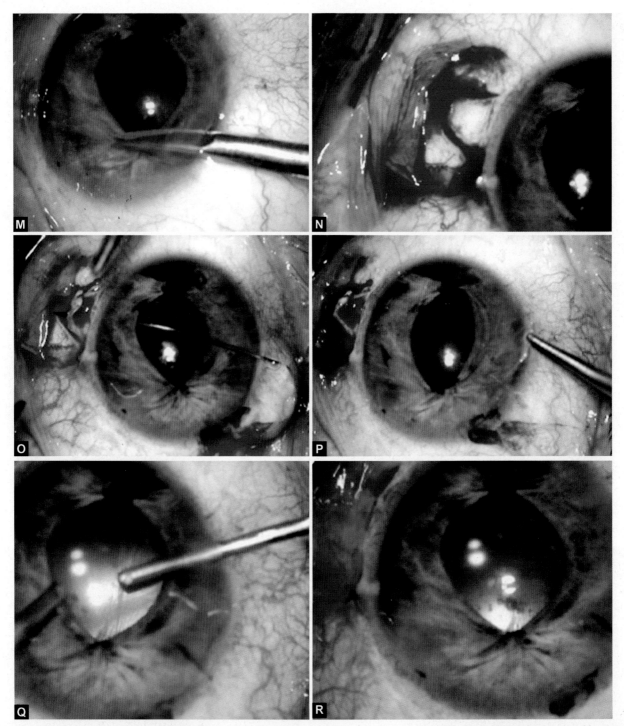

Figs 9A to R: Surgical sequence of male patient who suffered blunt trauma that caused traumatic mydriasis and cataract with ruptured posterior capsule that was operated urgently without Intraocular lens implantation and came to the author´s hospital with maximum traumatic mydriasis, fibrous appearance of the iris and aphakia with capsular support only on the left half. (A) Slit-lamp view. Only left half capsular support and very wide mydriasis. (B) Surgical microscopic view of the same eye in inverted position. (C) Paracentesis with 20G MVR knife. (D) Anterior vitrectomy. It is very important not to leave vitreous in the anterior segment to avoid traction or IOL tilting. (E) Holding and tractioning the iris with microforceps. (F and G) Lady´s bag suturing on the pupillary margin close to 180° through paracentesis and traspassing the cornea with the 10-0 polypropylene long needle suture on the contralateral side. (H) Pulling of the suture with hook or iris retractor through the paracentesis to make loop for slip suture. (I to M) The same maneuvers are repeated superiorly. (N) Partial thickness scleral flap for scleral fixation of PC IOL. (O) The needle leaves the eye at about 1 to 1.5 mm. (P) IOL is introduced after the haptic is sutured. (Q) Viscoelastic aspiration. (R) Pupil of right size and good esthetic appearance is obtained

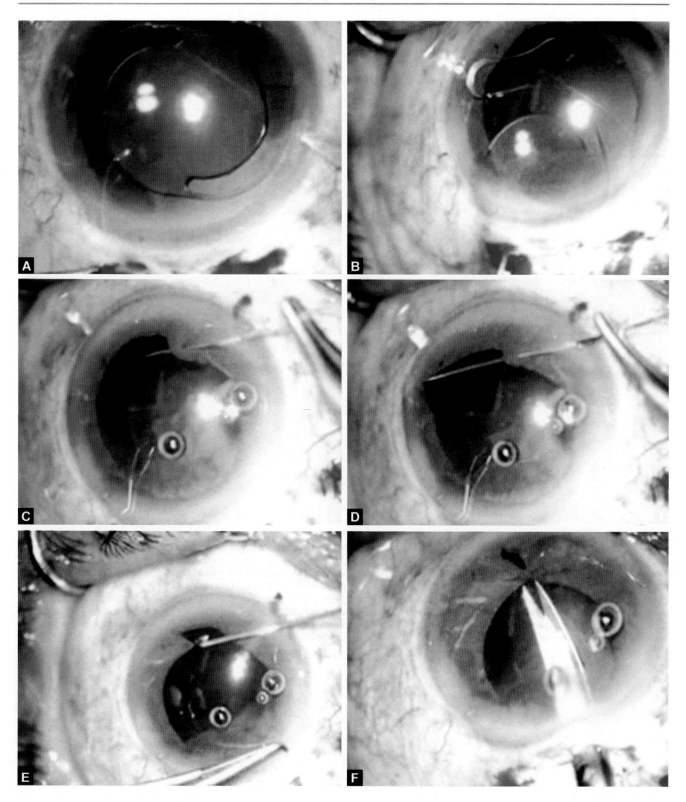

Figs 10A to F

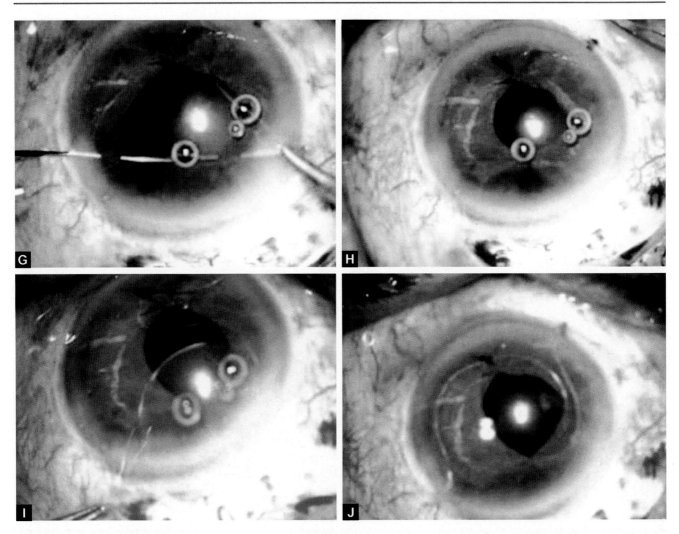

Figs 10A to J: Patient who was previously done traumatic cataract removal with implantation of an Anterior Chamber Intraocular Lens. Result was not satisfactory due to the large pupil of a larger diameter than the IOL, causing photophobia, diplopia and poor quality vision in general. There were vitreous strands in the Anterior Chamber. The surgical sequence is illustrated in the following figures. (A) Large traumatic mydriasis and Anterior Chamber Intraocular Lens. (B) Removal of anterior Chamber Intraocular Lens. (C) Long needle of Polypropylene suture is passed through paracentesis and crosses the iris at 0.5 mm of the pupil margin in h-7. Previous to this step anterior vitrectomy was done and viscoelastic placed in the anterior chamber. (D) The needle crosses the iris from below at h-4 and leaves the eye through the limbus. (E) Iris hook is used to pull the suture to create loop or slip knot. (F) Vannas scissors cut sutures at the knot. (G to H) The same maneuver is repeated superiorly. (I) Implantation of the same AC IOL the patient had. (J) Centered pupil of about 3.5 mm

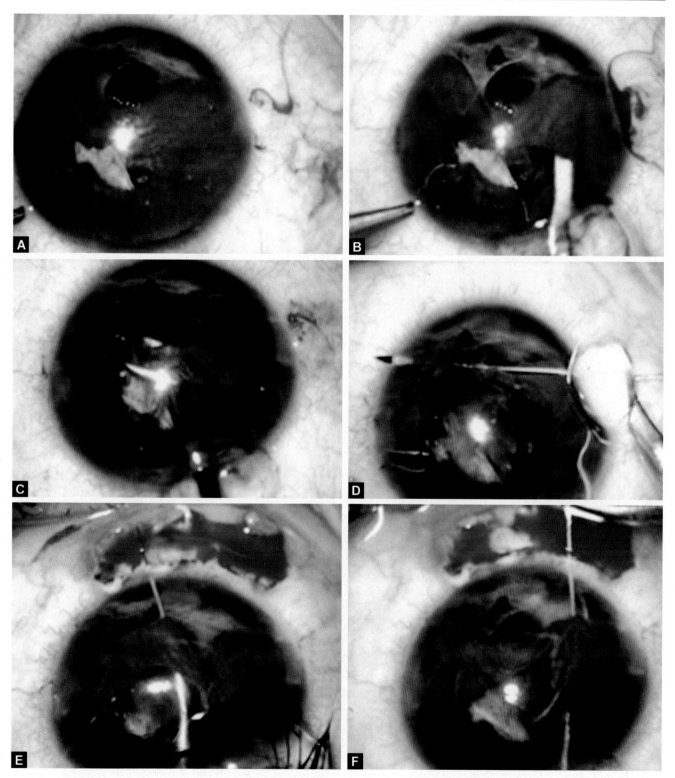

Figs 11A to F

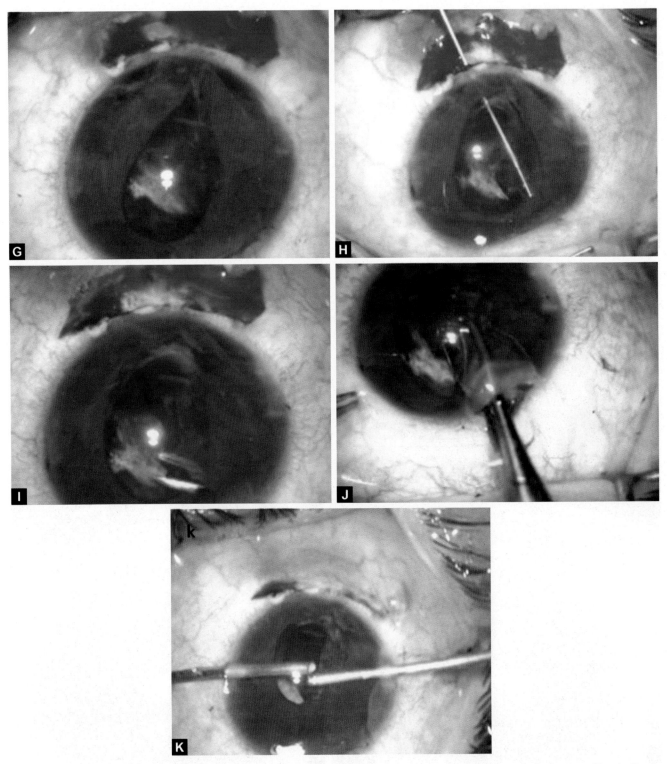

Figs 11A to K: Anterior Segment disorganization after trauma. Extensive iris dialysis and atrophy. Strong posterior synechiae to fibrotic opacified capsular remnants. Surgical sequence of iris reconstruction, posterior capsulotomy (Membranectomy) and Intraocular lens implantation. (A) Anterior Segment disorganization after trauma. (B) Synechiotomy with iris spatula. (C) Synechiolysis with microscissors. (D) Suture of ruptured iris with 10-0 long needle polypropylene suture. (E to I) Iris dialysis repair by suturing iris base to its anatomical position with 10-0 long needle polypropylene suture. (J) Foldable 3 pieces acrylic Posterior Chamber Intraocular lens Implantation. (K) Viscoelastic aspiration. Satisfactory result regarding iris repair and IOL placement

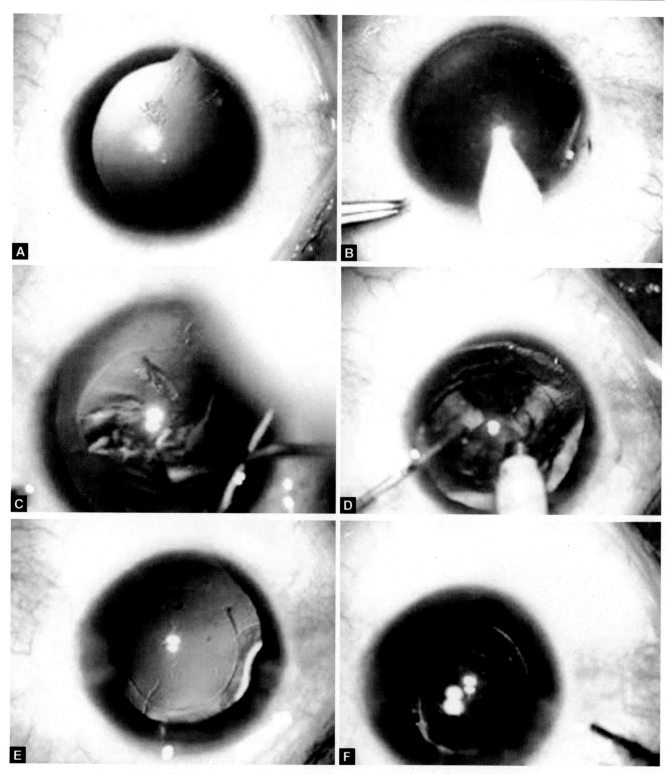

Figs 12A to F

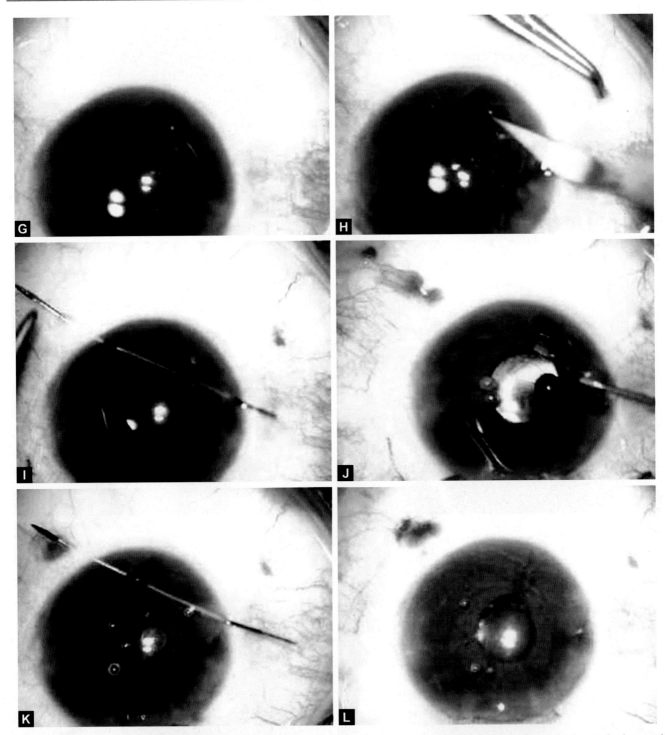

Figs 12A to L: Congenital typical Iris coloboma and cataract. Phacoemulsification, implantation of Posterior Chamber Intraocular lens and Pupilloplasty is performed. Surgical sequence. (A) Congenital typical Iris coloboma and cataract. (B) 2.8 mm incision for coaxial Phacoemulsification. (C) Capsulorhexis with needle cystotome. (D) Coaxial Phacoemulsification. (E) Clean capsular bag, capsulorhexis and coloboma can be seen. (F) Posterior Chamber IOL is implanted. (G) After closing the pupil with intracameral miotic, the IOL edge is seen inferiorly. This would cause diplopia in this patient. (H) Oblique paracentesis is made in position for the pupilloplasty. (I) 10-0 polypropylene suture long needle is passed through the iris at h-8 and h-5 to create anatomically round pupil. (J) Pulling the suture with hook. The pupil acquire a round shape. (K) A second slip stitch is placed in the middle iris stroma to avoid a second pupil formation inferiorly. (L) Final appearance with round esthetically satisfactory result

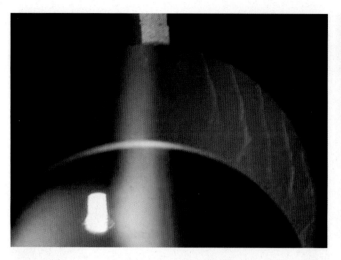

Fig. 13. Severe lens subluxation. The zonules are visible decreased in number and very relaxed

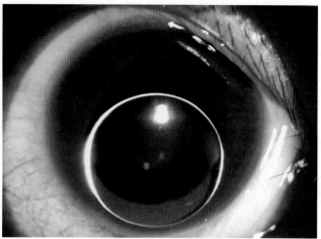

Fig. 14: Microphakic lens luxated to the anterior chamber

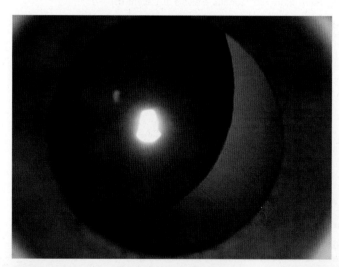

Fig. 15: Typical lens subluxation in patient with Marfan Syndrome. There is supero-temporal displacement of the lens, zonules look stretched

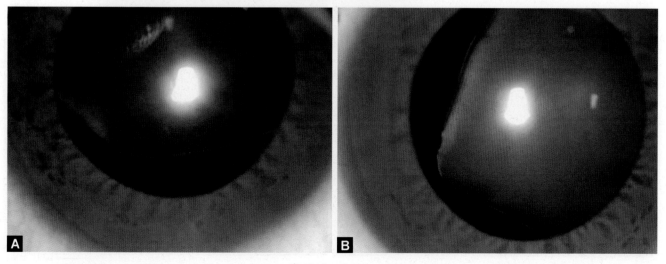

Figs 16A and B: Right and Left eye of patient with Marfan Syndrome. Less typical form in shape of lens colobomas

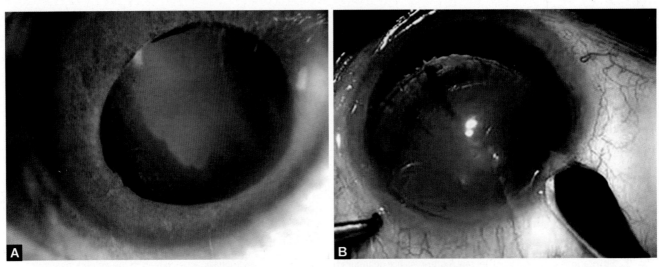

Figs 17A and B: Traumatic lens subluxation and cataract. Vitreous is prolapsed to the Anterior Chamber displacing the pupil inferiorly (A). More than 180° zonular dialysis in patient (B)

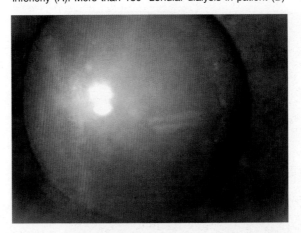

Fig. 18: Lens Pseudoexfoliation is one of the main causes of zonular weakness, and is frequently associated to complications during cataract surgery

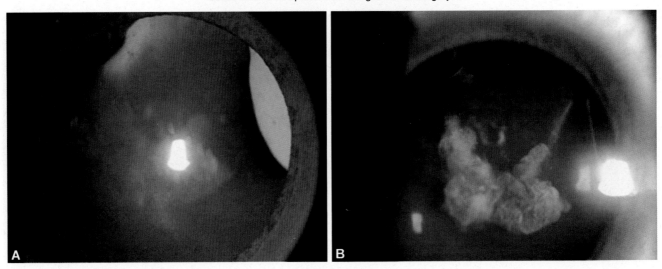

Figs 19A and B

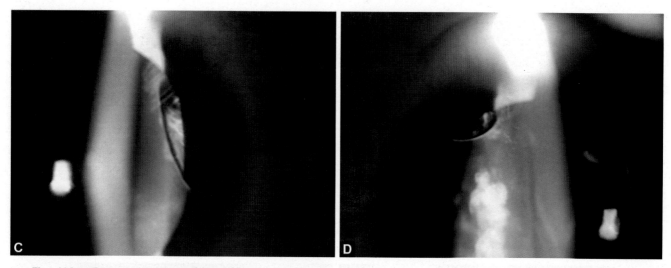

Figs 19A to D: Lens Colobomas with shape of two notches. Zonules are missing on the coloboma area and can only be observed at their limits. Congenital cataract is also present in this 12 years old male patient

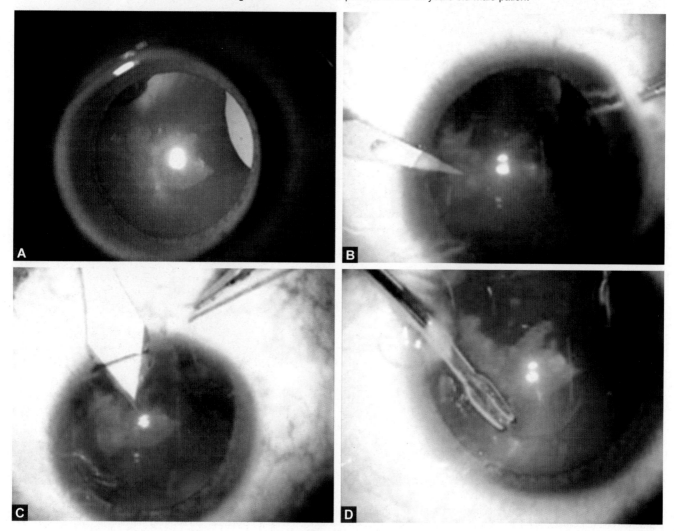

Figs 20A to D

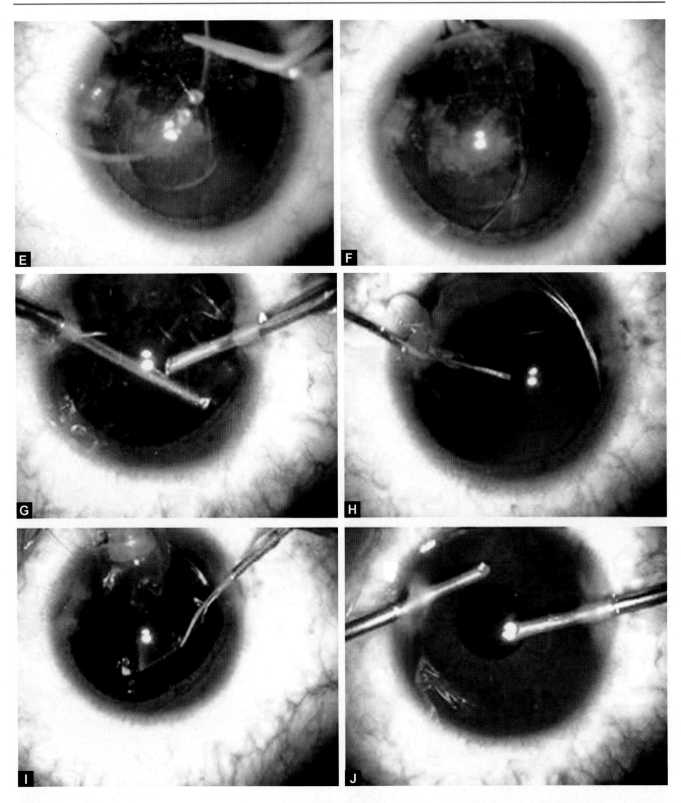

Figs 20A to J: Lens coloboma. Endocapsular tension ring implantation, Phaco and IOL implant. (A) Lens colobomas and cataract. (B) Paracentesis. (C) Clear corneal incisión. (D) Capsulorhexis. (E) Capsular tension ring. (F) Capsular tension ring implantation with fórceps. (G) Biaxial Phaco. (H) Viscoelastic. The ring can be seen inside the capsular bag. (I) IOL implantation with injector. (J) Viscoelastic aspiration

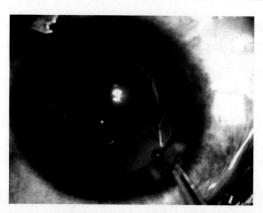

Fig. 21: In cases of severe lens subluxation the Capsular Tension Ring can be implanted inside the capsular bag after passing it through a loop of Polypropylene 10-0 suture and the complex Capsular Bag- Lens can be sutured to the sclera providing centering and stability to the lens

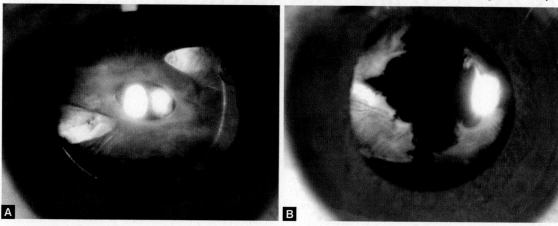

Figs 22A and B: Marked phymosis of the capsulorhexis with severe capsular shrinkage and haptics displacement centrally. (B) Same patient after relaxing cross shaped shots with yag laser. Notice that the haptics returned to their normal position

the Anterior Segment and the vitreous is compromised in a certain degree. And most important, the support structure for the Intraocular Lens for its correct placement in the capsular sack may be absent or unstable.

The capsulo-zonular complex affections although not routine, are observed with a relative frequency in the eye surgeon's practice, so it is of great importance to know their management and to be qualified to face these patients.

The Ectopia of the crystalline lens depending on the severity is denominated subluxation when there is a partial displacement, but the crystalline lens still remains in the pupillary space. If there is a total displacement of the crystalline lens outside of the patelar fossa of the lens and the lens is in the Anterior Chamber, floating freely in the vitreous or on the retina it is known as Luxation. The so called Colobomas of the crystalline lens refer to notches or irregularities observed in the equatorial border of the crystalline lens; there is not real lack of tissue, but lens deformation due to lack of zonular pull.

BIBLIOGRAPHY

1. Chang DF, Campbell JR. Intraoperative floppy iris syndrome associated with tamsulosin. J Cataract Refract Surg. 2005;31:664-73.

2. Fernández de Castro LE, Sandoval HP, Solomon KD, Vroman DT. Iris Cerclage Suture Technique for Traumatic Mydriasis. British Journal of Ophthalmology 2006;90:253-394.

3. Hammill MB, Quayle WH. Iris repair after a catastrophic laser in situ keratomileusis complication. J Cataract Refract Surg. 2005;31:2216-20.

4. Lam DS, Young AL, Leung AT, Rao SK, Fan DS.Scleral Fixation of a Capsular Tension Ring for severe Ectopia Lentis. J Cataract Refract Surg. 2000 Apr;26(4):609-12.

5. McCannel MA. A retrievable suture for anterior uveal problems. Ophthalmic Surg.1976;7:98-103.

6. Menapace R, Findl O, Georgopoulos M, Rainer G, Vass C, Schmetterer K. The Capsular Tension Ring: Designs, applications and techniques. J Cataract Refract. Surg. 2000 Jun;26(6):898-912.

7. Osher RH, Snyder ME, Cionni RJ. Modification of the Siepser slip knot technique. J Cataract Refract Surg. 2005;31:1098-100.

8. Villar-Kuri J, Monteegro-Tapia T. El Libro del Cristalino de las Américas. Anillo endo exocapsular para el manejo de la ectopia lentis. Livraria Santos Editora 2007.Chapter 20: 185-94.

333

Chapter 56

Primary Phacoemulsification Combined with Drainage Angle Viscodissection in the Management of Chronic Narrow Angle/Angle-Closure Glaucoma (CNAG/CACG) and Co-existent Cataract

P Cikatricis, TKJ Chan (UK)

Terms Chronic narrow-angle glaucoma (CNAG) and Chronic angle-closure glaucoma (CACG) refer to an eye where the anterior chamber drainage angle progressively narrows. Although there may be a number of reasons for this narrowing, if the peripheral iris remains apposed to the Trabecular meshwork for any length of time (chronic appositional closure) it is likely that a more permanent adhesions occur-peripheral anterior synechiae (PAS). In such eye, portions (even the whole circumference in extremis) of the anterior chamber drainage angle are closed permanently by PAS.

Subsequent rise in the Intraocular pressure (IOP), if maintained, is followed by glaucomatous optic neuropathy. Thus, even though the underlying cause for the narrowing is removed (e.g. pupillary block after surgical/laser peripheral iridectomy (PI) or cataract extraction in lens induced secondary angle-closure, so called 'phacomorphic effect'), the angle may remain closed and the IOP may remain high.

Therefore, there are variable results in long term intraocular pressure control after medical and surgical management of acute/chronic angle-closure/narrow-angle glaucoma.

This chapter is setting out to describe an innovative technique called Viscodissection of angle which is applied to break the PAS. It is safe and easy to perform as an additional step in a standard phacoemulsification-type cataract surgery, requiring no special extra equipment. For an experienced cataract surgeon there is virtually no learning curve.

A well-described procedure, surgical Goniosynechialysis, uses dedicated surgical time and a specialized instrument-irrigating cyclodialysis spatula- to physically break PAS from the angle, thus separating a possibly small segment of PAS with an anterior-to-posterior movement. This should restore the trabecular meshwork function. Angle Visco-dissection is relatively atraumatic, as well as a more effective alternative. It uses the physical effect of viscoelastic to open up the PAS along the whole 360 degree angle circumference during phacoemulsification cataract surgery. It is commonly believed that goniosynechialysis is successful only if the synechiae have been present for less than 1 year. Moreover, it may be impossible to perform it around 360 degrees. It has a higher rate of possible complications such as mild to severe hemorrhage from the iris or trabeculum, inflammation possibly with fibrin exudation, iridodialysis, choroidal hemorrhage, choroidal detachment and shallow anterior chamber.

Note: The authors of this chapter conducted a retrospective pilot study (case series) of acute or chronic narrow-angle/angle-closure glaucoma in patients with co-existent cataract from 1999 to 2007. Patients had undergone no previous glaucoma surgery except laser peripheral iridotomies. The subjects were divided into two groups, total of 49 eyes in 37 patients. Group one, the control group, consisted of 14 eyes of 11 patients, and group two, the study group, consisted of 35 eyes of 26 patients. Patients in group one underwent standard clear corneal temporal incision phaco, and patients in group two underwent phaco combined with biscodissection of the anterior chamber. All phaco surgeries in the study were performed by one experienced surgeon (TKJC) and were uneventful.

The study found that group two had significantly lower IOP than group one at all follow-up visits. Group two also had significantly lower post-operative medication use. (In group one, the control group, the patients were on mean 2.15 medications to control the IOP (range 0-5) and the mean preoperative IOP was 22 mm Hg. At the last follow-up, at a mean of 83 months, nine eyes in that group needed treatment with the mean of 1.36 post-operative anti-glaucoma medications. IOP was also lower at the last post-operative visit, at a mean of 18 mm Hg. One patient in group one had

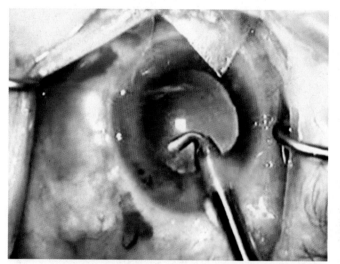

Fig. 1: Finalizing the irrigation and aspiration of the soft lens matter

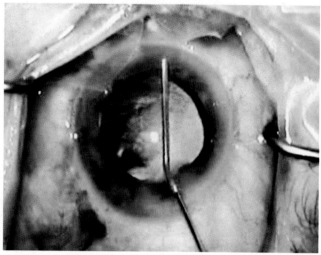

Fig. 4

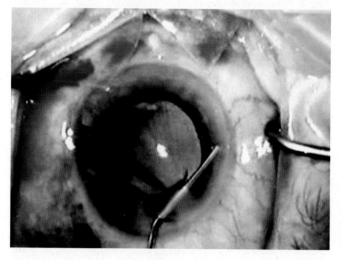

Fig. 2

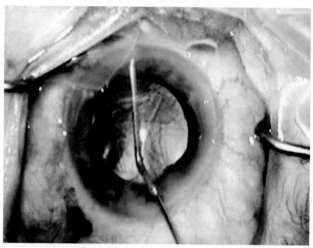

Fig. 5

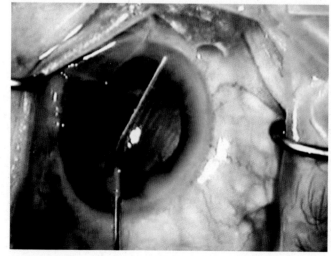

Fig. 3

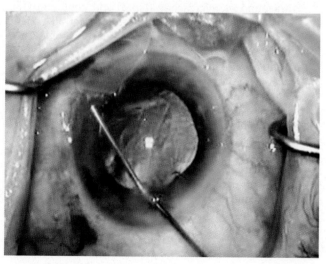

Fig. 6

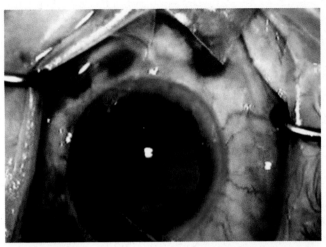

Fig. 7

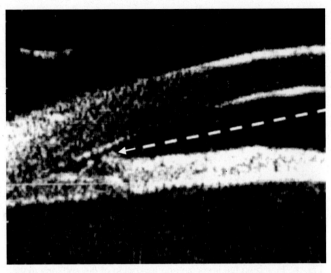

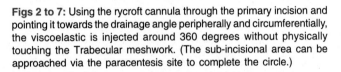

Figs 2 to 7: Using the rycroft cannula through the primary incision and pointing it towards the drainage angle peripherally and circumferentially, the viscoelastic is injected around 360 degrees without physically touching the Trabecular meshwork. (The sub-incisional area can be approached via the paracentesis site to complete the circle.)

Fig. 8: Pre-operative Ultrasound biomicroscopy (UBM) with shallow anterior chamber, appositional angle closure and clearly visible Peripheral Anterior Synechiae (arrow)

postoperative transient cystoid macular edema; there were no other postoperative complications in that group.

In group two, the study group, *the mean value of pre-operative medication use was 1.46 (range 0-5 medications), and the mean postoperative medication usage was only 0.06 (range 0-1). The mean preoperative IOP was 23 mm Hg (range 12-46), and IOP had been reduced to 14 mm Hg (range 9-19)* after at a mean follow-up of 53 months - at last follow-up, only two eyes needed anti-glaucoma treatment, and one drug each, to control their intraocular pressure. No permanent complications were noted.

THE PROCEDURE

1. Ultrasound biomicroscopy (UBM) and gonioscopy are required before and after the procedure for all patients with history of angle closure, either acute or chronic. These will confirm the presence/absence of PAS (and phacomorphic effect of the lens) and thus suitability of this procedure. After the procedure, these investigations will ascertain if it was successful.

2. Pre-operative lowering of IOP is recommended e.g. Acetazolamide (Diamox) or Hyperosmotics (e.g. Mannitol) to avoid expulsive hemorrhage due to incision-induced hypotonia and rupture of an artery.

3. The primary corneal incision should be placed slightly more centrally rather than limbally to gain better control during the procedure.

4. The timing for angle viscodissection is after the irrigation and aspiration of the soft lens matter and before the IOL is implanted into the capsular bag. Firstly, the viscoelastic is injected centrally to reform the anterior chamber and inflate and protect the capsular bag. Then, using the rycroft cannula through the primary incision and pointing it towards the drainage angle peripherally and circumferentially, the viscoelastic is injected around 360 degrees without physically touching the Trabecular meshwork. The sub-incisional area can be approached via the paracentesis site to complete the circle. It is like doing 'icing on the cake' effect literally to cover the whole 360 degrees around the angle. This should then break all the PAS and open the angle using only the viscoelastic as an instrument for gentle goniosynechialysis, the main driving force being its gravity.

5. Meticulous aspiration/removal of all viscoelastic (extra care taken for the peripheral drainage angle) after implantation of IOL in the capsular bag is essential to prevent high spikes of IOP post-operatively avoiding the occlusion of the drainage angle by the remnants of viscoelastic.

6. After the completion of the standard phacoemulsification surgery the angle can be visualized with a goniolens to assess the opening of the angle.

7. All the anti-glaucoma therapy should be stopped after the procedure to challenge the eye and find out if the procedure has worked.

8. It is recommended to use Acetylcholine intraocular solution (Miochol) to constrict the pupil at the end of the procedure and thus preventing reformation of PAS. Intensive topical steroid is also recommended (e.g. 2 hourly initially during the first week) to decrease the inflammatory response.

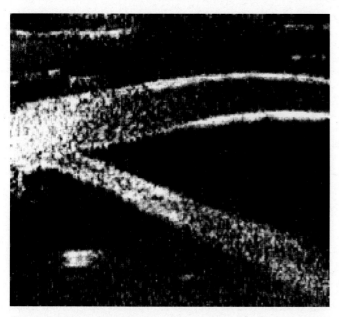

Fig. 9: Post-operative UBM of the same patient with deeper anterior chamber, broken and separated PAS and wide open angle

BIBLIOGRAPHY

1. Choong YF, Irfan S, Menage MJ. Acute angle closure glaucoma: an evaluation of a protocol for acute treatment. Eye 1999;13:613-16.
2. Gunning FP, Greve EL. Lens extraction for uncontrolled angle closure glaucoma. J Cat Refract Surg 2000;26:1012-16.
3. Jacobi PC, Dietlein TS, Luke C, et al. Primary phacoemulsification and intraocular lens implantation for acute angle closure glaucoma. Ophthalmology. 2002;09:1597-603.
4. Pereira FAS, Cronemberger S. Ultrasound biomicroscopic study of anterior segment changes after phacoemulsification and foldable intraocular lens implantation. Ophthalmology 2003;110:1799-806.
5. Salmon JF. The management of acute angle closure glaucoma. Eye 1999;13:609-10.
6. Teekhasaenee C, Ritch R. Combined phacoemulsification and goniosynechialysis for uncontrolled chronic angle closure glaucoma after acute angle closure glaucoma. Ophthalmology 1999;106:669-74.
7. Varma D, Adams WE, Phelan PS and Fraser SG. Viscogonioplasty in patients with chronic narrow angle glaucoma. Br J Ophthalmology 2006;90:648-49.
8. Varma D, Baylis O, Wride N, Phelan PS and Fraser SG. Viscogonioplasty: An effective procedure for lowering intraocular pressure in primary angle closure glaucoma. Eye 2007;21:472-75.

Chapter 57

Aspheric IOL Technology: Basic Principles and Clinical Application

Boris Malyugin (Russia)

In many cases the decline of visual function as well as loss of accommodation are related to crystalline lens changes with age. The goal of modern lenticular surgery is not only to increase visual function but also restore contrast sensitivity, make the eye emmetropic, accommodating with minimal or no aberrations. Incorporating aspheric IOLs in cataract surgery and refractive lens exchange practice is a logical and promising solution.

Basic Definitions

Aberrations fall into two classes.

Chromatic Aberrations

Where a system disperses the various wavelengths of light. These are axial, or longitudinal and lateral, or transverse, chromatic aberrations.

Monochromatic Aberrations

Monochromatic aberrations are produced without dispersion. These include the aberrations at reflecting surfaces of any colored light, and at refracting surfaces of monochromatic light of single wavelength. These include: piston, tilt, defocus, spherical, coma, astigmatism, curvature of field, image distortion.

Piston and tilt are not actually true optical aberrations, as they do not represent or model curvature in the wavefront. If an otherwise perfect wavefront is "aberrated" by piston and tilt, it will still form a perfect, aberration-free image, only shifted to a different position. Defocus is the lowest order true optical aberration.

In optics, *spherical aberration* (SA) is a deviation from the norm resulting in an image imperfection that occurs due to the increased refraction of light rays. The latter happens when rays strike a lens near its edge, in comparison with those that strike nearer the center. Spherical aberration is a symmetrical fourth-order aberration.

A perfect lens (Fig. 1) focuses all incoming rays to a point on the optic axis. A real lens with spherical surfaces (Fig. 2) suffers

from spherical aberration: it focuses rays more tightly if they enter it far from the optic axis than if they enter closer to the axis. It therefore does not produce a perfect focal point (Fig. 3). As a result the the contrast decreases and image details are blurred (Smith W., 2000).

When the normal healthy eye is fixed on the target, aberrations caused by the oblique light rays falling in the eye (i.e. coma and astigmatism) are diminished. In contrary this does not happen with spherical aberration. Among different types of high-order aberrations spherical aberration is one of the most significant.

A spherical aberration depends upon the focal length, aperture, shape, and distance of an object from the visual axis. The effect of spherical aberration induction is proportional to the fourth power of the diameter and inversely proportional to the third power of the focal length, so it is much more pronounced at short focal ratios.

Spherical Aberration and the Human Eye

Spherical aberrations can be induced in an optical system with multiple surfaces such as the human eye, which has four refracting surfaces (the anterior/posterior cornea and the anterior/posterior crystalline lens). The human visual system suffers from a small amount of spherical aberration, which rises as the pupil's size increases.

The lower-order aberrations (eg, astigmatism, myopia, hyperopia) and higher-order aberrations (eg, coma, spherical aberration) can be measured with a wavefront aberrometer by shining a small spot of light onto the retina and measuring the amount that is reflected from within the eye with the Hartmann-Shack sensor. The calculations then performed with the computer software program, which decomposes wavefront aberrations into a set of Zernike polynomials (Carvalho L., et al. 2002). Other types of the aberrometers are based on the Tscherning principle or ray tracing method.

Both anterior and posterior surfaces of the cornea as well as the crystalline lens contribute to the aberration of a wavefront passing through the eye (Kelly J, et al 2004). The cornea induces

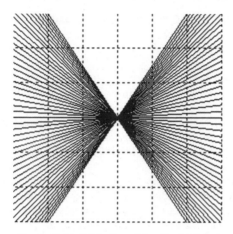

Fig. 1: Light distribution at the focal point of an "ideal" (aspheric) lens

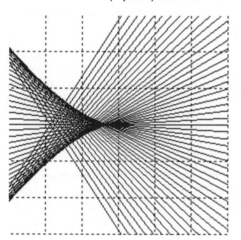

Fig. 2: Light distribution at the focal point of "conventional" spheric lens

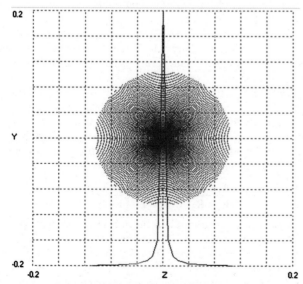

Fig. 3: Light density distribution at the lens focal point—Point spread function(PSF)

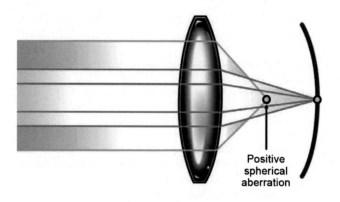

Fig. 4: Positive spherical aberration IOL (conventional optic)

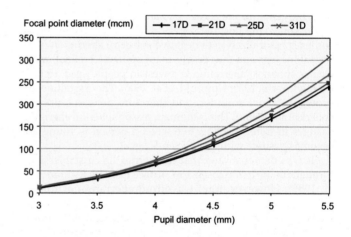

Fig. 5: Relationships between focal point and pupil diameters calculated for different optical powers of biconvex spheric IOL

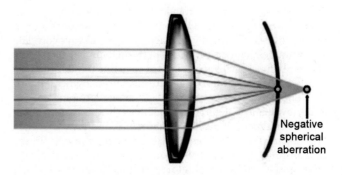

Fig. 6: Negative spherical aberration IOL (aspheric optic)

339

positive spherical aberration, although the relaxed natural lens induces negative spherical aberration (Smith G, et al 2001; Sicam V, et al, 2006).

The ideal asphericity for the anterior surface of the cornea to eliminate spherical aberration for a distant object would be a prolate ellipsoid with Q-value equals to -0.528. In reality corneal asphericity (Q-value) of the human eye averages -0.27 μm (0.00 to -0.50) with a wide variance (Kiely P., et al. 1982; Wang L., et al. 2003).

An important clinical point is that, even if the anterior cornea did have a Q-value of -0.528, it would only be free of spherical aberration for an object at infinity. An object at any distance other than infinity will result in spherical aberration (Holladay J., 2007).

With newer instruments – Pentacam (Oculus) and Visante OCT (Carl Zeiss Meditec) it was shown that the normal cornea is flatter in the central 2 mm, becomes steeper from 2 to 4 mm, and then begins to flatten beyond 4 mm. To accurately represent the true corneal shape the simple ellipsoid is not adequate, and we must use a figured ellipsoid in which the Q-value is not a constant but an equation that varies as one moves radially from the center of the cornea (Holladay J., 2007).

In youth, the positive spherical aberration of the prolate cornea is neutralized with negative spherical aberration of the crystalline lens and thus results in an optimized retinal image. Ocular spherical aberration is lowest in people aged 15 to 20 (Wang L., et al. 2005; Holzer M. et al. 2006). The crystalline lens grows, becomes rounder, and therefore develops positive spherical aberration. This is the main reason spherical aberration changes in time, it is negative when a person is young and becomes positive with age (Sicam V., et al., 2006).

It was demonstrated that the cornea has a stable shape throughout life in the absence of surface diseases (Guirao A., et al. 1999). However, total wavefront aberration of the eye increases more than threefold between 20 and 70 years of age (Artal P., et al. 2002). This is because the spherical aberration of the crystalline lens increases (from negative to positive) as a function of age (Glasser A., Campbell M. 1998).

As the eye ages, the crystalline lens grows, becomes rounder, and therefore develops positive spherical aberration itself, which adds to rather than offsets the average positive corneal spherical aberration. The individual variations however are wide.

Spherical Aberration and Visual Functions

Traditional spherical IOLs provide clear optical media improving a patient's Snellen acuity. Surgeons are aware that conventional measurements of Snellen visual acuity do not always correlate with how well patients can see to perform their daily activities. The term «functional vision» is used to define the ability to see clearly in varying levels of light during daily activities.

Contrast sensitivity testing is assuming a prominent place in our evaluation of surgical modalities. It reflects functional vision, correlates with visual performance, and provides a key to understanding optical and visual processing of images (Evans D., Ginsburg A. 1985). It was found that contrast sensitivity plays a major role in varied circumstances such as driving difficulty (McGwin G., et al. 2000) and crash involvement (Owsley

C., et al. 2001), falls (Lord SR, Dayhew J., 2001) activities of daily living and visual impairment (Rubin G., et al., 2001), as well as the performance of pilots in aircraft simulators (Ginsburg A., et al. 1982).

Contrast sensitivity declines with age, even in the absence of ocular pathology. The pathogenesis of this visual decline involves changes in spherical aberration of the crystalline lens.

Many investigators revealed that spherical aberration increases as contrast sensitivity decreases (Valois R., Valois K., 1988; Glasser A., Campbell M., 1998, 1999; Guirao A., Artal P., 2000).

Several researchers have demonstrated with image simulation how, together, certain higher-order aberrations can provide clearer images than lower amounts of other aberrations (Cheng X., et al. 2003, 2004; Marsack J., et al. 2004; Chen L., et al. 2005; Charman W. 2006). Suggestions that residual positive spherical aberration when the pupil constricts is beneficial refer to studies of Top Gun pilots who have an average of +0.1 μm SA (Levy Y., et al., 2005).

It is well-established fact that patients can usually tolerate an interval between -0.15 and +0.01D/mm of spherical aberration for a 6-mm pupil (Dietze H., Cox M., 2004; Legras R. et al., 2004). Different types of aberrations balances each other. According to McClellan J., et al. (2002) humans do not perceive chromatic aberration because they are balanced by achromatic higher-order aberrations in the eye.

Spherical Aberration Reduction

Due to spherical aberration rays of light spread across several points on the focal plane and along the optical axis. Thus the intensity of the light as well as its lateral and axial resolution are decreased, the image loses the details and become distorted (Monks C., 2004).

To influence spherical aberration of the optical system one has to change the curvature of its refractive surfaces. In the human eye this could be done with either corneal refractive surgery or lens exchange.

Various methods can minimize spherical aberration and improve an image's quality. Mathematical formulae are used to calculate an appropriate series of lenses that will reduce spherical aberration.

One can calculate parameters that minimize spherical aberration. For example, in a design consisting of a single lens with spherical surfaces and a given object distance "o", image distance "i", and refractive index "n", one can minimize spherical aberration by adjusting the radii of curvature R_1 and R_2 of the front and back surfaces of the lens such that

$$\frac{R_1 + R_2}{R_1 - R_2} = \frac{2(n^2 - 1)}{n + 2}\left(\frac{i + o}{i - o}\right)$$

Spherical aberrations can be minimized using special aspheric lenses. In the latter outer optic edges have a different curvature than in the center. The result is a sharp, clear image.

We have to keep in mind that "ideal" images without any aberrations are not possible to achieve. There is a limit in decrease of the focal point diameter due to wave nature of light.

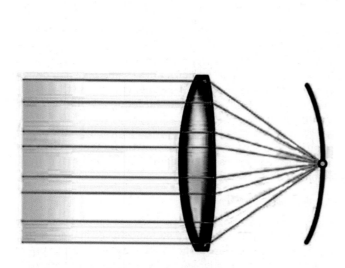

Fig. 7: Aberration-free IOL

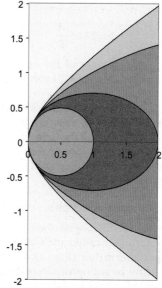

Fig. 8: Planar sections through of the spheric (dark blue), elliptic (purple), parabolic (blue) and hyperbolic (brown) IOL anterior surfaces

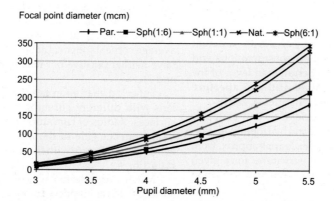

Fig. 9: Relationships between focal point and pupil diameters in different types of IOL refractive surfaces. IOL optic power – 20 D. IOL with parabolic surfaces focal parameters: 10.5 mm from the corneal side and 45 mm from the retinal side. IOL with spheric surfaces (ratio 1:6): anterior radius of curvature 9.96 mm, posterior - 59.76 mm. Symmetrical equiconvex IOL: both radii of curvature 16.9 mm. Natural lens: curvature radius of anterior surface – 10 mm, posterior surface -6 mm. Spheric IOL (ratio 6:1): anterior radius of curvature 58.8 mm, posterior -9.8 mm

According to the diffractive theory minimal diameter (d) of the light dot on the plane depends on the light diffraction on the aperture having diameter D. This is described with the formula:

$$d = 2.44\,f\,\frac{\lambda}{D}$$

where "f" – is a focal distance of the optical system, "λ" – wavelight length. For example: f = 20 mm, λ = 0.55·10^{-3} mm, D = 4 mm, that gives d = 6.7 mm.

To decrease the diameter of the light dot less than a diffractive limit is not possible even in case when the laws of the geometrical optics converges all the light rays in one dot. With the help of the aspheric lens spherical aberration cannot be avoided completely but rather diminished to the level, which is clinically insignificant.

Intraocular Lenses and Aberrations

Conventional spherical IOLs, with their bi-, equi-convex or convex-plano design, add rather than offset to the positive corneal spherical aberration (Fig. 4). That is why their implantation results in suboptimal visual quality due to increased spherical aberrations with poor point spread and modulation transfer (MTF) functions (Mester U. et al. 2003).

The distribution of curvatures between the lens' anterior and posterior surfaces affects the amount of spherical aberration induced by the IOL. Convex-plano lenses induce the lowest amount of spherical aberration, followed by equiconvex lenses and plano-convex lenses (Atchison D., 1991). IOL with more curved anterior surface induce lower amounts of positive spherical aberration. The amount of induced spherical aberration rose as the IOL' dioptric power increases with low-powered IOLs induce less spherical aberration (Smith G., Atchison D., 1997).

Clinical studies comparing Acrys of lenses with different optic design confirmed these theoretical considerations and found slight differences in spherical aberration in favor of the more curved anterior design but only at 6-mm aperture diameters (Bellucci R., et al. 2004; Taketani F., et al. 2005).

The optics of modern IOLs are made of several materials including PMMA, silicone, hydrophobic and hydrophilic acrylic. Each material has its own refractive index (varies approx. from 1.41 to 1.55) and consequently its own curvatures for a given power. They are both affect the amount of spherical aberration induced by the IOL's implantation.

The higher the refractive index, the lower the curvature. One may therefore expect IOLs with a high refractive index to induce less spherical aberration. This is a clinically proven fact (Bellucci R., et al. 2004; Martin R., Sanders D., 2005; Rohart C., et al. 2006).

The surgeon has to be aware that with low-powered lenses, the resulting spherical aberration of the eye will be close to the corneal spherical aberration. With high-powered lenses, as the curvature of the IOL's anterior surface diminishes there is subsequent increase in positive spherical aberration (Fig. 5).

Figure 5 represents calculated relationships between the pupil diameter and focal point diameter in the eyes with convex-plano IOL. For the purpose of calculations parameters of the anterior convex IOL surface were chosen to achieve minimally possible diameter of light dot on the retina for the 3.0 mm pupil diameter. Then pupil diameter was increased and the diameter of the focal point calculated.

According to physical optics, the amount of spherical aberration depends on the curvature of the refractive surfaces and the total dioptric power of the optical system (Atchison D. 1991). That means that the IOLs of the same material, design and optical power introduced in different eyes with variable axial length and corneal power will induce slightly different amount of aberrations.

With very high-powered spherical lenses, the induction of positive SA could decrease contrast sensitivity but simultaneously increase the depth of focus and may be will favor the near vision.

Aspheric IOLs Concepts

To enhance image quality it is necessary to diminish spherical aberration. In technical optical systems this can be done with the help of the lens combination compensationg aberrations of each other. Fot intraocular lenses the only way is to change the design and curvature of the refractive surfaces.

Specially designed aspheric intraocular lenses implanted during cataract surgery can compensate for the cornea's positive spherical aberration. This will optimize image quality and contrast, while minimizing the induction of asymmetrical aberrations and yield optimal overall optical performance of the eye mitigating adverse effects on the depth of field and relative MTF. One of the additional advantages of IOLs with modified prolate optical surfaces is enhanced retinal image and better posterior segment evaluation.

The available aspheric IOLs possess varying degrees of negative spherical aberration. Some are designed to offset the average corneal spherical aberration fully or partially, the others have neither positive nor negative spherical aberration (Figs 6 and 7).

Spherical aberration can also be reduced using asymmetric lens with different curvatures of the anterior and posterior surfaces. Radius of curvature from the object side must be less than from the side of the image. Maximal reduction can be achieved in this case with the convex-plano lens with curvature ratio 1:6.

Much more effective way of SA reduction is to use aspheric surfaces such as elliptic, parabolic or hyperbolic. Calculations of ray tracing with complex surfaces can be done with computer modeling. Figure 8 represents the sections of all the above-mentioned surfaces together with the spherical one.

Elliptical and parabolic IOL surfaces can significantly decrease spherical aberration. The reduction is proportional to the IOL optical power. Hyperbolic surfaces allow for the most effective aberration reduction.

Figure 9 represents the example of relationships between focal point diameter and pupil diameter for different versions of IOL refractive surfaces. Parameters of the model eye are: anterior corneal curvature 7.7 mm, posterior corneal curvature 6.8 mm, cornea refractive index 1.3777, aqueous humor

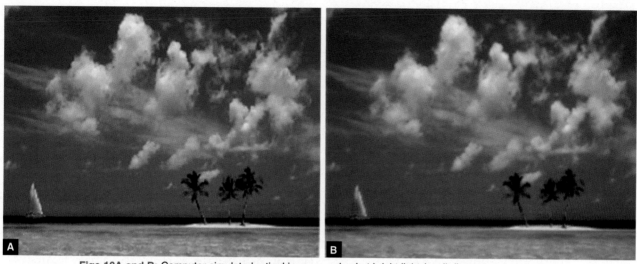

Figs 10A and B: Computer simulated retinal image received at bright light (pupil diameter 3.0 mm) of the with eye A) aspheric IOL (with hyperbolic surface) and B) spheric IOL

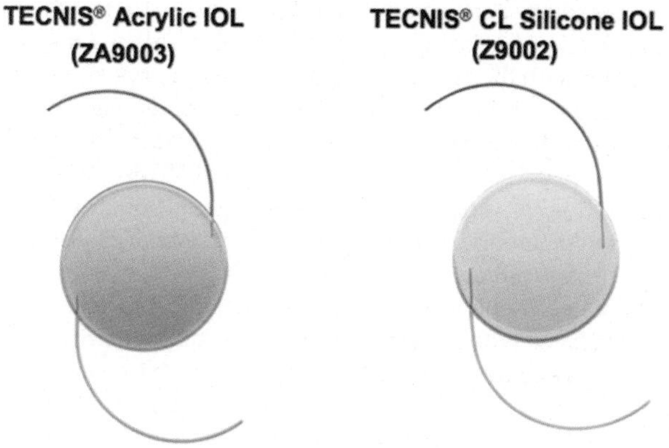

TECNIS® Acrylic IOL (ZA9003)

TECNIS® CL Silicone IOL (Z9002)

Fig. 11: Tecnis aspheric lenses (AMO, Inc.)

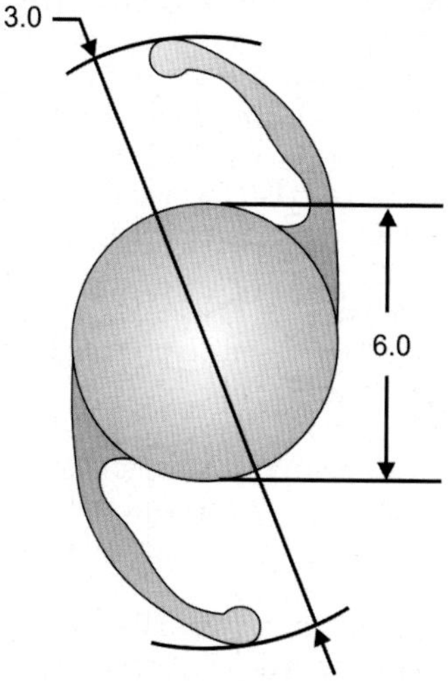

Fig. 12: Acrysof IQ lens (Alcon)

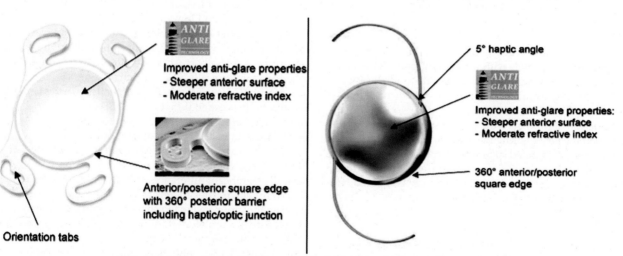

Figs 13A and B: Akreos AO (A) and SofPort (B) intraocular lenses (Bausch & Lomb)

refractive index 1.336, and distance from the anterior surface of the cornea to the retina – 23.5 mm. IOL optic diameter is 6.0 mm, coefficient of refraction 1.505 (in all cases). The light source is located in infinity.

The ability to use aspheric lenses clinically arises from the two main points. First, modern micro-incision cataract surgery introduces minimal or zero new corneal aberrations. Second, the optical quality of IOLs' surfaces far surpass those of the cornea.

Computer modeling illustrates the possibility to achieve with aspheric IOL image quality much higher than that with conventional optic IOL (Figs 10A and B).

An aspheric lens has the smaller focal point. That makes these lenses "more sensitive" to axial displacement. The latter happens when optical power of the IOL is not correct. Image quality in this situation will decrease more than with the regular spheric lens.

Tecnis IOL

Tecnis IOL (AMO, Inc.) is the first biconvex lens with a modified, aspheric, anterior prolate surface with -0.27μm spherical aberration to compensate for the average positive corneal spherical aberration calculated from the data taken from the general population (Z [4,0] = +0.27 ± 0.02 μm) (Fig. 11).

It is available on an acrylic (Tecnis ZA9003) or silicone (Tecnis Z9002) platforms with optic diameter 6.0 mm and overall length of 13 mm. Both are three-piece angulated foldable lenses that can be injected into the eye. The lenses acrylic model features the Optiedge design to minimize potential dysphotopsia and posterior capsular opacification.

The clinical benefits of Tecnis Z9000 platform are better low-contrast visual acuity, photopic and mesopic contrast sensitivity than achieved with spherical IOLs (Mester U. et al. 2003; Packer M et al. 2004; Kershner R 2003; Bellucci R. et al. 2004, 2005).

Tecnis design produces favorable theoretical and clinical results. Nevertheless optical laboratory studies have revealed the lens' potential limitations with it's decentration and tilt (Dietze H, Cox M, 2005; Altmann G et al, 2005).

Acrysof IQ

Acrysof IQ lens (Alcon Laboratories, Inc.) is a single-piece, hydrophobic, acrylic IOL with a modified posterior surface. This is the only aspheric lens that incorporates both the UV and blue light filtering chromofores. It is 9% thinner than the regular Acrysof lens (Fig. 12).

The design of this lens with -0.2 μm spherical aberration is based upon the idea of bring the average pseudophakic eye to a slightly positive targeted spherical aberration (approximately + 0.07 μm). This compansatory strategy results in an improvement of night-driving simulation test compared with a conventional monofocal spherical lens.

Akreos AO/SofPort AO

Akreos AO/Sofport AO lenses (Bausch & Lomb) does not add or subtract spherical aberration. Akreos AO is made of hydrophilic acrylic material while Sofport AO lens is made of second-generation silicone. Both have aspheric anterior and posterior surfaces with 0 μm spherical aberration and does not contribute to preexisting higher-order aberrations (Fig. 13).

Bausch and Lomb advanced optics IOLs are designed with uniform power from the center to the periphery. The main idea is to provide predictable and reliable visual results in most clinical conditions independent of the zonular weakness and/or capsular bag position, and misalignment of the pupil.

Clinical Studies of Aspheric IOLs

Aspheric IOLs have been shown to improve optical performance and contrast sensitivity compared with conventional spherical IOLs. Several clinical studies have demonstrated improved quality of vision with reduced ocular spherical aberration (Packer M., et al., 2002, 2004; Mester U., et al., 2003; Kershner R. 2003; Kennis H., et al., 2004; Denoyer A., et al. 2006; Lanzagorta-Aresti A., et al., 2005; Martinez P. et al., 2005; Bellucci R., et al. 2005; Munoz G., et al. 2006; Franchini A. 2006).

In the study performed by the AMO, Inc. patients who had no residual spherical aberration with the Tecnis lens were compared with those who had 0.30 to 0.40 μm of postoperative spherical aberration with spherical IOLs. Simulated night driving tests showed that patients who received the Tecnis IOL identified a pedestrian 0.5 seconds sooner at a speed of 55 mph than those implanted with a spherical IOL. These results suggest that the correction of spherical aberration not only improves vision but also increases patients' safety.

As stated by FDA experts mean spherical aberration in the eyes implanted with the Tecnis IOL are "not different from zero." The improvement in contrast sensitivity approximately 0.3 log units or 40% to 50% improved retinal image contrast were determined with this type of IOL. The FDA supported the labeling of the Tecnis lens for improved functional vision that is likely to provide a meaningful safety benefit to elderly drivers.

In the studies conducted by Malyugin B. (2006) and Takhchidi K., et al. (2007) aspheric Akreos AO outperoremed IOLs with conventional optics (Akreos Adapt and Acrysof) in contrast sensitivity testing and low contrast BCVA.

Altmann G. et al. (2005) using ray-tracing software and a pseudophakic eye model, calculated that the optical performance of Sofport AO was better than its conventional, spherical counterpart (LI61U; Bausch & Lomb).

Sofport AO also performed better than the Tecnis lens when decentration exceeded 0.15, 0.30, or 0.38 mm with 3-, 4-, or 5-mm pupils, respectively. Decentration of the Sofport AO had less negative impact on depth of field or defocus.

In the study conducted by Nichamin L. (2006), the Sofport AO lens was compared to a negatively aspheric IOL. Few clinically significant differences in both lenses' performance in vivo were shown. The differences in logMAR UCVA and BCVA between the groups were too small to be clinically meaningful. The negatively prolate IOL, did provide better low-contrast BCVA than the Sofport AO lens under mesopic conditions (at 1.5 cycles per degree only), both with and without glare.

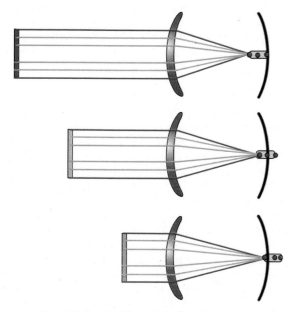

Fig. 14: Depth of focus in intermediate vision

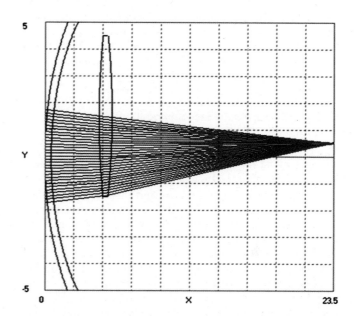

Fig. 15: Ray tracing in the eye in case of vertical IOL displacement (1.5 mm from the optical axis)

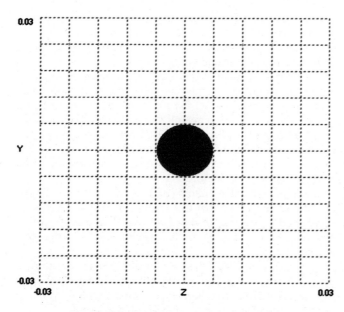

Fig. 16: Retinal image. IOL positioned centrally

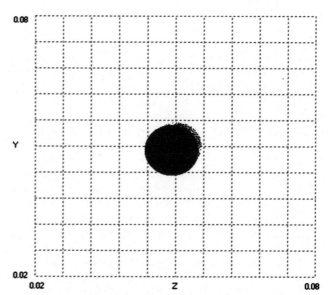

Fig. 17: Retinal image. IOL decentered by 0.25 mm

Mester U. et al. (2003) as well as Artal P. et al. (2004) showed that the contrast sensitivity function continued to improve from 3 months to 1 year after the Tecnis aspheric IOL implantation.

Thus when assessing the outcomes such as visual acuity and contrast sensitivity function we have to keep in mind both rapid and long-term (up to 1 year) phases of neural adaptation. The studies performed before the 1-year mark, when the the brain has not yet been adapted to the improved image, do not necessarily reflect the patient's final outcome.

Depth of Focus (Pseudoaccommodation) with Aspheric IOLs

One of the theoretical limitations of aspheric IOLs regards depth of focus. Correcting the corneal spherical aberration improves the contrast of the retinal image. A question is whether aspheric IOLs also reduces depth of focus and therefore renders the pseudophakic eye more vulnerable to defocus image errors.

Figure 14 represents schematically the relationships of the depth of focus and spherical aberrations. The distant object is seen through central rays (blue) falling on the cornea. When the object is getting closer, it is seen through medium (purple) and peripherial (green) rays. Without positive spherical aberration, all rays are focused on the single focal point (blue) that goes behind the retina when the object is getting closer.

Marcos S et al. (2005) analyzed optical quality (MTF) and simulated retinal images of the model eyes with Tecnis lens. They demonstrated that the through-focus behavior of the Tecnis at lower ranges of defocus (± 0.75D) was either better than or similar to that of spherical IOLs. With greater negative defocus, however, spherical IOLs performed better. The investigators concluded that eyes achieving BSCVA with spherical IOLs should perform near tasks better than those achieving BSCVA with aspheric IOLs.

In contrary, Piers P et al (2004) using an adaptive optics simulator in four normal, young patients, showed comparable visual performance for defocus as large as -1.00 D with both a spherical and an aspheric IOLs.

Tabernero J, Artal P et al (2006) developed ray-tracing model for predicting the optical performance of different types of IOLs after cataract surgery. They have found that at best focus, visual performance with the Tecnis lens was better. For different values of defocus, however, the aspheric lens performed better or similarly to the conventional spherical lens (CeeOn). This finding indicates that the aspheric IOL (Tecnis) generally improves retinal contrast at best focus and also for small values of defocus. In other words, actual pseudoaccommodation with aspheric lenses is not compromised.

This is the reason some surgeons (McDonald J., 2007) prefer to correct the presbyopic vision of healthy patients by implanting not multifocal but rather the aspheric monofocal IOLs bilaterally. He advocates to implant Sofport AO in subjects' near eyes first and target a postoperative refraction of between -0.75 and -1.50D. Postoperative refraction in their distance eyes is targeted from plano to -0.50D. As a result in a subjective survey, 100% of the patients reported that they did not wear spectacles for intermediate vision, and 73% said that they did not wear spectacles for near or distance vision.

Spherical aberration does not increase depth of focus. The only difference between spheric and aspheric lenses is at the best focus, where the aspheric surface comes to a single point and the spherical lens does not. The difference is not in the depth of focus, but in the clarity of best focus (Holladay J., 2007).

Effect of Decentration on IOL Performance

Perfect IOL centration on the visual axis is difficult to measure and achieve. An IOL that appears perfectly centered at the slit-lamp may actually be off axis by as much as 0.5 mm. Lining up an IOL with the center of a pupil, does not ensure the lens' centration on the visual axis. The average offset between the visual axis and the pupil's center has measured 0.37 ± 0.24 mm (Rynders M., et al. 1995).

Moreover the location of the pupillary center varies with dilation (Altmann G., et al. 2005); the center shifts an average of 0.19 mm.

IOL decentration leads to image degradation. Figure 15 illustrates the ray tracing in the schematic eye after IOL decentration 1.5 mm up from the optical axis. The distance to the light source is 33 cm. Note that retinal image is moved at the same direction as the IOL.
(1.5 mm from the optical axis)

Different degrees of calculated retinal image degradation with spherical IOL (optical power +20 D, pupil diameter 3.0 mm; light source located in infinity) decentration are presented on Figures 16 to 24.

Aspheric IOL decentration from the visual axis can cause image degradation more significant than in case of spheric IOL. Decentration of an aspheric IOL overshadow the lens apparent benefits and may induce defocus, astigmatism, and coma, which would degrade the retinal image quality.

Decentration of an aspheric IOL with negative spherical aberration produces a hyperopic refractive error along with asymmetric aberrations. At the same time equally decentered spherical IOL produces a myopic shift (Altmann G et al, 2005).

According to J.Holladay et al (2002) calculations of the MTF the Tecnis needed to be centered within 0.4 mm and tilted less than 7° in order to exceed the optical performance of a conventional spherical IOL.

Piers P. with collaborators (2004) used polychromatic eye model and concluded that the Tecnis lens would need to be decentered by 0.8 mm or tilted at least 10° before its optical performance would be worse than a spherical IOL of the same power.

Sarver E, et al. (2007) to study the effect of decentration on the performance of conventional (Soflex) and aspheric (Sofport AO, Tecnis) IOLs used schematic eye model with fixed 5 mm pupil. They have found that spherical IOLs decentered by 0.5 and 1.0 mm induced 14 to 25 times more coma and astigmatism than similarly decentered IOLs with zero spherical aberration. IOLs with negative spherical aberration induced even higher degrees of coma and astigmatism versus IOLs with zero

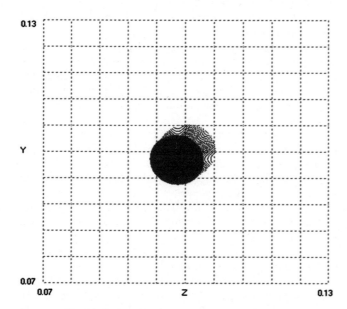

Fig. 18: Retinal image. IOL decentered by 0.5 mm

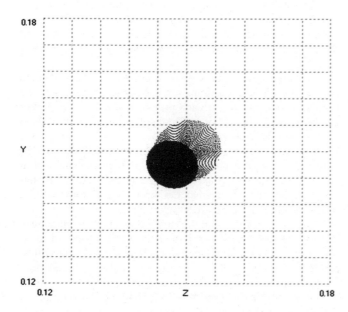

Fig. 19: Retinal image. IOL decentered by 0.75 mm

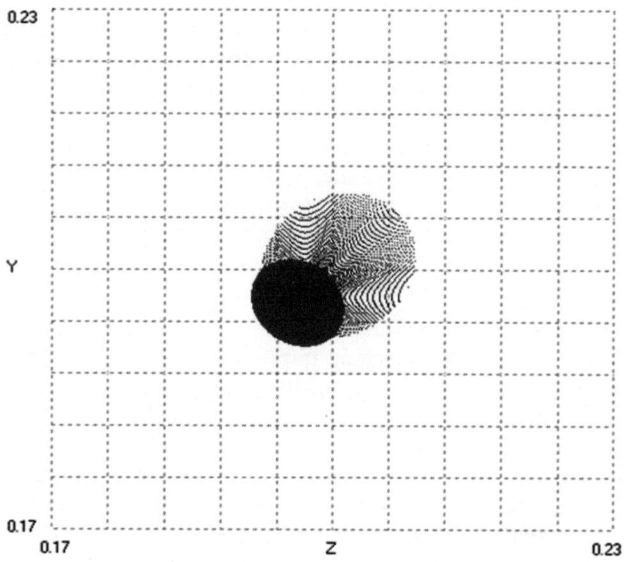

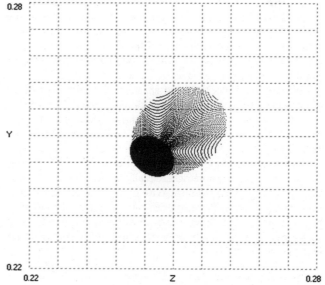

Fig. 20: Retinal image. IOL decentered by 1.0 mm

Fig. 21: Retinal image. IOL decentered by 1.25 mm

spherical aberration (23 to 50 times as much) when both were decentered by 0.5 and 1.0 mm.

Most of the clinical observations of IOL decentration and tilt fall below either of the aforementioned levels. In patients with senile miosis, the adverse effects of IOL decentration may be limited.

Spherical aberration can be compensated with spectacle correction. Nevertheless, asymmetrical aberrations such as coma that is induced by the decentered IOL with negative spherical aberration can not be corrected with glasses.

Pupillary Size and Aspheric IOLs

Studies have shown rising values of spherical aberrations in phakic eyes with increasing pupillary diameter (Castejon-Mochon J., et al. 2002; Wang Y., et al. 2003) (Fig. 25). This is also important in pseudophakic eyes with aspheric IOLs.

Kohnen T, Kasper T (2007) designed a study to evaluate higher-order aberrations as a function of the pupil's diameter. The median pupillary size in pseudophakic patients measured with the digital infrared pupillometer (Procyon P2000SA) under highly mesopic luminance (6.61 lux) was about 3.2 mm and it increased under mesopic illumination (0.88 lux) to 4.05 mm. Under low mesopic luminance (0.07 lux), the median pupillary diameter was about 5.0 mm.The researchers found statistically significantly lower values of Z(4,0) for all calculated pupillary diameters (3 to 6 mm) for the Tecnis IOL group as compared to the conventional optics IOL (Sensar) group. The absolute amount of the differences for small pupils (3 and 4 mm) was minor, but it rose as the pupil's size grew (5 and 6 mm).

For total higher-order aberrations (third- to fifth-order RMS), statistically significant differences were found in the aspheric group only with a pupillary diameter of 6 mm. It was concluded that that patients with larger pupils can derive a greater benefit from aspheric IOLs than people with smaller pupils.

Figure 26 shows the light scattering in different pupil diameters for the conventional spheric and aspheric IOLs. Pupil dilatation gives increased diameter of the light dot at the focal point in all cases. But the magnitude is different in different optic design.

In the presence of small pupils, the Acrysof IQ, Tecnis, Sofport AO, and any spherical IOL all perform about the same in terms of contrast sensitivity. With pupils of 4 mm and larger, however, the correction of anterior corneal spherical aberration begins to make a difference in both image quality and visual performance, as shown by contrast sensitivity testing (Mester U, Kaymak H., 2006).

Contraindications and Limitations of Aspheric IOLs

Myopic laser ablation tends to increase the eye's spherical aberration. In these cases IOLs with negative spherical aberration seems to be are appropriate.

But patients who previously underwent laser ablative corneal surgery are especially at risk for problems with a negatively aspheric IOL (Oliver K., et al. 1997; Chen C., et al.

2002; Wang L., Koch D. 2003). It can be difficult for ophthalmologists to determine the optical center of these patients' corneas and to match it with the IOL.

Conversely, negative aspheric IOLs should be used with caution in patients with negative corneal asphericity. In patients who have highly prolate corneas it will induce negative spherical aberration. Negative aspheric IOL should be avoided in patients following laser refractive surgery to treat hyperopia.

Preoperative testing should include pupillometry under mesopic and scotopic conditions, because in patient with senile miosis the benefit of an aspheric IOL may be limited. Small pupil may reduce the impact and advantages of an aspheric IOL on the visual performance.

Surgeons should avoid implanting negatively aspheric IOLs in the sulcus or in clinical situations that may increase the risk of IOL decentration. In clinical situations with compromised zonular or capsular integrity, optical effect of an aspheric IOL can be minimal or even negative.

The modulation transfer function of IOLs with zero spherical aberration is not affected by 0 to 1.0 mm of decentration. MTF of spherical and aspheric IOLs is adversely affected by 0.5 to 1.0 mm of decentration.

Customizing Aspheric IOLs

The manufacturers of aspheric IOLs have proposed that their implantation will give cataract patients super vision. This is the goal which did not achieved at this particular time.

The customized approach currently being accepted by most of the surgeons is to measure the corneal spherical aberration over a 6-mm zone and match this value with the aspheric IOL design to choose the one with the closest negative spherical aberration.

By using topographers with special software to calculate corneal wavefront measurements, the surgeons can select the optimal aspheric IOL for each pseudophakic eye. The target can be a small amount of residual spherical aberration or no residual spherical aberration.

IOLs with neutral asphericity (Sofport AO/ Akreos AO) may be most appropriate in patients with highly asymmetrical corneal aberrations (e.g. forme fruste pellucid marginal degeneration or keratoconus). On those patients they will not induce additional higher-order aberrations.

There is no doubts that the surgeon will have to customize selection of the lens for each patient. Probably a wider range of IOLs to correct different degrees of spherical aberration will be needed.

The Optimal Residual Spherical Aberration

What is the optimal ocular spherical aberration we should target with aspheric IOLs?

There are different opinions regarding the optimal, residual, postoperative spherical aberration in pseudophakic patient. Based upon studies in young individuals with supernormal vision some researches, for example, Artal P, et al. (2005) suggest that it should be zero.

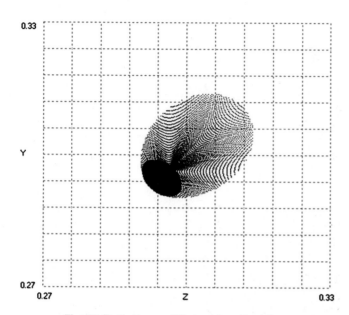

Fig. 22: Retinal image. IOL decentered by 1.5 mm

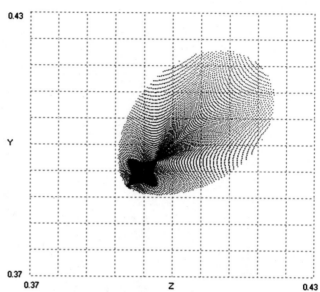

Fig. 24: Retinal image. IOL decentered by 2.0 mm

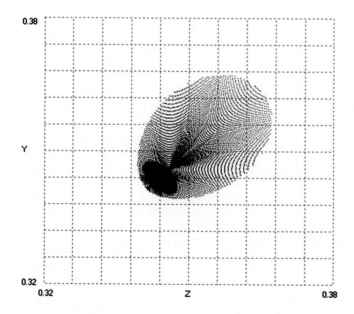

Fig. 23: Retinal image. IOL decentered by 1.75 mm

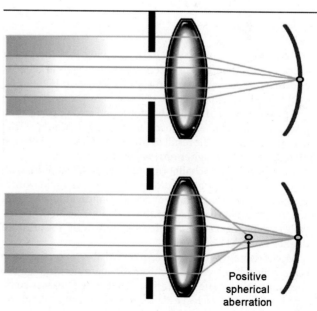

Positive
spherical
aberration

Fig. 25: Pupil diameter and spherical aberration induction in the
pseudophakic eye

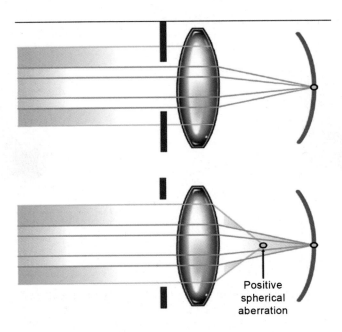

Fig. 26: Focal point diameters calculated for IOLs with symmetrical convex surfaces (A) and asymmetrical parabolic surfaces (B). Square side equals to 100 microns

According to Holladay J (2007) knowing that the ocular spherical aberration is nearly zero when the eye is at its peak performance does not necessarily prove that zero is the ideal target, especially as people age.

Applegate R, et al (2003) did not found strong correlation between spherical aberration and visual acuity. This phenomenon may be the result of complex interactions between different individual higher-order aberrations.

Amesbury E. and Schallhorn S. (2003) found that pilots with a UCVA of 20/12 or better did not have fewer higher-order aberrations comparing to a young control individuals without such supernormal vision. According to Levy Y. et al. (2005) the whole eye spherical aberration for eyes with a UCVA of 20/15 or better was +0.11 ± 0.07 µm.

Modest amounts of positive spherical aberration may also decrease the adverse effects of chromatic aberration and higher-order monochromatic aberration. That is the reason some investigators prefer to leave slight, residual, positive spherical aberration, which they believe may play a role in neural processing and adaptation.

In contrary, according to Holladay J (2007) there is no benefit to leaving any positive spherical aberration in the optical system, because it degrades the image and reduces patients' near vision as their pupils constrict. Some patients may benefit from a small amount of residual negative spherical aberration in order to achieve better unaided near vision.

DISCUSSION

Wavefront imaging that came from refractive surgery, opened a new era of understanding the human eye's higher-order aberrations. It was established that spherical aberration is present in the cornea as well as the crystalline lens in their native states in the human eye. Spherical aberration can be also induced iatrogenically by keratorefractive or lenticular surgeries. The cornea's curvature, pupil's size and the lens' shape, all influence spherical aberration.

The refractive goal of cataract surgery should be to eliminate or at least minimize all of the optical aberrations of the eye, including spherical aberration. Advances in IOL technology have incorporated the reduction of spherical aberration into the clinical practice.

Cataract patients have to be evaluated preoperatively as potential candidates for refractive surgery. Wavefront aberrometry helps to identify patients who have significant amounts of spherical aberration prior to the cataract surgery. This allows the surgeon to choose the specific IOL depends on the individual corneal shape. Ongoing research will reveal the full benefits of spherical aberration correction with IOLs.

BIBLIOGRAPHY

1. Altmann GE, Nichamin LD, Lane SS, Pepose JS. Optical performance of 3 intraocular lens designs in the presence of decentration. J Cataract Refract Surg 2005;31:574-85.

2. Amesbury EC, Schallhorn SC. Contrast sensitivity and limits of vision. Int Ophthalmol Clin 2003;43:31-42.

3. Applegate RA, Marsack JD, Ramos R, Sarver EJ. Interactions between aberrations to improve or reduce visual performance. J Cataract Refract Surg. 2003;29:1487-95.

4. Artal P, Chen L, Fernandez EJ, et al. Neural compensation for the eye's optical aberrations. J Vis 2004;4:281-87.

5. Artal P, Villegas EA, Alcon E, Benito A. Better than normal visual acuity does not require perfect ocular optics. Invest Ophthalmol Vis Sci. 2005;46:E-Abstract 3615.

6. Atchison DA. Design of aspheric intraocular lenses. Ophthalmic Physiol Opt. 1991;11:137-46.

7. Bellucci R, Morselli S, Piers P. Comparison of wavefront aberrations and optical quality of eyes implanted with five intraocular lenses. J Refract Surg 2004;20:297-306.

8. Bellucci R, Scialdone A, Buratto L, et al. Visual acuity and contrast sensitivity comparison between Tecnis and AcrySof SA60AT intraocular lenses: a multicenter study. J Cataract Refract Surg 2005;31:712-17.

9. Carvalho LA, Castro JC, Carvalho LA. Measuring higher order optical aberrations of the human eye: techniques and applications. Braz J Med Biol Res. 2002;35:1395-1406.

10. Castejon-Mochon JF, Lopez-Gil N, Benito A, Artal P. Ocular wave-front aberration statistics in a normal young population. Vision Res. 2002;42:1611-17.

11. Charman WN. The Charles F. Prentice Award Lecture 2005: optics of the human eye: progress and problems. Optom Vis Sci. 2006;83:335-45.

12. Chen CC, Izadshenas A, Rana MAA, Azar DT. Corneal asphericity following hyperopic laser in situ keratomileusis. J Cataract Refract Surg. 2002;28:1539-45.

13. Chen L, Singer B, Guirao A, et al. Image metrics for predicting subjective image quality. Optom Vis Sci. 2005;82:358-369.

14. Cheng X, Bradley A, Thibos LN. Predicting subjective judgment of best focus with objective image quality metrics. J Vis. 2004;4:310-21.

15. Cheng X, Thibos LN, Bradley A. Estimating visual quality from wavefront aberration measurements. J Refract Surg. 2003;19:S579-S84.

16. Denoyer A, Roger F, Majzoub S, Pisella PJ. Quality of vision after cataract surgery in patients with prolate aspherical lens. J Fr Ophtalmol. 2006;29:157-63.

17. Dietze HH, Cox MJ. Correcting ocular spherical aberration with soft contact lenses. J Opt Soc Am A Opt Image Sci Vis. 2004;21:473-85.

18. Dietze HH, Cox MJ. Limitations of correcting spherical aberration with aspheric intraocular lenses. J Refract Surg 2005;21(suppl):541-46.

19. Evans DW, Ginsburg AP. Contrast sensitivity predicts age-related differences in highway sign discriminability. Human Factors. 1985;27(12):637.

20. Franchini A. Comparative assessment of contrast with spherical and aspherical intraocular lenses. J Cataract Refract Surg. 2006;32:1307-19.

21. Ginsburg AP, Evans DW, Sekule R, Harp SA. Contrast sensitivity predicts pilots' performance in aircraft simulators. Am J Optom Physiol Opt 1982;(1):105-09.

22. Glasser A, Campbell MC. Biometric, optical and physical changes in the isolated human crystalline lens with age in relation to presbyopia. Vision Res. 1999;39:1991-2015.

23. Glasser A, Campbell MCW. Presbyopia and the optical changes in the human crystalline lens with age. Vision Res. 1998;38:209-29.

24. Guirao A, Artal P. Corneal wave aberration from videokeratography: accuracy and limitations of the procedure. J Opt Soc Am A Opt Image Sci Vis 2000;17:955-65.

25. Guirao A, Gonzales C, Redondo M, et al. Average performance of the human eye as a function of age in the normal population. Invest Ophthalmol Vis Science 1999;40:203-13.

26. Holladay J. Spherical aberration: the next frontier. Cataract and Refractive Surgery Today. April, 2007.

27. Holladay JT, Piers PA, Kozanyi G, et al. A new intraocular lens designed to reduce spherical aberration of pseudophakic eyes. J Refract Surg. 2002;18: 683-701.

28. Holzer MP, Goebels S, Aufarth GU. Total, corneal and internal aberrations of the human eye. Paper presented at: The DOC; May 27, 2006; Nuremburg, Germany.

29. Kelly JE, Mihashi T, Howland HC. Compensation of corneal horizontal/vertical astigmatism, lateral coma, and spherical aberration by internal optics of the eye. J Vis 2004;4:262-71.

30. Kennis H, Huygens M, Callebaut F. Comparing the contrast sensitivity of a modified prolate anterior surface IOL and of two spherical IOLs. Bull Soc Belge Ophtalmol 2004;294:49-58.

31. Kershner RM. Retinal image contrast and functional visual performance with aspheric, silicone, and acrylic intraocular lenses. Prospective evaluation. J Cataract Refract Surg. 2003;29:1684-94.

32. Kiely PM, Smith G, Carney LG. The mean shape of the human cornea. Opt Acta 1982;29:1027-40.

33. Kohnen T, Kasper T. At what pupil size does the aspheric matter? Cataract and Refractive Surgery Today. April, 2007.

34. Lanzagorta-Aresti A, Palacios-Pozo E, Taboada-Esteve JF, et al. Contrast sensitivity to intraocular lens Tecnis Z-9000. Arch Soc Esp Oftalmo 2005;80:651-58.

35. Legras R, Chateau N, Charman WN. Assessment of just-noticeable differences for refractive errors and spherical aberration using visual simulation. Optom Vis Sci. 2004; 81:718-28.

36. Levy Y, Segal O, Avni I, Zadok D. Ocular higher-order aberrations in eyes with supernormal vision. Am J Ophthalmol. 2005;139:225-28.

37. Lord SR, Dayhew J. Visual risk factors for falls in older people. J Am Geriatr Soc 2001;49(5):508-15.

38. Malyugin B. Aspheric optic versus conventional optic: functional and aberrometric results // Presented at the Congress of the ASCRS, San Francisco, USA, 2006.

39. Marcos S, Barbero S, Jimenez-Alfaro I. Optical quality and depth-of-field of eyes implanted with spherical and aspheric intraocular lenses. J Refract Surg 2005;21:223-35.

40. Marsack JD, Thibos LN, Applegate RA. Metrics of optical quality derived from wave aberrations predict visual performance. J Vis 2004;4:322-28.

41. Martin RG, Sanders DR. A comparison of higher order aberrations following implantation of four foldable intraocular lens designs. J Refract Surg 2005;21:716-21.

42. Martinez PA, Palacin MB, Castilla CM, et al. Spherical aberration influence in visual function after cataract surgery: prospective randomized trial. Arch Soc Esp Oftalmo 2005;80:71-78.

43. McClellan JS, Marcos S, Prieto PM, Burns SA. Imperfect optics may be the eye's defence against chromatic blur. Nature. 2002;417:174-76.

44. McDonald J. Aspheric IOLs for Continuous Vision (Cataract and Refractive Surgery Today. April, 2007.

45. McGwin G Jr, Chapman V, Owsley C. Visual risk factors for driving difficulty among older drivers. Accid Anal Prev. 2000;32(6):735-44.

46. Mester U, Dillinger P, Anterist N. Impact of a modified optic design on visual function: clinical comparative study. J Cataract Refract Surg. 2003;29:652-60.

47. Mester U, Kaymak H. Spherical aberration and functional vision with the Acrysof IQ Aspheric Natural IOL. Paper presented at: The ASCRS/ASOA 2006 Symposium & Congress; March 18, 2006; San Francisco, CA.

48. Monks C. Optical spherical aberration correction. GIT Imaging and Microscopy. March 2004;2-3.

49. Munoz G, Albarran-Diego C, Montes-Mico R, et al. Spherical aberration and contrast sensitivity after cataract surgery with the Tecnis Z9000 intraocular lens. J Cataract Refract Surg 2006;32:1320-27.

50. Nichamin LD. Contrast sensitivity with an aberration-free IOL compared to conventional and negatively aspheric IOLs. Paper presented at: The XXIV Congress of the ESCRS; September 12, 2006; London, England.

51. Oliver KM, O'Bratt DPS, Stephenson CG, et al. Anterior corneal optical aberrations induced by photorefractive keratectomy. J Refract Surg. 1997;13:246-54.

52. Owsley C, Stalvey BT, Wells J, et al. Visual risk factors for crash involvement in older drivers with cataract. Arch Ophthalmol 2001;119(6):881-87.

53. Packer M, Fine IH, Hoffman RS, Piers PA. Improved functional vision with a modified prolate intraocular lens. J Cataract Refract Surg 2004;30:986-92.

54. Packer M, Fine IH, Hoffman RS, Piers PA. Prospective randomized trial of an anterior surface modified prolate intraocular lens. J Refract Surg 2002;18:692-96.

55. Piers PA, Fernandez EJ, Manzanera S, et al. Adaptive optics simulation of intraocular lenses with modified spherical aberration. Invest Ophthalmol Vis Sci 2004;45:4601-10.

56. Rohart C, Lemarinel B, Thanh HX, Gatinel D. Ocular aberrations after cataract surgery with hydrophobic and hydrophilic acrylic intraocular lenses: comparative study. J Cataract Refract Surg 2006;32:1201-05.

57. Rubin GS, Bandeen-Roche K, Huang GH, et al. The association of multiple visual impairments with self-reported visual disability: SEE project. Invest Ophthalmol Vis Sci 2001;42(1)64-62.

58. Rynders M, Lidkea B, Chisolm W, Thibos LN. Statistical distribution of foveal transverse chromatic aberrations, pupil centration, and angle w in a population of young adult eyes. J Opt Soc Am A 1995;12:2348-57.

59. Sarver EJ, Li Wang, Koch DD. The Effect of Decentration on Higher-Order Aberrations.(Precisely placing aspheric IOLs is important for improving patients' visual quality. Cataract and Refractive Surgery Today. April, 2007.

60. Sicam VA, Dubbelman M, van der Heijde RG. Spherical aberration of the anterior and posterior surfaces of the human cornea. J Opt Soc Am A Opt Image Sci Vis. 2006;23:544-49.

61. Smith G, Atchison DA. The Eye and Visual Optic Instruments. Cambridge University Press: Cambridge; 1997.

62. Smith G, Cox MJ, Calver R, Garner LF. The spherical aberration of the crystalline lens of the human eye. Vision Res. 2001;41:235-43

63. Smith WJ. Modern optical engineering. 3rd ed. New York, NY: McGraw-Hill, 2000.

64. Tabernero J, Piers P, Benito A, et al. Predicting the optical performance of eyes implanted with IOLs to correct spherical aberration. Invest Ophthalmol Vis Sci 2006;47:4651-58.

65. Taketani F, Yukawa E, Yoshii T, et al. Influence of intraocular lens optical design on high-order aberrations. J Cataract Refract Surg 2005;31:969-72.

66. Takhchidi K, Malyugin B, Demiancehnko S. Akreos AO vs Acrysof: visual and aberrometric results // Presented at the XXIV Congress of the ESCRS, London, 2006.

67. Valois RL, Valois KK. Spatial Vision. Oxford, England: Oxford University Press, 1988.

68. Wang L, Dai E, Koch DD, Nathoo A. Optical aberrations of the human anterior cornea. J Cataract Refract Surg. 2003;29:1514-21.

69. Wang L, Koch DD. Anterior corneal optical aberrations induced by laser in situ keratomileusis for hyperopia. J Cataract Refract Surg. 2003; 29:1702-08.

70. Wang L, Santaella RM, Booth M, Koch DD. Higher-order aberrations from the internal optics of the eye. J Cataract Refract Surg. 2005;31:1512-19.

71. Wang Y, Zhao K, Jin Y, et al. Changes of higher order aberration with various pupil sizes in the myopic eye. J Refract Surg. 2003;19(2 suppl):S270-S74.

Chapter 58

1.8 mm C-MICS Phaco Chop with the Stellaris System

Boris Malyugin (Russia)

INTRODUCTION

Incision minimization is the natural evolution of the cataract surgery. This allows for reduction of operative trauma, decreases the possibility of infection and maximizes visual acuity restoration.

The standard practice today is coaxial phacoemulsification with incisions starting from 2.0 mm and wider, more often 2.75 mm in length. MICS or micro incision cataract surgery – the term introduced by J.Alio several years ago as opposed to the standard technique is considered by most of the surgeons as the technique utilizing the incisions 2.0 mm or less.

By performing cataract removal through smaller incisions, the surgeons are able to provide their patients with earlier visual rehabilitation and stabilization as well as higher quality of vision.

In a growing field of refractive cataract surgery there is trend to microincision procedures that will increasingly be required. The MICS technique is truly astigmatically neutral, which makes it ideal for refractive lens exchange, and it is associated with less likelihood for postoperative wound leakage compared with a larger incision procedure so that the risk of endophthalmitis is theoretically reduced.

There is also less risk of intraoperative complications. Quicker cataract surgery through smaller incisions uses less phaco power. Surge suppression helps to reduce capsular ruptures due to sudden chamber shallowing and posterior capsule "trampolining". There is less risk of burns, corneal edema and endothelial cell loss.

MICS is not an absolutely new surgical technique but rather the modification of the existing procedures. Currently two versions of MICS are available: B-MICS (biaxial) and C-MICS (coaxial). The biaxial technique described more than 20 years ago (Shearing, 1985) is still not widely adopted by the ophthalmic surgery community. The main reasons for this include the high risk of chamber instability, necessity to decrease fluidic parameters, and the absence of protective effect of a silicone sleeve introduced between vibrating US needle and the corneal wound.

Surgical Equipment

In 2007, Bausch & Lomb entered the market with the new Stellaris™ Vision Enhancement system (Fig. 1). This is a new generation of the phaco systems designed especially for the MICS procedures

The most useful characteristics of Stellaris include a compact, portable and easier to set up design. The high definition touch screen interface provides step–by–step illustrated instructions for setting up the machine. It is possible to monitor the surgery via the screen of the system (Fig. 2).

An advance to coaxial MICS has been enabled by new ultrasound technology and power modulation software. The Stellaris platform features CustomControl™ Software II, which is sophisticated software providing precise control of power modulation along with tremendous flexibility for safe and efficient cataract removal. Hyperpulse can be set up to 250 pps. Complementing its efficiency benefits is a new six-crystal handpiece for the Stellaris. This lightweight, ergonomic instrument has an increased stroke length for improved mechanical cutting, and it operates at 28.5 kHz to provide more effective cavitational energy relative to higher frequency handpieces.

New US needle is specially designed for the 1.8 mm incision coaxial surgery (Fig. 3). Thin walled transparent silicone sleeve allows for the infusion volume similar to a standard needle/sleeve combination.

Perfectly balanced EQ (equalized) fluidics and phaco power is obtained with either flow or vacuum based pump systems (AFM- Advanced Flow Module, VFM- Vacuum Fluidics Module), allowing the surgeon to choose according to his preferences (Fig. 4). In the flow mode, the Advanced Flow Module is a single module, which allows surgeons to switch between flow and vacuum modes as needed during surgery.

The Stellaris features anti surge technology with non-compliant tubing made of the more rigid material and with thicker walls. StableChamber™ tubing system minimizes and virtually eliminates post occlusion surges in high fluidics settings. Chamber stability is further enhanced by a micromesh filter,

353

which removes nuclear particles larger than 0.5 mm and prevents lens particles from clogging the aspiration line and allowing the flow and vacuum to be maintained as a constant. With the new tubing, surgeons can perform high vacuum phaco and maintain positive IOP with a deep and stable chamber even on occlusion break. In addition a bypass valve opens during surges monitored with advanced sensors to pull fluid from the irrigation bottle but not from the anterior chamber.

Added features of the Stellaris platform include an all electric system with no need for nitrogen tanks and external gas lines, a wireless, Bluetooth®-controlled foot pedal and voice confirmation of input changes (Fig. 5). The system is also equipped for direct Internet connection to B&L for online troubleshooting assistance, via the TruLink™ Customer Support Network.

Stellaris can be used for standard small-incision coaxial surgery but was designed primarily to optimize MICS using either a biaxial or coaxial technique.

1.8 mm C-MICS Surgical Technique

The modern concept in phacoemulsification is no longer based on the primary role of the US energy but rather on the optimal combination of the mechanical cutting, ultrasonic emulsification and vacuum aspiration. Before 1993 Divide & Conquer and *in situ* Fracture were the golden standards of phacoemulsification. It took several minutes of sculpting trenches or grooves before actually fracturing the lens nucleus into quadrants, requiring significant amounts of the ultrasonic energy to be delivered as well as causing pressure on the lens zonular apparatus.

This was until Dr K Nagahara described his revolutionary technique which he called Phaco Chop. His analogy of cataract splitting and wood chopping is currently widely accepted by the ophthalmic surgeons. Nowadays the array of chopping techniques modified by several authors include the Quick Chop technique, combined trenching and chopping (Stop & Chop), different variations of horizontal and vertical chopping, etc. Commonly referred to as "phaco chop", they are faster, more efficient and safer than traditional techniques based on sculpting and cracking.

Multiple designs of the choppers initially described as a "modified lens hook" are currently available. Some of them are longer, others are shorter, with sharp or blunt edges, stick or blade-like tip shapes, with different angles of attack.

What is common to all of the above mentioned techniques and instrumentation is the main surgical principle. The surgical approach involves using the US needle to hold and stabilize the nucleus with high vacuum and the second instrument (chopper) is buried in the nucleus and acts as an axe, causing its split first in a half and then into quarters or even smaller pieces according to the hardness of the lens material.

I personally prefer the micro coaxial approach. With Stellaris a new needle/sleeve combination designed to fit gently through a 1.8 mm incision provides inflow volume comparable to that achieved with traditional coaxial tips. The flexible sleeve walls also guarantee a perfect seal against the incision to eliminate outflow from the eye. In addition, the sleeve wall is designed to deliver more infusion laterally to minimize repulsion of nuclear fragments from the tip and improve followability.

The fluidics system of the Stellaris is also optimized for safe, efficient, and controlled microcoaxial surgery with components that include advanced pump technology and StableChamber high-vacuum, flow resistant, evacuation tubing.

Chamber stability is excellent therefore surgeons can use high vacuum settings to maximize holding force and emulsification efficiency. High vacuum settings are great for holding the nucleus and it fragments during phaco chop maneuvers. Increased flow and vacuum improve evacuation efficiency with no repulsion of the lens fragments and reduce the phaco energy needed to emulsify the lens. There was no need to raise the irrigating fluid bottle above its usual height or to use any adjunctive devices to increase infusion in order to maintain anterior chamber stability.

We conducted a study in order to assess the safety and efficacy of surgery using the new Stellaris system. Seventy five patients (75 eyes) were operated utilizing the 1.8 mm C-MICS technique.

Differential Approach

As it was already mentioned, numerous methods of nucleus disassembly have been described. As the nucleus densities are variable in size and density, there is no one universal technique that fits all clinical situations. My current concept is to use a spectrum of techniques of nucleus division and emulsification which I have found helpful in my own surgical practice. Patient selection is an essential factor in determining the best surgical technique. I divide my patients in one of three categories:

1. *Soft nucleus:* This kind of nucleus is impossible to chop because it can not withstand the high vacuum levels. That is why it has a tendency to be fragmented before the phaco tip can be fixated by the US needle to initiate the chop.

2. *Moderately dense nucleus:* It is most suitable for the quick chop technique. After performing continuous curvilinear capsulorhexis and introducing the US handpiece in the anterior chamber, the anterior soft portion of epinuclear material is aspirated without ultrasound. Then the US needle is impaled in the lens nucleus, holding it with high vacuum while the second instrument (chopper) is used to chop it. Vertical chopping is preferable because in this case more peripheral placement of the chopper and subsequent risk of anterior capsule rupture are greatly avoided. When the chopper is pulled towards the phaco tip, I activate a short burst of ultrasound. Just before contact of two instruments, they are then separated sufficiently to create the fracture. After chopping the nucleus into two halves it is rotated clockwise and each half divided into two or three quadrants, depending on the lens hardness. The latter are removed with the ultrasound-assisted phaco aspiration technique when minimal US energy is used, only to assist aspiration. The mechanical force of the chopper that mashes the smaller nucleus pieces in the phaco tip at this stage of the operation further decreases the small amount of ultrasound needed.

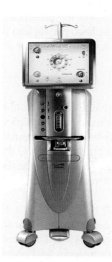

Fig. 1: Stellaris Vision Enhancement System (Bausch & Lomb) general view

FOOTPEDAL

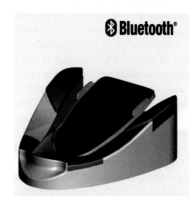

- Wireless technology
- **Dual linear-** Simultaneous control of US and aspiration
- Programmable
- Ergonomically designed

Fig. 2: New design US needle with sleeve for 1.8 mm coaxial phaco

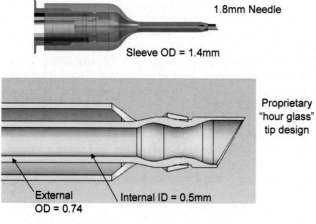

1.8mm Needle

Sleeve OD = 1.4mm

Proprietary "hour glass" tip design

External OD = 0.74

Internal ID = 0.5mm

- The flexible sleeve fits gently with the corneal 1.8 mm incision and enables significantly more flow than bimanual choppers
- It guarantees a perfect seal and eliminates outflow for the wound

Fig. 3: Wireless footpedal

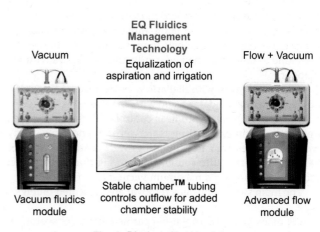

Vacuum

EQ Fluidics Management Technology
Equalization of aspiration and irrigation

Flow + Vacuum

Vacuum fluidics module

Stable chamber™ tubing controls outflow for added chamber stability

Advanced flow module

Fig. 4: Display with video inlay

355

3. *Dense or very dense nucleus*: The Stop & Chop technique first described by P Koch (1994) works best in this situation. First the central groove is created and the nucleus is cracked in half. Then each half is chopped into smaller bite-size pieces. By making a central groove, the surgeon creates room for the subsequently chopped fragments to ease their mobilization from within the capsular bag.

In cases of a very dense nucleus the posterior nucleus contains bridging leathery bands that prevent its complete separation. When operating on a hard brown lenses, I prefer to use the stop and chop technique. First I make a very deep central groove until the red reflex can be visible through the remaining posterior nucleus layers. I have found it very convenient to work with the microcoaxial tip in the deep groove. More over, as the sleeve is transparent and I can visualize lens tissue through it, this gives an additional margin of safety. Then I crack the lens in two parts. After rotating 90 degrees, each half of the nucleus is sliced into 4-6 peaces each (depending on the lens hardness, more fragments are needed in extremely hard nuclei). Using dual linear foot pedal control, I can achieve a tremendous grasping force that results in immediate emulsification and rapid evacuation of the nucleus fragments.

Using the Stellaris, even hard fragments are attracted rapidly to the phaco tip and easily aspirated. Although proponents of torsional phaco may point out that longitudinal ultrasound causes repulsion of nuclear fragments, I believe that phenomenon only occurs if the fluidic parameters are not properly selected so that there is not enough vacuum to achieve efficient aspiration. At the final step, when removing the remaining small nucleus fragments, I position my US needle at the center of the pupil below the level of the iris. This positions the needle at the optimal distance from the most delicate anterior chamber structures. I prefer not to move the US handpiece but rather to wait for the fragments to move directly to the needle from time to time assisting and conducting the pieces with the chopper.

All my surgeries with Stellaris were performed through a 1.6 × 1.8 mm trapezoidal incision with an infusion bottle height of 100 cm and using dual linear control. Ultrasound settings were 30% maximum, 80 pulses per second, and a 50% duty cycle, and aggressive vacuum settings were used, consisting of 400 mm Hg during ultrasound, 550 mm Hg during irrigation and aspiration, and the maximum vacuum rise time of "1".

The main steps of nucleus removal are presented on Figs 6 to 14.

For many years, I do not use separate settings for sculpting, chopping and removal of epinucleus. It is unnecessary to restrict myself to preset parameters. I prefer to set the highest limits of the US and flow, where I am absolutely confident rock-stable anterior chamber and sufficient power to emulsify the lens nucleus is guaranteed. Dual linear foot pedal control allows me to be very flexible in changing my instant surgical parameters depending on the intraoperative environment and stage of the surgery.

The microcoaxial approach makes it easier to operate in an eye with a hard nucleus because the smaller phaco needle penetrates more readily into a dense lens compared with a standard tip. With a small diameter US needle it is easier to engage and aspirate the epinucleus material with less chance of accidental aspiration and rupture of the posterior capsule.

Intraocular visualization is improved when operating in eyes with small pupils and the presence of the silicone sleeve between the vibrating phaco needle and the incision enhances corneal thermal protection to ensure a watertight incision postoperatively.

IOL Considerations

The previously available IOLs that could be delivered through a sub-2 mm incision suffered from multiple drawbacks, including fragility, poor stability within the capsular bag, problems with halos and glare, and a high risk of PCO due to the absence of a sharp edge optic design. These limitations have been successfully overcome with the introduction of the Akreos MI60 (MI60) IOL.

The Akreos MI60 IOL (MI60) is a single-piece implant constructed of a time-tested hydrophilic acrylic material with a good refractive index (1.458). The aberration-free optic is biconvex with aspheric anterior and posterior surfaces having uniform power from center to edge. It is available in dioptric powers ranging from +10.0 to +30.0 D in 0.5 D increments. Optic diameter and overall length vary depending on the dioptric power. Three overall lengths ensure optimal in-the-bag fit across the spectrum of capsular bag sizes from myopes to hyperopes.

The Akreos MI60 IOL is designed to maintain intraocular stability and prevent posterior capsule opacification (PCO). Its haptics provide four-point fixation in the capsular bag and have flexible tips that bend as the capsular bag contracts. As a result, the Akreos MI60 is able to resist the forces of capsular bag contraction and does not tilt or vault, but remains centered within the capsular bag over time. A 10° angulation of the haptics ensures early flattening against the posterior capsule, and 360° capsular contact is reinforced by the optic's continuous posterior square edge.

In all my C-MICS cases Akreos MI60 IOL was implanted with a wound-assisted technique through a 1.8 mm incision. The new lens is easy to load and deliver, and using a wound-assisted implantation technique, surgeons will find they are able to maintain a sub-2 mm final incision after only a short learning curve.

Results

The study enrolled 75 eyes that had a mean nuclear density of 2.85 ± 0.27. Average US power was $13\pm1.4\%$, average phaco time 22.8 ± 4.2 sec, elapsed phaco time 3.46 ± 0.76 sec.

Good clinical outcomes were achieved in the wide range of cataract hardness. The postoperative visual acuity results were favorable. At the first visit, 1 to 2 days after surgery, mean UCVA was 0.67 and mean BCVA was 0.83. By 1 week, mean UCVA had improved to 0.74 and mean BCVA was 0.85. Although the initial series of 50 eyes is preliminary and small, the results are very impressive.

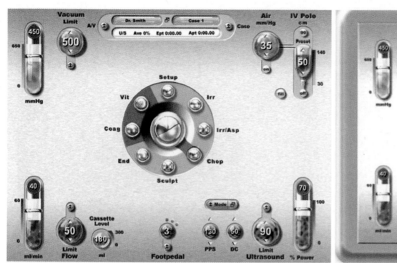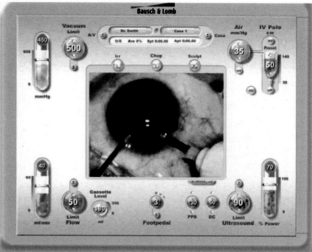

Fig. 5: Fluidics management technology of Stellaris with Stable Chamber™ tubing

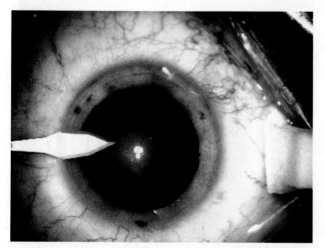

Fig. 6: Clear corneal incision with 1.6x1.8 mm trapezoidal metal keratome

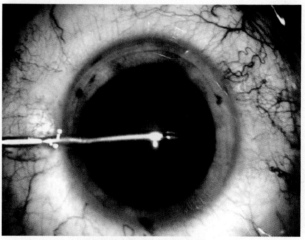

Fig. 7: Continuous curvilinear capsulotomy with forceps

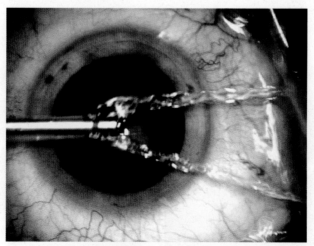

Fig. 8: High volume infusion is achieved with the
new needle/sleeve combination

357

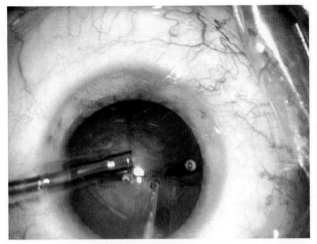

Fig. 9: Nucleus is divided into two halves with the chop maneuver

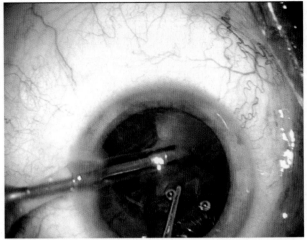

Fig. 12: Removal of nuclear quadrants

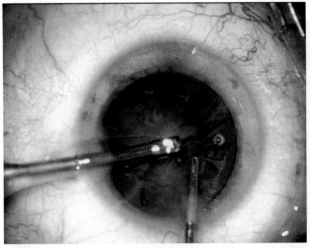

Fig. 10: Removal of nuclear quadrants

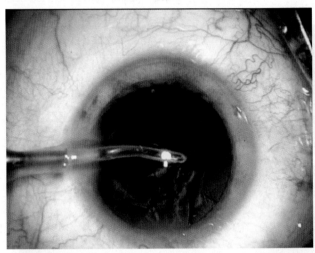

Fig. 13: Irrigation-aspiration with single use curved-coaxial handpiece (B&L)

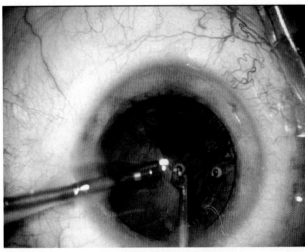

Fig. 11: Removal of nuclear quadrants

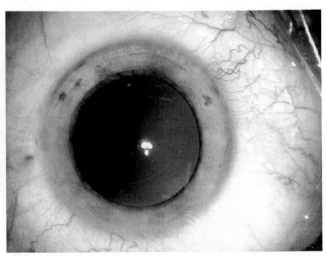

Fig. 14: Lens emulsification is completed

CONCLUSION

Transition to the new technique as well as the new equipment is always challenging. The C-MICS chop technique is more difficult than many other techniques, and it is suitable only for bimanual phaco surgeons. At the same time it is fast, allows reducing phaco time, minimizing corneal endothelial damage caused by excessive ultrasonic energy and also lessens the stress of the lens zonular apparatus.

The evolution of the modern phaco technique eliminates or substantially decreases US reliance. The efficiency of the combination of the hyperpulse with excellent fluidics and chamber stability is so obvious that the use of transverse oscillations of the phaco tip seem to add little or nothing to the overall efficiency and safety profile of the procedure. The learning curve with Stellaris was very short and most intuitive.

The Stellaris Vision Enhancement System is advanced technology that enables coaxial surgery through a 1.8 mm incision to be performed safely and effectively regardless of lens density. An ultrasound needle and sleeve system designed specifically for coaxial MICS provides sufficient inflow, and in conjunction with the advanced fluidics system of the Stellaris, ensures safe, surgeproof surgery. Followability is excellent so that surgery is completed efficiently using energy comparable to that delivered when performing a coaxial procedure through a larger incision. This experience supports the conclusion that coaxial MICS with the Stellaris Vision Enhancement System is friendly to the eye, the patient, and the surgeon. This is an invaluable addition to the ophthalmic surgeon armamentarium.

BIBLIOGRAPHY

1. Alio J, et al. Outcomes of microincision cataract surgery versus coaxial phacoemulsification. Ophthalmology 2005;112:1997-2003.
2. Koch P. Simplifying Phacoemulsification. Safe and efficient methods of cataract surgery. SLACK Inc, 1997;223.
3. Kohnen T (ed). Modern Cataract Surgery. S Karger AG 2002;244.
4. Kurz S, Krummenauer F, Gabriel P, Pfeiffer N, Dick HB. Biaxial microincision versus coaxial small-incision clear cornea cataract surgery. Ophthalmology 2006;113:1818-26.
5. Shearing SP, Relyea RL, Loaiza A, Shearing RL. Routine phacoemulsification through a one-millimeter nonsutured incision. Cataract 1985;2:6-11.
6. Yao K, Tang X, Ye P. Corneal astigmatism, higher order aberrations, and optical quality after cataract surgery: microincision versus small incision. J Ref Surg 2006;22(9 Suppl):S1079-82.

Chapter 59

Lens Laser Combination Surgery

Arun C Gulani (USA)

SPECIFICS

Topical anesthesia, Sutureless On-Axis incision, Elegant, small incision, vision-directed surgery

Concept

Always maintain elegant, least interventional surgery to aim for best and fastest vision outcomes- Principles of Corneoplastique.

Steps Seen in Images

- The Dystrophic, scarred cornea with Advanced Cataract and shallow AC with High Hyperopia.
- Anterior Lamellar Keratectomy was commenced to remove the bulk of the Dystrophic corneal scar
- Viscoat was used to coat the anterior cornea for visibility to commence capsulorhexis
- The capsulorhexis being performed

- Hydrodissection with Nuclear flip into AC
- Lateral engaging of Phaco tip (supra-capsular)- Gulani LaLop technique (Lateral Lollipop)
- I and A for complete cortical removal
- IOL deployed and unfolding into the capsular bag
- Incision hydration with suture less closure

Advantages

Instead of subjecting such patients to triple procedure of PKP with cataract surgery and resulting in less than perfect vision and that too with highly interventional surgery and lifetime of restrictions, this patient saw 20/40 next day.

A month later I performed Excimer laser on her cornea to correct her residual scars and ammetropia along with astigmatism. She sees 20/20 in this eye and looks like any normal cataract case if seen on slit-lamp.

These are the principles of Corneoplastique™

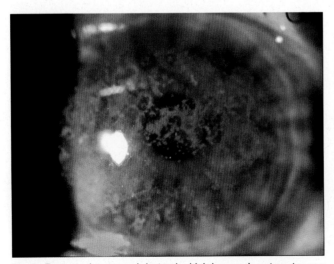

Fig. 1: Preoperative corneal dystrophy high hyperopia cataract preop

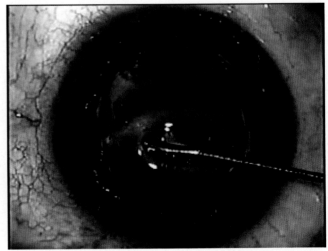

Fig. 2: Visco coating for visibility for capsulorhexis

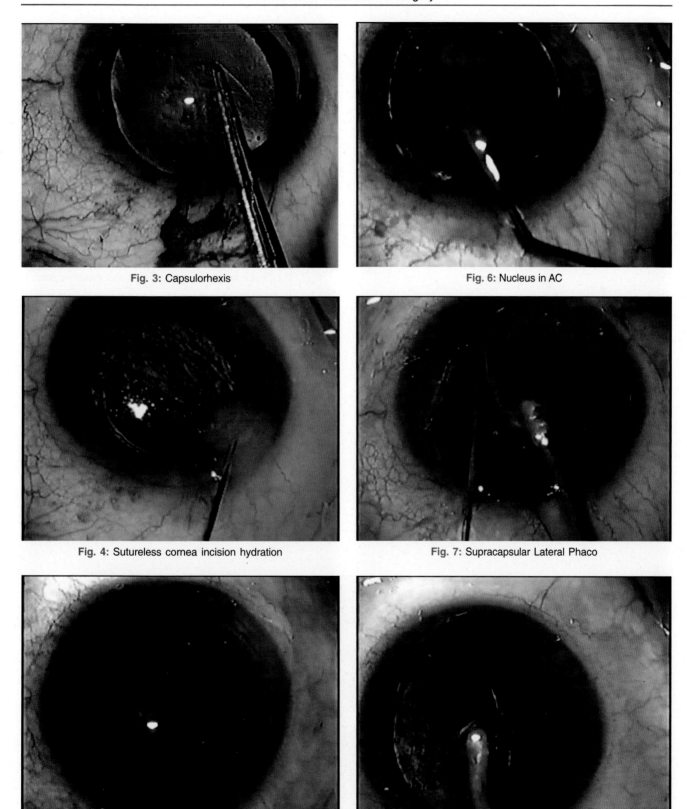

Fig. 3: Capsulorhexis

Fig. 6: Nucleus in AC

Fig. 4: Sutureless cornea incision hydration

Fig. 7: Supracapsular Lateral Phaco

Fig. 5: Hydrodissection for nuclear flip

Fig. 8: IA for complete cortical clean-up

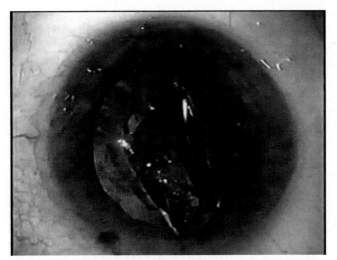

Fig. 9: IOL deployed

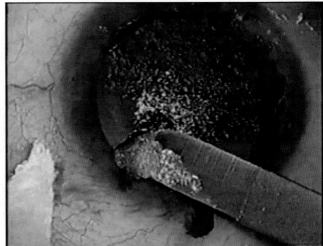

Fig. 12: Lamellar keartectomy for visibility and debulking scar

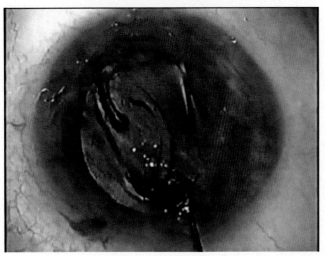

Fig. 10: IOL in the bag

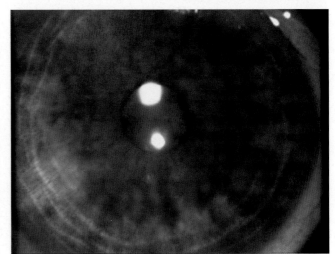

Fig. 13: Postop 2025 Vision

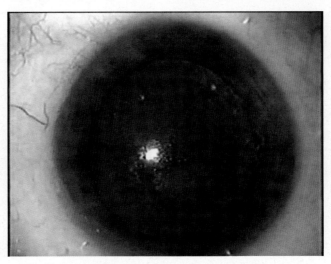

Fig. 11: Corneal dystrophy high hyperopia cataract in surgery

Chapter 60

The AT LISA Toric Multifocal IOL
The Customization of Microincision Phaco-refractive Surgery

Carlo F Lovisolo (Italy)

AT LISA is an acronym given by Zeiss-Meditec to its family of multifocal IOLs, which sums up the technical key features of the optical platform. L stands for Light distributed asymmetrically between distant (65 %) and near focus (35 %) to provide a spectacle-free lifestyle; I for Independency from pupil size due to the diffractive-refractive microstructure of the optic; S for Smooth steps for a lens diffractive grate surface without sharp angles for ideal optical imaging quality with reduced light scattering (SMP technology), to limit the photic symptoms caused by simultaneous vision; A is for Aberration correcting optimized aspheric optic for better contrast sensitivity and sharper vision.

The 366 D single piece plate haptic model is based on the Acri-Smart platform, the first successful micro-incision IOL for cataract surgery previously designed and marketed by AcriTEC (Henningsdorf, Germany). It is made in hydrophilic acrylate (25% H_2O) with hydrophobic surface. The available dioptric powers range from 0.0 to +32.0 D, while the near addition is +3.75 D at IOL plane. The optic size is 6.0 mm, the overall length 11.0 mm and the haptic angulation is 0°. It may be implanted through an astigmatically neutral microincision of 1.5 mm (Fig. 1).

Outside the eye, with computer simulation from an optical bench—artificial eye as compared to the performance of an emmetropic presbyopic eye (Figs 2A to C) and in clinical practise (Fig. 2D),[1-4] the AT LISA platform provides excellent near and distance vision, with an effective intermediate vision and a low level of disturbing visual phenomena.

The outstanding performance of the AT LISA in terms of optical quality has been reported.[3] On average, more than 90% of patients show a complete independence from glasses for all tasks. RMS values for intraocular aberrations with a pupil diameter of 5 and 6 mm are usually better than those obtained in eyes implanted with standard spherical monofocal IOLs. Overall spherical aberration, in particolar, typically shows values around zero (Fig. 3A) The split of the incoming optical radiation to different focus points inevitably causes a decrease of contrast sensitivity in multifocal and bifocal IOLs due to the simultaneous overlapping of out-of-focus images. Nevertheless, normal range contrast sensitivity values have been demonstrated[1,2,4] in photopic and mesopic conditions. Moreover, the competitive analysis against other multifocal IOLs available on the market shows the superior performance of the AT LISA IOL (Fig. 3B) Studies consistently report low levels of halos, glare and other visual phenomena, such as night driving problems with the AT LISA.

Residual astigmatism is a well known detrimental factor to the postoperative quality of vision with multifocal IOLs. A double Sturm conoid through the retina creates a less than tolerable dispersive interference among the focal lines, which degrades the optical quality. Moreover, a phenomenon called merional aniseikonia, i.e. the unequal magnification of the retinal images, may contribute to an unpleasant distortion in spatial perception. Incisional or excimer laser surgeries are therefore usually combined. However, the poor accuracy of the limbal relaxing incisions for cylinder corrections higher than 2.00 diopters and the costs, the risks, the delayed recovery and the difficulties in managing the aberrations with custom LASIK and PRK have stimulated the industry to provide a piece of technology that combines the toric correction to the multifocal optic. The AT LISA toric 466TD has finally filled the gap (Fig. 4A). By maintaining the same aspheric diffractive-refractive posterior surface of the AT LISA family, the toric correction is put on the anterior surface by using the Acri Comfort technology, which already showed unrivaled rotational stability and the exceptional results from the intraocular compensation of high, even extreme, astigmatic errors (Fig. 4B). The cylinder correction ranges from +1.0 to +12.0 D in 0.5 D increments. More than 2 years results for the AT LISA toric show that it provides excellent functional outcomes and patient satisfaction. Since the AT LISA is the only multifocal IOL that can be inserted througha microincision of 1.5 mm, it minimizes the chance of surgically induced astigmatism.

Keys to successful implantation include an efficient preliminary workflow, with sophisticated technologies like aberrometry, corneal topography and tomography (to detect irregular astigmatism like forme fruste keratoconus), OCT and fundus perimetry to carefully evaluate suspect macular, optic nerve disorders and amblyopic eyes, tear function test to detect

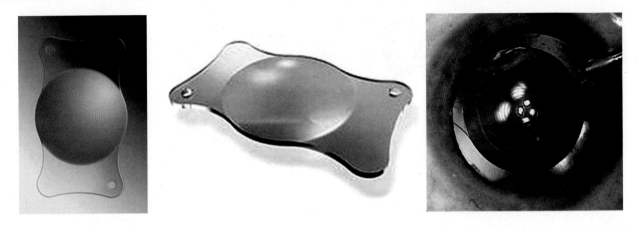

Fig. 1

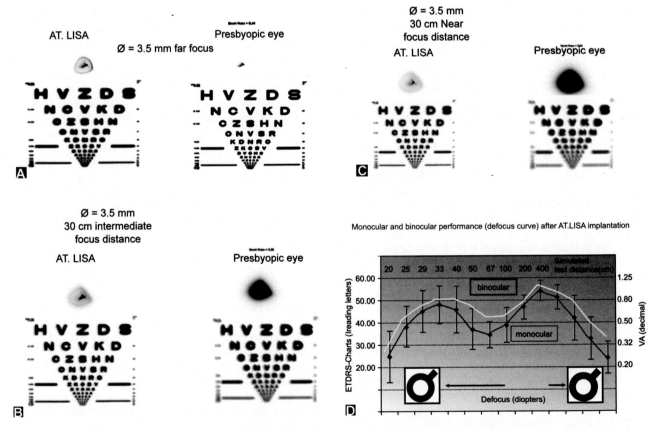

Figs 2A to D

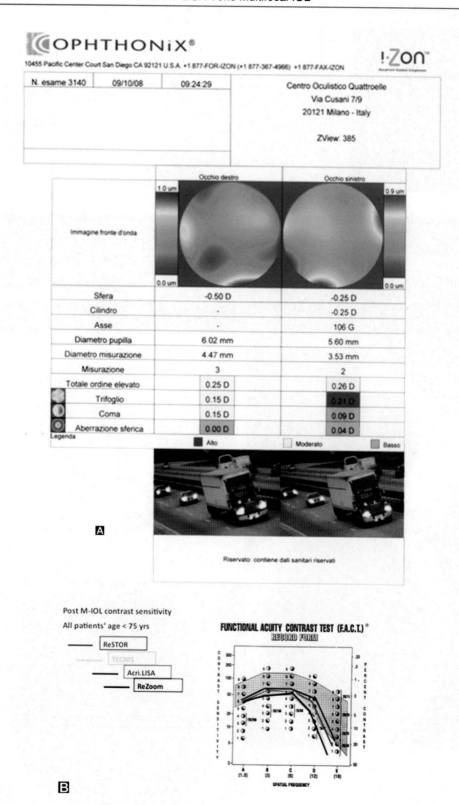

Figs 3A and B

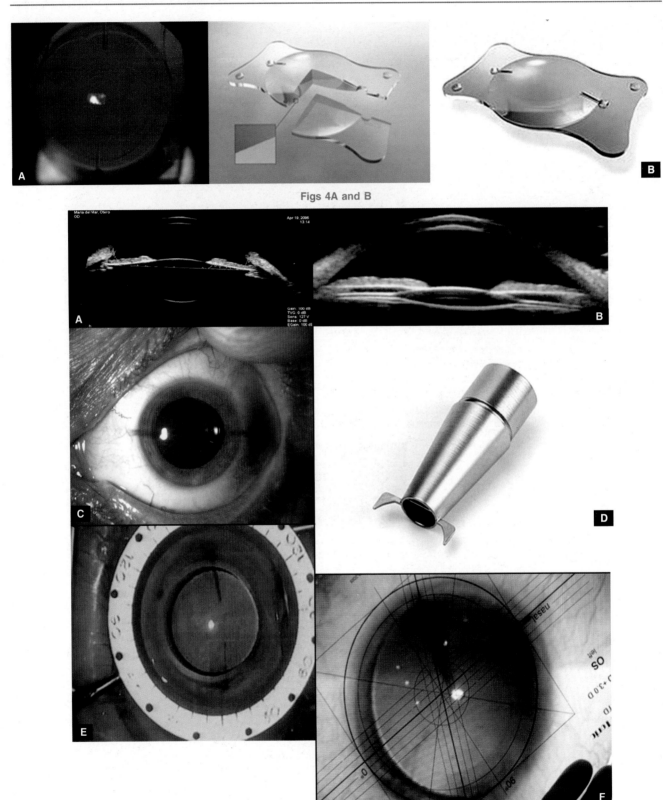

Figs 4A and B

Figs 5A to F

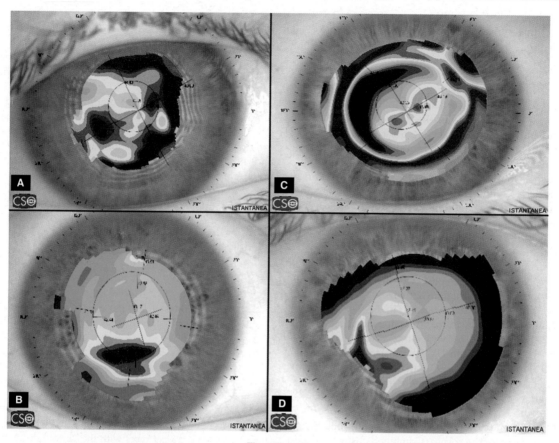

Figs 6A to D

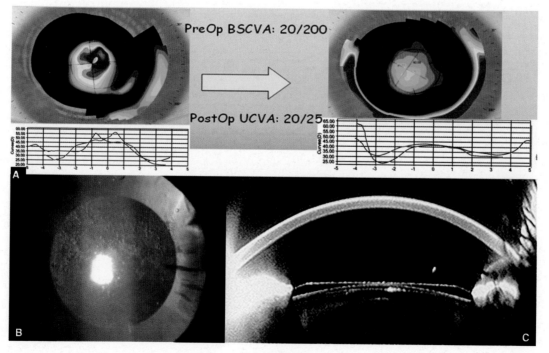

Figs 7A to C

dry eye, high precision optical biometry (IOLMASTER), an adjusted formula and very high frequency echography (Figs 5A and B) to precisely calculate the effective lens position (ELP), specially in the hyperopic population, to obtain emmetropia. Intraoperatively, the position of the reference marks placed horizontally at the slit lamp with special instruments (Figs 5C and D) are checked with a videokeratographic image. With the patient lying at the surgical table, the surgeon marks the steep axis with the help of a Mendez ruler (Fig. 5E) Coaxial or bimanual microincision cataract surgery is required to guarantee the astigmatic neutrality. A regular rhexis of 5 to 5.5 mm and a zealous viscoelastic gel removal are needed. At the end of surgery, the perfect alignment of the IOL's steep meridian lines with the corneal markings is double checked by the surgeon and the assistant who overlaps a transparent leaf provided by the company to the surgical monitor (Fig. 5F).

Some challenging cases, many of them previously considered as absolute contraindications to multifocal IOL implantation, can now be managed with the 466TD AT LISA. Residual ammetropia with high astigmatism after lamellar or penetrating keratoplasty, for instance (Fig. 6A), stable ectatic corneal disorders like pellucid marginal degeneration or early stages of keratoconus stabilized with intrastromal ring segments or collagen cross-linking with UV-A and riboflavin (Fig. 6C), post-trauma corneal scars (Fig. 6D) can be excellent candidates provided that the astigmatism is regular in the pupillary area.

Challenging postkerato-refractive surgery cases may also be faced,[5] at the condition that the original photoablative treatment is well centred and respectful of the physiologically prolate shape profile of the cornea. Combined custom ablation touch ups are often needed, as well as adequate expertise to calculate the IOL power.

The case presented in (Fig. 7A) showed an excessively prolate and irregular cornea after termokeratoplasty for hyperopic correction. The AT LISA was calculated and implanted six months after a topo-linked transepithelial surface ablation was performed to restore the physiological shape of the anterior surface of the cornea.

466TD AT LISA was very helpful in managing a case of unilateral iatrogenic cataract induced by an undersized toric ICL (Figs 7B and C) in a 33-year-old patient with a myopic astigmatism. The fellow eye's unaided vision was 20/20 for far and J1 for near. Postoperative disparity of accommodation from unilateral multifocality was well tolerated and the patient did not complain of significant loss of quality of vision in the AT LISA toric aphakic eye as compared to the toric ICL phakic fellow eye.

REFERENCES

1. Alfonso J, Fernández-Vega L, Señaris A, et al. Prospective study of the AT. LISA bifocal intraocular lens. J Cataract Refract Surg 2007;33:1930-35.

2. Kaymak H, Mester U. First results with a new aberration-correcting bifocal intraocular lens. Ophthalmologe 2007;104:1046-51.

3. Alió J, Elkady B, Ortiz D, et al. Clinical outcomes and intraocular optical quality of a diffractive multifocal intraocular lens with asymmetrical light distribution. J Cataract Refract Surg 2008;34:942-48.

4. Mai C, Torun N, Friederici L, et al. Bilateral results from a new diffractive multifocal lens. In: DOG. Berlin, Germany; 2008.

5. Lovisolo C. Special cases with the Toric Acri LISA multifocal IOL. Presented at the XXVI congress of the ESCRS, Berlin 2008.

Chapter 61

Capsular Bag Refilling Using Capsulotomy-Capturing Intraocular Lens

Okihiro Nishi, Kayo Nishi, Yutaro Nishi, Shiao Chang (Japan)

INTRODUCTION

Refilling the lens capsule with an injectable material, while preserving capsular integrity including zonules and ciliary muscles, offers a potential to restore ocular accommodation.[1,2] (Fig. 1) The greatest technical challenge in this procedure was primarily preventing the leakage of injectable IOLs.[3-6]

To prevent leakage, we developed a silicone plug to seal the capsular opening.[7,8] (Fig. 2) We could confirm some accommodation in the young macaca monkeys. Figure 3 shows the Scheimpflug photographies of the eye of a monkey before and after surgery, showing evidence of some accommodation being obtained. After application of 4% pilocarpine, there is thickening of the lens with steepening of the anterior capsule and shallowing of the anterior chamber, both before and after surgery, although the findings were much less marked after surgery.

From these experiments, we have concluded that refilling the lens capsule is technically quite feasible. It is suggested that the process may restore ocular accommodation in humans. However, there are some essential problems to overcome: Refining and simplifying the technique; Prevention of anterior capsule opacification (ACO) and posterior capsule opacification (PCO); Reducing surgically-induced astigmatism because the unilateral CCC, though tiny, caused a great astigmatism (unpublished data).

Here, I will demonstrate a completely new concept and novel lens refilling procedure that may solve these problems. We had this concept already in 1989[9] and resumed the technique, because endocapsular balloon technique and the capsular plug technique will not be supposed to be applied clinically, and the technique will solve the problems mentioned above.

REFILLING THE LENS CAPSULE WITH CAPSULOTOMY-CAPTURING INTRAOCULAR LENS

IOL

The IOL shape is similar to that of a conventional IOL, but the optic has small narrow grooves over its entire circumference (Fig. 4). The CCC edge is put in this groove, which chokes the IOL, preventing leakage of the injected material. Figure 5 illustrates the procedure. Figure 6 shows the most recent foldable version of the IOL.

Surgical Procedure

As in conventional cataract surgery, CCC, around 4 mm in diameter, is created in the middle of the anterior capsule. After phacoemulsification aspiration, viscoelastics are injected into the capsular bag in the usual manner. The folded IOL is introduced entirely into the capsular bag. A sinskey hook is introduced underneath the IOL, and the IOL is lifted by the hook, so that the optic edge groove of the lower half of the IOL is captured by the lower half of the CCC. The lower half of the groove is captured almost automatically while lifting the lower half of the IOL, because the IOL is firmly fixed in the middle by both haptics remaining in the capsular bag. Then, the viscoelastics are completely removed by aspiration, during which an I/A cannula is introduced underneath the upper half of the IOL, which is now outside of the capsular bag. Viscoelastics are injected into the anterior chamber onto the IOL. The upper half of the IOL is then captured by the CCC by pushing the IOL downward and posteriorly at the middle part of the IOL optic edge with a push-pull hook until the upper IOL clears the upper CCC edge to be captured. A small portion of the CCC edge at the optic groove is now hooked with the sinskey hook and pulled slightly to introduce the injection cannula. The injectable material, actually a mix of two liquid silicones is then injected into the capsular bag. It polymerizes in 2h *in vitro*.

RESULTS AND DISCUSSION

We have refilled many pig cadaver eyes and rabbit eyes using this technique (Figs 7-10). After the IOL was correctly captured by the CCC, there was no leakage of the injected silicone. Thus, the appropriate size for the CCC, not too small to capture but not too large to capture firmly the IOL, is crucial for surgical success. If the CCC is appropriately sized, the procedure is highly reproducible. We marked a 5 mm circle on the cornea

369

using a Hoffer optic zone marker for 5 mm, according to the technique described by Wallace,[10] and used this mark as a guide for an appropriate CCC diameter around 4 mm.

Expected Mechanism of Accommodation

The expected mechanism of accommodation involves forward-movement of the IOL and thickening of the lens.

These expected mechanisms are based on two recent studies. Nawa and his coworkers[11] demonstrated the accommodation-amplitude obtained per 1 mm forward movement of the IOL. For this purpose, a ray-focusing equation for pseudophakic eyes was established using the ray-tracing method with dedicated computer software. It was found that the amplitude depends on axial length and corneal power (Table 1). In eyes with an axial length of 21 mm and an IOL with 30 diopters, 1 mm forward movement yields 2.3 D of accommodation. Accordingly, in an eye with a length of 23 mm and 24 diopters, 1.6 D of accommodation will be obtained, while only 0.8 D will be obtained with values of 27 mm and 11 diopters. These findings indicate that improvements may be obtained with the recently developed accommodating IOL such as the crysta lens or 1CU, specifically in hyperopic eyes with a short axial length.

van der Heijde and co-workers[12] measured micro-fluctuations of steady-state accommodation using ultra-sonography, and demonstrated that fluctuations in accommodation are mainly caused by fluctuations of lens thickness. They found that on average, the lens increases by about 56 μm in thickness per diopter during fluctuation. That means that 3 diopters could be obtained by about 0.17 mm change in thickness.

Enhancement of Accommodation-Amplitude and PCO-Prevention by Dual-Optic

To prevent PCO and possibly to augment accommodation-amplitude being attained, we have drafted a dual-optic concept, as Figure 11 shows. First, a conventional foldable IOL with sharp edges and the enhanced haptic angulation is implanted into the capsular bag. It has a concave optic with a minus dioptric power, which may imperatively give a greater

power to the anterior optic, achieving emmetropia. During accommodation, the anterior capsule moves forward, while the posterior capsule stays relatively unmoved, so that an anterior optic with a greater power may enhance the accommodation-amplitude attained. A large angulation of the haptic will press the sharp optic edge against the posterior capsule to create a strong compression on it for the prevention of PCO. The injected silicone mix will additionally press the IOL onto the posterior capsule. As an alternative technique, the same CCC-capturing IOL can be implanted after a posterior CCC is performed (Fig. 12). Then, a CCC-capturing IOL is introduced into the capsular bag which contains the IOL being implanted previously and captured by the anterior CCC, as already described. To refill the bag, silicone mix is injected between two IOLs that are captured by the anterior and posterior CCCs.

Summary

To summarize, the novel anterior capsule-supported IOL is technically quite feasible. Some accommodation might be obtained by forward-movement and thickening of the lens. We will test this procedure in primate eyes. Anterior and posterior capsule opacification at least in the optical axis can be avoided. Postoperative emmetropia is supposed to be achieved more easily due to the predetermined optic. One of the advantages is that postoperative in vivo power change may be possible using an adjustable IOL.

In conclusion, restoration of accommodation by refilling the lens capsule is a goal of refractive cataract surgery. Technical feasibility has been repeatedly demonstrated by obtaining some useful accommodation in primates and will be further facilitated by modern technology. Capsular opacification is one of the essential problems to be overcome. The technique shown here may provide a breakthrough for possible clinical application to refilling of the lens capsule.

Table 1: The relationship between AL and dioptric power of an MA30BA IOL and amount of accommodation per 1.0 mm forward movement							
	Axial Length (mm)						
Parameter	21.0	22.0	23.0	24.0	25.0	26.0	27.0
IOL power (IOL)	30.0	27.0	24.0	20.0	17.0	14.0	11.0
Accommodation per 1.0 mm forward IOL movement (D)	2.3	1.9	1.6	1.3	1.1	0.9	0.8

(Preprinted by permission of J Cataract Refract Surg.[11])

REFERENCES

1. Ludwig K. Physiological premises of current concepts regarding restoration of accommodation. In: Current aspects of human accommodation II (Guthoff R; Ludwig, K, Eds), Kaden, Heidelberg 2003;39-48.
2. Kessler J. Experiments in refilling the lens. Arch Ophthalmol 1964;71:412-17.
3. Parel J-M, Gelender H, Treffers WF, Norton EWD. Phaco-ersatz. Graefes Arch Clin Exp Ophthalmol 1986;224:165-73.
4. Nishi O. Refilling the lens of the rabbit eye after endocapsular cataract surgery. Folia Ophthalmol (Japan) 1987;38:1615-18.
5. Nishi O, Nakai Y, Yamada Y, Mizumoto Y. Amplitudes of accommodation of primate lenses refilled with two types of inflatable endocapsular balloons. Arch Ophthalmol 1993;111:1677-84.
6. Haefliger E, Parel J-M. Accommodation of an endocapsular silicone lens (PhakoErsatz) in the aging rhesus monkey. J Refract Corneal Surg 1994;10:550-55.
7. Nishi O, Nishi K, Mano C, Ichihara M, Honda T. Controlling the capsular shape in lens refilling. Arch Ophthalmol 1997;115:507-10.

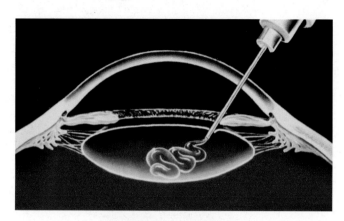

Fig. 1: Schematic illustration of the lens refilling procedure (*Courtesy of DJ Apple*)

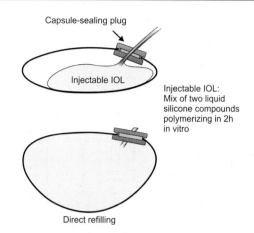

Fig. 2: Lens refilling technique using a silicone plug (Reprinted by permission of Archives of Ophthalmology[7])

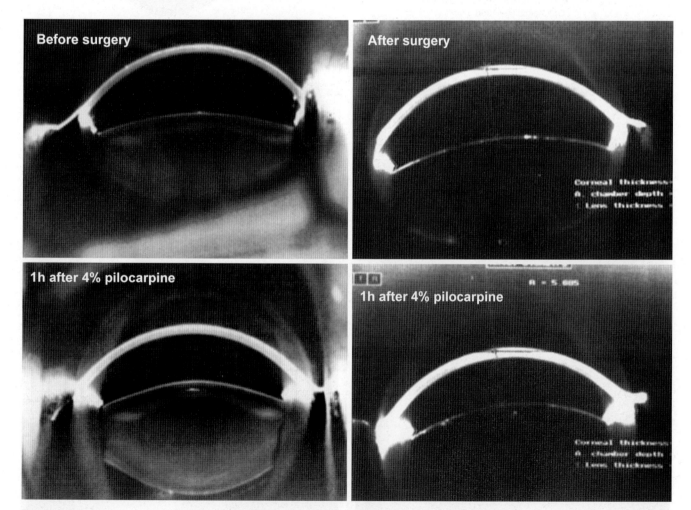

Fig. 3: Scheimpflug photographs of a monkey eye before and after refilling the lens capsule. Note that there was thickening of the lens with steepening of the anterior capsule and shallowing of the anterior chamber. After surgery (right), there were similar findings, though less remarkable. Note also that there were discontinuous zones in the lens before surgery, while the refilled lens was optically empty due to the silicone compound

Anterior Capsule-Supported IOL for Sealing CCC

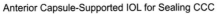
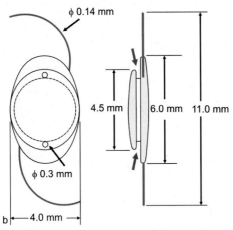

φ 0.14 mm

4.5 mm   6.0 mm   11.0 mm

φ 0.3 mm

b   4.0 mm

Nishi O, Nishi K, Graefe's Archives of Clin. Exp
Ophthalmology 1990

Fig. 4: Anterior capsule-supported IOL for sealing CCC. The arrows show the small, narrow grooves at the optic (Reprinted by permission of Graefe's Archives of Clinical and Experimental Ophthalmology[9])

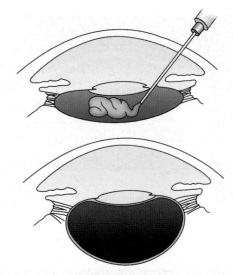

Fig. 5: Surgical lens refilling procedure using anterior capsule-supported IOL (Reprinted by permission of Graefe's Archives of Clinical and Experimental Ophthalmology[9])

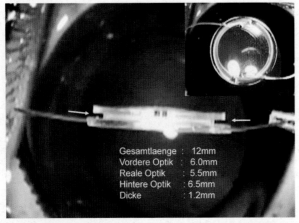

Gesamtlaenge : 12mm
Vordere Optik : 6.0mm
Reale Optik : 5.5mm
Hintere Optik : 6.5mm
Dicke : 1.2mm

Fig. 6: Anterior capsule-supported foldable IOL and its dimensions

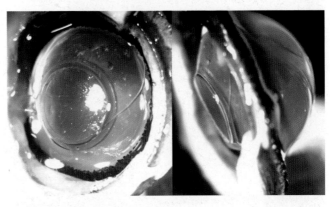

Fig. 7: A well-refilled pig cadaver capsule. The anterior capsule-supported IOL was firmly fixed, and there was no leakage of the material injected

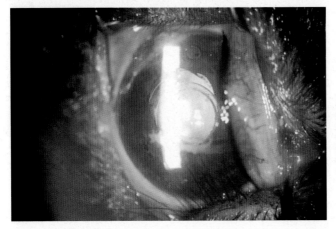

Fig. 8: A refilled rabbit crystalline lens three weeks after surgery. Note that the IOL was firmly and securely fixed. There was no leakage of the injected silicone compound. Posterior synechia

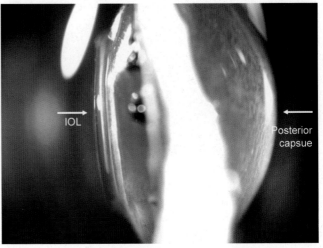

IOL   Posterior capsue

Fig. 9: An enucleated rabbit lens refilled

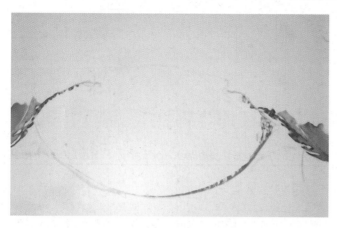

Fig. 10: Histopathological findings of an enucleated rabbit lens refilled three weeks after surgery

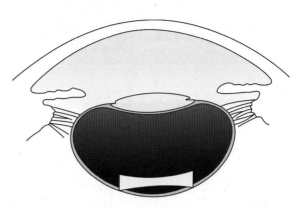

Fig. 11: Dual optic refilling concept I. The concave posterior IOL with a minus power and sharp edges is pressed on the posterior capsule, so that LEC migration might be prevented

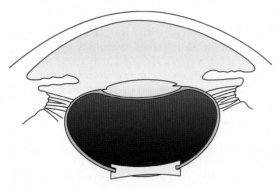

Fig. 12: Dual optic refilling concept II. The concave posterior IOL optic is captured by the posterior CCC. The posterior visual axis is expected to remain PCO-free

8. Nishi O, Nishi K. Accommodation amplitude after lens refilling with injectable silicone by sealing the capsule with a plug in primates. Arch Ophthalmol 1998;116:1358-61.

9. Nishi O, Sakka Y. Anterior capsule-supported intraocular lens. A new lens for small incision surgery and for sealing the capsular opening. Graefe's Arch Clin Exp Ophthalmol 1990;228:582-88.

10. Billotte C, Berdeaux G. Adverse clinical consequences of neodymium; YAG laser treatment of posterior capsule opacification. J Cataract Refract Surg 2004;30:206-471.

11. Nawa Y, Ueda T, Nakatsuka M, et al. Accommodation obtained per 1.0 mm forward movement of a posterior chamber intraocular lens. J Cataract Refract Surg 2003; 29:2069-72.

12. van der Heijde GL, Beers APA, Dubbelman M. Micro-fluctuations of steady-state accommodation measured with ultrasonograhy. Ophthalmol Physiol Opt 1996;16:216-21.

Chapter 62

Laser Cataract Surgery

Kumar J Doctor, Shilpa Kodkany, P Kaushik (India)

INTRODUCTION

Cataract surgery is the most common intraocular surgery performed today worldwide and ultrasound phacoemulsification is the preferred technique among cataract surgeons. Reduced phacoenergy and heat, smaller incisions, improved visual outcomes and efficiency—these are the goals driving advances in cataract phacoemulsification technology. The most negative factor in ultrasound phacoemulsification is the increase in water temperature, which causes an inflammatory response and potential injury to the incision and to the intracameral structures like corneal endothelium, iris, and posterior capsule. To solve these problems, different types of lasers have been developed. Current studies favor the infrared wavelength, particularly the erbium:YAG (Er:YAG) laser (wavelength 2940 nm) and the neodymium:YAG (Nd:YAG) laser (wavelength 1064 nm).

HOW DOES LASER PHACO WORK?

Both the Er:YAG laser and the Nd:YAG laser use the acoustic effect to fragment cataracts. The energy required by laser surgery is reported to be much lower than that generated by ultrasound, and this could be a significant advantage of the new technology. The principal difference between these 2 lasers is the level of water absorption; i.e. the absorption with the Er:YAG laser is very high and with the Nd:YAG, very low. This determines the manner in which they function. The Er:YAG laser beam can be focused directly on the cataract, and the high tissue water level shields the adjacent tissues from injury. The Nd:YAG laser beam is not totally absorbed at the desired point, and may damage adjacent structures. Hence, Er:YAG laser is more popularly used and many multicentric clinical trials have been conducted to study the safety and efficacy of this procedure of *laser phacoemulsification*.

The Er:YAG laser was initially investigated for cataract surgery by Peyman and Katoh and Tsubota in the 1980s (Fig. 1).

Technique of Er:YAG Laser Phaco

The laser procedure is performed using a bimanual technique. The Phacolaser is connected to an optical fiber made of zirconium fluoride and a nontoxic biocompatible quartz tip and the fluidics system from the Sovereign® phacoemulsification system

(AMO). The procedure begins with creation of a 1.2 mm incision in the temporal cornea and a 1.0 mm corneal incision at the 2 o'clock position. The phaco needle is inserted into the first incision with the optical fiber and connected to the aspiration system. The chopper with an irrigation system, which is specifically designed for this surgery, is introduced through the smaller incision. The laser needle has an external diameter of 0.9 mm and an internal diameter of 0.7 mm. A modified needle opening facilitates aspiration of the cortex fragments; there is no need to change the probe to an irrigation/aspiration (I/A) tip, as usually occurs during ultrasound. The 200 μm diameter optical fiber is placed inside the chopper 0.5 mm from the needle opening (which differs from procedures to date) to facilitate suctioning of the cataract fragments and improve the efficacy of the emulsification (Fig. 2).

The Er:YAG laser (wavelength 2940 nm), provides maximal water absorption. Erbium radiation is absorbed at all fluencies better than other types of radiation. It has a short penetration depth, 1.0 μm, which produces a small volume of ablated tissue, improving efficacy and minimizing the thermal effects. In addition, the Er:YAG laser has a lower ablation threshold and a greater photovaporization rate than other infrared systems such as the Nd:YAG laser. The Er:YAG laser ablates lens material directly, which may be more effective than disrupting lens material indirectly as with the Nd:YAG laser, which uses a target or photofragmentation chamber.

Advantages of Er:YAG Phaco over Ultrasound Phaco

Erbium laser phacoemulsification is a surgical method that makes the emulsification of softer nuclei under clinical conditions possible with a low rate of complications. For higher nucleus hardnesses, technical and surgical parameters have to be optimized. Advantages of erbium laser phacoemulsification compared to ultrasonic phacoemulsification are less energy transmission into the eye, no heating of anterior chamber, impossibility of corneal burns and easier access in eyes that are deep into the orbit.

Disadvantages of Er:YAG Phaco

The difficulties incurred with the laser surgical procedure depend on cataract hardness and result in longer surgical times,

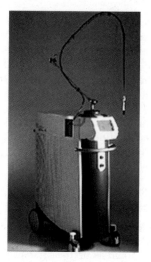

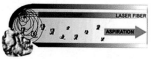

TITAN / TIP

Wordwide unique laser cataract surgery system

- Laser - phaco - MICS
- No heat at hand piece tip, no corneal burns possible
- Microincision cataract surgery (1.4 mm/1.2 mm in preparation)

Fig. 1

Fig. 2

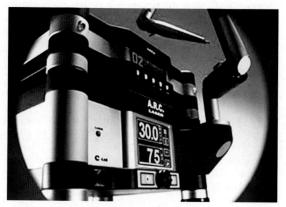

Fig. 3

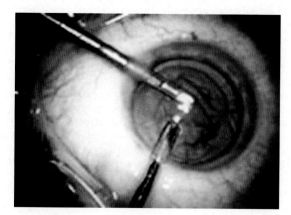

Fig. 4

especially with cataract densities of 3+ and 4+. At these levels, the intraocular irrigation time, including phacoemulsification and I/A is longer in patients who had laser surgery than in those who had an ultrasound procedure. The greater hydrodynamic trauma results in greater endothelial cell loss, the development of corneal edema, and the delay in visual recovery.

Complications include subclinical cystoid macular edema (CME) diagnosed by fluorescein angiography. Irreversible corneal edema, rupture of posterior capsule rupture, elevated IOP level.

Nd:YAG Laser Phacoemulsification
ARC Laser Corporation Dodick Photolysis

The Dodick Photolysis system, introduced in June 2000, uses Q-switched Nd:YAG laser energy instead of standard ultrasound waves to break up the cataract. The Nd:YAG laser (1,064 nm) systems employ plasma formation and shock wave generation to produce photolysis of lens material. The shock wave results from the impact of laser radiation on a titanium plate. How it works: First, the surgeon creates a 1.4 mm incision. Surgeons generally use a groove and crack technique with the laser, sculpting in a bimanual fashion and cracking as soon as possible. Alternatively, a prechopping technique may be used as taught by Jack Dodick, MD. He also creates a separate 0.9 mm incision for the infusion probe. He then inserts the laser aspiration probe through the first incision. The probe delivers laser energy via a quartz fiber onto a titanium target at the end of the probe. When the laser energy hits the titanium target, it creates shockwaves—the effect is like a 'mini earthquake'. It generates laser shock waves at 200 to 400 nanoseconds by striking a titanium target at the end of the aspirating hand piece. The system includes *Venturi fluidics, a touch-screen control panel* and an *ultrasound hand piece* port for cataracts that are too dense for laser phaco (Figs 3 and 4).

A significant disadvantage of the system is that it doesn't work well on dense nuclei. The total time that the tip is in the eye varies with the grade of nucleus, from 2.15 minutes for 1+ nuclear sclerosis to 9.8 minutes for 3+ nuclear sclerosis.

FDA-APPROVED

The only FDA-approved laser system is the Dodick Photolysis, Q-switched Nd:YAG system (ARC Laser Corp).

Nonetheless, laser is safe and efficacious. It provides cold phaco and small incisions, among other advantages. The addition of ultrasound capabilities to laser machines allows surgeons to switch back and forth between modalities for denser cataracts.

Conclusions

Laser phacoemulsification with either Er:YAG or Nd:YAG do help in reducing the energy levels in the eye, they work well while dealing with soft cataracts but for hard cataracts their efficacy and safety are still questionable.

BIBLIOGRAPHY

1. Erbium:YAG laser emulsification of the cataractous lens. J Cataract Refract Surg. Duran S, Zato M 2001;27(7): 1025-32.
2. Erbium:YAG laser phacoemulsification. Comparison of 2 different application systems. Ophthalmology. German. Wetzel W 2001;98(4):376-79.
3. J Cataract Refract Surg. Laser cataract surgery: technique and clinical results. Verges C, Llevat E 2003;29(7): 1339-45.
4. Klin Monatsbl Augenheilkd. Links [Erbium laser phaco-emulsification—a clinical pilot study] Hoh H, Fischer E 1999;214(4):203-10.
5. Temperature measurements during phacoemulsification and erbium:YAG laser phacoablation in model systems. J Cataract Refract Surg 1996;22(3):372-78.

Chapter 63

Micro-biaxial Cataract Surgery Combined with Posterior Vitrectomy

Arturo Pèrez-Arteaga (Mexico)

PHYSICAL BASIS

The objective for the anterior segment surgeon must be to perform the lens extraction but also to facilitate the vitreous-retinal surgeon his subsequent work, leading only smooth conditions and avoiding obstacles. To perform this objective the cataract surgeon must keep in mind that important conditions must exist at the end of the phacoemulsification:

1. Clear view of the posterior segment.
2. Stable anterior chamber with absence of leakage, more important at the possibility to work with contact lenses. To visualize the posterior segment.
3. Nice dilated pupil. Taking care of the uveal tissue during phacoemulsification is a considerable detail.
4. Integrity of posterior capsule to aloud a closed environment in the vitreous cavity during the Pars Plana Vitrectomy (PPV).
5. If there is a rupture in the posterior capsule there will be an increase in the difficulty of performing PPV and also in the possible damage to anterior segment structures like corneal endothelial cells; this possibility can take place sometimes during the surgery and some others in the postoperative period; in those conditions, silicon oil or recurrent hemorrhage can direct touch the cornea. Anyway, silicon oil is able to migrate to the anterior segment even without a rupture in the posterior capsule.

The single formula with the objective to facilitate the posterior segment surgeon to perform his work after we finished the phacoemulsification procedure is to obtain a stable anterior chamber with transparent structures (Fig. 1).

Coaxial vs Biaxial

In coaxial and microcoaxial surgery the incisions are longer than in biaxial surgery and much more in comparison to micro-biaxial techniques (microphakonit). Smaller incision means less leakage, and so, more stability of the anterior chamber with the only objective to help the posterior segment surgeon during the intraoperative maneuvers (Fig. 1).

Step by Step

We suggest the surgical steps in this order:
1. Perform biaxial cataract (or clear lens) extraction. If it´s possible with 700 micron technique, much better.
2. Suture or sutureless PPV
3. IOL implantation with model and power calculation according to the required conditions of previous PPV.

Incisions

1. Perform the minimal invasive incisions. Try to reach the 700 micron technology. You will obtain minimal leakage (Fig. 2).
2. Perform first the non-dominant hand incision. Fill the anterior chamber with viscoelastic (Fig. 3) and perform the incision for the dominant hand (Fig. 4).
3. Do not perform any other incision. Less invasive, best behavior of the anterior chamber.

Capsulorhexis

1. Perform all the maneuvers with both hands. Because these kinds of eyes sometimes have absence of red reflex, the surgeon must search the point of reflection of the capsule with the microscope light, and place the eye in this axis to obtain a better view (Fig. 5). Performing the capsular surgery with bimanuallity, your non- dominant hand is directing the eye to the best light angle, while the dominant hand is performing the capsular movements.
2. Hold the eye with the visco cannula through the non-dominant incision (you can inject visco any time you need) and insert cystitome with your dominant hand. Be sure to look always the light reflex over the anterior capsule (Fig. 6).
3. Perform microcapsulorhexis using both hands. Learn to use the light reflex to see the capsule. Use your non-dominant hand to hold the eye, orient it to the best angles of light source and to inject visco. Learn to forget about the need of red reflex (Fig. 7).

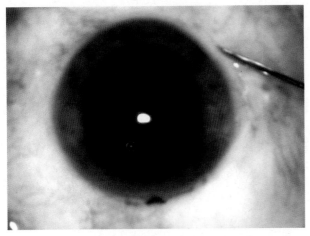

Fig. 1: Eye in aphaquia performed with biaxia technique ready to start PPV for vitreous hemorrhage

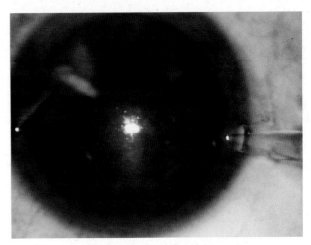

Fig. 4: Dominant hand incision

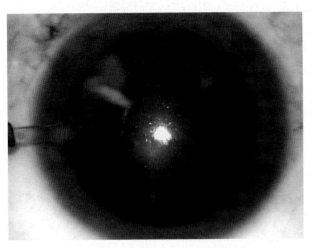

Fig. 2: Non-dominant hand incision

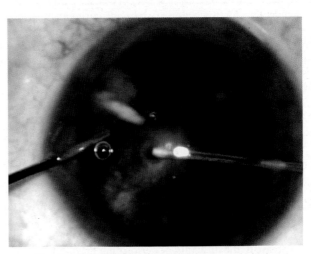

Fig. 5: Notice the light reflex over the capsule in the absence of red reflex

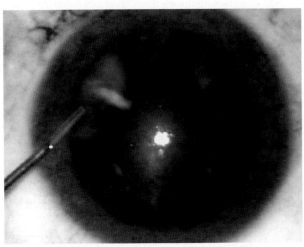

Fig. 3: Anterior chamber stability with visco

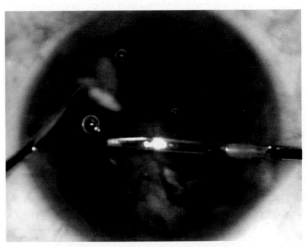

Fig. 6: Bimanual microcapsulorhexis

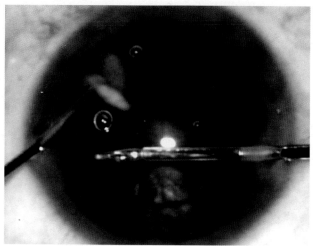

Fig. 7: Bimanual microcapsulorhexis

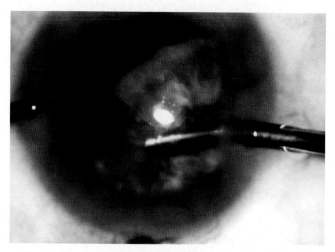

Fig. 10: 700 micron phaco outside the capsular bag. Notice the absence of red reflex

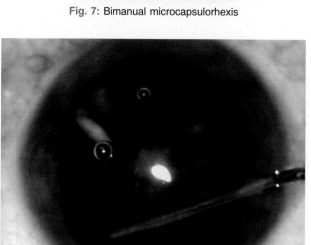

Fig. 8: Hydrodissection using dominant hand

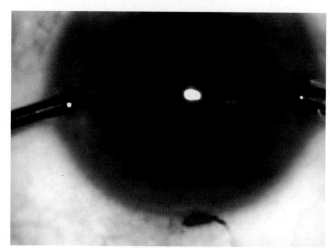

Fig. 11: Finishing biaxial phaco

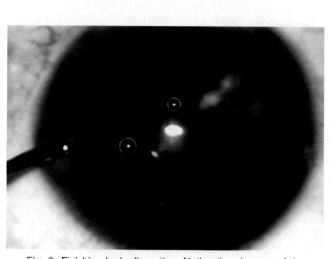

Fig. 9: Finishing hydrodissection. Notice the absence of the golden ring

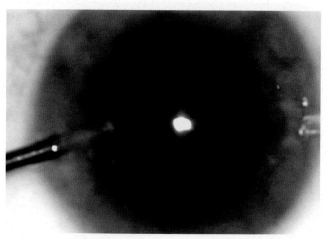

Fig. 12: Anterior chamber open with irrigation on, while changing

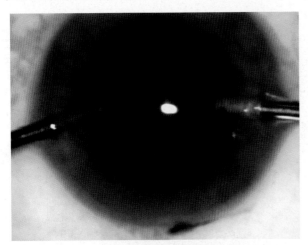

Fig. 13: Irrigation-Aspiration in biaxial approach in absence of red reflex

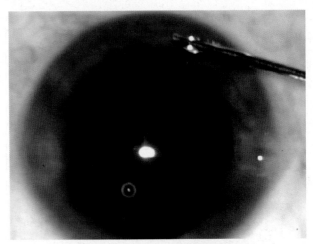

Fig. 16: Anterior chamber full of viscoelastic material

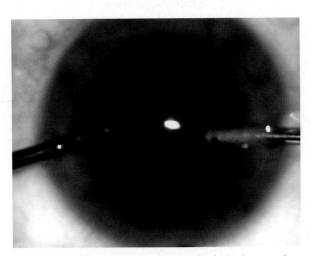

Fig. 14: Complete IA. Notice the margin of anterior capsule

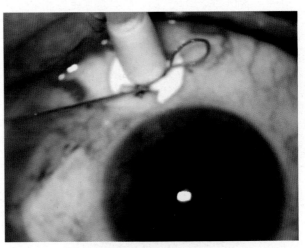

Fig. 17: Irrigation on through pars plana

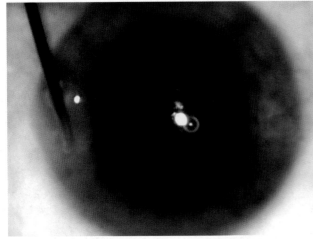

Fig. 15: Easy stromal edema with 700 micron incisions

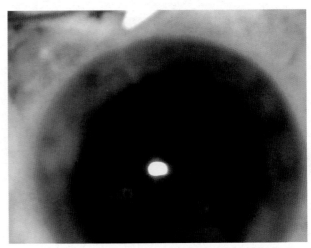

Fig. 18: Anterior chamber stability while performing PPV

Fig. 19: PPV over 700 micron phaco

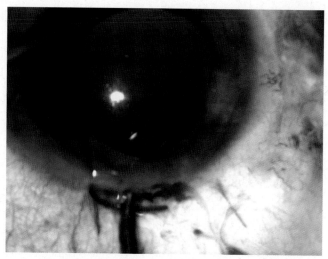

Fig. 21: Bimanual control of superior loop implantation

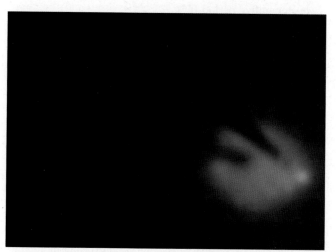

Fig. 20: Endolaser application through contact lens
and 700 micron phaco

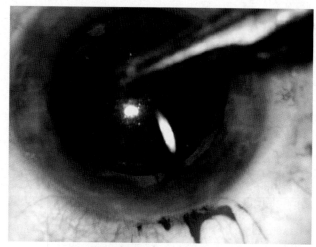

Fig. 22: Clear cornea suture collocation

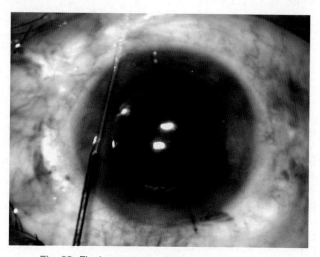

Fig. 23: Final appearance. Notice the IOL in the bag

Hydrodissection

1. Use both incisions; you can have two different angles of attack (Fig. 8).
2. Move the eye to see with light reflex your capsulorhexis margin.
3. Be careful; avoid too much pressure. You are not able to see the posterior wave because there is not red reflex (Fig. 9). You can feel comfortable when you are able to rotate the nucleus.

Phacoemulsification

1. Try to perform all the maneuvers outside the capsular bag at the iris plane. There is not red reflex to be used as reference (Fig. 10).
2. If you find difficulties to perform phaco outside the capsular bag, beaware of the depth of your movements and instruments because the posterior capsule is difficult to be seen.
3. Move the eye with bimanuallity searching the light reflex (Fig. 11)

Irrigation/Aspiration

1. When finish phacoemulsification change to I/A instruments avoiding a collapse of the anterior chamber. A lack of stability in the anterior segment can lead to some posterior segment complications undesirable for the posterior segment surgeon (Fig. 12).
2. I/A maneuvers are difficult because of absence of red reflex (Fig. 13). Again move the eye with both hands to the best place to visualize the cortical material and the posterior capsule (Fig. 14). Take advantage of bimanuallity.
3. Close the incisions with stromal edema and place visco in the anterior chamber. High density visco can be a good option if the surgeon notices some leakage. Be aware to cause any chamber collapse (Fig. 15).
4. Be sure about the chamber stability before start PPV (Figs 1 and 16).

The anterior segment surgeon must stay inside the OR while the vitreous-retinal surgeon is performing PPV. Do not leave, stay and see how our patient is doing. Start to plan IOL implantation according to the events ongoing during the posterior segment procedure.

Pars-Plana Vitrectomy

1. The posterior segment surgeon will find very easy to place the irrigating piece if the eye has a good IOP. With low IOP there are many difficulties. A no-leakage anterior chamber is the key for the success in this maneuver (Figs 1, 15 and 16).
2. Be sure that the anterior chamber remains wide open without any leakage while starting PPV; be aware of this before the collocation of pre-corneal lens (Fig. 17).
3. Be sure about the eye stability while performing complete PPV (Fig. 18).
4. Take care about the integrity of the posterior capsule in particular if silicon oil is implanted in the vitreous cavity and perform PPV as usual (Figs 19 and 20).

IOL Implantation

1. Choose the IOL power and model according to the events during PPV.
2. Fill again the anterior chamber with visco until you feel comfortable with the amplitude of the anterior segment and the intraocular pressure.
3. Try to use the smallest incision size.
4. Be gentle with the eye. Keep in control the intraocular pressure. The eye has not now the "cushion" of the vitreous body.
5. May be it can be better to implant with forceps, in order to avoid increase the IOP with injector (Fig. 21).

Final Steps

1. Utilize suture (Fig. 22). No matter how small your implantation incisión can be. The eye has not vitreous body, so it has less resistance.
2. Create again stromal edema in all incisions.
3. Check the IOP before finish. Check it frequently in the postoperative period (Fig. 23).

BIBLIOGRAPHY

1. Bimanual microphaco for posterior polar cataracts. Aravind Haripriya, Srinivasan Aravind, Kavitha Vadi, Govindappa Natchiar. Journal of Cataract and Refractive Surgery 2006;32(6):914-17.
2. Cataracts associated with posterior segment surgery. Giacomo Panozzo, Barbara Parolini.Ophthalmology Clinics of North America 2004;17(4):557-68.
3. Combined microphakonit and 25-gauge transconjunctival sutureless vitrectomy. Amar Agarwal, Soosan Jacob, Athiya Agarwal. Journal of Cataract and Refractive Surgery 2007;33(11):1839-40.
4. Combined pars plana vitrectomy and lens management in complex vitreoretinal disease. Chaughry NA, Cohen KA, Flynn HW, Murray TG. Semin Ophthalmol 2003;18:132-41.
5. Combined pars plana vitrectomy and phacoemulsification to restore acuity in patients with chronic uveitis. Sofia Androudi, Muna Ahmed, Tito Fiore, Periklis Brazitikos, C. Stephen Foster. Journal of Cataract and Refractive Surgery 2005;31(3):472-78.
6. Combined phacoemulsification and pars plana vitrectomy: Clear corneal versus scleral incisions: Prospective randomized multicenter study. Heiligenhaus A, Holtkamm A, Koch J, et al. Journal of Cataract and Refractive Surgery 2003;29:1106-12.
7. Combined phacoemulsification, foldable intraocular lens implantation, and 25-gauge transconjunctival sutureless vitrectomy. Jong-uk Hwang, Young Hee Yoon, Deok-Soo Kim, June-Gone Kim 2006;32(5):727-31.
8. Combined phacoemulsification, intraocular lens implantation, and vitrectomy for eyes with coexisting cataract and vitreoretinal pathology. Demetriades AM, Gottsch JD, Thomsen R, et al. Am J Ophthalmol 2003;135:291-96.
9. Combined phacoemulsification, parsplana vitrectomy, and foldable intraocular lens implantation. Lam DCS, Young AL, Rao SK, et al. J Cataract Refract Surg 2003; 29:1064-69.
10. Comparison of clear corneal phacoemulsification combined with 25-gauge transconjunctival sutureless vitrectomy and standard 20-gauge vitrectomy for patients with cataract and

vitreoretinal disease. Cheng-Jong Chang, Yun-Hsiang Chang, Shang-Yi Chiang, Le-Tien Lin. Journal of Cataract and Refractive Surgery 2005;31(6)1198-1207.

11. Cool phaco in combined phacoemulsification and vitrectomy surgery. Nawrocki J, Michalewska Z, Cisiecki S. Klin Oczna. 2006;108:16-19.

12. In vivo analysis of wound architecture in 700 µm microphakonit cataract surgery. Amar Agarwal, Dhivya Ashok Kumar, Soosan Jacob, Athiya Agarwal. "Journal of Cataract and Refractive Surgery 2008;34(9):1554-60.

13. Phacoemulsification and Acri. Smartintra-ocular lens implantation combined with vitreoretinal surgery. Gian Maria Cavallini, Alessandro Pupino, Cristina Masini, Luca Campi, Simone Pelloni. Journal of Cataract and Refractive Surgery 2007;33(7):1253-58.

14. Phacovitrectomy: Expanding indication. David HW. Steel. Journal of Cataract and Refractive Surgery 2007;33(6):933-36.

15. Presbyopic phacovitrectomy. Ling R, Simcock P, McCoombes J, Shaw S. Br J Ophthalmol 2003;87:1333-35.

16. Sutureless single-port transconjunctival pars plana limited vitrectomy combined with phacoemulsification for management of phacomorphic glaucoma. Tanuj Dada, Sanjeev Kumar, Ritu Gadia, Anand Aggarwal, Viney Gupta, Ramanjit Sihota. Journal of Cataract and Refractive Surgery. 2007;33(6): 951-54.

17. Vitrectomy and lensectomy in the management of posterior dislocation of the lens fragments. Patrick Watts, James Hunter, Catey Bunce. Journal of Cataract and Refractive Surgery 2000;26(6):832-37.

Chapter 64

Multifocal IOLs

D Ramamurthy, Chitra Ramamurthy (India)

Modern cataract surgery has become the most frequently performed Refractive Surgery today. Multifocal IOLs has become an important addition in our quest to provide freedom from glasses for all ages at all distances.

OPTICS OF MULTIFOCAL IOLs

All these multifocal IOL works on the principle of simultaneous image perception with images from distance, near and intermediate (in case of Refractive Multifocals) (Fig. 1) brought into simultaneous perception and the direction of gaze and object of regard determines which image is in focus and which is out of focus. It is because of the defocused light rays falling on the Retina, which contributes the unwanted noise, compared to the signal which creates the focused image (Fig. 2) that dysphotopsia like glare, halos and night vision difficulties (Figs 3 and 4) arise.

TYPES OF MULTIFOCAL IOLs

Since the initial introduction of these lenses there have been significant advances in the technology. In the Refractive Multifocal IOLs we have the Array (Fig. 5), Rezoom (Fig. 6) and MF4 (Fig. 7) lenses. While the Array and Rezoom are distant dominant lenses with an add power of +3.50 diopters the MF4 is a near dominant lens with an add power of +4D.

In the diffractive multifocal IOLs we have the Tecnis (Fig. 8) (+4 D add) Restor (Fig. 9) (+4 D and +3 D add) and the Acrilisa (Figs 10 and 11) (+3.75 D). While the Tecnis is currently a 3 piece lens on silicone platform, single piece hydrophobic version of these lenses are likely to become available shortly. The Restor is a Diffractive/Refractive IOL with the diffractive rings being present only in the central 3.6 mm. Acrilisa is a plate haptic, hydrophilic IOL with a +3.75 D add in it. A Toric version (Fig. 12) of this IOL is also available. All these diffractive IOLs have asphericity incorporated in them.

COUNSELING FOR MULTIFOCAL IOLs

Mention always relative independence from spectacles with multifocals and also warn about problem of dysphotopsia which most often disappear with time and after bilateral implantation.

Pre-selection of Patients

1. Do not take up patients who are obsessive about their vision and freedom from glasses.
2. Normal eyes with potential for vision of 20/30 or better after surgery.
3. Normal healthy Retina. Routine OCT may be performed to evaluate the Macula. Figs 13 and 15 show relatively normal macula on fundus photography but the corresponding OCT images Figs 14 and 16 show significant macula problems which could compromise the outcome. Hence routine OCT evaluation of the macula before multifocal IOL implantation must be carried out.
4. Less than 1 D of corneal astigmatism or measures to reduce astigmatism must be employed intra or postoperatively.
5. Ambient pupillary size of 2.5 mm or more.
6. Patients with significant cataracts and hyperopes are easiest to satisfy.

Surgical Steps and Results

1. Good quality atraumatic phacoemulsification with predictable refractive outcomes.
2. 360° overlap of the Rhexis margin on the optic of the IOL (Figs 17 and 18) to ensure good centration.
3. Complete cortical clean up and PC polishing.
4. Intact posterior capsule.

POST-SURGICAL MANAGEMENT

1. Add topical NSAIDs in addition to steroids at least for a month after surgery.
2. Take care of the tear film.
3. Address the residual Refractive error if significant by glasses, laser vision correction or limbal relaxing incision.
4. Perform YAG capsulotomy if PCO causes deterioration of vision.
5. Ensure the Macula is healthy.

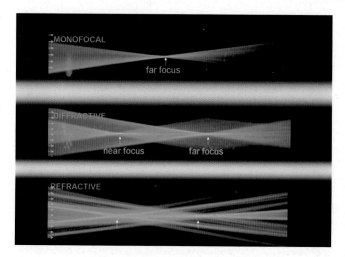

Fig. 1: Optical principles of IOLs

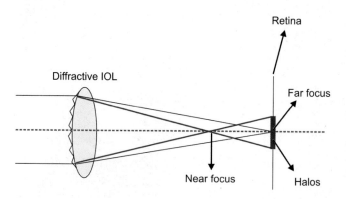

Fig. 2: Signal and noise with multifocals

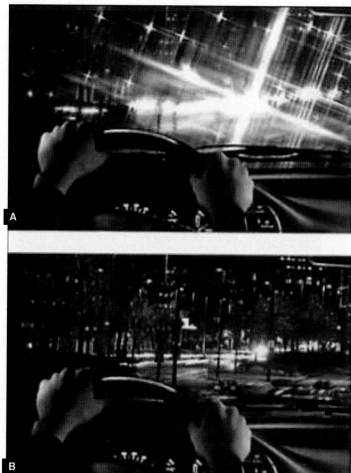

Figs 3A and B: Night vision

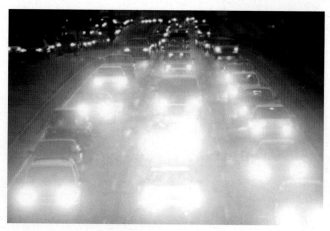

Fig. 4: Night vision

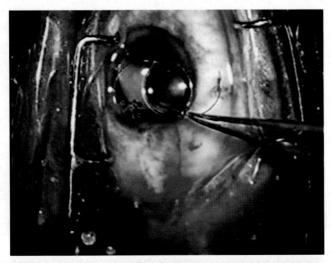

Fig. 5: Array

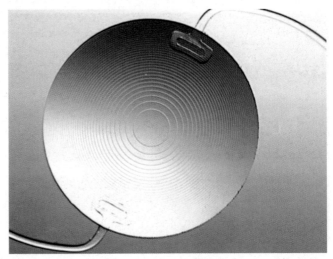

Fig. 8: Tecnis

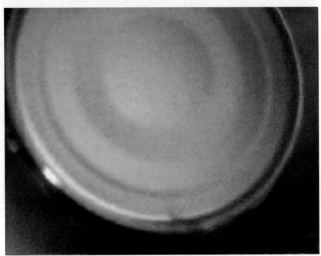

Fig. 6: Rezoom

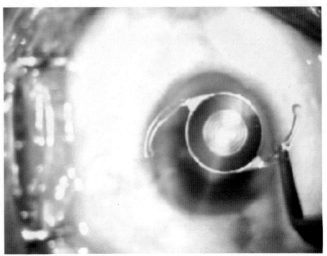

Fig. 9: Restor

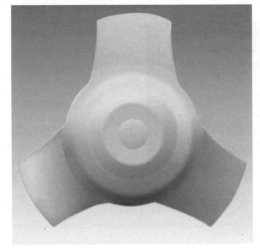

Fig. 7: MF4

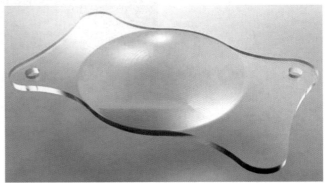

Fig. 10: Acrilisa

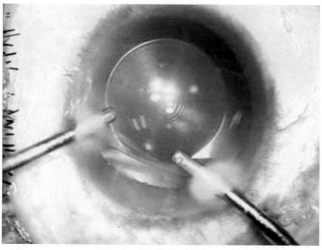

Fig. 11: Acrilisa in the bag

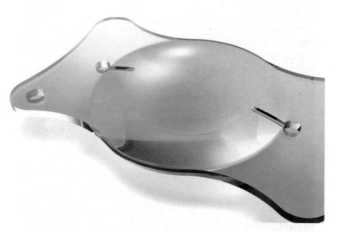

Fig. 12: Toric

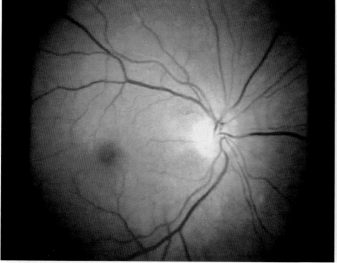

Fig. 13: Normal looking fundus

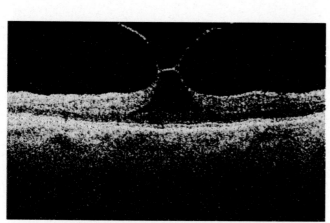

Fig. 14: Significant vitreo retinal changes

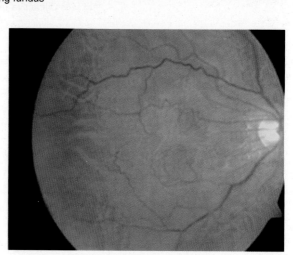

Fig. 15: Mild kinking of vessels

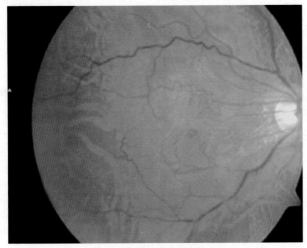

Fig. 16: Epiretinal membrane

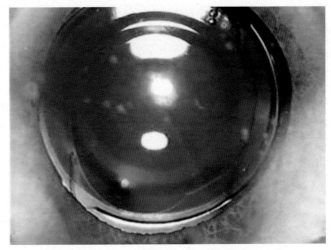

Fig. 17: Refractive multifocal with 360 degree overlap

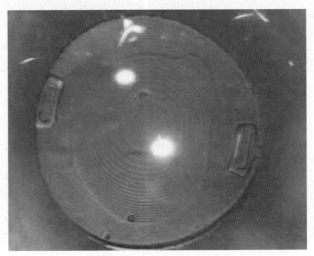

Fig. 18: Diffractive multifocal with 360 degree overlap

Chapter **65**

Cataract Surgery in Post RK Cases

Arun C Gulani (USA)

In many cases (since patients with Radial Keratotomies are now in their cataractous ages). They shall need cataract surgery. Here too, plan to maximize all optical imperfections so you always plan for the most effective vision by performing the least amount of intervention for the patient and help them gain maximum advantage for their vision.

You can plan for cataract surgery in such a way that you can address not only their hazy vision due to the cataract but also their refractive errors, i.e. hyperopia with appropriate IOL power calculations.

For their associated problems, i.e. Presbyopia and or astigmatism you may select multifocal lens implants, Toric lens implants, etc.

I have had good success with ReStor Lens implants in such patients thus optimizing their eye (like a camera) from within the eye first and then getting ready for Laser vision surgery to address three more aspects:

1. Residual refractive error
2. Astigmatism
3. Increase the optical zone to excellent visual outcomes without glasses (remember most RK surgeries were done with small optical zones).

Do not get too anxious about having to perform cataract surgery on a post-RK eye. I would suggest the following tips:

1. Select the site of entry based on astigmatism axis and available space between two radial incisions
2. Low flow techniques. I use low flow phacoemulsification/ Aqualase or phacochop techniques to keep the pressure in the eye down as you work
3. Do not move the phaco tip (**Gulani Phaco-Feed** technique) and instead feed the cataract and epi cortex via the second hand into the phaco so as to minimize incisional torsion.
4. Always **remember** that these patients were once myopic in refraction (even though today they are presenting with hyperopia) and still have the myope's ocular anatomy, so all the risks of cataract surgery in myopia [namely retinal issues] still apply.

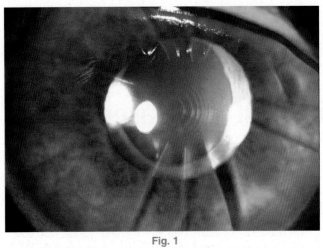

Fig. 1

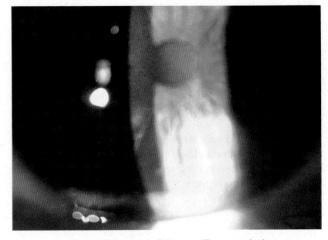

-1 Myopia -2 Astgm: RK Cornea S/P Phaco-IOL

Fig. 3

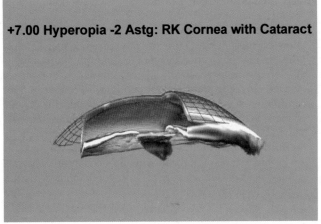

+7.00 Hyperopia -2 Astg: RK Cornea with Cataract

Fig. 2

Fig. 4: Cataract in RK case (Preoperative)

Index